Metabolism in Cancer

Metabolism in Cancer

Edited by Meryl Brody

hayle medical

New York

Hayle Medical,
750 Third Avenue, 9th Floor,
New York, NY 10017, USA

Visit us on the World Wide Web at:
www.haylemedical.com

ISBN: 978-1-63241-837-1

Cataloging-in-Publication Data

Metabolism in cancer / edited by Meryl Brody.
p. cm.
Includes bibliographical references and index.
ISBN 978-1-63241-837-1
1. Cancer cells--Metabolism. 2. Cancer cells--Molecular aspects. 3. Metabolism.
4. Cancer. I. Brody, Meryl.
RC269.7 .M48 2020
616.994 07--dc23

Table of Contents

Preface

Over the recent decade, advancements and applications have progressed exponentially. This has led to the increased interest in this field and projects are being conducted to enhance knowledge. The main objective of this book is to present some of the critical challenges and provide insights into possible solutions. This book will answer the varied questions that arise in the field and also provide an increased scope for furthering studies.

Cancer metabolism is an important area of research in cancer biology that is based on the principle that cancer cells have altered metabolic activities, which support the acquisition and maintenance of malignant properties. Research in this domain strives to understand the mechanism by which metabolism becomes reprogrammed in cancer cells and how such metabolic changes can be exploited for therapeutic benefit. An important theme in cancer metabolism is the cellular fitness provided by reprogrammed activities that enable a selective advantage during tumorigenesis. Due to this, cancer cells grow and proliferate at elevated levels, and survive under stressful conditions. Altered bioenergetics, redox balance and enhanced biosynthesis are some processes that provide benefit to the malignant cell and hence holds potential as therapeutic targets. This book includes some of the vital pieces of work being conducted across the world, on various topics related to cancer metabolism. It presents the complex subject of cancer metabolism in the most comprehensible language. It is meant for students who are looking for an elaborate reference text in this domain.

I hope that this book, with its visionary approach, will be a valuable addition and will promote interest among readers. Each of the authors has provided their extraordinary competence in their specific fields by providing different perspectives as they come from diverse nations and regions. I thank them for their contributions.

Editor

1

Metabolic profiling of triple-negative breast cancer cells reveals metabolic vulnerabilities

Nathan J. Lanning[1*], Joshua P. Castle[2], Simar J. Singh[3], Andre N. Leon[1], Elizabeth A. Tovar[2], Amandeep Sanghera[3], Jeffrey P. MacKeigan[2,4], Fabian V. Filipp[3] and Carrie R. Graveel[2*]

Abstract

Background: Among breast cancers, the triple-negative breast cancer (TNBC) subtype has the worst prognosis with no approved targeted therapies and only standard chemotherapy as the backbone of systemic therapy. Unique metabolic changes in cancer progression provide innovative therapeutic opportunities. The receptor tyrosine kinases (RTKs) epidermal growth factor receptor (EGFR), and MET receptor are highly expressed in TNBC, making both promising therapeutic targets. RTK signaling profoundly alters cellular metabolism by increasing glucose consumption and subsequently diverting glucose carbon sources into metabolic pathways necessary to support the tumorigenesis. Therefore, detailed metabolic profiles of TNBC subtypes and their response to tyrosine kinase inhibitors may identify therapeutic sensitivities.

Methods: We quantified the metabolic profiles of TNBC cell lines representing multiple TNBC subtypes using gas chromatography mass spectrometry. In addition, we subjected MDA-MB-231, MDA-MB-468, Hs578T, and HCC70 cell lines to metabolic flux analysis of basal and maximal glycolytic and mitochondrial oxidative rates. Metabolic pool size and flux measurements were performed in the presence and absence of the MET inhibitor, INC280/capmatinib, and the EGFR inhibitor, erlotinib. Further, the sensitivities of these cells to modulators of core metabolic pathways were determined. In addition, we annotated a rate-limiting metabolic enzymes library and performed a siRNA screen in combination with MET or EGFR inhibitors to validate synergistic effects.

Results: TNBC cell line models displayed significant metabolic heterogeneity with respect to basal and maximal metabolic rates and responses to RTK and metabolic pathway inhibitors. Comprehensive systems biology analysis of metabolic perturbations, combined siRNA and tyrosine kinase inhibitor screens identified a core set of TCA cycle and fatty acid pathways whose perturbation sensitizes TNBC cells to small molecule targeting of receptor tyrosine kinases.

Conclusions: Similar to the genomic heterogeneity observed in TNBC, our results reveal metabolic heterogeneity among TNBC subtypes and demonstrate that understanding metabolic profiles and drug responses may prove valuable in targeting TNBC subtypes and identifying therapeutic susceptibilities in TNBC patients. Perturbation of metabolic pathways sensitizes TNBC to inhibition of receptor tyrosine kinases. Such metabolic vulnerabilities offer promise for effective therapeutic targeting for TNBC patients.

Keywords: Triple-negative breast cancer, Metabolism, Rate-limiting enzymes, Receptor tyrosine kinase, Tyrosine kinase inhibitor, Metabolic inhibitor

* Correspondence: nlannin@calstatela.edu; Carrie.Graveel@vai.org
[1]California State University, Los Angeles, 5151 State University Drive, Los Angeles, CA 90032, USA
[2]Van Andel Research Institute, 333 Bostwick Ave, NE, Grand Rapids, MI 49503, USA

Background

Triple-negative breast cancer

Triple-negative breast cancer (TNBC) accounts for 15–20% of invasive breast cancers. TNBC is characterized by the lack of estrogen receptor (ER) and progesterone receptor (PR) expression and human epidermal growth factor receptor 2 (HER2) amplification. TNBCs are associated with advanced stage at diagnosis and poorer outcome compared to other breast cancer subtypes [1]. Characteristic TNBC clinical features include a peak in recurrence risk within the first 3 years, a weak relationship between the tumor size and lymph node metastasis, and a peak of cancer-related death in the first 5 years [2]. At the molecular level, TNBC has significant overlap with the basal-like subtype as approximately 80% of TNBCs are classified as basal-like [1]. Currently, TNBCs are treated with cytotoxic combination chemotherapy. Even though TNBC patients have significantly higher rates of pathologic complete response compared to non-TNBC, TNBC patients have decreased 3-year progression-free survival and overall survival rates [1, 3]. Hence, there is a vital need for a comprehensive understanding of the molecular basis of TNBC progression and emerging treatment approaches.

TNBC is a highly heterogeneous disease at the molecular level, and this heterogeneity likely underlies the variable treatment responses in patients. Recent studies involving comprehensive gene expression analysis revealed extensive molecular heterogeneity within TNBC cases and identified four to six distinct molecular TNBC subtypes [4, 5]. These subtypes have unique expression signatures and ontologies and are defined as basal-like, mesenchymal and luminal androgen receptor subtypes. To identify novel treatment strategies for TNBC patients, it is essential that we understand the unique and common molecular features of these TNBC subtypes.

Current treatment options for TNBC patients are restricted to chemotherapy; however, receptor tyrosine kinases (RTK) are promising druggable targets due to their high expression in TNBC. The epidermal growth factor receptor (EGFR) and MET receptor are highly expressed in multiple TNBC subtypes with EGFR overexpression in 54% of basal breast cancers (predominantly TNBC). Additionally, EGFR is a biomarker for identification of basal breast cancers [6–10]. Similarly, MET is associated with poor clinical outcome in breast cancer [11–15], and high MET expression correlates with TNBC [16, 17]. Previously, we demonstrated that the MET inhibitor cabozantinib inhibited TNBC growth, invasion, and metastasis [18]. Recently, we determined that combined MET and EGFR inhibition was highly effective at abrogating tumor growth in patient-derived TNBC tumorgrafts and significantly decreased the variability in treatment response compared to monotherapy with MET or EGFR inhibitors [19]. These results highlight that MET and/or EGFR inhibition may be a highly effective treatment strategy for TNBC patients. Metabolic alterations are now widely understood to support the cancer phenotype, and RTKs such at MET and EGFR have been implicated in driving some of these the metabolic alterations [20–25].

Metabolic characteristics of TNBC

Particular metabolic characteristics of TNBC have been investigated, and overall TNBC cell models and patient samples are characterized by elevated glycolysis. Along these lines, a genome wide screen identified a small subset of metabolic genes, including core glycolytic and oxidative phosphorylation (OXPHOS) genes, whose suppression was lethal in a TNBC cell model [26]. Compared to ER+ breast cancer cell lines, MDA-MB-231 and MDA-MB-468 TNBC cell models are reported to harbor high glycolytic flux and low OXPHOS activity [27] and are more primed to switch to a glycolytic program in the context of limited oxygen than non-transformed cells [28]. In patient samples, high glucose transporter, GLUT1, expression is observed in TNBC compared to non-TNBC tumors [29]. GLUT1 may also enhance invasion by localizing to the invasive edge of in vivo tumor models [30]. Mechanistically, high MYC expression in TNBC cell models suppresses expression of the glycolytic inhibitor, thioredoxin-interacting protein, TXNIP, resulting in increased glycolytic flux [31]. In addition, a siRNA screen revealed that TNBC cell line models are dependent on elevated glycolysis through the LDHB (lactate dehydrogenase B) as opposed to their non-TNBC counterparts [32].

Recent evidence indicates that the metabolic characteristics of TNBC correlate with therapeutic response. The glycolytic potential of TNBC cells may be associated with chemotherapeutic resistance as exposing TNBC cell models to increasing concentrations of glucose increases proliferation and decreases the efficacy of metformin-induced apoptosis [33, 34]. Additionally, PKM2, a glycolytic enzyme associated with high tumoral glycolytic flux [35], may confer some resistance to doxorubicin treatment in vitro and in MDA-MB-231 orthotopic breast cancer models [36]. Other studies demonstrate that stimulation of mitochondrial activity and concurrent inhibition of mitochondrial respiratory complex I [37] or a combination of glycolytic and mitochondrial inhibitors [38] effectively kills TNBC cells and TNBC xenografts.

Collectively, the above studies demonstrate a clear role for altered metabolism supporting the aggressive TNBC phenotype. Much like the genetic and signaling heterogeneity found in cancers in general and TNBC in particular [39], metabolic heterogeneity also likely exists in TNBC patients [40, 41] and cell models [33, 42] and likely drives differential responses to therapeutics. Therefore, comprehensive and systematic investigations into the metabolism of TNBC and TNBC cell models are necessary in order to gain insight into the best therapeutic strategies. Some previous approaches referenced above undertook genome-wide siRNA screening approaches or utilized computational approaches [43]. In the present study, we provide detailed metabolic analyses of the commonly used MDA-MB-231, MDA-MB-468, Hs578T, and HCC70 TNBC cell line models, which represent the two major basal-like subtype and the mesenchymal subtypes [4]. We determined the basal and maximal metabolic rates, as well as the metabolic rates in response to EGFR and MET inhibitors in these TNBC lines. We also measure viability in response to chemical modulation of five metabolic pathways. Finally, we report the viability effects of suppressing each KEGG metabolic pathway in combination with EGFR (erlotinib) or MET (INC280) inhibition in these cell lines. Overall, these results provide a more thorough view of the metabolic landscape of TNBC and the effect of RTK inhibition on TNBC metabolism.

Methods

Cell culture

All cells were purchased from ATCC. MDA-MB-231, MDA-MB-468, Hs578T, and HCC70 cells were cultured in DMEM (ThermoFisher) supplemented with 10% fetal bovine serum. hTERT-HME1 cells were cultured in MEBM (Lonza) supplemented with hEGF, insulin, hydrocortisone, and BPE (Lonza).

Metabolomics profiling

For metabolite quantification, cells were seeded in triplicate (n = 3) in 6-well plates with DMEM supplemented with 10% FBS. After 24 h, the media was removed and replaced with fresh media. Upon reaching 70% confluency, cells were washed twice with phosphate buffered saline (PBS, 46-013-CM, Corning) and lifted from culture wells using 0.25% Trypsin/2.21 mM EDTA (25-053-CI, Corning). Cells were then washed with PBS containing 10% FBS followed by 0.9% NaCl (Sigma, S9888). Cell pellets frozen in liquid nitrogen before storage at 193 K.

Frozen cell pellets were thawed on ice for 10 min before addition of 1 mL cold extraction solvent containing acetonitrile/isopropanol/water (3:3:2) at 253 K. Samples were then vortexed (15 s × 5) and frozen on dry ice for 20 mins and the freeze/thaw/vortex cycle repeated twice. Samples were dried via vacuum centrifugal evaporation and stored at −80 °C before analysis.

Dried samples were derivatized first by addition of 10 μL of MOX Reagent (20 mg/mL methoxyamine-hydrochloride in dry pyridine (TS-45950, Thermo Fisher Scientific) followed by 90-min incubation in a digital heating shaking drybath at 303 K and 1100 rpm. Next, 90μL N-Methyl-N-(trimethylsilyl)trifluoroacetamide (MSTFA, Sigma 394,866) was added and samples were incubated at 310 K and 1000 rpm for 30mins before centrifugation for 5 min at 14,000 rpm/277 K. The supernatant was transferred to an auto sampler vial for gas chromatography-mass spectrometry (GC-MS) analysis.

Derivatized samples were analyzed on a Triple Quadrupole GC-MS (TSQ8000, Thermo Fisher Scientific) equipped with a TG-5MS (30 m × 0.25 mm i.d. × 0.25 μm, 26098-1420, Thermo Fisher Scientific) capillary column and run under electron ionization at 70 eV. The GC was programed with an injection temperature of 523 K and splitless injection volume of 1 μl. The GC oven temperature program started at 232 K for 1 min, rising to 523 K at 10 K/min with a final hold at this temperature for 6 min. The GC flow rate with helium carrier gas was 1.2 mL/min. The transfer line temperature was set at 563 K and ion source temperature at 568 K. A range of 50–600 m/z was scanned with a scan time of 0.25 s.

Metabolites were identified using TraceFinder software v 3.3 (Thermo Fisher Scientific) based on in-house libraries of metabolite retention time and fragmentation patterns. Identified metabolites were quantified using the total ion count peak area for specific mass ions, and standard curves generated from reference standards run in parallel. The mean, standard deviation, and 95% confidence interval were calculated for each cell line and treatment condition. ANOVA with student's t test was used to compare treatment conditions within each cell line.

Metabolic flux analysis

For all metabolic flux analyses, a Seahorse 96 XFe was used. Twenty-four hours prior to metabolic flux analyses, cells were cultured in identical media (10 mM glucose, 2 mM glutamine, 1 mM pyruvate). Cells were plated at a density of 40,000 cells per well in a Seahorse 96-well assay plate 16 h prior to analysis. For basal and maximal metabolic profiles, four independent experiments were performed, each with three biological replicates and five technical replicates. For basal metabolic profiles in the context of RTK inhibitor treatment, three biological replicates each with five technical replicates were performed, and cells were treated with 10 μM erlotinib or INC280/capmatinib (Selleck Chemicals) for 18 h prior to metabolic rate analysis. After metabolic rate analyses, extracellular acidification rate (ECAR) and oxygen consumption rate (OCR) measurements were normalized to CyQUANT (Invitrogen) measurements cell count measurements in each well. For basal rate measurements, ECAR and OCR measurements were spaced 6 min apart. For maximal rate measurements, basal rates were measured twice at an interval of 6–7 min, followed by carbonyl cyanide-p-trifluormethoxyphenylhydrazone (FCCP)

(1 μM final concentration) injection, mixture, and measurement 6–7 min later, followed another measurement 6–7 min later, followed by 2-deoxyglucose (2-DG, 100 mM final concentration) or rotenone + antimycin (1 μM each final concentration) injection, mixture, and measurement 6–7 min later, followed by a final measurement 6–7 min later. Maximal rate data are representative experiments displayed as averages of three biological replicates with error bars representing standard deviation.

Cell viability in response to metabolic modulators

Cells were plated at a density of 2500 cells per well in 96-well plates in growth media. Cells were treated with vehicle or the following concentrations of chemicals: 25 mM 2-DG, 200 μM 6-aminonicotanimide (6-AN), 1 μM rotenone, 10 mM metformin, and 1 mM 5-Aminoimidazole-4-carboxamide ribonucleotide (AICAR). After 48 h of treatment, viability was measured by CellTiter-Glo (Promega). Two independent experiments, each containing six biological replicates, were performed. Data are from one representative experiment and provided as averages with error bars representing standard deviation.

siRNA screen

Screen design

All small interfering RNAs (siRNAs) were from Qiagen (Additional file 1: Table S1) and were transfected into cells with siLentFect (BioRad, 1 μl per ml, for transfection efficiency for each cell line, see Additional file 2: Figure S1A). Rate-limiting enzymes were collated through KEGG annotation (http://www.genome.jp/kegg/), the Rate-Limiting Enzyme Regulation Database (http://rle.cbi.pku.edu.cn/home.cgi, [44]), and literature searches and categorized according to KEGG. Genes and metabolic categories and pathways are provided in Additional file 3: Table S2 according these KEGG-based annotations. For the siRNA screen, cells were transfected with control (non-targeting) siRNAs or siRNAs targeting the above-described rate-limiting enzymes, then treated with either DMSO, INC280, or erlotinib (Additional file 2: Figure S1A). Cells were plated in 96-well assay plates at 2500 cells per well. Sixteen hours later, cells were transfected with a pool of two siRNAs per gene. Twenty-four hours post-transfection, fresh media was added containing 10 μM INC280, 10 μM erlotinib, or 0.1% DMSO (the final DMSO concentration in wells containing INC280 or erlotinib). The screen was carried out in duplicate for each siRNA and each condition (DMSO, INC280, or erlotinib) in each cell line. Seventy-two hours post-transfection (48-h post-drug treatment), cell viability was assessed by CellTiter-Glo (Promega).

Screen analysis

The siRNA screen was performed in duplicate, and sensitivity index (below) values were derived from replicate averages. Replicates resulting in a variance larger than 0.04 were not considered for further analysis. To determine which siRNAs resulted in the greatest loss of viability in combination with INC280 or erlotinib compared to DMSO, a variation on the sensitivity index (SI) equation developed by Hoffman and Gardner (1983) was used to estimate the effect of siRNA knockdown on drug sensitivity [45]. The SI value for each siRNA was calculated using the following equation:

$$SI = \left(\frac{R_c}{C_c} \times \frac{C_d}{C_c}\right) - \left(\frac{R_d}{C_c}\right).$$

In this equation, R_c is the average viability in drug-untreated (DMSO) wells transfected with siRNA targeting rate-limiting enzymes, R_d is the average viability in drug-treated wells (INC280 or erlotinib) with siRNA targeting rate-limiting enzymes, C_c is the average viability in drug-untreated (DMSO) wells with control (non-targeting) siRNA, and C_d is the average viability in drug-treated (INC280 or erlotinib) wells with control (non-targeting) siRNA [46]. The SI ranges from −1 to 1, with negative values indicating an antagonistic effect on drug performance and positive values indicating a sensitizing effect. This is accomplished by comparing the predicted effect of drug and siRNA exposure ($R_c/C_c \times C_d/C_c$) to the observed effect of combined exposure (R_d/C_c). Although the SI allows for rapid analysis of siRNA screening data that surpasses the power observed in simple fold-change analysis, it does not allow for the calculation of a p value, as it does not consider probability distribution [46, 47]. As a result, the top 10% of sensitizing siRNAs was used in metabolic pathway analysis. These resulting genes were grouped into KEGG-annotated Metabolic Categories for each drug treatment in each cell line and into KEGG-annotated Metabolic Pathways for each drug treatment.

Results

Metabolomics profiles of TNBC cell lines

To understand the diversity of metabolic activity in TNBC, we examined multiple TNBC cell lines that are representative of several TNBC subtypes identified by Lehmann et al. [4]. These cell lines correspond to the two major basal-like subtypes and a mesenchymal-like subtype. This included Hs578t (mesenchymal stem-like; basal B), MDA-MB-231 (mesenchymal stem-like; basal B), MDA-MB-468 (basal-like 1; basal A), and HCC-70 (basal-like 2, basal A) cells (Additional file 2: Figure S1B). To produce initial metabolic profiles of TNBC, we measured the basal glycolytic and mitochondrial oxidative metabolism rates in four TNBC cell models (MDA-MB-231, MDA-MB-468, HS578t, HCC70) and one immortalized, non-transformed mammary gland epithelial cell model (hTERT-HME1) (Additional file 2: Figure S1C).

We profiled pool sizes of 43 central carbon metabolites of subconfluent TNBC cell lines in exponential growth phase. In addition, we quantified pool size changes following treatment with small molecule inhibitors of the RTKs MET and EGFR. Both MET and EGFR were prominently expressed in the assayed cell lines. Hierarchical clustering of metabolic profiles of TNBC cell lines reveals molecular heterogeneity between the TNBC mesenchymal-like and basal-like subtypes (Fig. 1). Pool size measurements showed common clusters of low TCA cycle and elevated amino acid metabolites of mesenchymal-like MDA-MB-231 and Hs578 which were distinct from the basal-like MDA-MB-468 and HCC70 cell lines (Fig. 1a, Additional file 4: Table S3). Drug perturbations of amino acid pool sizes demonstrated similar response of mesenchymal-like subtype MDA-MB-231 and Hs578 cell lines to both, INC280 or erlotinib, treatment (Fig. 1b). Clusters of each subtype and cell line were well separated by metabolic profiles and drug responses showing that each subtypes had major similarities but each breast cancer cell line also had distinct components. The TCA cycle organic acid α-ketoglutaric acid is significantly reduced upon INC280 treatment with p values below 0.05 for all tested TNBC cell lines. Similarly, TCA cycle and central carbon metabolites aspartic acid, fumaric acid, and malic acid are significantly reduced upon erlotinib treatment with p values below 0.05 for all cell lines. In addition, the MDA-MB-231 cell lines show significant perturbation of amino acid metabolism for both inhibitors. Interesting, the MDA-MB-231 cell line stands out for its strong metabolic perturbation affecting TCA cycle metabolites, many amino and keto acids (Fig. 1b).

TNBC basal metabolic profiles

MDA-MB-231 and MDA-MB-468 cells exhibited similar glycolytic rates (extracellular acidification rate, ECAR) compared to HME1 cells, while HS578t and HCC70 cells displayed approximately 1.5 and two times the glycolytic rate of HME1 cells, respectively (Fig. 2a, c). MDA-MB-231 and HS578t cells exhibited slightly elevated oxygen consumption rates (OCR) compared to HME1 cells, whereas MDA-MB-468 and HCC70 displayed approximately four times the oxygen consumption rate of HME1 cells (Fig. 2b, c). Determining each cell lines' relative ECAR/OCR ratio provides a relative index of which metabolic program each cell line utilizes more in the basal state (Fig. 2d). HME1 cells utilize relatively more basal glycolytic than oxidative metabolism, as do Hs578T and MDA-MB-231 cells. HCC70 cells utilize relatively similar basal glycolytic and oxygen metabolism, while MDA-MB-468 cells utilize relatively more oxygen metabolism than

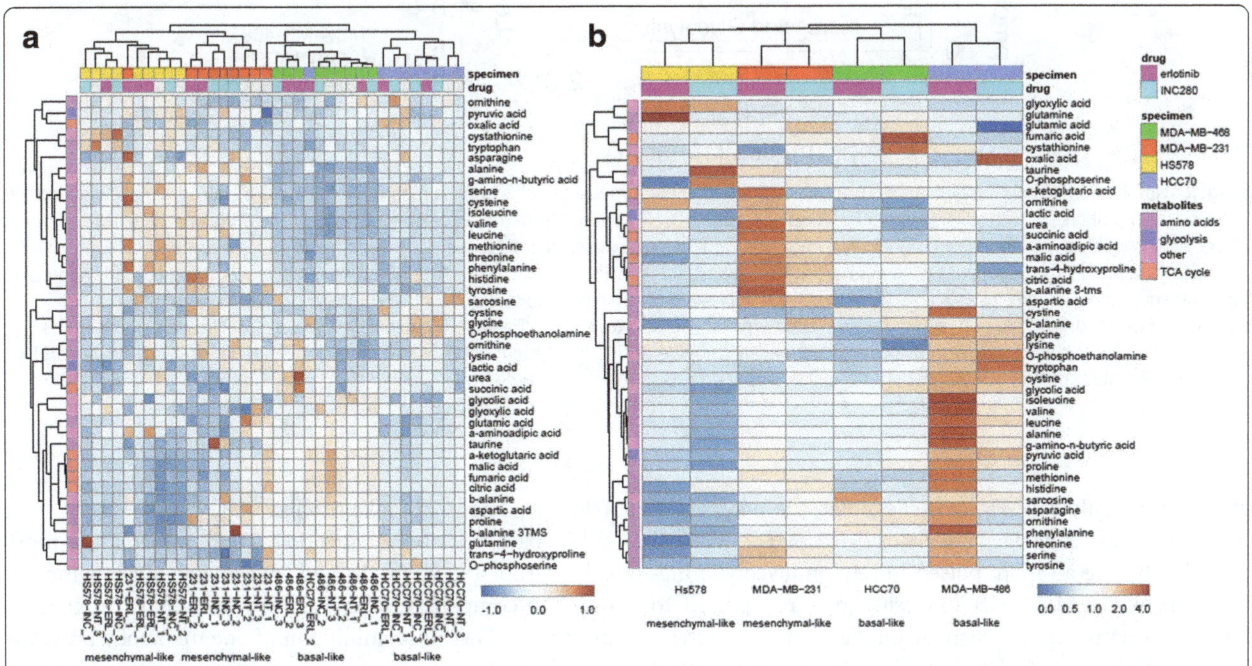

Fig. 1 Metabolomics profiling of TNBC cell lines. Hierarchical clustering of metabolic profiles of TNBC cell lines reveals molecular heterogeneity between subtypes. **a** Pool size measurements show common clusters of low TCA cycle and elevated amino acid metabolites of mesenchymal-like subtype cell lines MDA-MB-231 and Hs578 vs basal-like subtypes HCC70 and MDA-MB-456. **b** Clustering of drug responses of TNBC cell lines (average ratios of metabolite concentrations in conditions INC280/vehicle and erlotinib/vehicle are plotted for each set of biological triplicates). Drug perturbations of reduced amino acid pool sizes show similar response of reduced amino acid pool sizes upon receptor tyrosine kinase inhibitor treatment of mesenchymal-like subtype MDA-MB-231 and Hs578 cell lines. INC280/capmatinib was used to inhibit proto-oncogene MET receptor tyrosine kinase, and erlotinib was used to inhibit receptor tyrosine kinase and growth factor receptor EGFR in TNBC cell lines

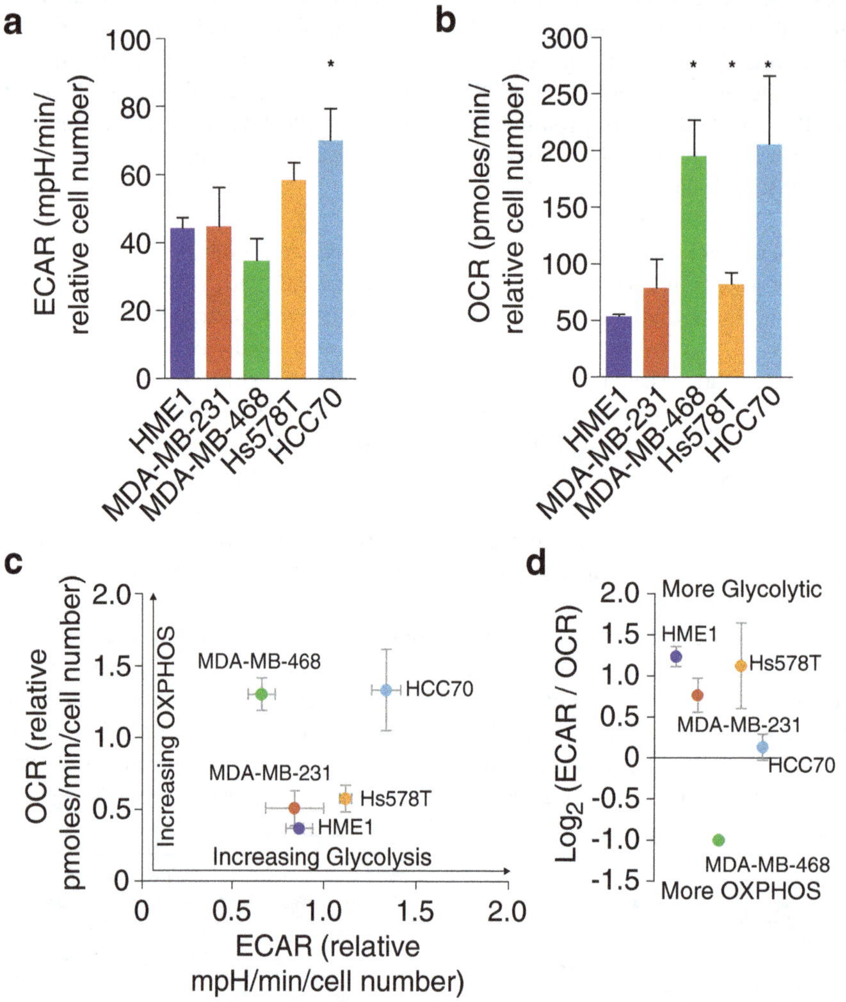

Fig. 2 TNBC basal metabolic profiles. **a** Cells were maintained in uniform media for 24 h prior to measuring ECAR. ECAR values were normalized to total cell numbers for each cell line in the ECAR assay. Data are ECAR averages from four experiments, each with five biological replicates. Error bars represent SEM. Asterisks indicate significance compared to HME1 cell values ($p \leq 0.05$). **b** Cells were maintained in uniform media for 24 h prior to measuring OCR. OCR values were normalized to total cell numbers for each cell line in the OCR assay. Data are OCR averages from four experiments, each with three biological replicates. Error bars represent SEM. Asterisks indicate significance compared to HME1 cell values ($p \leq 0.05$). **c** Relative ECAR and OCR data from **a** and **b** were plotted simultaneously to reveal overall relative basal metabolic profiles for each cell model. **d** The ECAR/OCR ratio of the data in **d** was log2 transformed to provide an index of each cell model's comparative utilization of glycolytic and oxidative metabolism

glycolytic metabolism (Fig. 2d). Together, the analyses of basal metabolic rates indicate that HME1, MDA-MB231, and Hs578T are all more poised to rely on glycolytic metabolism, while MDA-MB-468 cells are more poised to rely on oxidative metabolism in the basal state. Interestingly, in the basal state, HCC70 cells exhibited the greatest glycolytic and oxidative metabolism rates (Fig. 2a–c), but also exhibited the most balance between these rates (Fig. 2d). Understanding basal metabolic rates and the relative metabolic index may provide insight into which metabolic program specific cancers or cancer cell models may be especially sensitive (Fig. 4).

TNBC maximal metabolic profiles

While basal metabolic rates (Fig. 2) are informative, most cells harbor the ability to alter one metabolic program in order to compensate when another metabolic program is perturbed. Therefore, inhibition of one metabolic program (e.g., glycolysis) allows measurement of the maximal capability of the other metabolic program (e.g., oxidative metabolism) (Fig. 3a). To determine the maximal glycolytic and oxygen consumption metabolic capabilities (Additional file 5: Figure S2A, B) in these TNBC cell models, we measured respiration arrest-induced maximal glycolytic rates and depolarization-induced maximal

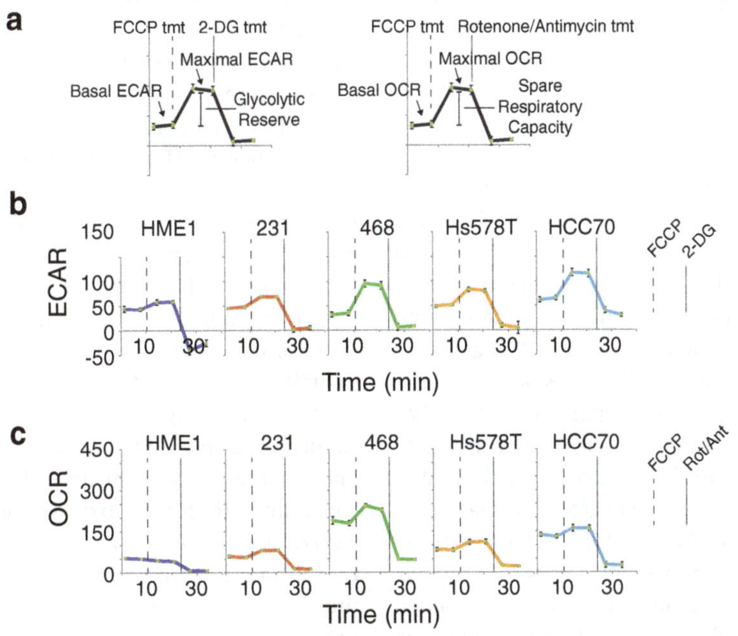

d

	Glycolytic Reserve		Spare Respiratory Capacity	
	Rate Increase	Percent Increase	Rate Increase	Percent Increase
HME1	14.6	33%	-8.8	-17%
MDA-MB-231	22.3	48%	23.3	41%
MDA-MB-468	60.0	179%	50.4	27%
Hs578T	30.8	61%	28.3	34%
HCC70	52.5	82%	26.4	20%

Fig. 3 TNBC maximal metabolic profiles. **a** Schematic indicating derivation of maximal metabolic rates, glycolytic reserve, and spare respiratory capacity from the experiments in (**a**) and (**b**). **b** Cells were maintained in uniform media prior to measuring ECAR. ECAR was measured twice in the basal state, and then twice again following each metabolic inhibitor treatment (1 μM FCCP, 50 mM 2-deoxyglucose) at 7 minute intervals. ECAR values were normalized to a measurement of total cell numbers for each cell line in the ECAR assay. Data are ECAR averages from one representative experiment, with error bars representing SD. **c** Cells were maintained in uniform media prior to measuring OCR. OCR was measured twice in the basal state, and then twice again following each metabolic inhibitor treatment (1 μM FCCP, 1 μM rotenone + 1 μM antimycin) at 7 minute intervals. OCR values were normalized to a measurement of total cell numbers for each cell line in the OCR assay. Data are OCR averages from one representative experiment, with error bars representing SD. **d** Glycolytic reserve (derived from **b**) and spare respiratory capacity (derived from **c**) calculations. Data are expressed as actual rate unit increase and percent increase over basal rates. Rate increases were calculated by subtracting the basal rate values from the maximal rate values. Percent increases were calculated by dividing the rate increase values by the basal values

OXPHOS rates (Fig. 3b, c). The MDA-MB-231 cell line and the non-transformed mammary gland epithelial cell model, HME1, exhibited the least metabolic flexibility, as demonstrated by only moderate adjustments in ECAR and OCR (changes in values post-FCCP addition, Fig. 3b) and subsequent calculated glycolytic reserve and spare respiratory capacity rates (Fig. 3c). Interestingly, these two cell lines also displayed very modest basal metabolic rates (Fig. 2). Hs578T maximal ECAR and OCR were moderately elevated above basal rates, above those of HME1 and MDA-MB-231 but below MDA-MB-468 and HCC70. Both MDA-MB-468 and HCC70 maximal ECAR were nearly double basal rates, with HCC70 displaying the greatest glycolytic capacity. MDA-MB-468 and HCC70 maximal OCR were moderately elevated above basal rates, and MDA-MB-468 displayed the greatest capacity for oxidative metabolism. From these measurements, glycolytic reserve and spare respiratory capacity can be calculated (Fig. 3a). While all cell models displayed some glycolytic reserve, HCC70 and MDA-MB-468 cells exhibited the greatest glycolytic reserves (Fig. 3d). MDA-MB-468 also exhibited the greatest spare respiratory capacity (Fig. 3d). These data indicate that each of the TNBC cells possesses a measure of metabolic flexibility as defined by their abilities to increase ECAR or OCR when the one program is perturbed, with MDA-MB-468 cells exhibiting the greatest metabolic flexibility.

TNBC response to metabolic modulators

To further characterize the metabolic profiles of these cell models, we assessed the effects on viability following treatment with metabolic modulators at concentrations commonly utilized in published literature (Fig. 4). These experiments evaluated the effects of the 5′ adenosine monophosphate-activated protein kinase (AMPK) activator [5-aminoimidazole-4-carboxamide-1β riboside (AICAR)] [48], the glycolytic inhibitor 2-deoxy-glucose (2DG) [49], the pentose phosphate inhibitor 6-amino-nicotinamide (6-AN) [50], the mitochondrial complex I inhibitor rotenone [51], and the AMPK activator/Complex I inhibitor metformin [52, 53] (Fig. 4a). Similar to the metabolic rate investigations above, the TNBC models exhibited heterogeneous responses to these treatments; however, from these results, some interesting patterns were observed (Fig. 4b–f). Each TNBC model exhibited an approximately 40–60% loss of viability in response to the glycolytic inhibitor 2-DG. Interestingly, HME1 cells, which exhibited the greatest bias towards basal utilization of glycolytic metabolism (Fig. 2e), were most affected by 2-DG treatment, as well as the pentose phosphate inhibitor 6-AN (Fig. 4b). Conversely, MDA-MB-468 cells, which exhibited the greatest bias towards basal utilization of oxidative metabolism (Fig. 2e), were most affected by the electron transport chain inhibitor, rotenone (Fig. 4d).

Also of note, Hs578T cells exhibited enhanced proliferation in response to AICAR while other cell lines exhibited variable decreases in viability compared to control. While AICAR and metformin are both commonly used as AMPK activators, they activate AMPK via disparate mechanisms. However, metformin and rotenone both perturb oxidative phosphorylation through respiratory chain complex I (RCI) inhibition. Our results reveal more similar viability effects between metformin and rotenone (common RCI inhibitors) than between metformin and AICAR (common AMPK activators) (Fig. 4b–f).

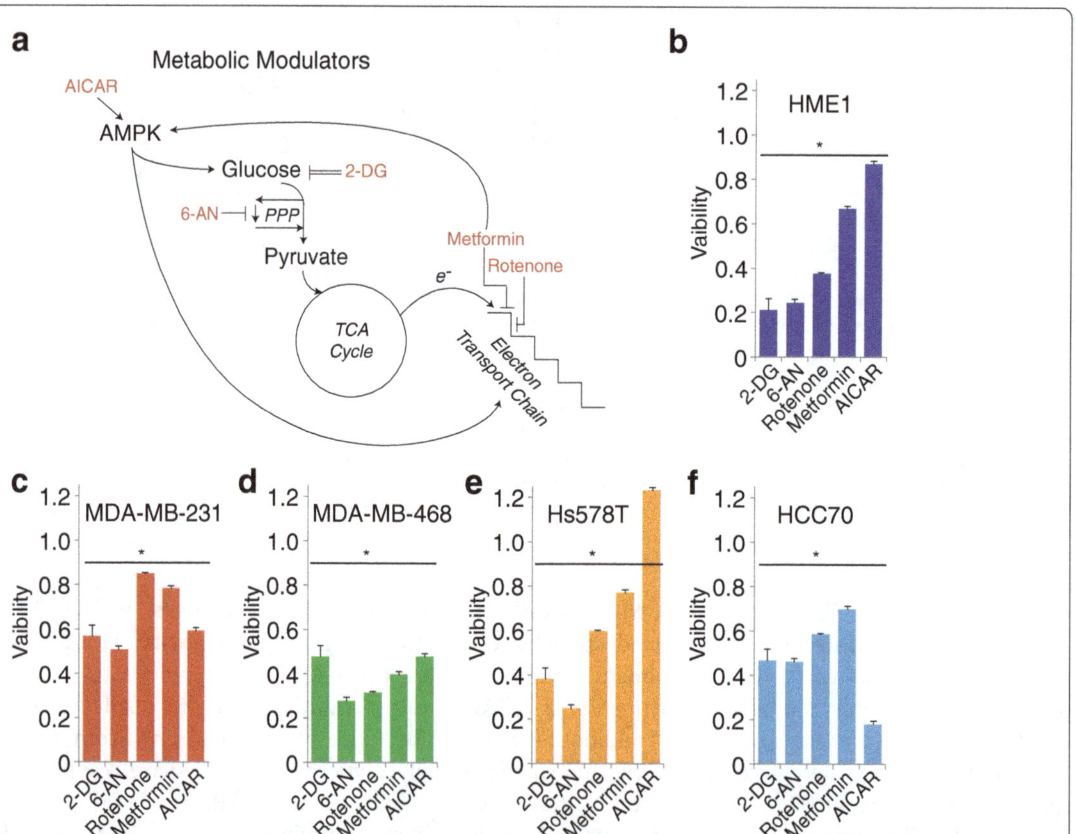

Fig. 4 TNBC response to metabolic modulators. **a** Schematic of metabolic pathways and the points at which chemical inhibitors or activators act. **b–d** Viability measurements of cells following 48 h of treatment with indicated chemicals: 25 mM 2-DG, 200 μM 6-AN, 1 μM rotenone, 10 mM metformin, and 1 mM AICAR. Data are viability averages from one representative experiment with error bars representing SD. Asterisks represent significance compared to vehicle control ($p \leq 0.01$)

Comprehensive analysis of rate-limiting enzymes and RTK inhibition

EGFR and MET receptors are known to drive tumorigenic progression, and RTKs are known to regulate metabolic signaling pathways [54]. To investigate the effects of EGFR and MET inhibition on TNBC metabolism, we measured ECAR and OCR in TNBC cells treated with the EGFR inhibitor erlotinib and the MET inhibitor INC280 (capmatinib). As in the above analyses, the TNBC cell models displayed heterogeneous responses to the tyrosine kinase inhibitors (TKIs). We observed that MET and EGFR inhibition had little effect on the glycolytic and oxidative metabolism rates of basal A/B subtype MDA-MB-468 or HCC70 cell lines (Fig. 5a). In contrast, in both mesenchymal-like MDA-MB-231 and Hs578T cell lines, both MET and EGFR inhibition strongly perturbed both glycolysis and oxidative metabolism (Fig. 5a). Importantly, comparing these data to a principal component analysis of our metabolomics data revealed that metabolic changes of mesenchymal-like MDA-MB-231 and Hs578T cell lines upon drug treatment recapitulated the observed changes of metabolic fluxes (Fig. 5b). Both cell lines show perturbation of the top two principal components (reflecting 84.9% of the data) in the same direction and magnitude. In contrast, major principle components of metabolic perturbations do not change for basal-like subtype MDA-MB-468 or HCC70. Despite the metabolic responses of MDA-MB-231 and Hs578T cell lines to INC280 vs erlotibib based on amino acid and TCA cycle metabolism of mesenchymal-like cell lines are in agreement, glycolytic rates show differential perturbation. Among the assessed TNBC cell lines, mesenchymal-like subtypes showed strong, consistent perturbations, despite underlying heterogeneity of breast cancer subtypes.

To more comprehensively investigate the metabolic consequences of EGFR and MET inhibition in TNBC models, we performed a siRNA screen in each cell line targeting all 323 rate-limiting enzymes in the human KEGG metabolic pathways and Rate Limiting Enzyme Regulation databases. This compliment of enzymes was divided into 11 major metabolic categories representing 89 metabolic pathways (Additional file 3: Table S2). The siRNA screen was performed in duplicate in each cell line in cells treated with vehicle (DMSO), INC280, or erlotinib. A sensitivity index was applied to viability measurements to determine the effect of siRNA knockdown

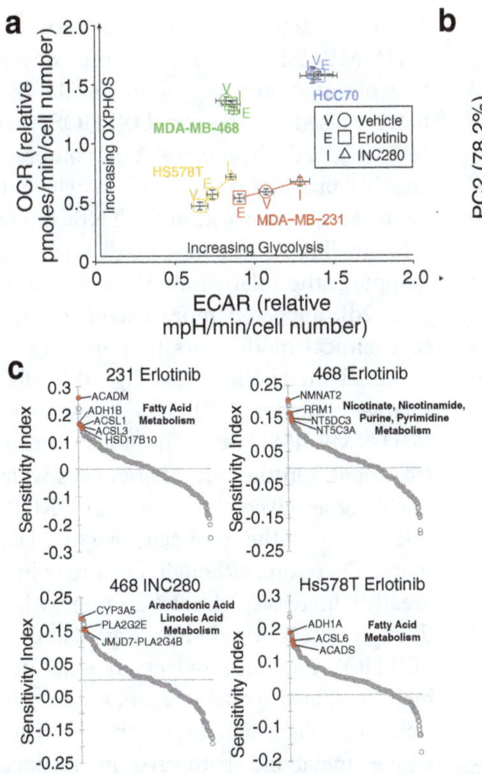

Fig. 5 RTK-dependent TNBC sensitization to metabolic pathway perturbation. **a** Metabolic rate response to RTK inhibitors. 40,000 cells per well were plated in Seahorse 96-well assay plates. Cells were treated for 24 h with the DMSO, erlotinib, or INC280, and then ECAR and OCR were measured as described in Methods. **b** Principle component analysis of drug responses. Mesenchymal-like subtype MDA-MB-231 and Hs578 cell lines show largest perturbations. **c** RNAi screen results for selected TKI treatments which induce sensitivities to knockdown of common metabolic pathway genes

on drug sensitivity, and therefore identifies genes whose knockdown preferentially reduces viability in TNBC cells treated with a TKI vs vehicle alone (see Methods, Additional file 6: Table S4). Eight of the 11 major metabolic categories were represented in the sensitivity index to varying levels for each TNBC model and each TKI (Additional file 7: Figure S3, see also Additional file 6: Table S4, Additional file 8: Table S5). Notably, lipid metabolism was prominent (represented > 15% of hits) in each TNBC model treated with INC280 or erlotinib, while amino acid metabolism was also prominent in each TNBC model treated with INC280. Evaluating individual significant rate-limiting enzymes in each group revealed potential sensitivities associated with specific TKI for some TNBC subtypes (Fig. 5c). MDA-MB-231 and Hs578T cells treated with erlotinib were sensitive to knockdown of fatty acid genes, while MDA-MB-468 cells treated with the same TKI were sensitive to knockdown of specific nucleotide metabolism pathways. INC280 sensitized MDA-MB-468 cells to knockdown of arachidonic and linoleic acid metabolism rate limiting enzymes. Interestingly, a broader analysis of metabolic pathways across cell TNBC subtypes in response to TKI treatments identified additional sensitivities. The top ten metabolic pathways identified by the sensitivity index displayed significant overlap between the TKI treatments (Additional file 7: Figure S3, see also Additional file 8: Table S5). Additionally, within this set of common pathways, three pathways which are engaged to counteract oxidative stress were enriched in the screen results (Glutathione metabolism, cytochrome P450 metabolism, and non-P450 drug metabolism pathways). These results suggest that even with the molecular heterogeneity that is present in TNBC, there are common metabolic programs that can be targeted in TNBC subtypes. Taken together, these data shows that targeting pathways such as fatty acid metabolism, pyrimidine metabolism, or oxidative stress relief pathways in combination with MET or EGFR inhibition may represent an effective therapeutic strategy.

Discussion

In this study, we characterized the metabolic heterogeneity of TNBC and identified a core set of metabolic pathways that are common among the TNBC subtypes, yet observed diverse metabolic profiles among TNBC cell lines. Genetic and signaling heterogeneity is observed in most solid cancers, and studies have indicated that there is a particularly high level of genomic heterogeneity among TNBC patients [39]. These observations of heterogeneity have been borne out in metabolic analyses of TNBC as well. Analyses of TNBC patient tissues have demonstrated heterogeneity of glycolytic and mitochondrial protein expression [40, 41, 55]. TNBC cell lines have also exhibited heterogeneity with respect to glutamine metabolism [42] and response to the metabolic modulator, metformin [33, 34]. Therefore, the heterogeneity evident between TNBC cell lines in our detailed metabolic characterization extends these previous findings. Metabolic pool sizes and drug responses revealed common patterns between TNBC subtypes but also highlighted cell line-specific responses (Fig. 1). Importantly, drug responses of metabolic rates and principle metabolic components identified a theme of metabolic capacity and adaptability as major difference of mesenchymal-like vs basal-like subtypes (Fig. 5) [56]. Basal-like cell lines are metabolically most active with the highest OCR and ECAR (Fig. 2c), resulting in low, depleted metabolic pool sizes (Fig. 1a). Mesenchymal-like cell lines have significantly lower OXPHOS allowing them to modulate and adaptively respond to the drug challenges (Fig. 5a, b). The HCC70 cell is an example of extremely high OCR and ECAR that allows for minimal adjustment to drug challenges. The unique metabolic profiles (Figs. 1, 2, and 3) response to chemical modulators (Fig. 4) and sensitivities to combined RTK, and metabolic pathway inhibition (Fig. 5) provides platforms which can help place the responses of these TNBC cell line models in previous and future studies into a broader metabolic context. For example, previous work demonstrated that MDA-MB-468 cells are more sensitive to metformin than MDA-MB-231 cells. Here, we provide a potential basis for that observation as we found MDA-MB-468 cells to be more poised to rely on OXPHOS than MDA-MB-231 cells (Fig. 2d). Therefore, this comprehensive metabolic analysis provides a platform in which to identify therapeutic sensitivities within the TNBC metabolic landscape.

In the TNBC cell models that we evaluated, an index mapping, the relative affinities for basal metabolic rates (Fig. 2d), appeared more useful for predicting response to chemical modulators (Fig. 4) than did an analysis of maximal metabolic rates (Fig. 3). Cells which displayed relatively higher OXPHOS rates than glycolytic rates (MDA-MB-468) were the most sensitive to rotenone treatment. On the other hand, cells which displayed relatively higher glycolytic rates than OXHPOS rates (HME1, Hs578T) were the most sensitive to 2-DG and 6-AN treatment. Therefore, although a cell may harbor the ability to greatly increase glycolytic rate when OXPHOS is disrupted (MDA-MB-468, Fig. 3a, d), its higher basal OXPHOS rate may reflect an absolute requirement for high, sustained oxidative metabolism. Therefore, it is possible that cells which display the ability to upregulate alternative metabolic pathways in response to metabolic insults still remain dependent on the metabolic pathways which they preferentially utilize in the basal state.

In addition to glycolytic and mitochondrial oxidative metabolism alterations, TNBC patient samples display evidence of altered glutamine metabolism compared to HER2 positive cancers [57]. TNBC cancer cell line models enhance glutamine uptake and metabolism, which are associated with epigenetic changes favoring expression of pro-tumorigenic genes [58, 59]. Other studies provide evidence of altered amino acid metabolism in TNBC. MDA-MB-231 and MDA-MB-468 cells exhibit elevated serine metabolism protein expression compared to HER2 positive cell lines, an observation that is shared in patient samples [60, 61]. Metabolomics analyses of patient samples identified lower amino acid levels in TNBC patients compared to healthy controls [62]. A folate metabolism enzyme may also serve as a biomarker for TNBC in distinct ethnic populations [63]. Finally, altered lipid metabolism appears to play a part in TNBC. Patient TNBC and non-TNBC tissues can be discriminated based on markers of lipid metabolism [64, 65], and MDA-MB-231 and MDA-MB-468 cells are effectively induced to undergo apoptosis upon suppressing expression of the lipogenic transcription factors, SREBP1/2 [66]. Recent metabolomics analyses identified metabolites associated with the Warburg effect, and the oxidative stress response, and specific metabolite signatures associated with different driver mutations [67]. Metabolomics have also identified potential global differences in breast cancer-associated metabolites between patients of different races [61], and miRNA-associated thiamine homeostasis specific to TNBC patient samples [68].

RTKs are promising drug targets due to their high expression in TNBC. The success of trastuzumab in $HER2^+$ breast cancer underscores the potential of targeting tyrosine kinases yet, in spite of this promising start, monotherapy with tyrosine kinase inhibitors (TKIs) has had limited success in the clinic. In this study, we evaluated the effects of RTK inhibition on metabolic pathways in TNBC. This analysis highlighted the unique metabolic dependencies in our TNBC models, but also revealed reveal a core set of metabolic pathways that are universally affected by TKI treatment. Collectively, TNBC cells were commonly sensitized to inhibition of redox homeostasis, fatty acid metabolism, and nucleotide metabolism by erlotinib and INC280 treatment. The metabolomics results provide a mechanistic basis for the lipid metabolism sensitivity identified in the RLE siRNA screen. Flux analyses of multiple cancers demonstrate that altering TCA cycle flux significantly impinges upon lipid metabolism [69]. Therefore, the sensitivities to lipid metabolism RLE knockdown could be predicted by the concurrent changes in amino acid metabolites. Glutathione metabolism, cytochrome P450 metabolism, and non-P450 drug metabolism pathways, each of which ameliorate oxidative stress, were enriched in the siRNA screen, highlighting the importance of redox homeostasis in this context. Clinically, redox pathways have been shown to be upregulated in TNBC vs ER+ tumors [70] and heightened glycolytic metabolism may be regulated in part by oxidative stress in TNBC cells [71]. Our data provide additional impetus for co-targeting these metabolic and kinase pathways in TNBC patients [72]. siRNAs targeting fatty acid metabolism and specifically arachidonic acid metabolism genes were also common hits in the screen. Expression of fatty acid metabolism enzymes have previously been associated with TNBC metastasis [64] and survival rates [65]. Arachidonic acid metabolism itself may also be linked to cytochrome P450 metabolism in breast cancers [72]. Interestingly, suppression of tryptophan metabolism enhances INC280 treatment (Additional file 7: Figure S3). A previous investigation of BT549 TNBC cells demonstrated a link between tryptophan metabolism-dependent kynurenine production and breast cancer cell anoikis resistance, particularly in ER negative cell [73]. Because the data in Fig. 3d show that MDA-MB-468 cells have very little relative glycolytic activity while maintaining high OXPHOS activity, it would be reasonable to expect less effects from suppression of carbon metabolism RLEs. The data in Additional file 2: Figure S3 bear this out as carbon metabolism RLE knockdown has the least effect on MDA-MB-468 cells. A potential mechanism for this observation may be the KRAS mutational status of MDA-MB-468 cells which is not shared by the other TNBC lines under study. A previous study has demonstrated that some KRAS-driven cancers cells significantly upregulate OXPHOS metabolism [74]. Finally, MET or EGFR inhibition collectively sensitized TNBC cells to knockdown of pyrimidine and purine metabolism enzymes. Interestingly, a significant proportion of the siRNA hits driving enrichment of these metabolic pathways in our study are 5′-nucleotidases and nucleotide kinases. These results suggest that regulation of nucleotide phosphorylation plays an important role in determining sensitivity to RTK inhibitors in TNBC. Therefore, small molecules disrupting nucleotide phosphorylation dynamics may prove effective at enhancing RTK inhibition in TNBC.

Conclusions

The findings in this study provide comprehensive information on the metabolic background of TNBC subtypes, their unique and common metabolic dependencies, and how they respond to metabolic insults. These results provide a valuable resource for investigators who utilize these TNBC cell lines. Additionally, our siRNA analysis establishes a comprehensive analysis of metabolic rate-limiting enzymes and identifies erlotinib- and INC280-sensitized pathways. Overall, this comprehensive metabolic analysis demonstrates the metabolic heterogeneity within TNBC and identifies therapeutic sensitivities that may be exploited in treating TNBC patients.

Additional files

Additional file 1: Table S1. Genes targeted and siRNA sequences used in siRNA screen. (XLSX 57 kb)

Additional file 2: Figure S1. RNAi screen, cell lines, and metabolic rates. (A) Schematic of RNAi screen (left) and transfection efficiency under screen conditions (right). (B) Characteristics of each cell line used in this study. (C) Schematic representing biological compartments and metabolic pathways assessed for metabolic rates. (PDF 957 kb)

Additional file 3: Table S2. Genes and metabolic categories and pathways used in siRNA screen. Rate-limiting enzymes were collated through KEGG annotation (http://www.genome.jp/kegg/), the Rate-Limiting Enzyme Regulation Database (http://rle.cbi.pku.edu.cn/home.cgi, [51]), and literature searches and categorized according to KEGG. (XLSX 25 kb)

Additional file 4: Table S3. Quantitation of metabolic pool sizes, ratios for cell lines, and drug responses with statistical values. Total ion count integrated over peak area for metabolite-specific mass ion validated by multiple precursor-product ion combinations. Mean, standard deviation, and ANOVA with student's t test compares triple-negative breast cancer (TNBC) cell lines and treatment with INC280 or erlotinib vs control vehicle (DMSO). (XLSX 52 kb)

Additional file 5: Figure S2. OCR and ECAR measurement explanation. (A) i. Normally functioning cellular respiration utilizes electrons in the form of NADH and FADH2 to pass down the electron transport chain (ETC) gradient. These redox reactions in the ETC pump hydrogen ions from the mitochondrial matrix into the mitochondrial inner membrane space (IMS), providing an electrochemical gradient which in turn powers ATP synthase-dependent ATP production. ii. FCCP is a lipid-soluble ionophore that allows hydrogen ions to escape the IMS, functionally uncoupling the ETC from ATP synthase-mediated ATP production. iii. In order to restore FCCP-mediated depletion of ATP levels, glycolytic flux increases to maximum capacity. iv. In order to maintain a minimal hydrogen ion gradient in the IMS, mitochondrial complex IV activity increases to maximum capacity, thus inducing maximum oxygen consumption. (B) The order of metabolic rate measurements and metabolic toxin treatment for maximal rate measurements. i. Basal glycolytic rate. ii. Respiration arrest-induced maximal glycolytic rate. iii. Glycolytic arrest. iv. Basal OXPHOS rate. v. Depolarization-induced maximal OXPHOS rate. vi. OXPHOS arrest. (PDF 997 kb)

Additional file 6: Table S4. Drug response and sensitivity index for siRNA treatment of triple-negative breast cancer (TNBC) cell lines.. (XLSX 128 kb)

Additional file 7: Figure S3. Sensitization to metabolic pathway perturbation. (A) Graphical representation of the proportion which each metabolic category (Table S2) was represented in the top 10% sensitivity index scores. (B) The combined top ten pathways as defined by high-scoring sensitivity index genes for each TKI (INC80 or erlotinib). (PDF 801 kb)

Additional file 8: Table S5. Top 10% scoring siRNAs in the siRNA screen for each condition. (XLSX 27 kb)

Abbreviations

2-DG: 2-deoxyglucose; 6-AN: 6-aminonicotanimide; AICAR: 5-Aminoimidazole-4-carboxamide ribonucleotide; AMPK: 5′ adenosine monophosphate-activated protein kinase; DMSO: Dimethyl sulfoxide; ECAR: Extracellular acidification rate; EGFR: Epidermal growth factor receptor; ER: Estrogen receptor, ESR1; HER2: Human epidermal growth factor receptor 2, NEU, ERBB2; INC280: Capmatinib, MET small molecule inhibitor; KEGG: Kyoto Encyclopedia of Genes and Genomes; MET: Hepatocyte growth factor receptor; OCR: Oxygen consumption rate; OXPHOS: Oxidative phosphorylation; PR: Progesterone receptor, PGR; RCI: Respiratory chain complex I; RTK: Receptor tyrosine kinase; SI: Sensitivity index; siRNA: Small interfering RNA; TKI: Tyrosine kinase inhibitor; TNBC: Triple negative breast cancer

Funding

This work was supported by NIH National Cancer Institute grants CA159709 (NJL) and CA154887 (F.V.F.), The Frederik and Lena Meijer Student Internship Program (JC), The Van Andel Foundation (JM, CRG), The Breast Cancer Research Foundation (CRG), Health Science Research Institute Grant (F.V.F.), and University of California Cancer Research Coordinating Committee research grant CRN-17-427258 (F.V.F.).

Authors' contributions

NJL participated in study conception and design, carried out all experiments except metabolomics experiments, analyzed all data, and wrote the manuscript. JPC and EAT participated in assay development and RTKi experiments. ANL analyzed RNAi screen data. JPM participated in study conception, design, and coordination, and data analysis. SJS and AS extracted, derivatized, and quantitated metabolites. FVF designed and analyzed metabolomics experiments and conducted data interpretation and writing of the manuscript. CRG conceived of the study, participated in study design, coordination, and data analysis, and wrote the manuscript. All authors read and approved the final manuscript.

Competing interests

The authors declare that they have no competing interests.

Author details

[1]California State University, Los Angeles, 5151 State University Drive, Los Angeles, CA 90032, USA. [2]Van Andel Research Institute, 333 Bostwick Ave, NE, Grand Rapids, MI 49503, USA. [3]Systems Biology and Cancer Metabolism, Program for Quantitative Systems Biology, University of California Merced, 2500 North Lake Road, Merced, CA 95343, USA. [4]College of Human Medicine, Michigan State University, 15 Michigan St. NE, Grand Rapids, MI 49503, USA.

References

1. Foulkes WD, Smith IE, Reis-Filho JS. Triple-negative breast cancer. N Engl J Med. 2010;363:1938–48.
2. Dent R, Trudeau M, Pritchard KI, Hanna WM, Kahn HK, Sawka CA, Lickley LA, Rawlinson E, Sun P, Narod SA. Triple-negative breast cancer: clinical features and patterns of recurrence. Clin Cancer Res. 2007;13(15 Pt 1):4429–34.
3. Liedtke C, Mazouni C, Hess KR, André F, Tordai A, Mejia JA, Symmans WF, Gonzalez-Angulo AM, Hennessy B, Green M, Cristofanilli M, Hortobagyi GN, Pusztai L. Response to neoadjuvant therapy and long-term survival in patients with triple-negative breast cancer. J Clin Oncol. 2008;26:1275–81.
4. Lehmann BD, Bauer JA, Chen X, Sanders ME, Chakravarthy AB, Shyr Y, Pietenpol JA. Identification of human triple-negative breast cancer subtypes and preclinical models for selection of targeted therapies. J Clin Invest. 2011;121:2750–67.
5. Burstein MD, Tsimelzon A, Poage GM, Covington KR, Contreras A, Fuqua SAW, Savage MI, Osborne CK, Hilsenbeck SG, Chang JC, Mills GB, Lau CC, Brown PH. Comprehensive genomic analysis identifies novel subtypes and targets of triple-negative breast cancer. Clin Cancer Res. 2015;21:1688–98.
6. Koenders PG, Beex LV, Geurts-Moespot A, Heuvel JJ, Kienhuis CB, Benraad TJ. Epidermal growth factor receptor-negative tumors are predominantly confined to the subgroup of estradiol receptor-positive human primary breast cancers. Cancer Res. 1991;51:4544–8.
7. Sainsbury JR, Farndon JR, Needham GK, Malcolm AJ, Harris AL. Epidermal-growth-factor receptor status as predictor of early recurrence of and death from breast cancer. Lancet (London, England). 1987;1:1398–402.
8. Singletary SE, Baker FL, Spitzer G, Tucker SL, Tomasovic B, Brock WA, Ajani JA, Kelly AM. Biological effect of epidermal growth factor on the in vitro growth of human tumors. Cancer Res. 1987;47:403–6.
9. Toi M, Osaki A, Yamada H, Toge T. Epidermal growth factor receptor expression as a prognostic indicator in breast cancer. Eur J Cancer. 1991;27:977–80.
10. Cheang MCU, Voduc D, Bajdik C, Leung S, McKinney S, Chia SK, Perou CM, Nielsen TO. Basal-like breast cancer defined by five biomarkers has superior prognostic value than triple-negative phenotype. Clin Cancer Res. 2008;14: 1368–76.
11. Ghoussoub RA, Dillon DA, D'Aquila T, Rimm EB, Fearon ER, Rimm DL. Expression of c-met is a strong independent prognostic factor in breast carcinoma. Cancer. 1998;82:1513–20.
12. Camp RL, Rimm EB, Rimm DL. Met expression is associated with poor outcome in patients with axillary lymph node negative breast carcinoma. Cancer. 1999;86:2259–65.
13. Tolgay Ocal I, Dolled-Filhart M, D'Aquila TG, Camp RL, Rimm DL. Tissue microarray-based studies of patients with lymph node negative breast

carcinoma show that met expression is associated with worse outcome but is not correlated with epidermal growth factor family receptors. Cancer. 2003;97:1841–8.
14. Edakuni G, Sasatomi E, Satoh T, Tokunaga O, Miyazaki K. Expression of the hepatocyte growth factor/c-Met pathway is increased at the cancer front in breast carcinoma. Pathol Int. 2001;51:172–8.
15. Lengyel E, Prechtel D, Resau JH, Gauger K, Welk A, Lindemann K, Salanti G, Richter T, Knudsen B, Vande Woude GF, Harbeck N. C-Met overexpression in node-positive breast cancer identifies patients with poor clinical outcome independent of Her2/neu. Int J Cancer. 2005;113:678–82.
16. Graveel CR, DeGroot JD, Su Y, Koeman J, Dykema K, Leung S, Snider J, Davies SR, Swiatek PJ, Cottingham S, Watson MA, Ellis MJ, Sigler RE, Furge KA, Vande Woude GF. Met induces diverse mammary carcinomas in mice and is associated with human basal breast cancer. Proc Natl Acad Sci. 2009;106:12909–14.
17. Ponzo MG, Lesurf R, Petkiewicz S, O'Malley FP, Pinnaduwage D, Andrulis IL, Bull SB, Chughtai N, Zuo D, Souleimanova M, Germain D, Omeroglu A, Cardiff RD, Hallett M, Park M. Met induces mammary tumors with diverse histologies and is associated with poor outcome and human basal breast cancer. Proc Natl Acad Sci U S A. 2009;106:12903–8.
18. Sameni M, Tovar EA, Essenburg CJ, Chalasani A, Linklater ES, Borgman A, Cherba DM, Anbalagan A, Winn ME, Graveel CR, Sloane BF. Cabozantinib (XL184) inhibits growth and invasion of preclinical TNBC models. Clin Cancer Res. 2016;22:923–34.
19. Linklater ES, Tovar EA, Essenburg CJ, Turner L, Madaj Z, Winn ME, Melnik MK, Korkaya H, Maroun CR, Christensen JG, Steensma MR, Boerner JL, Graveel CR. Targeting MET and EGFR crosstalk signaling in triple-negative breast cancers. Oncotarget. 2016;7(43):69903–15.
20. Wellen KE, Thompson CB. A two-way street: reciprocal regulation of metabolism and signalling. Nat Rev Mol Cell Biol. 2012;13:270–6.
21. De Rosa V, Iommelli F, Monti M, Fonti R, Votta G, Stoppelli MP, Del Vecchio S. Reversal of warburg effect and reactivation of oxidative phosphorylation by differential inhibition of EGFR signaling pathways in non-small cell lung cancer. Clin Cancer Res. 2015;21(22):5110–20.
22. Bian Y, Yu Y, Wang S, Li L. Up-regulation of fatty acid synthase induced by EGFR/ERK activation promotes tumor growth in pancreatic cancer. Biochem Biophys Res Commun. 2015;463:612–7.
23. Li X, Lu Y, Lu H, Luo J, Hong Y, Fan Z. AMPK-mediated energy homeostasis and associated metabolic effects on cancer cell response and resistance to cetuximab. Oncotarget. 2015;6:11507–18.
24. Borlak J, Singh P, Gazzana G. Proteome mapping of epidermal growth factor induced hepatocellular carcinomas identifies novel cell metabolism targets and mitogen activated protein kinase signaling events. BMC Genomics. 2015;16:124.
25. Natan S, Tsarfaty G, Horev J, Haklai R, Kloog Y, Tsarfaty I. Interplay between HGF/SF-met-Ras signaling, tumor metabolism and blood flow as a potential target for breast cancer therapy. Oncoscience. 2014;1:30–8.
26. Petrocca F, Altschuler G, Tan SM, Mendillo ML, Yan H, Jerry DJ, Kung AL, Hide W, Ince TA, Lieberman J. A genome-wide siRNA screen identifies proteasome addiction as a vulnerability of basal-like triple-negative breast cancer cells. Cancer Cell. 2013;24:182–96.
27. Pelicano H, Zhang W, Liu J, Hammoudi N, Dai J, Xu R-H, Pusztai L, Huang P. Mitochondrial dysfunction in some triple-negative breast cancer cell lines: role of mTOR pathway and therapeutic potential. Breast Cancer Res. 2014;16:434.
28. Diers AR, Vayalil PK, Oliva CR, Griguer CE, Darley-Usmar V, Hurst DR, Welch DR, Landar A. Mitochondrial bioenergetics of metastatic breast cancer cells in response to dynamic changes in oxygen tension: effects of HIF-1α. PLoS One. 2013;8:e68348.
29. Choi J, Jung W-H, Koo JS. Metabolism-related proteins are differentially expressed according to the molecular subtype of invasive breast cancer defined by surrogate immunohistochemistry. Pathobiology. 2013;80:41–52.
30. Estrella V, Chen T, Lloyd M, Wojtkowiak J, Cornnell HH, Ibrahim-Hashim A, Bailey K, Balagurunathan Y, Rothberg JM, Sloane BF, Johnson J, Gatenby RA, Gillies RJ. Acidity generated by the tumor microenvironment drives local invasion. Cancer Res. 2013;73:1524–35.
31. Shen L, O'Shea JM, Kaadige MR, Cunha S, Wilde BR, Cohen AL, Welm AL, Ayer DE. Metabolic reprogramming in triple-negative breast cancer through Myc suppression of TXNIP. Proc Natl Acad Sci U S A. 2015;112:5425–30.
32. McCleland ML, Adler AS, Shang Y, Hunsaker T, Truong T, Peterson D, Torres E, Li L, Haley B, Stephan J-P, Belvin M, Hatzivassiliou G, Blackwood EM, Corson L, Evangelista M, Zha J, Firestein R. An integrated genomic screen identifies LDHB as an essential gene for triple-negative breast cancer. Cancer Res. 2012;72:5812–23.
33. Wahdan-Alaswad R, Fan Z, Edgerton SM, Liu B, Deng X-S, Arnadottir SS, Richer JK, Anderson SM, Thor AD. Glucose promotes breast cancer aggression and reduces metformin efficacy. Cell Cycle. 2013;12:3759–69.
34. Zielinski DC, Filipp FV, Bordbar A, Jensen K, Smith JW, Herrgard MJ, Mo ML, Palsson BO, Mjorndal T, Pirmohamed M, Arrowsmith J, Arrowsmith J, Loffler W, Kilian R, Toumi M, Angermeyer MC, Passarelli MC, Jacob-Filho W, Figueras A, Begaud B, Martin K, Fourrier A, Haramburu F, Pirmohamed M, Park BK, Kuhn M, Ong SE, Manolio TA, Lee S, Lee KH, et al. Pharmacogenomic and clinical data link non-pharmacokinetic metabolic dysregulation to drug side effect pathogenesis. Nat Commun. 2015;6:7101.
35. Filipp F V. Cancer metabolism meets systems biology: Pyruvate kinase isoform PKM2 is a metabolic master regulator. J Carcinog. 2013;12.
36. Wang F, Yang Y. Inhibition of PKM2 sensitizes triple-negative breast cancer cells to doxorubicin. Biochem Biophys Res Commun. 2014;454:465–70.
37. Palorini R, Simonetto T, Cirulli C, Chiaradonna F. Mitochondrial complex I inhibitors and forced oxidative phosphorylation synergize in inducing cancer cell death. Int J Cell Biol. 2013;2013:243876.
38. Cheng G, Zielonka J, Dranka BP, McAllister D, Mackinnon AC, Joseph J, Kalyanaraman B. Mitochondria-targeted drugs synergize with 2-deoxyglucose to trigger breast cancer cell death. Cancer Res. 2012;72:2634–44.
39. Jiang T, Shi W, Natowicz R, Ononye SN, Wali VB, Kluger Y, Pusztai L, Hatzis C. Statistical measures of transcriptional diversity capture genomic heterogeneity of cancer. BMC Genomics. 2014;15:876.
40. Kim S, Kim DH, Jung W-H, Koo JS. Metabolic phenotypes in triple-negative breast cancer. Tumour Biol. 2013;34:1699–712.
41. Choi J, Kim DH, Jung WH, Koo JS. Metabolic interaction between cancer cells and stromal cells according to breast cancer molecular subtype. Breast Cancer Res. 2013;15:R78.
42. Timmerman LA, Holton T, Yuneva M, Louie RJ, Padró M, Daemen A, Hu M, Chan DA, Ethier SP, van't Veer LJ, Polyak K, McCormick F, Gray JW. Glutamine sensitivity analysis identifies the xCT antiporter as a common triple-negative breast tumor therapeutic target. Cancer Cell. 2013;24:450–65.
43. Yizhak K, Le Dévédec SE, Rogkoti VM, Baenke F, de Boer VC, Frezza C, Schulze A, van de Water B, Ruppin E. A computational study of the Warburg effect identifies metabolic targets inhibiting cancer migration. Mol Syst Biol. 2014;10:744.
44. Zhao M, Chen X, Gao G, Tao L, Wei L. RLEdb: a database of rate-limiting enzymes and their regulation in human, rat, mouse, yeast and E. coli. Cell Res. 2009;19:793–5.
45. Hoffman FO, Miller CW: Uncertainties in environmental radiological assessment models and their implications. 1983.
46. Ye F, Bauer JA, Pietenpol JA, Shyr Y. Analysis of high-throughput RNAi screening data in identifying genes mediating sensitivity to chemotherapeutic drugs: statistical approaches and perspectives. BMC Genomics. 2012;13(Suppl 8):S3.
47. Hamby DM. A comparison of sensitivity analysis techniques. Health Phys. 1995;68:195–204.
48. Corton JM, Gillespie JG, Hawley SA, Hardie DG. 5-aminoimidazole-4-carboxamide ribonucleoside. A specific method for activating AMP-activated protein kinase in intact cells? Eur J Biochem. 1995;229:558–65.
49. BROWN J. Effects of 2-deoxyglucose on carbohydrate metablism: review of the literature and studies in the rat. Metabolism. 1962;11:1098–112.
50. Koutcher JA, Alfieri AA, Matei C, Meyer KL, Street JC, Martin DS. Effect of 6-aminonicotinamide on the pentose phosphate pathway: 31P NMR and tumor growth delay studies. Magn Reson Med. 1996;36:887–92.
51. Singer TP, Ramsay RR. The reaction sites of rotenone and ubiquinone with mitochondrial NADH dehydrogenase. Biochim Biophys Acta. 1994;1187:198–202.
52. Owen MR, Doran E, Halestrap AP. Evidence that metformin exerts its anti-diabetic effects through inhibition of complex 1 of the mitochondrial respiratory chain. Biochem J. 2000;348(Pt 3):607–14.
53. Zhou G, Myers R, Li Y, Chen Y, Shen X, Fenyk-Melody J, Wu M, Ventre J, Doebber T, Fujii N, Musi N, Hirshman MF, Goodyear LJ, Moller DE. Role of AMP-activated protein kinase in mechanism of metformin action. J Clin Invest. 2001;108:1167–74.
54. Ward PS, Thompson CB. Metabolic reprogramming: a cancer hallmark even warburg did not anticipate. Cancer Cell. 2012;21:297–308.
55. Kim M-J, Kim D-H, Jung W-H, Koo J-S. Expression of metabolism-related proteins in triple-negative breast cancer. Int J Clin Exp Pathol. 2014;7:301–12.

56. Filipp FV, Ratnikov B, De Ingeniis J, Smith JW, Osterman AL, Scott DA. Glutamine-fueled mitochondrial metabolism is decoupled from glycolysis in melanoma. Pigment Cell Melanoma Res. 2012;25:732–9.
57. Cao MD, Lamichhane S, Lundgren S, Bofin A, Fjøsne H, Giskeødegård GF, Bathen TF. Metabolic characterization of triple negative breast cancer. BMC Cancer. 2014;14:941.
58. Simpson NE, Tryndyak VP, Beland FA, Pogribny IP. An in vitro investigation of metabolically sensitive biomarkers in breast cancer progression. Breast Cancer Res Treat. 2012;133:959–68.
59. Simpson NE, Tryndyak VP, Pogribna M, Beland FA, Pogribny IP. Modifying metabolically sensitive histone marks by inhibiting glutamine metabolism affects gene expression and alters cancer cell phenotype. Epigenetics. 2012; 7:1413–20.
60. Kim SK, Jung WH, Koo JS. Differential expression of enzymes associated with serine/glycine metabolism in different breast cancer subtypes. PLoS One. 2014;9:e101004.
61. Noh S, Kim DH, Jung WH, Koo JS. Expression levels of serine/glycine metabolism-related proteins in triple negative breast cancer tissues. Tumour Biol. 2014;35:4457–68.
62. Shen J, Yan L, Liu S, Ambrosone CB, Zhao H. Plasma metabolomic profiles in breast cancer patients and healthy controls: by race and tumor receptor subtypes. Transl Oncol. 2013;6:757–65.
63. López-Cortés A, Echeverría C, Oña-Cisneros F, Sánchez ME, Herrera C, Cabrera-Andrade A, Rosales F, Ortiz M, Paz-Y-Miño C. Breast cancer risk associated with gene expression and genotype polymorphisms of the folate-metabolizing MTHFR gene: a case-control study in a high altitude Ecuadorian mestizo population. Tumour Biol. 2015;36:6451–61.
64. Jung YY, Kim HM, Koo JS. Expression of lipid metabolism-related proteins in metastatic breast cancer. PLoS One. 2015;10:e0137204.
65. Kim S, Lee Y, Koo JS. Differential expression of lipid metabolism-related proteins in different breast cancer subtypes. PLoS One. 2015;10:e0119473.
66. Griffiths B, Lewis CA, Bensaad K, Ros S, Zhang Q, Ferber EC, Konisti S, Peck B, Miess H, East P, Wakelam M, Harris AL, Schulze A. Sterol regulatory element binding protein-dependent regulation of lipid synthesis supports cell survival and tumor growth. Cancer Metab. 2013;1:3.
67. Tang X, Lin C-C, Spasojevic I, Iversen ES, Chi J-T, Marks JR. A joint analysis of metabolomics and genetics of breast cancer. Breast Cancer Res. 2014;16:415.
68. Kim S, Rhee J, Yoo HJ, Lee HJ, Lee EJ, Lee JW, Yu JH, Son BH, Gong G, Kim SB, Singh SR, Ahn SH, Chang S. Bioinformatic and metabolomic analysis reveals miR-155 regulates thiamine level in breast cancer. Cancer Lett. 2015; 357:488–97.
69. Boroughs LK, DeBerardinis RJ. Metabolic pathways promoting cancer cell survival and growth. Nat Cell Biol. 2015;17:351–9.
70. Kanaan YM, Sampey BP, Beyene D, Esnakula AK, Naab TJ, Ricks-Santi LJ, Dasi S, Day A, Blackman KW, Frederick W, Copeland RL, Gabrielson E, Dewitty RL. Metabolic profile of triple-negative breast cancer in African-American women reveals potential biomarkers of aggressive disease. Cancer Genomics Proteomics. 2014;11:279–94.
71. Hart PC, Mao M, de Abreu ALP, Ansenberger-Fricano K, Ekoue DN, Ganini D, Kajdacsy-Balla A, Diamond AM, Minshall RD, Consolaro MEL, Santos JH, Bonini MG. MnSOD upregulation sustains the Warburg effect via mitochondrial ROS and AMPK-dependent signaling in cancer. Nat Commun. 2015;6:6053.
72. Go R-E, Hwang K-A, Choi K-C. Cytochrome P450 1 family and cancers. J Steroid Biochem Mol Biol. 2015;147:24–30.
73. D'Amato NC, Rogers TJ, Gordon MA, Greene LI, Cochrane DR, Spoelstra NS, Nemkov TG, D'Alessandro A, Hansen KC, Richer JK. A TDO2-AhR signaling axis facilitates anoikis resistance and metastasis in triple-negative breast cancer. Cancer Res. 2015;75:4651–64.
74. Viale A, Pettazzoni P, Lyssiotis CA, Ying H, Sánchez N, Marchesini M, Carugo A, Green T, Seth S, Giuliani V, Kost-Alimova M, Muller F, Colla S, Nezi L, Genovese G, Deem AK, Kapoor A, Yao W, Brunetto E, Kang Y, Yuan M, Asara JM, Wang YA, Heffernan TP, Kimmelman AC, Wang H, Fleming JB, Cantley LC, DePinho RA, Draetta GF. Oncogene ablation-resistant pancreatic cancer cells depend on mitochondrial function. Nature. 2014;514:628–32.

2

Hexokinase 2 is dispensable for T cell-dependent immunity

Manan M. Mehta[1], Samuel E. Weinberg[1], Elizabeth M. Steinert[1], Krishan Chhiba[1], Carlos Alberto Martinez[2], Peng Gao[3], Harris R. Perlman[1], Paul Bryce[1], Nissim Hay[4] and Navdeep S. Chandel[1*]

Abstract

Background: T cells and cancer cells utilize glycolysis for proliferation. The hexokinase (1–4) family of enzymes catalyze the first step of glycolysis. Hexokinase 2 (HK2) is one of the most highly upregulated metabolic enzymes in both cancer and activated T cells. HK2 is required for the development and/or growth of cancer in several cancer models, but the necessity of HK2 in T cells is not fully understood. The clinical applicability of HK2 inhibition in cancer may be significantly limited by any potential negative effects of HK2 inhibition on T cells. Therefore, we investigated the necessity of HK2 for T cell function. In order to identify additional therapeutic cancer targets, we performed RNA-seq to compare in vivo proliferating T cells to T cell leukemia.

Methods: HK2 was genetically ablated in mouse T cells using a floxed *Hk2* allele crossed to CD4-Cre. CD4+ and CD8+ cells from mice were characterized metabolically and tested in vitro. T cell function in vivo was tested in a mouse model of colitis, Th2-mediated lung inflammation, and viral infection. Treg function was tested by crossing *Hk2*-floxed mice to FoxP3-Cre mice. Hematopoietic function was tested by deleting HK2 from bone marrow with Vav1-iCre. RNA-seq was used to compare T cells proliferating in response to virus with primary T-ALL leukemia induced with mutant Notch1 expression.

Results: We unexpectedly report that HK2 is largely dispensable for in vitro T cell activation, proliferation, and differentiation. Loss of HK2 does not impair in vivo viral immunity and causes only a small impairment in the development of pathological inflammation. HK2 is not required for Treg function or hematopoiesis in vivo. One hundred sixty-seven metabolic genes were identified as being differentially expressed between T cells and leukemia.

Conclusions: HK2 is a highly upregulated enzyme in cancer and in T cells. The requirement for HK2 in various cancer models has been described previously. Our finding that T cells are able to withstand the loss of HK2 indicates that HK2 may be a promising candidate for cancer therapy. Furthermore, we identify several other potential metabolic targets in T-ALL leukemia that could spare T cell function.

Keywords: Hexokinase 2, T cells, Tregs, Leukemia, Colitis, LCMV

Background

T lymphocytes in the immune system and neoplastic cells in cancer are both highly proliferative cell types, relying on highly active metabolic pathways [1, 2]. T cells typically divide and expand in response to a specific antigen, while cancer cells exhibit uncontrolled proliferation. Nonetheless, similar molecular mechanisms underlie the ability of these different cell types to proliferate. Indeed, one of the major side effects of chemotherapies which target proliferating cancer cells is immunosuppression. One common mechanism utilized by both cancer and activated T cells to support their proliferation is an upregulation of glycolysis to provide intermediates for macromolecule synthesis [3, 4].

Glucose metabolism is essential for both normal T cell-mediated immunity and pathological T cell-mediated inflammation [5–11]. Studies have similarly shown that glucose metabolism is required for tumor growth in a variety of cancer models [12]. Furthermore, in the tumor microenvironment, evidence indicates that T cells and

* Correspondence: nav@northwestern.edu
[1]Department of Medicine, Northwestern University Feinberg School of Medicine, McGaw Pavilion, Rm. M-334, 240 East Huron Street, Chicago, IL 60611, USA

cancer cells may compete for glucose and that cancer cells may upregulate glycolysis in part to deprive T cells of glucose as a means to evade and suppress the immune system [13, 14]. These studies have led to interest in using anti-glycolytic agents for cancer therapy. Clearly, glucose metabolism is essential for both cancer and T cells. However, it is not clear if glucose is utilized differently in cancer and T cells and thus if glucose metabolism is a viable target for cancer therapy. Given that T cells also rely heavily on glucose, it is possible that anti-glycolytic therapy could lead to immunosuppression, leaving patients susceptible to infections. Furthermore, such immunosuppression would work at cross purposes with emerging cancer therapies such as check point blockade which rely on T cells. Therefore, any potential glycolytic target for cancer therapy should ideally spare T cell function.

One possible target for anti-glycolytic cancer therapy is hexokinase (HK), first committed step of glycolysis. HK can be expressed as four different isoforms, with HK1 being a somewhat ubiquitous isoform and HK2 existing as a more selectively regulated isoform [15]. Cancer cells highly upregulate HK2 compared to their normal tissue of origin and it is required for tumorigenesis in a variety of mouse cancer models, including breast and lung cancer and T cell leukemia [16–19]. However, HK2 is also highly upregulated in activated T cells [20, 21]. Furthermore, pan-hexokinase inhibition with 2-deoxyglucose (2DG) causes impaired differentiation of the inflammatory Th17 CD4+ T cell lineage and a shift from effector to memory cells in CD8+ T cells [20, 22, 23]. Presently, it is unknown whether the loss of HK2 would impair T cell-mediated inflammation and immunity.

In this study, we report that HK2 is largely dispensable in T cells for viral immunity and inflammation in several mouse models. Collectively, our data indicate that targeting HK2 may be a promising avenue for further research in cancer therapy, as it may spare T cell function while inhibiting cancer growth.

Methods

Mouse models

$HK2^{fl/fl}$ mice were previously generated [16]. HK2 WT, floxed (Fl), and null alleles were genotyped using the following primers: HK2-F (CCCCTTCGCTTGCCATTAC), HK2-R (TGTCTTGGCTCAGATGTGAC), and HK2-null (AACCACGACGCCCAATGATTTAG). CD4-Cre, Vav-iCre, FoxP3-YFP-Cre, CD45.1, and IL-$10^{-/-}$ mice were obtained from the Jackson Labs. Except where noted otherwise, approximately 2–4-month old adult mice of both sexes were used for experiments. Animals were not randomized to experimental groups, but were age-matched, sex-matched, and littermates where possible. No animals were excluded from analysis. Investigators were blinded to mouse genotypes for histological scoring but not blinded otherwise. All animals were housed and bred in the Northwestern animal vivarium, and procedures were approved by the Institutional Animal Care and Use Committee (IACUC) at Northwestern University.

T cell isolation and in vitro culture

Spleens from approximately 2–4-month old mice were mechanically disrupted through a 70 uM strainer in 2% FBS/PBS to yield splenocytes. CD4+ T cells and CD8+ T cells were isolated from splenocytes using a negative selection magnetic bead kit according to manufacturer's protocol (StemCell). Resulting T cells were activated 1:1 with CD3/CD28-coated beads (Gibco) and 20 ng/mL IL-2 (PeproTech) for 24–72 h in RPMI 1640 media, 10% fetal bovine serum (FBS), 10 mM HEPES, 2 mM glutamax, and 50 uM beta-mercaptoethanol with antibiotic/antimycotic. Oxygen consumption and extracellular acidification rate were measured as previously descried using a Seahorse XF96 analyzer (Agilent) [24]. For proliferation experiments, cells were stained with CFSE prior to activation according to manufacturer's protocol (Thermo Fisher). For low glucose experiments, dialysed fetal bovine serum was used and glucose was added as indicated. For experiments requiring conditions biased for certain lineages, activation was altered as follows. Cells were activated with 5:1 irradiated splenocytes (3000 rad) and 2.5 μg/mL soluble anti-CD3 (eBiosciences). Cytokines and blocking antibodies were added to promote Th1 (10 ng/mL IL-12, 10 μg/mL anti-IL-4), Th2 (300 ng/mL IL-4, 10 μg/mL anti-IL-12, 10 μg/mL anti-IFNγ), Th17 (2 ng/mL TGFb, 20 ng/mL IL-6), and Treg (2 ng/mL TGFb) differentiation. Th0 consisted of base media without any additional cytokines or blocking antibodies. IL-12 was obtained from PeproTech, anti-IL-4 and anti-IFNγ from BioLegend, IL-6 and anti-IL-12 from eBiosciences, and IL-4/TGFb from R&D. Cells split 1:2 after 3 days and supplemented with additional media and IL-2 for 2 days before analysis.

Glucose assays

HK activity and 2-DG uptake were measured on activated CD4+ and CD8+ T cells by commercially available kits (BioVision and Promega, respectively) according to manufacturer's instructions. HK lysates were flash frozen in liquid nitrogen prior to storage at – 80 °C.

Flow cytometry and sorting

Single-cell suspensions were resuspended in 2% FBS/PBS for surface staining, and the following antibodies were used as indicated (clone numbers in parenthesis): anti-CD4 (GK1.5, RM4–5), CD8 (53–6.7), CD45.2 (104), CD25 (PC61.5), CD69 (H1-2F3), CD44 (IM7), CD62L (MEL14), F4/80 (BM8), CD11c (N418), B220 (RA3-6B2), CD11b (M1/70), Gr-1 (RB6-8C5), NK1.1 (PK136),

TER-119 (TER-119), and CD19 (1D3). Viability was determined by exclusion of nucleic dye, either propidium iodide (Thermo Fisher), LIVE/DEAD Fixable Blue stain (Thermo Fisher), or Ghost Dye Red 780 (Tonbo). For intracellular cytokine staining, cells were pretreated with 50 ng/mL PMA (Sigma), 1μg/mL ionomycin (Sigma), and protein transport inhibitor cocktail (eBiosciences) for approximately 4 h (except in case of gp33 stimulation, which is performed as described below). For intracellular cytokines and transcriptions factors, cells were fixed with a Cell Fixation/Permeabilization Kit (BD) or FoxP3/Transcription Factor Staining Kit (eBiosciences) and stained with the following antibodies as indicated: anti-Tbet (O4–46), GATA3 (TWAJ), RORγt (B2D), FoxP3 (FJK-16 s), IFNγ (XMG1.2), IL-4(11B11), and IL-17a (17B7). Absolute counts were obtained by running samples with a known concentration of beads (Spherotech) or by counting cells on a Cellometer (Nexcelom). gp33 monomer (D(b)/LCMV.GP33.KAVYN FATM) was obtained from the NIH Tetramer Core Facility and tetramerized according to their provided protocol. All samples were run on LSR Fortessa or FACSymphony flow cytometers (BD) and data was analyzed using FlowJo software. Cells were sorted using the FASC Aria II (BD). Sorted cells were reanalyzed afterwards to ensure approximately 90% purity.

Protein extraction and western blot

Cells pellets were stored at − 80 °C until resuspension and lysis. Protein content was quantified by BCA assay. Four to twenty percent or Any kD polyacrylamide gels (Bio-Rad) were used to separate lysate proteins. Protein was then transferred to nitrocellulose membranes using Trans-Blot Turbo (Bio-Rad). Membranes were blocked using 5% milk/TBS for 1 h, washed with TBST, and then incubated in 5% BSA/TBST with anti-HK2 (Santa Cruz, product #6521, diluted approximately 1:500) and anti-β-actin (Sigma, catalog no. T9026/A2066; diluted 1:1000) or anti-GAPDH (Santa Cruz, clone C65, diluted 1:1000) overnight. HK1 and HK3 blotting performed similarly with antibodies from Cell Signaling (clone C35C4) and Abcam (catalog no. ab126217), respectively. Membranes were washed with TBST and incubated in appropriate secondary antibodies—donkey anti-goat or goat anti-rabbit IRDye 800CW (LI-COR, diluted 1:5000-1:10000 in 5% milk/TBST) and donkey anti-mouse or anti-rabbit IRDye 680RD (LI-COR, diluted 1:10,000 in 5% milk/TBST)—for 1 h at room temperature. Membranes were imaged using the Odyssey Fc Analyzer (LI-COR).

RNA isolation and real-time PCR

RNA was isolated using standard lab protocols. cDNA was generated using M-MLV Reverse Transcriptase (Invitrogen). Real-time PCR was performed on the CFX384 Real-Time System (Bio-Rad) using iQ SYBR Green Supermix (Bio-Rad) and 200 nM primers. Alternatively, low quantity RNA samples were analyzed using a one-step protocol (Tonbo CYBRFast 1-Step RT-qPCR Lo-Rox). Primers used as follows: HK2-F (GTGTGCTCCGAGTAAGGGTG), HK2-R (CAGGCAT TCGGCAATGTGG), HK1-F (AACGGCCTCCGTCA AGATG), HK1-R (GCCGAGATCCAGTGCAATG), HK 3-F (TGCTGCCCACATACGTGAG), HK3-R (GCCTG TCAGTGTTACCCACAA), Hmgcs2-F (GAAGAGAGC GATGCAGGAAAC), Hmgcs2-R (GTCCACATATTGG GCTGGAAA), Chdh-F (TTCGGCTGGATGGACATGA C), Chdh-R (CTGCTTACAAGTGTCTGGACC), Ldhb-F (CATTGCGTCCGTTGCAGATG), Ldhb-R (GGAGGAA CAAGCTCCCGTG), Prodh-F (GCACCACGAGCAGT TGTTC), Prodh-R (CTTTGTTGTGCCGGATCAGAG), Fbp1-F (CACCGCGATCAAAGCCATCT), Fbp1-R (AGG TAGCGTAGGACGACTTCA), b-Actin-F (CTAAGGCC AACCGTGAAAAG), b-Actin-R RPL-19-F (GAAGGTCA AAGGGAATGTGTTCAA), and RPL-19-R (TTTCGTGC TTCCTTGGTCTTAGA). Data was analyzed using ΔCT method by comparing genes of interest to the geometric mean of indicated housekeeping genes.

Colitis model and histology

$IL10^{-/-}$ mice were allowed to spontaneously develop colitis, typically between 8 and 14 weeks of age. Mice were euthanized if they lost greater than 20% of their body weight or if they developed rectal prolapse. $IL\text{-}10^{+/+}$ littermates were euthanized at approximately 13–15 weeks as controls. Colon, spleen, and mesenteric lymph nodes from euthanized mice were collected. Colons were fixed for 2 days in 10% neutral buffered formalin for H&E staining or immediately digested to isolate lamina propria cells as previously described [25]. Lymph nodes were mechanically disrupted in RPMI on scored plates to yield lymphocytes. Lymphocytes were analyzed by flow cytometry as described above. Fixed tissues were paraffin-embedded, sectioned, mounted, and stained with H&E by the Northwestern mouse histology core. Scoring was performed blinded according to established criteria [26].

OVA immunization and airway inflammation

OVA immunization and challenge was performed as previously described [27]. Six to eight-week old mice were sensitized to OVA by treating with intraperitoneal 10 mg OVA (Grade VI, Sigma-Aldrich) in alum (3 mg) or equal volume PBS/alum on days 0 and 14. On days 21–23, mice were challenged daily with 1% OVA/PBS aerosolized by nebulizer. Mice were euthanized on day 24, trachea was cannulated, and lungs were flushed with PBS + 10% FCS + 1 mM EDTA. Resulting BAL fluid was counted for total nucleated cell count, cells were cytospun onto slides, and supernatants were used for ELISA cytokine quantification. Differential counts were performed after staining slides with DiffQuik. Lung tissue was homogenized for RNA isolation (Qiagen) and analyzed by TaqMan probes according to manufacturer's protocol (Thermo Scientific, probe numbers mm00445259_m1, mm00439646_m1, mm00434204_m1, mm01168134_m1, and mm00439618_m1). Remaining lung tissue was fixed and H&E stained as described above.

LCMV infection, CD8+ T cell restimulation, and plaque assay
Adult mice were infected with 200,000 pfu LCMV-Armstrong intraperitoneally. Peripheral blood was acquired by retro-orbital bleeds on indicated days. Red blood cells were lysed in RBC lysis buffer (eBiosciences) and blood was analyzed by flow cytometry as described above. Mice were euthanized after 60 days post infection (DPI) and splenocytes were isolated as described above. One million splenocytes per sample were stimulated with 30 ng/mL exogenous gp_{33-41} peptide (KAVYNFATM, GenScript) for approximately 5 h in the presence of GolgiPlug (BD), after which surface staining, tetramer staining, and intracellular cytokine staining were performed as described above. Alternatively, mice were euthanized at three and eight DPI, and liver and spleens were removed. Eight DPI spleens were sorted for CD8+ T cells which were used for RNA-seq and metabolomics as described below. Liver was homogenized and used to determine viral load by plaque assay as described in detail by others [28]. Briefly, serial dilutions of liver homogenate were added to a monolayer of Vero cells and overlayed with 0.5% agarose for 5 days, stained with neutral red for 1 day, and PFUs were counted.

Bone marrow isolation and leukemic transformation
Peripheral blood counts were obtained by retro-orbital bleeds of mice and analysis on a HEMAVET (Drew). Bone marrow from adult mice was harvested by dissecting pelvis, femur, and tibia. Bones were centrifuged for 5 min at 5000 rcf in an 18G-punctured 500 uL tube nested in a 1.5 mL tube. Platinum-E cells were used to create Notch1-DE retrovirus by treating cells with MIGR1-Notch1-DE plasmid and using the jetPRIME manufacturer's protocol (plasmid and cell line gifted by Panagiotis Ntziachristos). Bone marrow was used with a CD117+ positive selection magnetic bead isolation kit (StemCell) to yield CD117+ cells. CD117+ cells were grown in Opti-MEM (Thermo Fisher) supplemented with 10 ng/mL IL-3 (PeproTech), 10 ng/mL IL-7 (PeproTech), 50 ng/mL SCF (PeproTech), 50 ng/mL Flt3L (PeproTech), and 20 ng/mL IL-6 (eBiosciences). Cells were infected with Notch1-DE retrovirus by adding virus to cells, centrifugation at 2500 rpm at 25 °C for 90 min, incubation at 37 °C for 4 h, and removal of virus replacing with previous media. Infection was repeated on the next day, after which cells were allowed to rest for 2 days. Seventy-five thousand lineage (CD4, CD8a, B220, CD11b, Gr-1, NK1.1, Ter-119)-negative, GFP+ cells were sorted and mixed with 750,000 bone marrow cells from CD45.1 mice resuspended in PBS. Cells were adoptively transferred into lethally irradiated (1000 rad) CD45.1 mice by retro-orbital injection. Mice were monitored over 6 weeks by analyzing peripheral blood with flow cytometry for CD45.2 + GFP + CD4 + CD8+ leukemic cells to ensure development of leukemia. Splenocytes were sorted for leukemic cells and analyzed by RNA-seq (described below).

RNA-seq data acquisition and analysis
RNA quality and quantity were measured using Agilent 4200 TapeStation using High Sensitivity RNA ScreenTape System (Agilent Technologies). SMART-Seq v4 Ultra Low Input RNA Kit (Takara Bio USA, Inc.) was used to generate full-length cDNA, and NextEra XT DNA sample preparation kit (Illumina Inc.) was used to prepare the final library. An Illumina NextSeq 500 (Illumina Inc.) was used to sequence library with single-end sequencing (1 × 75 cycles) using NextSeq 500 High Output reagent kit (Illumina Inc.). FASTQ reads were trimmed using Trimmomatic to remove end nucleotides with a PHRED score less than 30 and requiring a minimum length of 20 bp. Reads were then aligned to the mm10 genome using TopHat version 2.1.0 using the following options: --no-novel-juncs, --read-mismatches 2, --read-edit-dist 2, --max-multihits 20, and --library-type fr-unstranded. The generated bam files were then used to count the reads only at the exons of genes using htseq-count with the following parameters: -q -m intersection-nonempty -s no -t exon. The R package edgeR was used to determine significance of differentially expressed genes, only genes with > 2-fold change in expression and adjusted p value < 0.01 were considered significant and included in heatmap. Genes were filtered for involvement in metabolism based on the KEGG mmu01100 genes. Broad Institute GSEA software was used to perform a pre-ranked GSEA analysis using 3000 permutations and the Hallmark pathway database.

Metabolomics
Cell pellets were flash frozen in liquid nitrogen and stored at − 80 °C until metabolite extraction. Samples were thawed and pellets were resuspended in ice cold 80% methanol, freeze-thawed three times, and centrifuged at 18,000 rcf for 10 min at 4 °C. Supernatants were transferred to new tubes, dried, resuspended, and volume-adjusted so 500,000 cells' worth of metabolites were analyzed for targeted metabolomics. Samples were analyzed by High-Performance Liquid Chromatography and High-Resolution Mass Spectrometry and Tandem Mass Spectrometry (HPLC-MS/MS). Specifically, system consisted of a Thermo Q Exactive in line with an

electrospray source and an Ultimate3000 (Thermo) series HPLC consisting of a binary pump, degasser, and auto-sampler outfitted with a Xbridge Amide column (Waters; dimensions of 4.6 mm × 100 mm and a 3.5-μm particle size). The mobile phase A contained 95% (vol/vol) water, 5% (vol/vol) acetonitrile, 20 mM ammonium hydroxide, 20 mM ammonium acetate, pH = 9.0; and B was 100% acetonitrile. The gradient was: 0–1 min, 15% A; 18.5 min, 76% A; 18.5–20.4 min, 24% A; 20.4–20.5 min, 15% A; and 20.5–28 min, 15% A with a flow rate of 400 μL/min. The capillary of the ESI source was set to 275 °C, with sheath gas at 45 arbitrary units, auxiliary gas at 5 arbitrary units, and the spray voltage at 4.0 kV. In positive/negative polarity switching mode, an m/z scan range from 70 to 850 was chosen and MS1 data was collected at a resolution of 70,000. The automatic gain control (AGC) target was set at 1 × 106 and the maximum injection time was 200 ms. The top five precursor ions were subsequently fragmented, in a data-dependent manner, using the higher energy collisional dissociation (HCD) cell set to 30% normalized collision energy in MS2 at a resolution power of 17,500. Data acquisition and peak extraction/integration were carried out by Xcalibur 4.0 software and TraceFinder 2.1 software, respectively (Thermo Fisher). Low quality peaks were omitted from analysis. Resulting ion counts were normalized to total ion counts per sample and analyzed using multiple *t* tests with a Benjamini-Kreiger false discovery rate of 10%.

Statistical analyses

Data were analyzed statistically using Prism 7 (GraphPad), except RNA-seq data which was analyzed as described above. Statistical tests, error bar representations, *p* values, biological replicates, sample sizes, and independent experiments are specified in figure legends. Appropriate statistical tests were selected for each comparison based on type of data and assuming normality. Adjustments for multiple comparisons were performed when appropriate and are described in figure legends. Representative images of gels and histology are from at least three biological replicates. No outliers were removed from data analysis.

Results

HK2 is dispensable for T cells in vitro

To assess the necessity of HK2 for basic T cell function in vitro, we generated mice that have a conditional deletion of the *Hk2* gene in T cells by crossing CD4-Cre mice with mice harboring a floxed *Hk2* allele ($Hk2^{fl/fl}$). Resulting CD4-Cre, $Hk2^{fl/fl}$ mice are herein referred to as T-$Hk2^{-/-}$ mice. Spleens from the mice were removed and CD4+ and CD8+ cells were isolated and activated in vitro. As has been observed previously, CD4+ and CD8+ WT T cells highly upregulated *Hk2* transcript upon activation [20], but T cells from T-$Hk2^{-/-}$ mice had no increase in HK2 mRNA or protein upon activation (Fig. 1a, b, Additional file 1: Figure S1A–B, Additional file 2: Figure S2A). Importantly, there was no compensatory increase in HK1 or HK3 mRNA or protein in CD4+ or CD8+ cells from T-$Hk2^{-/-}$ mice (Fig. 1a, b, Additional file 1: Figure S1A–B). Surprisingly, total HK activity measured in activated CD4+ and CD8+ cells was not statistically different between WT and T-$Hk2^{-/-}$ mice. (Fig. 1c). Glucose uptake capacity was measured by the amount of 2-DG taken up by cells. 2-DG uptake was unaffected by HK2 deficiency in CD4+ and CD8+ T cells (Fig. 1d). Basal and maximal extracellular acidification rate (ECAR) is a surrogate measure of lactate production and glycolytic activity. ECAR was similar between activated T cells from WT and T-$Hk2^{-/-}$ mice (Fig. 1e). Oxygen consumption rate was also unchanged in activated CD4+ and CD8+ T cells (Fig. 1f). Overall, our data show that HK2 deficiency causes only small changes in T cell glucose usage.

In order to determine if HK2-deficient T cells had any functional deficits in vitro, we measured their ability to activate and proliferate after stimulation. Surprisingly, HK2-deficient CD4+ and CD8+ T cells had no decrease in expression of the activation markers CD25 or CD69 after 24 h (Fig. 2a, Additional file 3: Figure S3A). CD4+ T cells had no decrease in proliferation after 72 h as measured by CFSE staining, while CD8+ T cells consistently showed a small but insignificant deficit (Fig. 2b). Together, these data indicate that HK2 is not required for T cell viability, activation, or proliferation in vitro.

Another important function of T cells is their ability to differentiate into specialized subsets. We tested the ability of CD4+ cells to differentiate in vitro by skewing them towards Th1, Th2, Th17, and Treg lineages. No major impairment was observed between WT- and HK2-deficient T cells in any of these lineages as determined by viability and expression of lineage defining transcription factors (Fig. 3a–e, Addtional file 3: Figure S3C). We also compared the steady state levels of different cell types in the spleens of WT and T-$Hk2^{-/-}$ mice. We observed no differences in percent of CD4+, CD8+, naïve ($CD62L^{hi}CD44^{lo}$), memory ($CD44^{hi}$), Th1, Th2, Th17, or Treg cells in T-$Hk2^{-/-}$ mice (Fig. 3f–h, Additional file 4: Figure S4F, Additional file 3: Figure S3B). Furthermore, there were no observed differences in other immune cell numbers (Additional file 4: Figure S4G). Together, these data demonstrate that T-$Hk2^{-/-}$ mice do not have an impairment in T cell differentiation in vitro or at steady state in vivo.

The unexpected dispensability for HK2 in vitro lead us to hypothesize that perhaps HK2 is upregulated in T cells to maintain glycolysis during conditions of low glucose availability. To this end, we activated CD4+ T cells in vitro under various glucose concentrations, from

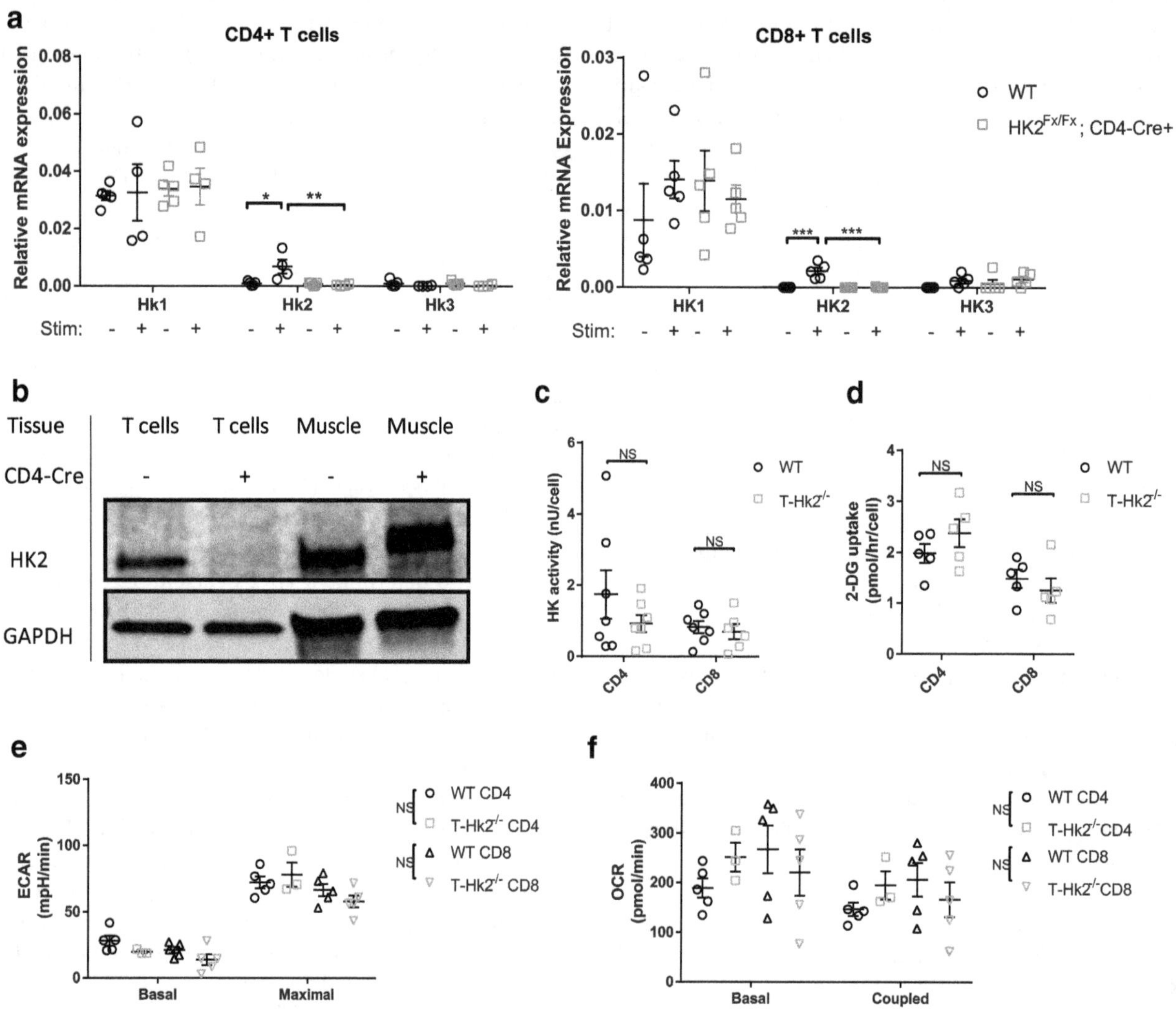

Fig. 1 HK2 is dispensable for T cell glycolysis. Naïve CD4+ and CD8+ T cells were enriched from splenocytes isolated from adult WT and T-Hk2$^{-/-}$ mice. T cells were activated in vitro with anti-CD3/28-coated beads for 24–72 h. **a** RNA expression of HK isoforms in CD4+ and CD8+ T cells after 24 h stimulation, compared to naïve unstimulated cells. Expression relative to β-actin and Rpl-19. Biological replicates, $n = 4$–5 (as indicated by individual data points) from at least two independent experiments **b** Western blot for protein expression of HK2 in muscle tissue or CD4+ T cells after 24 h stimulation. Representative of four independent experiments. **c**–**f** CD4+ or CD8+ T cells stimulated for 72 h and assayed for **c** total HK activity, **d** 2-DG uptake, **e** extracellular acidification rate (ECAR), and **f** oxygen consumption rate (OCR). **c**–**f** At least two independent experiments performed, biological replicates, $n = 3$–7 as indicated by individual data points. In all panels unless otherwise noted, error bars represent mean ± SEM, one-way or two-way ANOVA with Sidak multiple comparisons, $^*p < 0.05$; $^{**}p < 0.01$. NS = not significant

5.5 mM (physiological blood glucose) to 0 mM. Previous work has shown that activation and viability at 24 h should not be affected by low concentrations of glucose, but the complete absence of glucose will cause T cell death that can be rescued by pyruvate [24, 29]. Consistent with previous findings, we observed a sharp decline in viability and activation in WT T cells between 0.1 mM glucose and 0 mM glucose that was restored with 1 mM pyruvate (Additional file 4: Figure S4A–B). Remarkably, HK2-deficient T cells exhibited an identical response to glucose concentrations as WT T cells (Additional file 4: Figure S4A–B). Similarly, WT- and HK2-deficient T cells stimulated for 3 days under varying concentrations of glucose showed comparable viability, proliferation as measured by CFSE proliferation index, and proliferation as measured by cell number (Additional file 4: Figure S4C–E). These data demonstrate that *Hk2* is dispensable in vitro for T cell viability, activation, and proliferation even under limiting glucose levels.

HK2 deficiency mildly reduces T cell-mediated inflammation in vivo

It is possible that though we did not see any differences in vitro from loss of HK2, there could be differences in

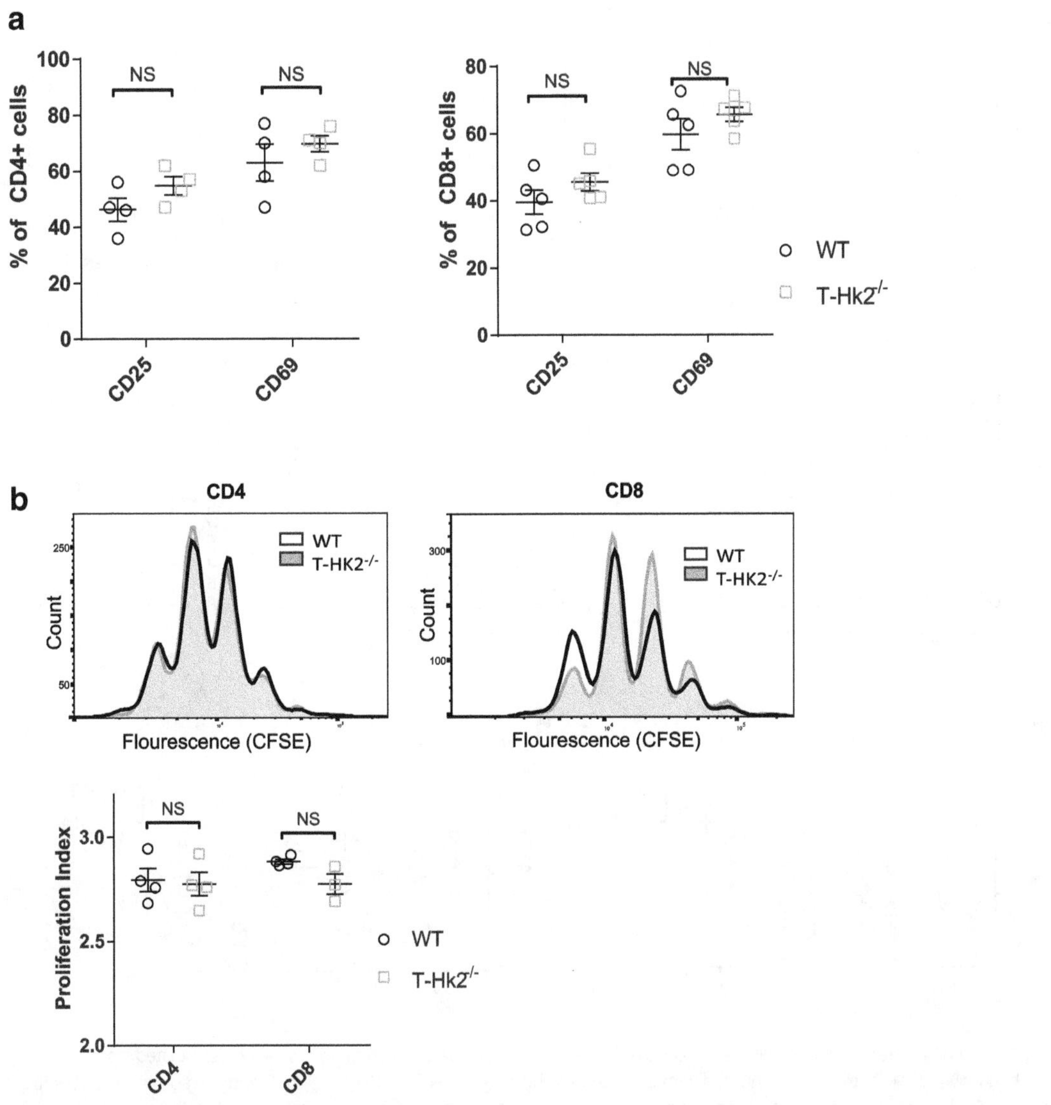

Fig. 2 HK2 is not required for T cell activation and proliferation. Naïve CD4+ and CD8+ T cells were enriched from splenocytes isolated from adult WT and T-Hk2$^{-/-}$ mice. T cells were activated in vitro with anti-CD3/28-coated beads for 24–72 h. **a** Percent of cells positive for indicated activation markers by flow cytometry gated on CD4+ (left) or CD8+ (right) cells after 24 h stimulation. Biological replicates, $n = 4$ from at least two independent experiments. **b** CFSE dilution in activated CD4+ and CD8+ T cells after 72 h of stimulation. Representative image of $n = 4$ biological replicates from at least two independent experiments. Quantified by proliferation index on right, $n = 3$–4 biological replicates as indicated by individual data points. In all panels unless otherwise noted, error bars represent mean ± SEM, one-way or two-way ANOVA with Sidak multiple comparisons, $*p < 0.05$; $**p < 0.01$. NS = not significant

vivo in T-*Hk2*$^{-/-}$ mice under inflammatory conditions. We tested whether HK2 deficiency in T cells would impair T cell-mediated inflammation by using a mouse model of colitis driven by IL-10 deficiency. IL10$^{-/-}$ mice spontaneously develop colitis in a T cell-dependent manner thought to be driven by Th1 and Th17 cytokine-producing cells [30–33]. We generated *Hk2*$^{fl/fl}$, CD4-Cre^{+}, and IL-10$^{-/-}$ mice that were globally deficient in IL-10 and had a T cell-specific HK2 deficiency (herein referred to as IL-10$^{-/-}$; T-*Hk2*$^{-/-}$). IL-10$^{-/-}$ mice and IL-10$^{-/-}$;T-*Hk2*$^{-/-}$ mice both developed mild colitis marked by lymphocytic infiltrate in the colon, a failure to gain weight, splenomegaly, and rectal prolapse (Fig. 4a–d). IL-10-sufficient littermate control mice showed no signs of disease. Interestingly, IL-10$^{-/-}$,T-*Hk2*$^{-/-}$ mice developed spontaneous rectal prolapse at a significantly lower rate than IL-10$^{-/-}$ mice, though weight change and splenomegaly were similar between the two (Fig. 4b–d). To further investigate differences in the inflammation between IL-10$^{-/-}$ mice and IL-10$^{-/-}$;T-*Hk2*$^{-/-}$ mice, we analyzed tissues by flow cytometry which showed increase cellularity in the mesenteric

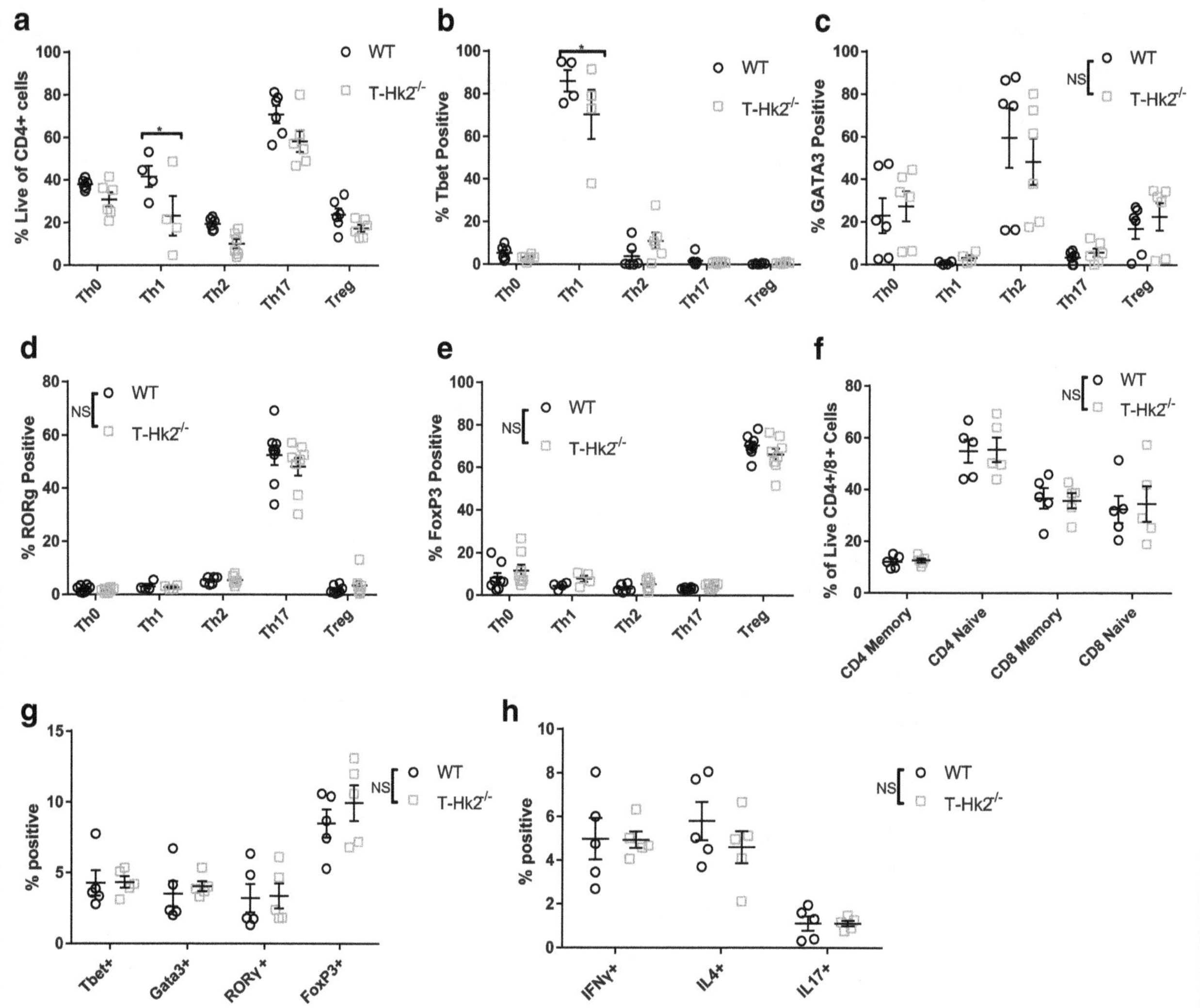

Fig. 3 HK2 is dispensable for T cell differentiation. **a**–**e** Naïve CD4+ T cells were enriched from splenocytes isolated from adult WT and T-Hk2$^{-/-}$ mice. Enriched naïve CD4+ T cells were stimulated with irradiated splenocytes under Th0, Th1, Th2, Th17, and Treg promoting conditions for 5 days. Percent of CD4+ T cells positive for viability or viable and positive for indicated transcription factor shown. Biological replicates, $n = 4$–8 (as indicated by individual data points) from at least two independent experiments. **f**–**h** Splenocytes were isolated from 8 to 12 week old WT and T-Hk2$^{-/-}$ mice to analyze steady state levels of various populations. **f** Percent of viable CD4+ or CD8+ cells that are CD62L^{hi}CD44^{lo} (naive) or CD44^{hi} (memory). Biological replicates, $n = 5$ mice. **g**–**h** Percent of viable CD4+ T cells positive for the indicated transcription factor (**g**) or cytokine (**h**). Biological replicates, $n = 5$ mice. In all panels unless otherwise noted, error bars represent mean ± SEM, two-way ANOVA with Sidak multiple comparisons, *$p < 0.05$; **$p < 0.01$. NS = not significant

lymph nodes and lamina propria of both IL10$^{-/-}$ mice and IL-10$^{-/-}$;T-*Hk2*$^{-/-}$ when compared to IL10$^{+/+}$ mice (Fig. 4e, f). There were no observed differences in CD4 +, CD8+, CD69+, IFNγ +, IL17+, or FoxP3+ cell numbers in the mesenteric lymph nodes of IL10$^{-/-}$ mice and IL-10$^{-/-}$;T-*Hk2*$^{-/-}$ mice (Fig. 4e, f). However, there was a mild decrease in CD4+ T cells in the lamina propria of IL-10$^{-/-}$;T-*Hk2*$^{-/-}$ mice (Fig. 4g). Overall, these data indicate that IL-10$^{-/-}$;T-*Hk2*$^{-/-}$ develop colitis, but with a lower severity than IL10$^{-/-}$ mice.

We also tested the necessity of HK2 in a mouse model of Th2 lung inflammation by sensitizing WT and T-*Hk2*$^{-/-}$ mice with ovalbumin/aluminum hydroxide (OVA/alum) and provoking airway inflammation subsequently with aerosolized OVA. Inflammation in the airway in response to OVA is known to be a Th2-driven process with a Th17 component [34]. Non-sensitized WT and T-*Hk2*$^{-/-}$ mice lacked any pulmonary inflammation after challenge with OVA while both WT and T-*Hk2*$^{-/-}$ sensitized mice developed significant inflammation (Fig. 5a). Bronchoalveolar lavage after OVA challenge showed both WT and T-*Hk2*$^{-/-}$ mice had an increase in BAL cellularity when compared to mice that were not previously sensitized (Fig. 5b). Absolute levels of T cells and eosinophils were increased in the BAL of both WT and *Hk2*$^{-/-}$ mice, but T-*Hk2*$^{-/-}$ mice had a

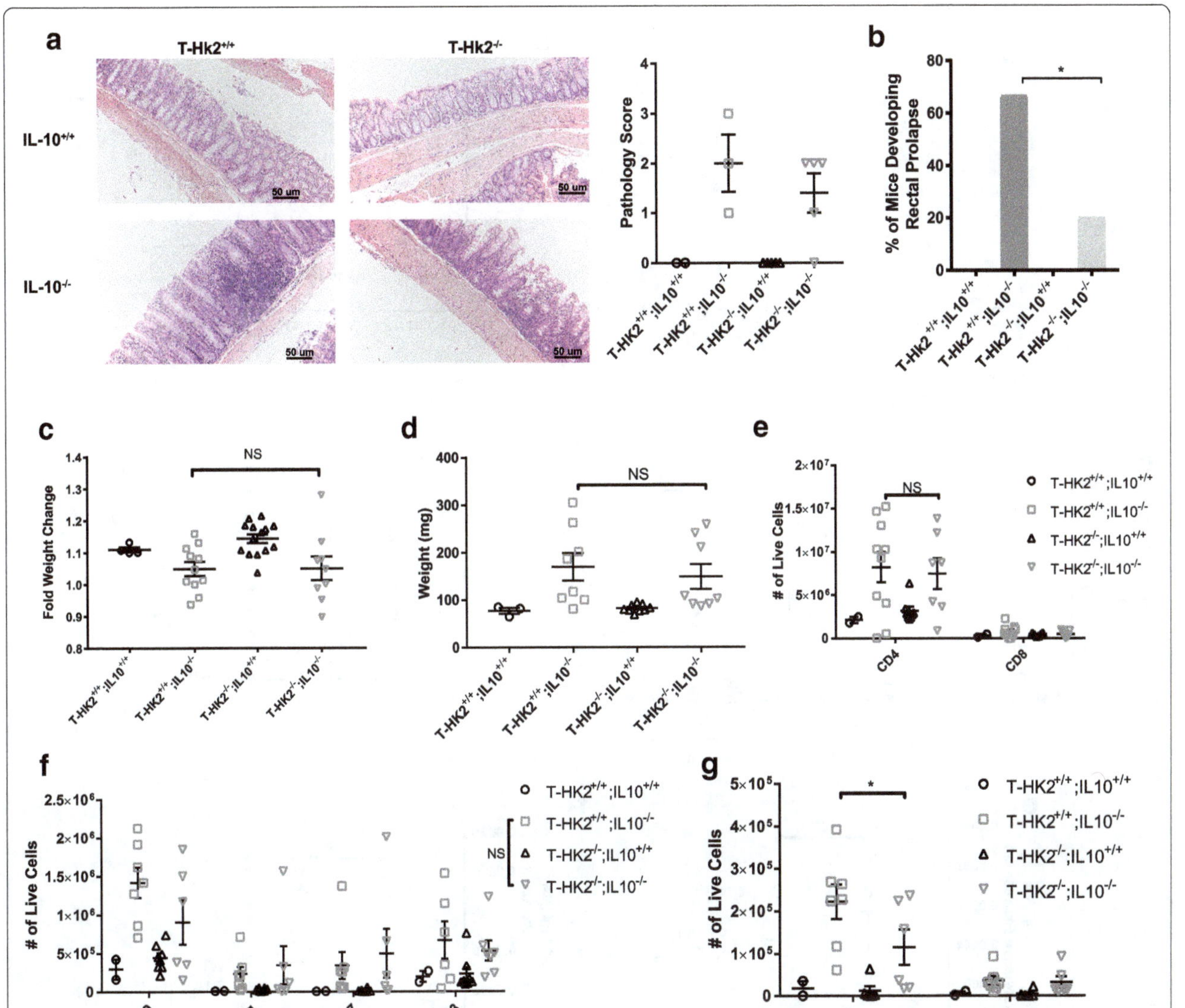

Fig. 4 HK2 deficiency reduces T cell-mediated colon inflammation in vivo. T-Hk2$^{-/-}$ mice were crossed to IL10$^{-/-}$ mice to induce colitis. Mice were euthanized at approximately 13–15 weeks of age or earlier if required due to weight loss or rectal prolapse. **a** H&E staining and scoring of large intestine section in indicated mice. Scale bars show 50 um, representative images shown. Biological replicates, $n = 2$–5 mice as indicated by individual data points. **b** Percentage of mice which spontaneously develop rectal prolapse by 15 weeks of age. Chi-squared test. $n = 4$, 12, 10, 10 mice (left to right). **c** Fold change in weight between week 9 and euthanasia. Biological replicates, $n = 4$–15 mice, as indicated by individual data points. **d** Spleen weight. Biological replicates, $n = 3$–11 mice as indicated by individual data points. **e-g** Total number of indicated cell type isolated from mesenteric lymph nodes (**e**, **f**; $n = 2$–10 mice, as indicated by individual data points) and colon lamina propria (**g**; $n = 2$–7 mice, as indicated by individual data points). In all panels unless otherwise noted, error bars represent mean ± SEM, at least three independent experiments performed, one-way or two-way ANOVA with Sidak multiple comparisons correction, $^{*}p < 0.05$; $^{**}p < 0.01$. NS = not significant

small decrease in eosinophils when compared to WT mice (Fig. 5b). Th2 cytokines in the BAL were increased in both WT and T-*Hk2*$^{-/-}$ mice (Fig. 5c). While T-*Hk2*$^{-/-}$ mice had cytokine levels that trended downward compared to WT mice, the decrease was not statistically significant. Whole lung RNA cytokine levels showed similar results with a significant increase in Th2 and Th17 cytokines in both WT and T-*Hk2*$^{-/-}$ mice when compared to unsensitized mice; IFNγ, a Th1 cytokine, was not increased (Fig. 5d–h). Furthermore, similar to BAL levels, RNA levels showed a descending trend in cytokine levels when comparing T-*Hk2*$^{-/-}$ mice to WT mice. However, again, the decrease in cytokine levels of T-*Hk2*$^{-/-}$ mice was not statistically significant, though the decrease in IL-17 approached significance ($p = 0.06$). Taken together, these results indicate that *Hk2* is not strictly required for development of Th2 inflammation, but its presence may modulate the extent of inflammation.

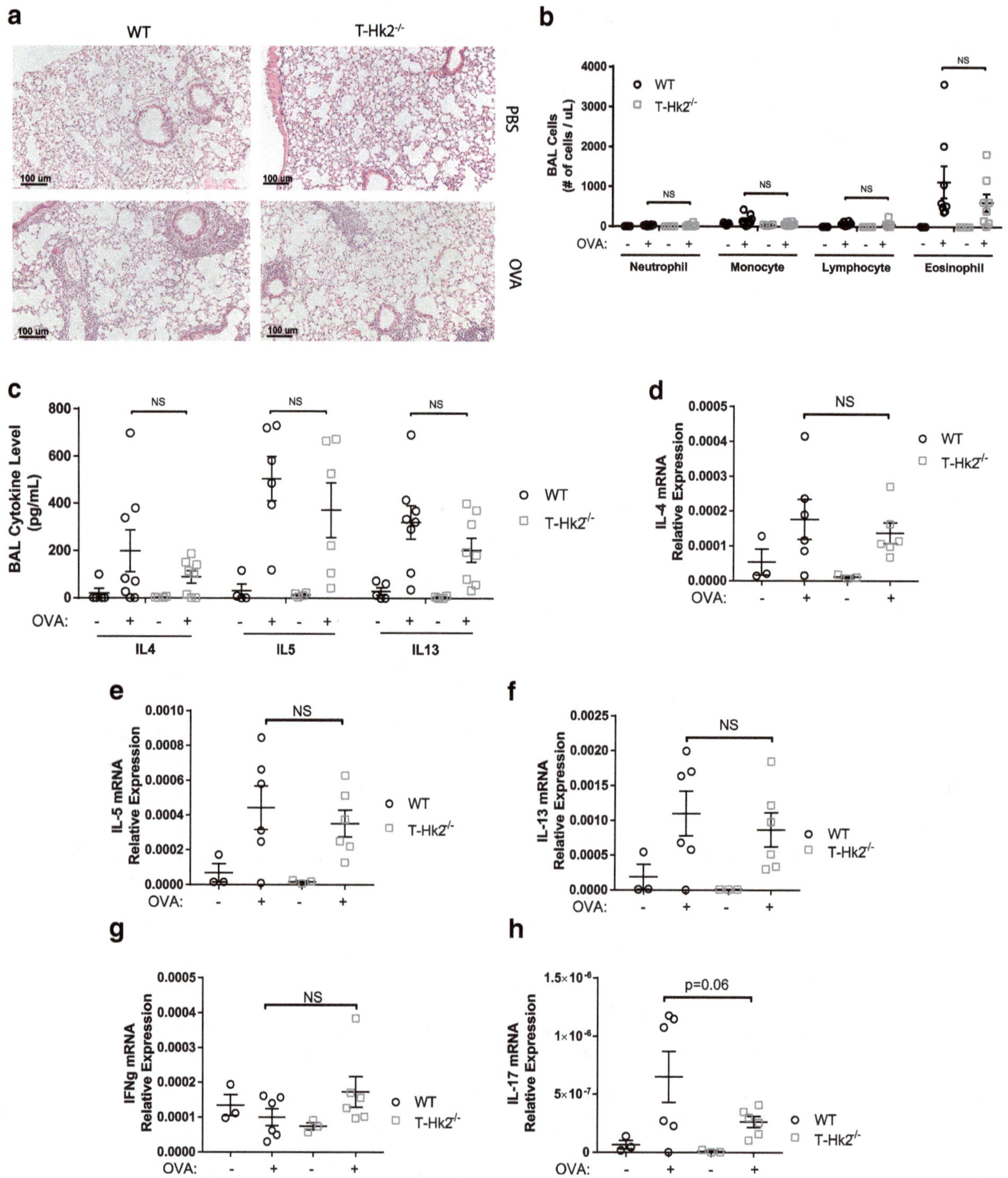

Fig. 5 HK2 deficiency impairs Th2-mediated lung inflammation in vivo. Six to eight-week old WT and T-Hk2$^{-/-}$ mice were pre-sensitized to OVA twice, 14 days apart with intraperitoneal injection of OVA/alum or PBS/alum. Twenty-one days after initial pre-sensitization, mice were challenged with aerosolized OVA daily for 3 days. Mice were euthanized for analysis on the fourth day. **a** H&E staining of lung tissue. Scale bars show 100 um, representative images shown from $n = 4$ mice. **b** Number of indicated cells present in BAL fluid (**c**) ELISA for indicated cytokines in BAL fluid. **b**, **c** Multiple *t* tests with Holm-Sidak correction for multiple comparisons. **d**–**h** RNA expression of indicated cytokine relative to β-actin. In all panels unless otherwise noted, error bars represent mean ± SEM, biological replicates, $n = 5, 8, 4, 8$ mice (left to right) from three independent experiments, unless otherwise noted, one-way ANOVA with Sidak multiple comparisons correction, $^{*}p < 0.05$; $^{**}p < 0.01$. NS = not significant

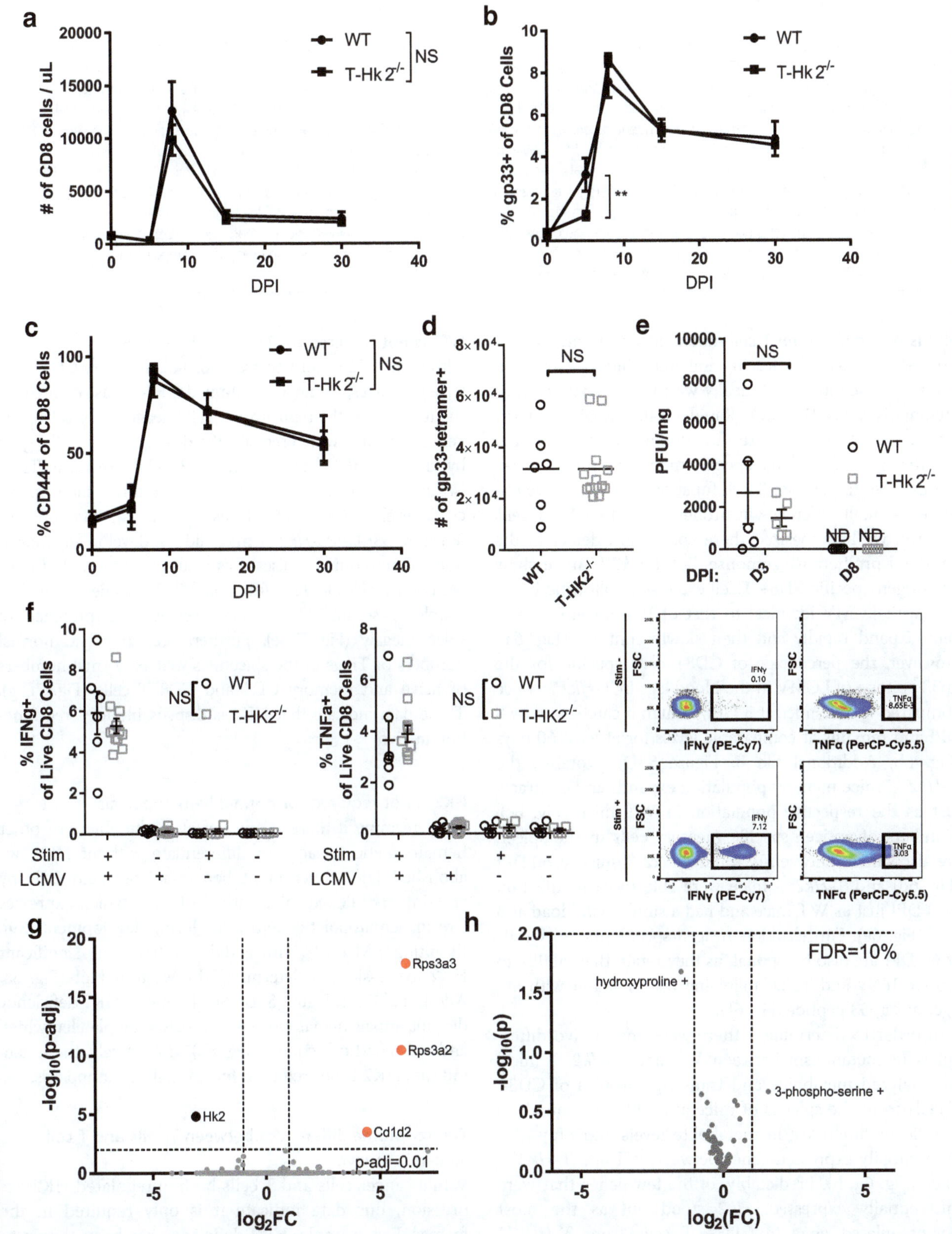

Fig. 6 (See legend on next page.)

(See figure on previous page.)
Fig. 6 HK2 is largely dispensable for immunity to LCMV. Eight to twelve-week old WT and T-Hk2$^{-/-}$ mice were injected intraperitoneally with 2×10^5 pfu LCMV. **a**–**c** T cell expansion was monitored over time by flow cytometry of peripheral blood. **a** Number of CD8+ cells. **b** Percentage of CD8+ cells positive for gp-33 tetramer (D(b)/LCMV.GP33.KAVYNFATM) or (**c**) CD44. Biological replicates, $n = 6$ WT, 14 T-Hk2$^{-/-}$ mice from three independent experiments. **d** Number of gp33-tetramer+ CD8+ T cells in spleen of WT and T-Hk2$^{-/-}$ mice at 60 DPI. Biological replicates, $n = 6$ WT, 12 T-Hk2$^{-/-}$ mice from two independent experiments, analyzed by unpaired Student's *t* test. **e** Viral load as measured by plaque assay from right lobe of liver from 3 and 8 DPI. Biological replicates, $n = 5$ mice from two independent experiments. **f** Splenocytes from uninfected mice and mice 60 DPI were stimulated in vitro for 5 h with 30 ng/mL $gp_{33–41}$ peptide or vehicle control and stained for IFNγ and TNFα secretion. Example gating shown on right. Biological replicates, $n = 4$ mice from two independent experiments. **g**, **h** RNA and metabolites were isolated from sorted splenic CD8+ T cells from WT and T-Hk2$^{-/-}$ mice 8 DPI. **g** Volcano plot of gene expression differences. Differentially regulated genes include those with greater than 2 fold change in expression and multiplicity adjusted *p* value < 0.01. **h** Volcano plot of metabolite concentration differences. Vertical dashed lines indicate 2 fold change in metabolite concentration. Horizontal dashed line indicates no discoveries made (False Discovery Rate of 0.1, two-stage Benjamini-Krieger method, $n = 5$ mice). In all panels unless otherwise noted, error bars represent mean ± SEM, two-way ANOVA with Sidak multiple comparisons correction (**a**–**c** includes repeated measures), $*p < 0.05$; $**p < 0.01$. NS = not significant. n.d. = not detected. DPI = days post injection

HK2 is not required for T cell-mediated viral immunity

To test the role of HK2 in viral immunity, we infected T-*Hk2*$^{-/-}$ mice intraperitoneally with lymphocytic choriomeningitis virus (LCMV). Rapid clearance of the virus after acute infection requires function of CD8+ T cells and maintenance of a LCMV-specific memory population requires CD4+ and CD8+ T cell function [35, 36]. As we observed a small difference in proliferation of CD8+ T cells in vitro, we hypothesized there could be a defect in the anti-viral proliferative response, but T-*Hk2*$^{-/-}$ mice show an antigen-specific CD8+ T cell expansion following infection with LCMV identical to that of WT mice; CD8+ T cells expand rapidly and then slowly contract (Fig. 6a). However, the percentage of CD8+ cells specific for the gp33 epitope of LCMV in the blood lags in T-*Hk2*$^{-/-}$ mice compared to WT mice at 5 DPI, though it catches up by 8 DPI and remains at comparable levels for at least 60 days (Fig. 6b, Additional file 3: Figure S3D). Notably, the T-*Hk2*$^{-/-}$ mice memory population expands and contracts just as the respective population in WT mice (Fig. 6c). Numbers of antigen-specific memory cells in the spleen are also similar between WT and T-*Hk2*$^{-/-}$ mice at 60 DPI (Fig. 6d) and T-*Hk2*$^{-/-}$ mice were able to clear infection by 8 DPI just as WT mice and had a similar viral load at 3 DPI (Fig. 6e). Furthermore, antigen-specific memory cells at 60 DPI are also functional, as they retain their ability to secrete IFNγ and TNFα following restimulation with exogenous gp33 peptide (Fig. 6f).

In order to determine if there were any in vivo differences in metabolism between WT and T-*Hk2*$^{-/-}$ mice, we analyzed metabolite and transcript profiles of CD8+ T cells from the spleens of mice at 8 DPI. We found no significant difference in metabolite levels and only four differentially expressed genes between WT and T-*Hk2*$^{-/-}$ mice (Fig. 6g, h). Predictably, of the few genes that were differentially expressed, *Hk2* stood out as the most downregulated gene in CD8+ T cells from T-*Hk2*$^{-/-}$ mice. Importantly, HK1 was unchanged in both WT- and HK2-deficient T cells. These data indicate that HK2 is dispensable for CD8+ T cell-mediated viral immunity.

HK2 is not required for Treg function in vivo

Although HK2 is not necessary for inflammatory CD4+ and CD8+ lineages, we next determined if HK2 was required for the function of the regulatory T cell lineage (Treg cells). We generated mice with Treg-specific deletion of the *Hk2* gene by crossing *Hk2*$^{fl/fl}$ mice with FoxP3-YFP-Cre mice. Tregs isolated from these mice (FP3-*Hk2*$^{-/-}$) did not show appreciable levels of *Hk2* mRNA transcript (Fig. 7a, Additional file 3: Figure S3E). FP3-*Hk2*$^{-/-}$ mice did not develop any indications of autoimmune disease as would be expected of mice with deficiencies in Treg function [37, 38], as determined by histology, serum ANA titers, weight, and presence of splenomegaly (Fig. 7b-e). Furthermore, they had normal numbers of Tregs in the spleen, as well as normal numbers of naïve and memory CD4 and CD8 T cells (Fig. 7f, g). These data indicate that HK2 is dispensable for Treg function in vivo.

HK2 is not required for normal hematopoiesis

To determine if there is any defect in the ability of other hematopoietic lineages to differentiate without HK2, we abolished HK2 function in hematopoietic stem cells by crossing *Hk2*-floxed mice with Vav1-iCre, which expresses Cre in hematopoietic stem cells during development [39]. Resulting BM-*Hk2*$^{-/-}$ mice did not have any significant HK2 expression as determined by western blot (Fig. 8a, Additional file 2: Figure S2B). Furthermore, HK2 deficiency did not impair hematopoiesis as assessed by platelet, white, and red blood cell counts (Fig. 8b). Collectively, these data indicate HK2 is not required for normal hematopoiesis.

Transcriptome differences between T cells and T cell leukemia in vivo

While cancer cells and T cells both upregulated HK2 expression, our data indicate it is only required in the former. For example, HK2 deficiency has been shown to decrease tumor burden in a mouse model of T cell acute lymphoblastic leukemia (T-ALL) [19]. Finding therapeutics that target neoplastic T cells while sparing normal T

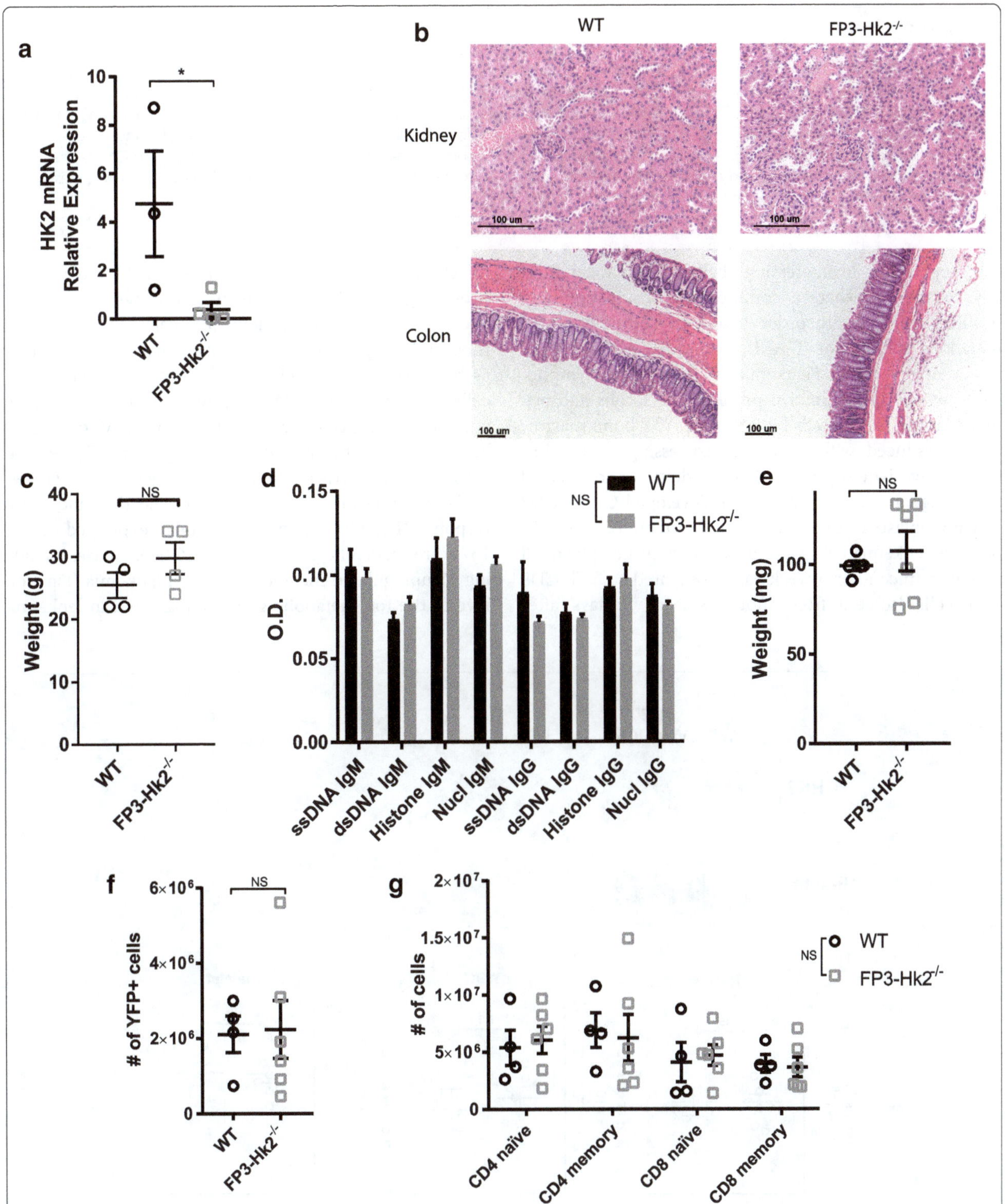

Fig. 7 (See legend on next page.)

(See figure on previous page.)
Fig. 7 HK2 is not required for Treg function in vivo. Mice with YFP+ HK2-deficient Treg cells were generated (FP3-Hk2$^{-/-}$ mice). **a** CD4+ cells from spleens of adult WT and FP3-Hk2$^{-/-}$ mice were stimulated under Treg promoting conditions and RNA was isolated from sorted YFP+ cells. Hk2 expression relative to β-actin ($n = 3$ WT, 4 FP3-Hk2$^{-/-}$). **b–g** WT and FP3-Hk2$^{-/-}$ mice were aged to 6 months. **b** Representative H&E stained sections of indicated tissues, $n = 4$ mice. Scale bars show 100 um. **c** Mouse weight; biological replicates, $n = 4$ mice. **d** Titer of indicated auto-antibodies in serum; biological replicates, $n = 4$ WT, 7 FP3-Hk2$^{-/-}$ mice. **e** Spleen weight; biological replicates, $n = 5$ WT, 6 FP3-Hk2$^{-/-}$ mice. **f** Number of splenic Treg cells and **g** percent of viable CD4+ or CD8+ T cells that are CD62L^{hi}CD44^{lo} (naive) or CD44^{hi} (memory); biological replicates, $n = 4$ WT, 6 FP3-Hk2$^{-/-}$ mice. In all panels unless otherwise noted, error bars represent mean ± SEM, experiments performed twice independently, single-tailed Student's t test or two-way ANOVA with Sidak multiple comparisons correction, $^{*}p < 0.05$; $^{**}p < 0.01$. NS = not significant

cells represents an interesting challenge in cancer therapy, as the two share a common origin and common proliferative goals. In order to identify other potential metabolic targets for T-ALL beyond HK2 that would preferentially inhibit leukemia while sparing lymphocytes, we compared in vivo proliferating T cells and primary mouse T-ALL cells by RNA-seq. WT bone marrow was transduced with retrovirus expressing a constitutively active Notch protein (Notch1-deltaE) and injected into congenic CD45.1 mice. Mice developed CD4 + CD8 + lymphoblasts in their blood and lymphoid organs. WT primary leukemia cells were isolated from the spleens of recipient mice after 6 weeks and compared to WT CD8 + T cells isolated from mouse spleens 8 days after infection with LCMV (Additional file 3: Figure S3F). A wide range of differentially expressed genes were identified between T cells and leukemic cells (Fig. 9). Three thousand three hundred thirty-one genes were identified as being significantly differentially expressed between T cells and leukemia (Fig. 9a), with leukemic samples enriched in expected gene sets such as Myc targets, beta-catenin pathway, and notch1 signaling (Fig. 9b). T cells were unsurprisingly enriched for gene sets involved in T cell processes such as allograft rejection and IFNγ response (Fig. 9b). Of the differentially expressed genes, 167 were metabolic genes in the KEGG database, including 61 upregulated metabolic genes in leukemia (Fig. 9c). Five of the top metabolic genes upregulated in leukemia

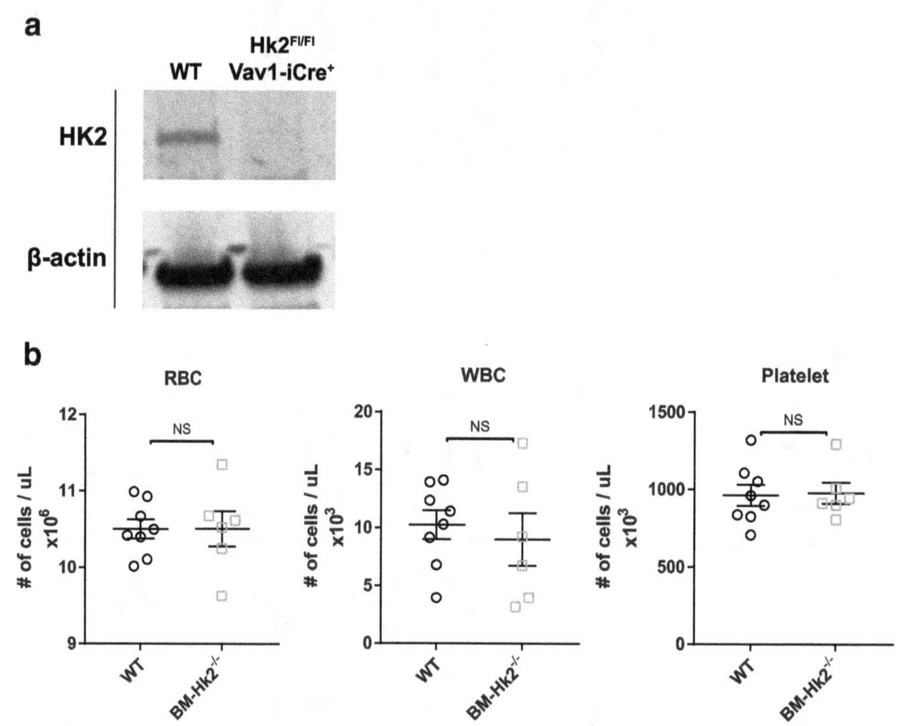

Fig. 8 HK2 is not required for normal hematpoiesis. Mice with HK2-deficient bone marrow were generated (Hk2$^{Fl/Fl}$;Vav1-iCre^{+}, referred to as BM-Hk2$^{-/-}$) **a** Western blot for protein expression of HK2 and β-actin in bone marrow. Representative of four independent experiments **b** Peripheral blood counts of indicated hematopoietic lineages in adult WT and Hk2$^{Fl/Fl}$; Vav1-iCre^{+} mice. $n = 8$ WT, 6 Hk2$^{Fl/Fl}$; Vav1-iCre^{+} mice. In all panels, biological replicates shown, at least two independent experiments performed, error bars represent mean ± SEM, unpaired t test, $^{*}p < 0.05$; $^{**}p < 0.01$. NS = not significant

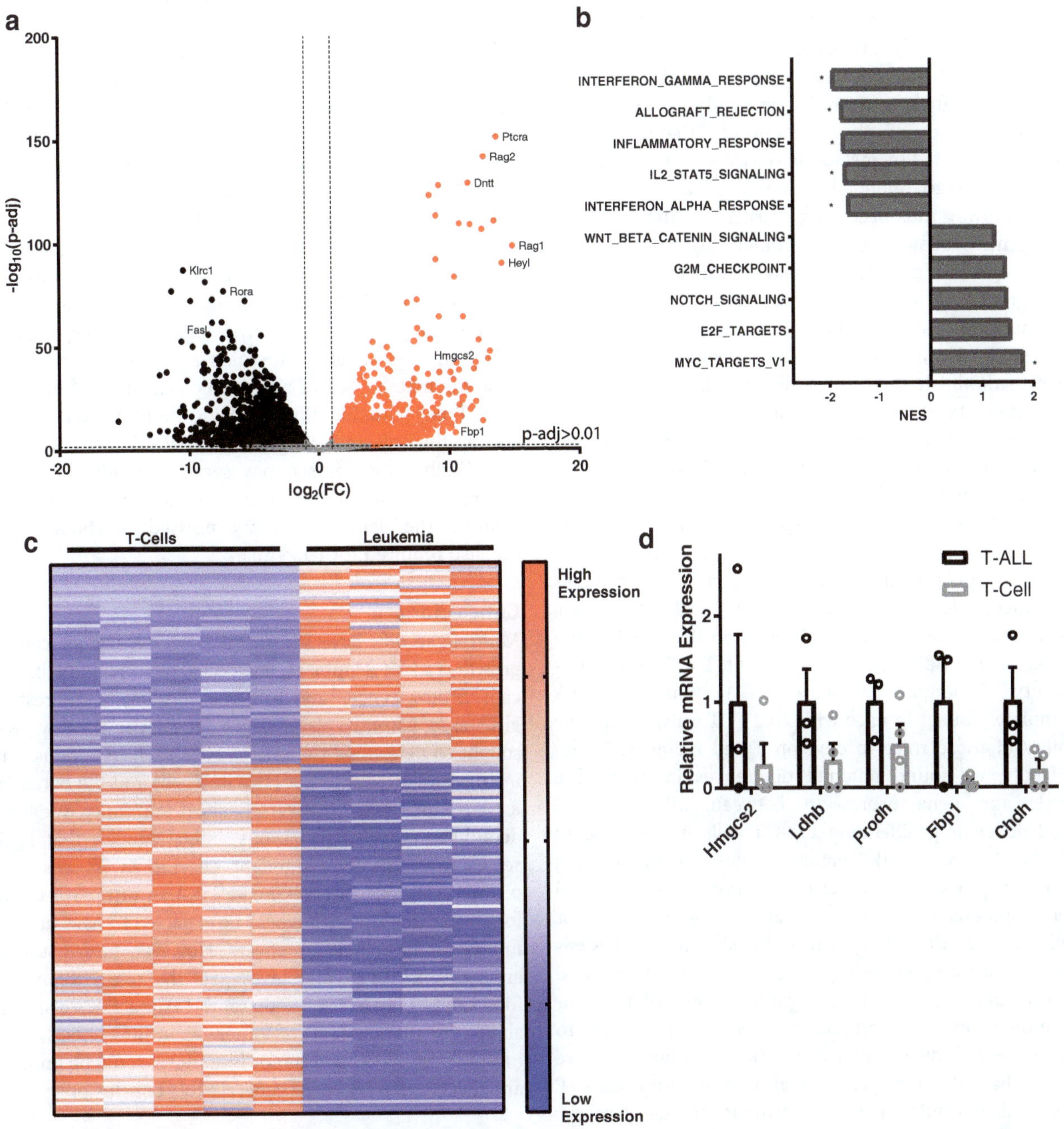

Fig. 9 Transcriptomic and metabolomic analysis reveals essential differences in metabolism of leukemia and lymphocytes. Sorted splenic CD8+ T cells from WT mice 8 days after LCMV infection, compared to sorted T-ALL cells from WT mice 6 weeks after adoptive transfer. RNA isolated from sorted cells and analyzed by RNA-seq **a** Volcano plot of gene expression differences. Differentially regulated genes include those with greater than 2 fold change in expression and multiplicity adjusted p value < 0.01. Blue dots are overexpressed in CD8+ T cells, red in T-ALL. **b** Hallmark pathways enriched in leukemia (positive values) and T cells (negative values) and their normalized enrichment score. Statistical significance shown by * (FWER $p < 0.05$). **c** Expression of differentially regulated metabolic genes from the KEGG database. **d** Expression of select metabolic genes by RT-PCR relative to β-actin and Rpl-19. Biological replicates, $n = 3$–4 mice, as indicated by individual data points

when compared to CD8+ T cells were Hmgcs2, Chdh, Fbp1, Prodh, and Ldhb. These genes consistently showed higher expression in leukemia cells when re-evaluated by RT-PCR (Fig. 9d). While some differences were statistically significant after t tests, no individual gene reached statistical significance on multiple comparisons correction. Taken together, these data reveal essential differences in T cell and T-ALL cell metabolism that may be harnessed to selectively inhibit leukemic proliferation.

Discussion

In the past decade, there has been a resurgence of targeting metabolism for cancer therapy. Cancer cells undergo metabolic reprogramming to acquire sufficient nutrients to fuel macromolecule synthesis for growth and proliferation [2, 4, 12]. However, the therapeutic window is limited by metabolic rewiring that cancer cells quickly undergo upon inhibition of a particular metabolic pathway thus becoming resistant to therapies targeting metabolism. Normal proliferating T cells, stem and progenitor cells also display features of metabolic reprogramming similar to cancer cells, further limiting the therapeutic index in targeting metabolism of cancer cells [1, 3, 11]. Moreover, targeting metabolism within T cells to diminish their proliferation and function could leave patients susceptible to life threatening infections while also rendering useless cutting-edge immunotherapies such as checkpoint blockade and CAR-T cells.

A similar metabolic feature of proliferating cancer cells and T cells is that they both highly upregulate glycolytic enzymes [4, 10, 11, 16–18]. HK2 is the one the most highly upregulated glycolytic enzymes in activated T cells and oncogenic transformed cells [16–18, 20, 21]. Thus, we were surprised with our observation that HK2 is dispensable for the essential function of T cells—viral immunity. Clearance of acute LCMV infection was completely intact in mice with *Hk2*$^{-/-}$ T cells, as was the ability of those mice to develop T cell memory. Unexpectedly, we found minimal differences in metabolite levels and gene expression between wild-type and HK2-deficient proliferating CD8 T cells in response to LCMV. Moreover, HK2 deficiency did not impair Treg function. Loss of HK2 also did not impair normal hematopoiesis indicating normal stem and progenitor cell function. Recent work has also shown that HK2 is required for angiogenesis [40], and this inhibition could theoretically further synergize with cancer cell HK2 inhibition to improve response to therapy. In contrast to the observed dispensability of HK2 in immunity, we found that HK2 may play a small role in pathological T cell-mediated inflammation. In a mouse model of colitis, HK2 deficiency conferred a limited degree of protection against inflammation. We speculate that the simplest explanation for this is that pathogenic T cells have a higher demand for glucose which HK2-deficient cells are unable to meet. Indeed, this effect has been observed in other models of inflammation, and 2-DG has been proposed as a potential therapeutic in autoimmune diseases [7, 8]. However, it is also possible the microenvironment specific to these models may play a potential role, and it is also possible that HK2 could have non-metabolic functions contributing to pathogenesis.

It is important to note that recent work from another group supports our finding of HK2 dispensability in T cells, but in a model of herpes virus infection [41]. However, while they propose a compensatory upregulation of HK1- in HK2-deficient T cells, we are unable to confirm that conclusion in our system. There was no observed compensatory increase in HK1 or HK3 expression at the RNA or protein level. Rather, we believe HK2 is dispensable because HK2-mediated glucose phosphorylation only constitutes a small percentage of total glucose phosphorylation in CD4+ and CD8+ T cells.

To identify other targets which could be utilized to selectively inhibit cancer cells, we compared the transcriptome and metabolome of proliferating T cell leukemia with T cells proliferating physiologically in response to infection. This analysis revealed striking differences in how the metabolism of a leukemic cell differs from that of a T cell and identified specific potential targets for cancer therapy, including Hmgcs2, Prodh, Ldhb, Fbp1, and Chdh. This dataset may serve as a significant resource for future studies in cancer therapy to determine if any of the identified highly expressed metabolic genes are also required for leukemia.

Conclusions

Multiple studies have shown HK2 is essential for cancer growth and development, including in models of breast cancer, lung cancer, and leukemia, leading to interest in HK2 as a potential drug target for cancer therapy. We sought to determine the role of HK2 in T cells, considering the high expression of HK2 in T cells and the potential for HK2 inhibition to adversely affect immunity. We have demonstrated through various animal models that HK2 serves as a mostly redundant enzyme in T cells. We propose that our findings make HK2 an attractive target for cancer therapy, as it would be expected to have limited immunosuppressive side effects. However, future studies are necessary to further investigate the role HK2 inhibition could play in cancer therapy. Testing HK2 dispensability in the context of other viral infections, other immune cell types, and tumor immunity would be important steps to making more generalizable conclusions.

Additional files

Additional file 1: Figure S1. HK isoform expression in Hk2−/− T cells. CD4+ and CD8+ T cells were enriched from splenocytes isolated from adult WT and T-Hk2−/− mice. T cells were activated in vitro with anti-CD3/28 coated beads for 72 h. HK isoform and β-actin protein expression in (A) CD4+ and (B) CD8+ T cells. Biological replicates, *n* = 4. (PDF 5200 kb)

Additional file 2 Figure S2. Uncropped Gel Images. HK2 and loading control expression in (A) activated CD4+ T cells and (B) bone marrow. (B) Combined exposure shown or (A) individual exposures shown as appropriate. (PDF 2760 kb)

Additional file 3 Figure S3. Example Gating Strategies. (A) Example live CD8+ T cell gating, and subsequent gating for evaluation of activation markers. Similar gating used for CD4+ T cells (B) Gating on single cells for mixed populations of CD4+ and CD8+ T cells followed by gating for

CD62L and CD44 expression (performed on CD4+ and CD8+ T cells separately). (C) Gating on live CD4+ cells for expression of transcription factors. (D) Gating on CD8+ cells for gp-33 tetramer. (E) Gating on CD4+ cells for YFP. (F) Gating on single cells for CD45.2 and GFP expression. (PDF 1300 kb)

Additional file 4: Figure S4. HK2 is dispensable for T cell function in glucose-limited conditions. Naïve CD4+ and T cells were enriched from splenocytes isolated from adult WT and T-Hk2−/− mice. T cells were activated in vitro with anti-CD3/28 coated beads. (A-B) CD4+ T cells activated in indicated glucose/pyruvate concentrations for 24 h. (B) Percent of CD4+ cells positive for viability and (C) percent of viable CD4+ cells expressing CD69 by flow cytometry. Biological replicates, $n = 6$ from 3 independent experiments (C-E) Enriched splenic CD4+ T cells activated for 72 h in media with 1 mM pyruvate and indicated glucose concentrations. CD4+ T cells analyzed by flow cytometry for (D) percent of cells positive for viability, (E) proliferation as measured by CFSE dilution, and (F) proliferation as measured by cell number. Biological replicates, $n = 4$ WT, 5 T-Hk2−/− from 2 independent experiments. (F-G) Splenocytes were isolated from 8 to 12 week old WT and T-Hk2−/− mice to analyze steady state levels of various populations by indicated marker, $n = 5$ mice. MP = macrophage, DC = dendritic cell, NK = natural killer cell, Neutro = neutrophil. In all panels, error bars represent mean ± SEM, two-way ANOVA with Sidak multiple comparisons correction, $^{*}p < 0.05$; $^{**}p < 0.01$. NS = not significant. (PDF 809 kb)

Abbreviations

2-DG: 2-deoxyglucose; DPI: Days post infection; ECAR: Extracellular acidification rate; Fl: Floxed; HK: Hexokinase; LCMV: Lymphocytic choriomeningitis virus; OCR: Oxygen consumption rate; OVA: Ovalbumin; T-ALL: T cell acute lymphoblastic leukemia

Acknowledgements

We would like to thank the Northwestern University flow cytometry core (RHLCC) and mouse histology core (MHPL). RNA sequencing was performed by the Northwestern High Throughput RNA-Seq Center, within the Division of Pulmonary and Critical Care. We thank Kiwon Nam and Hiam Abdala-Valencia for the processing of RNA sequencing samples. The following reagent was obtained through the NIH Tetramer Core Facility: D(b)/LCMV.GP33.KAVYNFATM. We thank Panagiotis Ntziachristos for his gifts of Notch1-DE plasmid and Platinum-E cells.

Funding

This work was supported by the NIH (R35CA197532 and 5P01HL071643-13) to N.S.C., NIH (T32 T32HL076139) to S.E.W., NIH (T32 CA009560) to M.M.M., and 101BX0007333 and R01 CA206167 to NH.

Authors' contributions

MMM designed and performed the experiments. NSC, NH, and SEW contributed intellectually to the experimental design and conception. ES contributed to colitis and LCMV experiments. PB and KC helped design and performed asthma experiments. CAM analyzed RNA-seq data. PG conducted LC-MS experiments. HRP designed and supervised serum ANA testing. All authors read and approved the final manuscript.

Competing interests

The authors declare that they have no competing interests.

Author details

[1]Department of Medicine, Northwestern University Feinberg School of Medicine, McGaw Pavilion, Rm. M-334, 240 East Huron Street, Chicago, IL 60611, USA. [2]Department of Biochemistry and Molecular Genetics, Northwestern University Feinberg School of Medicine, Chicago, IL 60611, USA. [3]Metabolomics Core Facility, Northwestern University Robert H. Lurie Comprehensive Cancer Center, Chicago, IL 60611, USA. [4]Department of Biochemistry and Molecular Genetics, University of Illinois at Chicago, Chicago, IL 60607, USA.

References

1. Pearce EL, Poffenberger MC, Chang CH, Jones RG. Fueling immunity: insights into metabolism and lymphocyte function. Science. 2013;342(6155):1242454.
2. DeBerardinis RJ, Chandel NS. Fundamentals of cancer metabolism. Sci Adv. 2016;2(5):e1600200.
3. Andrejeva G, Rathmell JC. Similarities and distinctions of cancer and immune metabolism in inflammation and tumors. Cell Metab. 2017;26(1):49–70.
4. Lunt SY, Vander Heiden MG. Aerobic glycolysis: meeting the metabolic requirements of cell proliferation. Annu Rev Cell Dev Biol. 2011;27:441–64.
5. Chang CH, Curtis JD, Maggi LB Jr, Faubert B, Villarino AV, O'Sullivan D, Huang SC, van der Windt GJ, Blagih J, Qiu J, et al. Posttranscriptional control of T cell effector function by aerobic glycolysis. Cell. 2013;153(6):1239–51.
6. Blagih J, Coulombe F, Vincent EE, Dupuy F, Galicia-Vazquez G, Yurchenko E, Raissi TC, van der Windt GJ, Viollet B, Pearce EL, et al. The energy sensor AMPK regulates T cell metabolic adaptation and effector responses in vivo. Immunity. 2015;42(1):41–54.
7. Yin Y, Choi SC, Xu Z, Perry DJ, Seay H, Croker BP, Sobel ES, Brusko TM, Morel L. Normalization of CD4+ T cell metabolism reverses lupus. Sci Transl Med. 2015;7(274):274ra218.
8. Yang Z, Fujii H, Mohan SV, Goronzy JJ, Weyand CM. Phosphofructokinase deficiency impairs ATP generation, autophagy, and redox balance in rheumatoid arthritis T cells. J Exp Med. 2013;210(10):2119–34.
9. Wang T, Marquardt C, Foker J. Aerobic glycolysis during lymphocyte proliferation. Nature. 1976;261(5562):702–5.
10. Michalek RD, Gerriets VA, Jacobs SR, Macintyre AN, MacIver NJ, Mason EF, Sullivan SA, Nichols AG, Rathmell JC. Cutting edge: distinct glycolytic and lipid oxidative metabolic programs are essential for effector and regulatory CD4+ T cell subsets. J Immunol. 2011;186(6):3299–303.
11. Gerriets VA, Rathmell JC. Metabolic pathways in T cell fate and function. Trends Immunol. 2012;33(4):168–73.
12. Shaw RJ. Glucose metabolism and cancer. Curr Opin Cell Biol. 2006;18(6): 598–608.
13. Chang CH, Qiu J, O'Sullivan D, Buck MD, Noguchi T, Curtis JD, Chen Q, Gindin M, Gubin MM, van der Windt GJ, et al. Metabolic competition in the tumor microenvironment is a driver of cancer progression. Cell. 2015;162(6):1229–41.
14. Ho PC, Bihuniak JD, Macintyre AN, Staron M, Liu X, Amezquita R, Tsui YC, Cui G, Micevic G, Perales JC, et al. Phosphoenolpyruvate is a metabolic checkpoint of anti-tumor T cell responses. Cell. 2015;162(6):1217–28.
15. Wilson JE. Isozymes of mammalian hexokinase: structure, subcellular localization and metabolic function. J Exp Biol. 2003;206(Pt 12):2049–57.
16. Patra KC, Wang Q, Bhaskar PT, Miller L, Wang Z, Wheaton W, Chandel N, Laakso M, Muller WJ, Allen EL, et al. Hexokinase 2 is required for tumor initiation and maintenance and its systemic deletion is therapeutic in mouse models of cancer. Cancer Cell. 2013;24(2):213–28.
17. Botzer LE, Maman S, Sagi-Assif O, Meshel T, Nevo I, Yron I, Witz IP. Hexokinase 2 is a determinant of neuroblastoma metastasis. Br J Cancer. 2016;114(7):759–66.
18. Wang L, Xiong H, Wu F, Zhang Y, Wang J, Zhao L, Guo X, Chang LJ, Zhang Y, You MJ, et al. Hexokinase 2-mediated Warburg effect is required for PTEN- and p53-deficiency-driven prostate cancer growth. Cell Rep. 2014;8(5):1461–74.
19. Kishton RJ, Barnes CE, Nichols AG, Cohen S, Gerriets VA, Siska PJ, Macintyre AN, Goraksha-Hicks P, de Cubas AA, Liu T, et al. AMPK is essential to balance glycolysis and mitochondrial metabolism to control T-ALL cell stress and survival. Cell Metab. 2016;23(4):649
20. Shi LZ, Wang R, Huang G, Vogel P, Neale G, Green DR, Chi H. HIF1alpha-dependent glycolytic pathway orchestrates a metabolic checkpoint for the differentiation of TH17 and Treg cells. J Exp Med. 2011;208(7):1367–76.
21. Tan H, Yang K, Li Y, Shaw TI, Wang Y, Blanco DB, Wang X, Cho JH, Wang H, Rankin S, et al. Integrative proteomics and phosphoproteomics profiling reveals dynamic signaling networks and bioenergetics pathways underlying T cell activation. Immunity. 2017;46(3):488–503.
22. Dang EV, Barbi J, Yang HY, Jinasena D, Yu H, Zheng Y, Bordman Z, Fu J, Kim Y, Yen HR, et al. Control of T(H)17/T(reg) balance by hypoxia-inducible factor 1. Cell. 2011;146(5):772–84.
23. Sukumar M, Liu J, Ji Y, Subramanian M, Crompton JG, Yu Z, Roychoudhuri R, Palmer DC, Muranski P, Karoly ED, et al. Inhibiting glycolytic metabolism enhances CD8+ T cell memory and antitumor function. J Clin Invest. 2013; 123(10):4479–88.

24. Sena LA, Li S, Jairaman A, Prakriya M, Ezponda T, Hildeman DA, Wang CR, Schumacker PT, Licht JD, Perlman H, et al. Mitochondria are required for antigen-specific T cell activation through reactive oxygen species signaling. Immunity. 2013;38(2):225–36.
25. Steinert EM, Schenkel JM, Fraser KA, Beura LK, Manlove LS, Igyarto BZ, Southern PJ, Masopust D. Quantifying memory CD8 T cells reveals regionalization of immunosurveillance. Cell. 2015;161(4):737–49.
26. Erben U, Loddenkemper C, Doerfel K, Spieckermann S, Haller D, Heimesaat MM, Zeitz M, Siegmund B, Kuhl AA. A guide to histomorphological evaluation of intestinal inflammation in mouse models. Int J Clin Exp Pathol. 2014;7(8):4557–76.
27. Bryce PJ, Mathias CB, Harrison KL, Watanabe T, Geha RS, Oettgen HC. The H1 histamine receptor regulates allergic lung responses. J Clin Invest. 2006; 116(6):1624–32.
28. Welsh RM, Seedhom MO. Lymphocytic choriomeningitis virus (LCMV): propagation, quantitation, and storage. Curr Protoc Microbiol. 2008;Chapter 15:Unit 15A. 11
29. Jacobs SR, Herman CE, MacIver NJ, Wofford JA, Wieman HL, Hammen JJ, Rathmell JC. Glucose uptake is limiting in T cell activation and requires CD28-mediated Akt-dependent and independent pathways. J Immunol. 2008;180(7):4476–86.
30. Berg DJ, Davidson N, Kuhn R, Muller W, Menon S, Holland G, Thompson-Snipes L, Leach MW, Rennick D. Enterocolitis and colon cancer in interleukin-10-deficient mice are associated with aberrant cytokine production and CD4(+) TH1-like responses. J Clin Invest. 1996;98(4):1010–20.
31. Chichlowski M, Sharp JM, Vanderford DA, Myles MH, Hale LP. Helicobacter typhlonius and Helicobacter rodentium differentially affect the severity of colon inflammation and inflammation-associated neoplasia in IL10-deficient mice. Comp Med. 2008;58(6):534–41.
32. Hoshi N, Schenten D, Nish SA, Walther Z, Gagliani N, Flavell RA, Reizis B, Shen Z, Fox JG, Iwasaki A, et al. MyD88 signalling in colonic mononuclear phagocytes drives colitis in IL-10-deficient mice. Nat Commun. 2012;3:1120.
33. Kuhn R, Lohler J, Rennick D, Rajewsky K, Muller W. Interleukin-10-deficient mice develop chronic enterocolitis. Cell. 1993;75(2):263–74.
34. Afshar R, Medoff BD, Luster AD. Allergic asthma: a tale of many T cells. Clin Exp Allergy. 2008;38(12):1847–57.
35. Shedlock DJ, Shen H. Requirement for CD4 T cell help in generating functional CD8 T cell memory. Science. 2003;300(5617):337–9.
36. Fung-Leung WP, Kundig TM, Zinkernagel RM, Mak TW. Immune response against lymphocytic choriomeningitis virus infection in mice without CD8 expression. J Exp Med. 1991;174(6):1425–9.
37. Zheng Y, Rudensky AY. Foxp3 in control of the regulatory T cell lineage. Nat Immunol. 2007;8(5):457–62.
38. Shrestha S, Yang K, Guy C, Vogel P, Neale G, Chi H. Treg cells require the phosphatase PTEN to restrain TH1 and TFH cell responses. Nat Immunol. 2015;16(2):178–87.
39. de Boer J, Williams A, Skavdis G, Harker N, Coles M, Tolaini M, Norton T, Williams K, Roderick K, Potocnik AJ, et al. Transgenic mice with hematopoietic and lymphoid specific expression of Cre. Eur J Immunol. 2003;33(2):314–25.
40. Yu P, Wilhelm K, Dubrac A, Tung JK, Alves TC, Fang JS, Xie Y, Zhu J, Chen Z, De Smet F, et al. FGF-dependent metabolic control of vascular development. Nature. 2017;545(7653):224–8.
41. Varanasi SK, Jaggi U, Hay N, Rouse BT. Hexokinase II may be dispensable for CD4 T cell responses against a virus infection. PLoS One. 2018;13(1): e0191533.

3

Elevated circulatory levels of leptin and resistin impair therapeutic efficacy of dacarbazine in melanoma under obese state

Parmanand Malvi, Balkrishna Chaube, Shivendra Vikram Singh, Naoshad Mohammad, Maleppillil Vavachan Vijayakumar, Snahlata Singh, Surbhi Chouhan and Manoj Kumar Bhat*

Abstract

Background: Obesity is associated with increased risk, poor prognosis and outcome of therapy, in various cancers. Obesity-associated factors or adipokines, especially leptin and resistin, are purported to promote growth, survival, proliferation, and invasiveness of cancer cells. However, the mechanistic link between these adipokines and therapeutic response in malignancies is not clearly understood.

Methods: ob/ob and db/db mouse models were used in this study to evaluate the role of leptin and resistin towards the outcome of dacarbazine (DTIC) therapy in melanoma. Unique in vitro approaches were employed to complement in vivo findings by culturing melanoma cells in the serum collected from the experimental mice.

Results: Here, we have shown the role of important adipokines leptin and resistin in growth and the outcome of DTIC therapy in melanoma. Both leptin and resistin not only enhance proliferation of melanoma cells but also are involved in impairing the therapeutic efficacy of DTIC. Leptin and resistin treatment caused an increase in the protein levels of fatty acid synthase (FASN) and caveolin 1 (Cav-1) respectively, through their stabilization in A375 cells. Further, it was observed that leptin and resistin impaired the response of melanoma cells to DTIC via upregulation of heat shock protein 90 (Hsp90) and P-glycoprotein (P-gp) respectively.

Conclusion: These findings unraveled the involvement of adipokines (leptin and resistin) in melanoma progression, and more importantly, in the outcome of DTIC therapy.

Keywords: Obesity, Leptin, Resistin, Melanoma, Chemotherapy, Weight-control interventions

Background

Obesity is characterized by increased accumulation of white adipose tissue in the body [1]. White adipose tissue secretes many cytokines and hormonal factors, which are collectively referred to as adipokines. In obese state, the secretion profile of adipose tissue is altered [2]. As a consequence of the alteration in secretion profile of adipose tissue, increased level of pro-inflammatory adipokines and a simultaneous decrease in anti-inflammatory adipokines is observed [3, 4]. Adipokines act through receptors or membrane-associated molecules, and mediate their effect by activating various cellular signaling pathways [5]. Altered levels of adipokines support cancer cells in terms of survival, growth, and proliferation, thereby promoting tumor development, angiogenesis, progression, and metastasis.

In addition to being an influential tumor-promoting factor, obesity has also been reported to have a critical impact on the outcome of therapeutic responses in certain cancers. Under the obese state, numerous key inflammatory and metabolic factors, and their pathways, are assumed to mediate the obesity-associated impairment of chemotherapeutic responses [6, 7]. The purported mechanisms underlying increased cancer risk in the obese state relate to multiple molecular and metabolic changes arising primarily

* Correspondence: manojkbhat@nccs.res.in; manojkbhat62@gmail.com
National Centre for Cell Science, Savitribai Phule Pune University Campus, Ganeshkhind, Pune 411 007, India

as a consequence of adipose tissue expansion. The obesity-related changes include elevated levels of hormones and growth factors such as insulin, insulin-like growth factor (IGF)-1, and sex steroid hormones; adipokine imbalances; and a chronic state of low-grade inflammation. The altered systemic and local microenvironments that occur as a consequence of the obesity not only increase the likelihood of tumor development and progression but also potentially create an unfavorable state for response to chemotherapeutic regimens [7]. The mechanistic studies on the impact of the obese phenotype towards the outcome of cancer therapy are still lacking. There is a need to reconsider the dosing pattern of chemotherapeutic drugs with the concomitant implication of interventions, which curtail adiposity.

The involvement of adipose tissue in impairing the therapeutic response in cancers has been reported [8–10]. However, very little is known about the specific role of adipokines in the outcome of cancer therapy. Adipokines such as leptin and resistin are found to be elevated in the serum of obese individuals [11]. Leptin is known to activate various signaling pathways including PI3K/Akt, JAK/STAT, and MAPK. Its role in growth and proliferation has been extensively explored in breast and prostate cancers [12, 13]. However, the specific role of leptin in modulating melanoma cell proliferation and the chemotherapeutic outcome is obscure. Another important adipokine, resistin, is known to promote cancer growth. There is a considerable amount of experimental and epidemiological evidences which suggest that resistin may have pathophysiological effects, particularly in some cancer types, in addition to its traditional roles in energy homeostasis [14]. Moreover, resistin is also known to promote drug resistance phenotype in certain malignancies [15]. Previously, study from our group has shown that obesity impairs the therapeutic outcome of dacarbazine (DTIC) in melanoma and induces drug-resistant phenotype by upregulating fatty acid synthase (FASN), caveolin (Cav)-1, and P-glycoprotein (P-gp) [7]. In the present study, we investigated the specific role of leptin and resistin in melanoma cell growth, proliferation, and the outcome of DTIC-based chemotherapy. Using appropriate in vivo and in vitro approaches, we have shown that these adipokines not only modulate the growth and proliferation of melanoma cells but also are responsible for impairment in the efficacy of DTIC.

Materials and methods

Cell lines and culture conditions

Murine melanoma cells B16F10 and B16F1, human melanoma cells A375, and murine preadipocyte cells 3T3-L1 were procured from American Type Culture Collection (ATCC, Manassas, VA, USA). All the cell lines were maintained at our in-house cell repository at National Centre for Cell Science (NCCS), Pune, India. All the cells were routinely cultured in Dulbecco's modified Eagles medium (Life Technologies, CA, USA) containing 25 mM glucose and supplemented with 10% heat-inactivated (56 °C for 30 min) fetal bovine serum (Hyclone, UT, USA, or Gibco, NY, USA), penicillin (100 U/ml), and streptomycin (100 μg/ml) (Invitrogen Life Technologies, CA, USA) and maintained at 37 °C in a 5% CO_2 humidified incubator (Thermo Fisher Scientific, OH, USA).

Chemicals and reagents

Dacarbazine, MCD, and geldanamycin (GA) were procured from Sigma (MO, USA), cerulenin was obtained from Calbiochem (CA, USA), and cycloheximide was purchased from ICN (CA, USA). Antibodies against Hsp90 (Rabbit polyclonal, sc-7947), TNF-α (Goat polyclonal, sc-1347), ob (leptin) (Rabbit polyclonal, sc-9014), and resistin (Goat polyclonal sc-16117) and HRP-conjugated secondary antibodies against rabbit, mouse, rat, and goat IgG were purchased from Santa Cruz Biotechnology, CA, USA. P-gp (Mouse monoclonal, cat.no. ab3364) antibody was purchased from Abcam, MA, USA. IL-6 (Rat monoclonal, cat no. 554400) antibody was purchased from BD Biosciences, NJ, USA. FITC and Rhodamine-conjugated secondary antibodies against mouse, rabbit, and goat IgG were purchased from KPL, Gaithersburg, Maryland, USA.

Cycloheximide chase experiment

Approximately 3×10^5 A375 cells were plated in 35-mm culture dishes. After 24 h, culture medium was replaced by DMEM medium supplemented with 1% FBS, and the cells were treated with leptin and resistin for 48 h. Next, cycloheximide (Chx) was added to the cells at a concentration of 100 μg/ml. Cells were further incubated for 0, 30, 60, and 120 min. Thereafter, cell lysates were prepared and subjected to Western blotting.

Rhodamine-123 efflux assay

To measure efflux of Rhodamine-123 (Rh-123), reflective of transport activity for P-gp, melanoma cells were seeded at a density of 3×10^5 cells in 35-mm culture dishes and allowed to adhere for 24 h. These cells were then grown in the presence or absence of leptin or resistin for 24 h. Cells were washed thrice with PBS and incubated for 30 min at 37 °C in PBS containing 2 μM Rh-123. The solution was removed and cells were detached from culture flask by incubating in trypsin-containing, Ca^{2+}-free, phosphate-buffered solution with 2 μM Rh-123. Trypsin digestion was stopped by adding cold PBS solution supplemented with 5% fetal bovine serum and 2 μM Rh-123.

Cell aliquots were prepared in 1.5 ml tubes and centrifuged at 3000 rpm for 5 min at 4 °C. The supernatant was aspirated out, 2-ml cold incubation solution was added into the tubes and kept at 4 °C. The loading of Rh-123 at this point was considered as 0-min time point. Thereafter, the efflux of Rh-123 was initiated by incubating the cells at 25 °C for 30 min. Next, the fluorescence intensity of Rh-123 was measured through a 530/30 nm bandpass using FACS Calibur, and the data were analyzed using CellQuest Pro software (BD Biosciences, NJ, USA).

MTT assay

Melanoma cells were plated at a density of 6×10^3 cells/well in 96-well plates and allowed to adhere. After 24 h, cells were treated with vehicle (PBS or ethanol), drugs, or adipokines as per the experimental requirements. After required treatment time points, medium was removed and 50 µl of MTT (methyl thiazol tetrazolium, 1 mg/ml in DMEM without phenol red) (Sigma, MO, USA) was added to each well and further incubated for 4 h at 37 °C. MTT is reduced by mitochondrial dehydrogenase activity in metabolically active cells to form insoluble formazan crystals. Formazan crystals were solubilized in 100 µl of isopropanol and absorbance was measured at 570 nm using 630 nm as a reference filter (MultiSkan Go, Thermo Fisher Scientific, OH, USA). The absorbance given by untreated cells was taken as 100% cell survival.

Long-term survival assay

B16F10, B16F1, and A375 cells were plated at an appropriate density of 1×10^3 cells/well in 6-well plates. Next day, cells were treated with vehicle or drugs or inhibitors as per the experimental requirements. After 48 h, the medium was removed and fresh medium was added. Cells were allowed to grow for 10 days with medium change every 2–3 days. Thereafter, cells were fixed with 3% paraformaldehyde for 10 min and stained with 0.05% crystal violet for 2 h at room temperature. Images were taken using a digital camera (Olympus, Tokyo, Japan). Quantitation of colonies was performed by using NIH Image J software (Image J Freeware; http://rsb.info.nih.gov/ij/). The survival of control cells was considered as 100%.

Experimental mice

Wild-type (WT)-ob, ob/ob, WT-db, and db/db mice (6–8 weeks aged, male or female) and C57BL/6J mice were used in the present study. WT-ob, ob/ob, WT-db, and db/db mice were procured from Jackson Laboratories (ME, USA) and were maintained in Experimental Animal Facility (EAF) at National Centre for Cell Science (NCCS), Pune, India. Mice were housed and maintained in animal quarters under environmentally controlled conditions (22 ± 2 °C) with a 12-h light/dark cycle and had free access to water and standard rodent pellet food (Golden feeds, New Delhi, India) *ad libitum*, unless otherwise stated. For developing diet-induced obesity, C57BL/6J mice were fed with high fat diet (HFD) as described previously [7]. All animal experiments were carried out as per the requirement and guidelines of the Committee for the Purpose of Control and Supervision of Experiments on Animals (CPCSEA), Government of India, and after obtaining permission of the Institutional Animal Ethics Committee (IAEC).

Calorie restriction (CR) in ob/ob and db/db mice, tumor challenge, DTIC administration, and follow-up

To study the impact of leptin on the outcome of DTIC therapy in melanoma, B16F10 melanoma isograft was induced in ob/ob and db/db mice by injecting cells (2×10^5) in 100 µl of PBS subcutaneously (sc). After the appearance of the palpable tumor, mice were divided into four groups. Group 1 mice were kept as control, group 2 mice were treated with DTIC, group 3 mice were kept on 50% caloric restrictions (CR), and group 4 mice were kept on CR followed by DTIC treatment (80 mg/kg intraperitoneally for 5 consecutive days as described previously) [7]. The detailed experimental plan is illustrated in Fig. 4a. Tumor volume was calculated using the formula: $0.52 \times \text{length} \times \text{width}^2$ and was followed up throughout the study. At the end of the experiment, mice were sacrificed by CO_2 euthanasia. Excised tumors volume and weight were recorded, and the samples were immediately preserved at − 80 °C until further use. To observe their survival rates, five mice from each group were followed up for an additional 60 days.

Serum biochemical analysis

Glucose level was measured using rapid glucose analyzer (Accu-Chek Sensor Comfort, Roche Diagnostics, Mannheim, Germany) by collecting blood through an approved tail cap method. For serum collection, blood was collected by orbital sinus puncture and centrifuged at 6000 rpm at room temperature. Triglycerides (TG), cholesterol, LDLc, and free fatty acids levels in fresh serum were estimated using colorimetric kits (Spinreact, Girona, Spain) as per the manufacturer's instructions. Insulin, leptin, and adiponectin levels in the serum were estimated by mouse-specific respective ELISA kits as per the manufacturer's protocol. Leptin, resistin, IL-6, and TNF-α levels in the serum were detected by indirect ELISA. Briefly, a standard curve was prepared with different concentrations of respective recombinant proteins. ELISA plates (Becton Dickenson, NJ, USA) were coated with serum samples collected from mice. Blocking was done using 2% BSA in phosphate buffered saline (PBS; pH = 7.4). After washing with PBS, samples were incubated with primary antibodies (1:100) for resistin, IL-6, and TNF-α specified for ELISA. Following washing, samples were incubated with HRP-conjugated secondary antibodies (1:200). ABTS [2,2′-azinobis-(3-ethylbenzothiazoline-6-sulfonic acid)] (Sigma, MO, USA) was used as a chromogenic substrate for HRP. After developing the color, absorbance was recorded at 405 nm.

Reverse transcription PCR (RT-PCR)

Total RNA from treated and untreated cells was extracted using TRIzol™ reagent (Invitrogen, Carlsbad, USA), according to the manufacturer's instructions. Cells (5×10^5) were seeded in 35-mm plates and allowed to adhere for 24 h. Treatment conditions are indicated in respective experiments. Cells were directly lysed in culture plate by adding 1 ml of TRIzol reagent, and passing the cell lysates several times through the pipette tip, and collected in a 1.5-ml tube. Homogenized samples were incubated at room temperature for 5 min, and 200 μl chloroform was added. The contents in tubes were mixed by gentle shaking and incubated for 2–3 min at room temperature. Next, the tubes were centrifuged at 12,000×g for 15 min at 4 °C. Following centrifugation, the upper colorless aqueous phase was collected in fresh tubes. RNA was precipitated from the aqueous phase by addition of 500 μl isopropanol. Tubes were incubated for 10 min at room temperature and centrifuged at 12,000×*g* for 10 min at 4 °C. Supernatant was removed, and RNA pellet was washed once with 1 ml of 75% ethanol in DEPC-treated water by mixing and centrifuging at 7500×*g* for 5 min at 4 °C. At the end, RNA pellets were briefly air dried and dissolved in DEPC-treated water at 55 °C for 10 min.

Culture of melanoma cells in serum collected from experimental ob/ob and db/db mice

Serum collected from experimental ob/ob, db/db, and their WT counterparts was pooled from respective groups. Approximately 1.5×10^2 B16F10 cells were plated in 24-well plates and allowed to adhere. After 24 h, DMEM containing 5% serum collected from experimental mice was added and cells were cultured chronically for 10 days. The medium was changed on every 2–3 days. Finally, cells were fixed with paraformaldehyde, stained with crystal violet, and images were taken (as described above).

Treatment with adipokines in vitro

To study the effect of leptin and resistin, recombinant human leptin and resistin (Sigma, MO, USA) were used to treat melanoma cells in vitro. A375 cells were plated in culture dishes or 6-well plates in DMEM containing 10% FBS. After 24 h, the medium was removed and cells were treated with varying concentrations (range 0.01–100 ng/ml) of leptin and resistin in DMEM containing 1% FBS for 24 or 48 h as per the experimental requirements. Treated cells were then analyzed by MTT assay or processed for immunoblotting or RT-PCR or confocal staining.

Immunodepletion of leptin and resistin from serum collected from mice

Serum from HFD C57BL/6 J mice was collected, and pooled (as described above). Leptin and resistin (or both together) were immunodepleted from the serum by incubating it with respective specific antibody (Santa Cruz Biotechnology, CA, USA), at 4 °C for overnight. Antigen-antibody complexes were precipitated using protein A/G-plus agarose beads (Santa Cruz Biotechnology, CA, USA) by incubating at 4 °C for 4 h. Next, the supernatant containing immunodepleted serum was collected by centrifuging the tubes at 10,000 rpm at 4 °C. Following validation of immunodepletion of leptin and resistin in the serum (Additional file 1: Figure S1A and S1B), B16F10 or B16F1 cells (3×10^5) seeded in 35-mm dishes were cultured in DMEM containing 5% immunodepleted serum. After 48 h, the cells were harvested and lysates were prepared for immunoblotting.

Statistical analysis

Statistical analysis was performed using Sigma Plot 12.0 (Systat Software Inc., CA, USA). All data were represented as the mean ± standard error of the mean (S.E.M.). All in vitro experiments were performed at least three times unless otherwise mentioned. For in vivo experiments involving more than two groups, one-way ANOVA was used, followed by the Tukey multiple comparison test. In vitro or in vivo data involving two experimental groups were analyzed using two-tailed unpaired Student's t test. The values of $p < 0.05$, $p < 0.01$, and $p < 0.001$ were considered as statistically significant (*), very significant (**), and highly significant difference (***) respectively, unless otherwise mentioned.

Results

Leptin and resistin impair the efficacy of DTIC in melanoma cells

Previously, we have reported that obesity impairs efficacy of DTIC in melanoma, which is mediated by FASN and Cav-1 [7]. To unravel the mechanism as to how obesity impairs the outcome of DTIC therapy in melanoma, we investigated the specific role of leptin and resistin as their levels in serum are elevated under obese condition. Firstly, to explore whether leptin and resistin could have any role in modulating the sensitivity of melanoma cells to DTIC, A375 cells were treated with DTIC in the presence or absence of leptin or resistin. We observed that leptin significantly impaired the response of A375 cells to DTIC as evident from the increase in IC_{50} of DTIC by ~5-fold (2592 μM) as compared to the control (461 μM) (Fig. 1a). Similarly, in A375 cells treated with resistin IC_{50} for DTIC increased to 2739 μM as compared to control (421 μM) (Fig. 1b).

Additionally, to verify the involvement of leptin in modulating the response of melanoma cells to DTIC therapy, B16F10 cells were cultured in the medium containing serum of genetically obese mice strains ob/ob (leptin

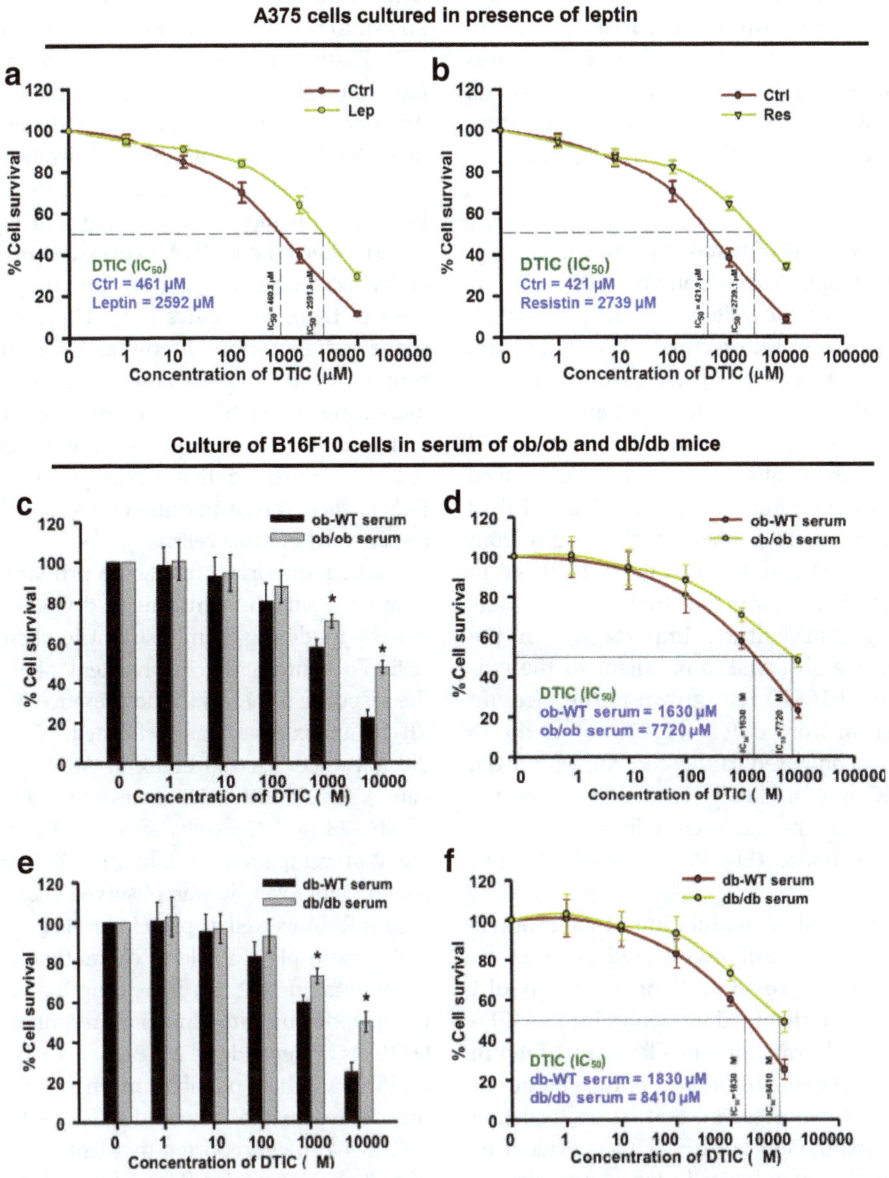

Fig. 1 Leptin and resistin impair the outcome of DTIC therapy in melanoma cells. **a**, **b** Effect of leptin (**a**) and resistin (**b**) on the outcome of DTIC in A375 cells. A375 (human melanoma) cells were plated in 96-well plates. After 24 h, cells were treated with 100 ng/ml of recombinant leptin or resistin in DMEM containing 1% FBS for 1 h. Then, cells were treated with DTIC at the indicated concentrations and incubated for 48 h. These cells were subjected to MTT assay, and IC_{50} of DTIC was calculated. **c**–**f** Effect of ob/ob and db/db serum factors on the survival of B16F10 cells upon DTIC treatment. B16F10 cells were chronically grown in medium containing 5% serum collected from ob-WT or ob/ob mice for 15 days. These cells were then subjected to DTIC treatment at the indicated concentrations, for 48 h, and MTT assay was performed. **c** Survival of B16F10 cells in DMEM containing ob-WT or ob/ob serum. **d** Measurement of IC_{50} values of DTIC in DMEM containing ob-WT or ob/ob serum. **e**, **f** B16F10 cells were chronically grown in medium containing 5% serum collected from db-WT or db/db mice for 15 days. These cells were then subjected to DTIC treatment at the indicated concentrations, for 48 h, and MTT assay was performed. **e** Survival of B16F10 cells in DMEM containing db-WT or db/db serum. **f** Measurement of IC_{50} value of DTIC in DMEM containing db-WT or db/db serum. The data are representative of experiments performed three times in triplicate. The results are given as means ± standard error of the mean. All the experiments were performed three times. Statistical analysis was performed using two-tailed unpaired Student's *t* test; $^*p < 0.05$; Ctrl, control; Lep, leptin; Res, resistin

deficient) or db/db (leptin receptor deficient). As compared to ob-WT serum, the cytotoxicity of DTIC was found to be impaired in ob/ob serum (Fig. 1c). Interestingly, the IC_{50} value of DTIC was increased (7720 μM) in cells grown in ob/ob serum as compared to those cultured in ob-WT serum (1630 μM) (Fig. 1d). Similarly, the response of melanoma cells to DTIC was found to be reduced in the presence of ob/ob serum when compared to that of db-WT serum (Fig. 1e). Higher IC_{50} value of DTIC was observed in melanoma cells grown in the serum of db/db mice (8410 μM), which contains very high circulatory leptin, as compared to control (1830 μM) (Fig. 1f).

Diminished circulatory level of leptin and resistin improves the efficacy of DTIC in melanoma cells

Further, to complement the role of leptin and resistin and other obesity-associated factors in cell growth, long-term cell survival assay was performed. Melanoma cells were cultured in the medium containing serum from ob/ob or db/db mice or the caloric restricted (CR), in the presence or absence of DTIC. Enhanced cell growth and proliferation was observed in B16F10 cells grown in the medium containing the serum from ob/ob or db/db mice as compared to those cultured in the medium containing serum from their WT counterparts in the long-term culture. Importantly, in the long-term culture, we observed impairment in the efficacy of DTIC in the B16F10 cells grown in the medium containing the serum from ob/ob (Fig. 2a, b) or db/db (Fig. 2c, d) mice as compared to the control. Moreover, the effect of DTIC was markedly rescued upon culturing these cells in the medium containing serum of calorically restricted ob/ob (Fig. 2a, b) or db/db mice (Fig. 2c, d).

To further check whether modulation of chemotherapeutic outcome by obesity-associated factors is dependent on leptin or resistin, B16F10 and B16F1 cells were cultured in the medium containing HFD-C57BL/6J serum which was immuno-depleted of leptin or resistin by respective antibodies either alone or together. Interestingly, we observed that leptin depletion significantly improved the efficacy of DTIC as evident by decrease in the number of colonies in long-term survival assay as compared to the cells grown in the medium containing the control serum [(B16F10: Fig. 2e, f) and (B16F1: Fig. 2g, h)]. Similarly, resistin depletion resulted in improved efficacy of DTIC in melanoma cells as compared to the cells grown in the medium containing the control serum [(B16F10: Fig. 2e, f) and (B16F1: Fig. 2g, h)]. Interestingly, upon simultaneous immunodepletion of both leptin and resistin, the effect of DTIC was prominently improved [(B16F10: Fig. 2e, f) and (B16F1: Fig. 2g, h)].

Leptin- and resistin-induced impaired response of melanoma cells to DTIC is mediated by FASN/Hsp90 and Cav-1/P-gp respectively

To get insights into the role of leptin and resistin in causing attenuation in the response to DTIC, we intended to analyze the status of FASN and Cav-1 which are upregulated in melanoma in the obese (HFD) mice [16], and are known to be involved in resistance to cancer chemotherapy [17]. Firstly, we checked the protein levels of FASN and Cav-1 in A375 cells upon treatment with leptin or resistin. An increased level of FASN was detected in A375 cells upon leptin treatment (Fig. 3a), while resistin treatment caused increase in the level of Cav-1 in A375 cells (Fig. 3b). Previously, it has been reported that leptin and resistin do not affect the mRNA expression of FASN and Cav-1 at transcription levels; however, they increase protein level of these molecules [18]. Therefore, these findings suggested that both leptin and resistin modulate the protein levels of FASN and Cav-1 respectively, likely by increasing the stability of these proteins. To verify this, cycloheximide chase experiment was performed in A375 cells. We observed that leptin promoted stabilization of FASN, whereas resistin caused Cav-1 stabilization (Fig. 3c, d, respectively) in these cells.

Another important molecule primarily responsible for pumping out the anticancer drugs from cancer cells thereby rendering them resistant to chemotherapy is P-gp [19]. To confirm the involvement of P-gp in decreasing the response to DTIC in the presence of leptin or resistin, Rh-123 efflux assay was performed. We noticed that leptin did not affect Rh-123 efflux in A375 cells (Fig. 3e, upper panel). On the other hand, resistin did increase the efflux of Rh-123 in A375 cells, which was reversed upon treatment of verapamil, an inhibitor of P-gp (Fig. 3e, lower panel). Moreover, it was observed that resistin increased P-gp mRNA as well as protein levels (Fig. 3f, g), suggesting that resistin plays a role in chemotherapeutic outcome in melanoma, in part, via increasing the expression of P-gp, while leptin-mediated impaired response of cancer cells to DTIC is independent of P-gp activity. This led us to explore another possible mechanism by which leptin contributes to the impaired DTIC action on melanoma cells. It has been reported that leptin modulates the levels of heat shock proteins (Hsps) [20, 21]. Moreover, Hsp90 is one of the major heat shock proteins known to contribute to drug-resistant phenotype [22, 23]. Therefore, we analyzed the involvement of Hsp90 and checked the expression of Hsp90 in melanoma cells upon treatment with leptin. We found that leptin treatment indeed increased transcript and protein levels of Hsp90 in A375 cells (Fig. 3h, i).

To confirm whether FASN and Hsp90 are involved in leptin-induced impairment in the response of melanoma cells to DTIC, we used their respective inhibitors.

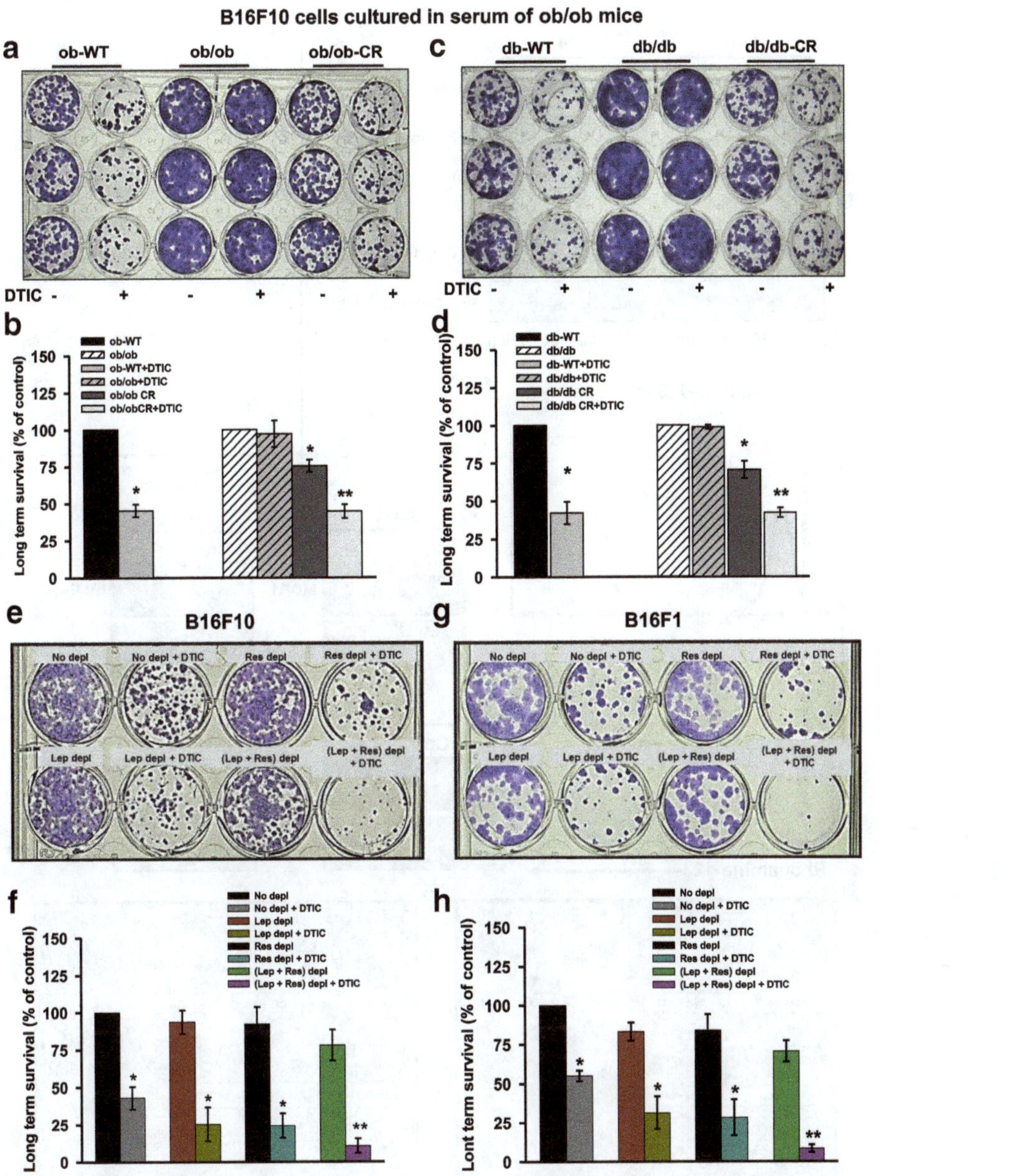

Fig. 2 Effect of obesity-associated serum factors on the long-term survival of B16F10 and B16F1 cells treated with DTIC. **a**, **b** B16F10 cells were chronically grown in the medium containing 5% serum collected from experimental ob/ob mice for 15 days. Thereafter, these cells were subjected to DTIC treatment for 48 h. Then, the medium was changed and fresh medium was added. The medium was changed every 2–3 days. **a** Representative image showing the long-term survival of B16F10 cells. **b** Bar graph showing the quantitation of number of surviving population from the image shown in **a**. **c**, **d** Similar experiment was performed in B16F10 cells chronically grown in the serum from db/db mice. After 10 days, the cells were stained with 0.05% crystal violet, and images were taken using Olympus digital camera. **e**–**h** B16F10 and B16F1 cells were cultured in serum (collected from C57BL/6J mice) which was immuno-depleted of leptin and or resistin for 48 h. Then, DTIC treatment was given, and cells were incubated for 48 h. Next, the medium was changed and fresh medium was added. **e** Representative image showing the long-term survival of B16F10 cells. **f** Bar graph showing the quantitation of number of surviving population from the image shown in **e**. **g** Representative image showing the long-term survival of B16F1 cells. **h** Bar graph showing the quantitation of number of surviving population from **g**. The data are representative of experiments performed two times at least in triplicates. The data were quantified using Image J software. The results are given as means ± standard error of the mean. Statistical analysis was performed using one-way ANOVA, followed by the Tukey multiple comparison test (for **b** and **d**), whereas two-tailed unpaired Student's *t* test was used (for **f** and **g**). *$p < 0.05$, **$p < 0.001$; Ctrl, control; Lep, leptin; Res resistin

Inhibition of FASN and Hsp90 individually by cerulenin and geldanamycin respectively increased the sensitivity of A375 cells to DTIC even in the presence of leptin (Fig. 3j). Moreover, combined inhibition of FASN and Hsp90 enhanced the effect of DTIC in A375 cells compared to single inhibitor treatment (Fig. 3j; Additional

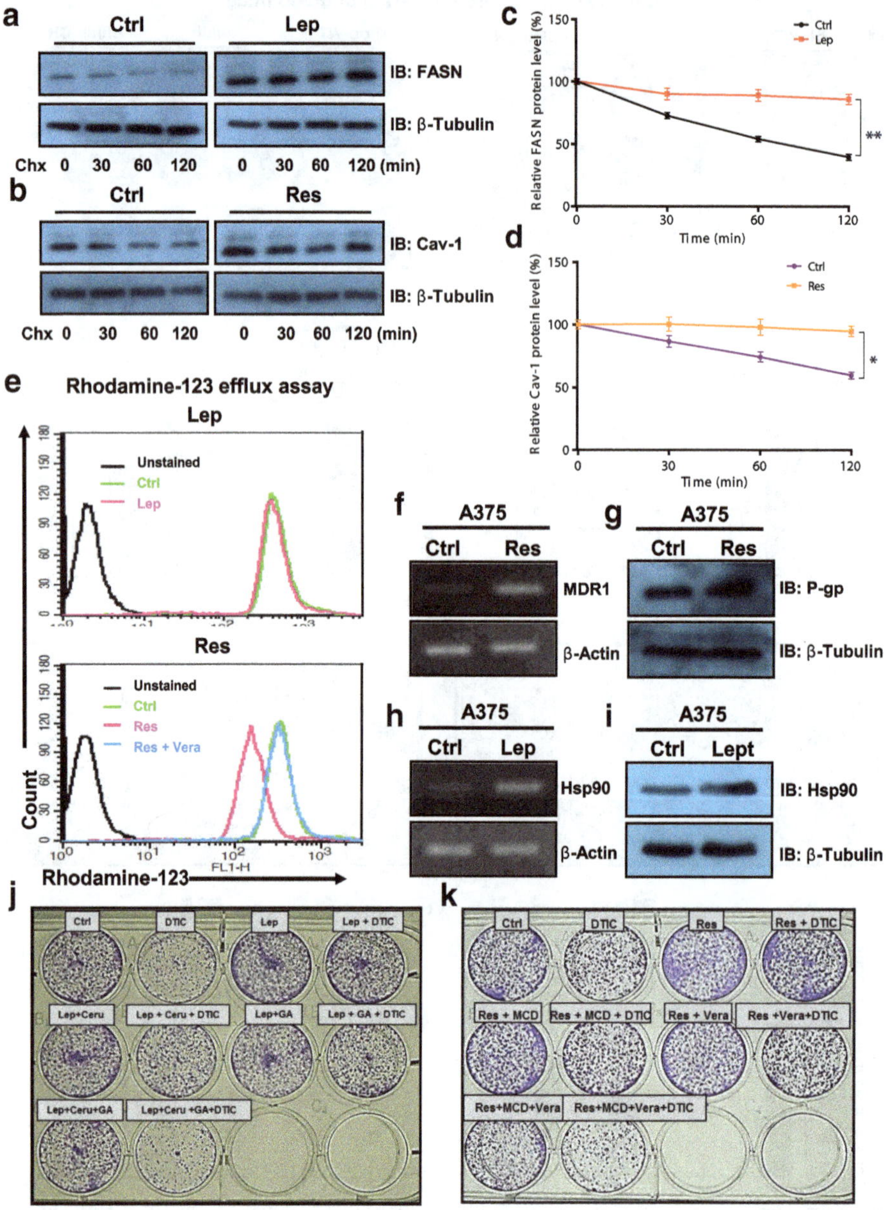

Fig. 3 Molecular events associated with leptin and resistin induced impaired outcome of DTIC therapy in melanoma cells. **a**, **b** A375 cells were treated with leptin or resistin at a concentration of 100 ng/ml in DMEM containing 1% FBS for 48 h as described in the "Materials and methods" section. Thereafter, cycloheximide (100 μg/ml) treatment was given for the indicated time points. Representative immunoblot of FASN (**a**) and Cav-1 (**b**) in A375 cells treated with leptin or resistin respectively. **c**, **d** Bar graph showing the quantitation of band intensity of FASN and Cav-1 immunoblots. **e** Rhodamine-123 efflux assay in A375 cells treated with leptin (upper panel) or resistin (lower panel). A375 (human melanoma) cells were plated in 12-well plates. After 24 h, cells were treated with 100 ng/ml of recombinant leptin in DMEM containing 1% FBS for 48 h. Thereafter, these cells were subjected to Rh-123 efflux assay via flow cytometry. **f**, **g** RT-PCR (**f**) and immunoblotting (**g**) analysis of MDR and P-gp respectively in A375 cells treated with resistin. **h**, **i** RT-PCR (**h**) and immunoblotting (**i**) analysis of HSP90 in A375 cells treated with leptin. **j**, **k** Representative image showing the long-term survival of A375 cells grown in the presence or absence of leptin (**j**) or resistin (**k**) together with inhibitors. The results are given as means ± standard error of the mean. All the experiments were performed three times. Statistical analysis was performed using two-tailed unpaired Student's *t* test for **c** and **d**. $^*p < 0.05$, $^{**}p < 0.001$; Ctrl, control; Lep, leptin; Res, resistin; Chx, cycloheximide; Ceru or C, cerulenin; GA or G, geldanamycin

file 1: Figure S2A). Similarly, to verify the role of Cav-1 and P-gp in impairing the response to DTIC by resistin, their inhibitors MCD and verapamil respectively were used. Inhibition of these molecules resulted in increased sensitivity of A375 cells to DTIC (Fig. 3k). Simultaneous inhibition of both of these molecules profoundly improved the anticancer effect of DTIC (Fig. 3k; Additional file 1: Figure S2B).

Elevated serum level of leptin and resistin is correlated with enhanced melanoma growth and impaired efficacy of DTIC in vivo

To corroborate the involvement of leptin in melanoma growth and in the outcome of DTIC treatment, we employed ob/ob and db/db mice. Leptin is an important adipocyte-secreted factor involved in controlling appetite. Due to lack of functional leptin and leptin receptor respectively, ob/ob and db/db mice are morbidly obese (despite fed on a normal fat diet) exhibiting higher level of fat accumulation. Thus, these mice serve as good models for the leptin-related studies.

To understand the involvement of leptin in melanoma progression, and the outcome of chemotherapy, ob/ob and db/db mice, as well as their WT counterparts, were ectopically isografted with B16F10 cells as shown in Fig. 4a. After the appearance of palpable tumors, DTIC was administered for 5 consecutive days and tumor progression was followed up until the termination of the experiment. We observed that DTIC treatment did not affect the serum levels of obesity-associated factors in ob/ob (Additional file 1: Table S1) and db/db mice (Additional file 1: Table S2) as well as in their WT littermates. As expected, DTIC significantly retarded tumor progression in respective WT counterparts, as evident by reduced tumor volume and weight (Fig. 4b–d, h–j). Surprisingly, therapeutic efficacy of DTIC was impaired in both ob/ob and db/db mice as is evident by the increase in tumor progression as compared to respective untreated controls (Fig. 4e–g, k–m).

In previous study, we have shown that shifting mice from HFD to ND has a profound impact on melanoma progression, which correlates with normalization in the body weight and in the levels of obesity-associated factors [18]. Therefore, to determine whether caloric restriction (CR) could improve the effect of DTIC in ob/ob and db/db mice, we subjected these mice to CR by reducing their feed by 50% as shown in Fig. 4a. In the present study, it was observed that CR itself reduced tumor progression in both ob/ob and db/db mice which correlated with the limited normalization in the levels of obesity-associated factors (Additional file 1: Table S1 and Table S2). More importantly, CR significantly improved the outcome of DTIC therapy in these mice (Fig. 4e–g, k–m).

Discussion

Obesity is associated with an elevation in the levels of many pro-inflammatory and proliferative factors, which contribute to increased growth and proliferation of cancer cells [24]. Furthermore, in vitro studies have revealed growth-promoting effect of serum from ob/ob mice on cultured melanoma cells [25]. Pro-inflammatory (such as IL-6 and TNF-α) and proliferative (like leptin and insulin) factors are considered as tumor growth favoring molecules [26–28]. Both leptin and resistin are two of the important adipokines, which are elevated in obesity. Although the involvement of leptin and resistin in malignancies such as breast and prostate cancers has been extensively studied, very little is known about their role in melanoma growth and chemotherapeutic outcome. For better understanding and management of obesity-promoted malignancies, the involvement of obesity-associated factors needs to be comprehensively investigated [29]. The present study is aimed at unraveling the specific role of leptin and resistin in melanoma growth and the chemotherapeutic outcome using appropriate in vitro and in vivo approaches.

As observed in our previous study, by controlling obesity, tumor growth is restricted partly through normalization in the serum levels of obesity-associated factors such as leptin and resistin [18]. It has been shown that leptin and resistin stimulate the Akt signaling in cancer cells [30, 31], and hyperactivated Akt pathway was associated with increased protein levels of FASN and Cav-1 [16]. Our in vitro studies show that treatment of melanoma cells with leptin or resistin leads to increased levels or activation of proteins which are associated with regulation of cellular growth and metabolism, indicating their involvement in promoting melanoma cell growth and proliferation, which is consistent with findings of other research groups [25, 32]. Previously, we have examined the effect of various concentrations of both leptin and resistin on cell survival [18]. As the data indicated in the study, the optimum dose response was found to be 100 ng/ml, which was used throughout the study. Owing to the limitations in replicating the physiological conditions precisely in cell based experiments, especially, when the availability and dynamics/kinetics of these cytokines vary in vitro and in vivo, it would be inappropriate to compare the level of these adipokines present in vivo with the concentration used in vitro. The levels of cytokines are, generally, maintained at steady level in vivo. On the other hand, considering the half-life and artificially maintained physiology, higher concentrations of adipokines are required under in vitro conditions. Therefore, to sustain the effect of these adipokines during the course of in vitro studies, we relied on higher concentrations. Also, there are number of studies which used similar concentration of these adipokines for other related studies [33–36].

From a molecular point of view, leptin and resistin specifically enhanced FASN and Cav-1 protein level respectively. Intriguingly, there was no change in the transcript level of FASN or Cav-1 in cells treated with leptin or resistin. However, cycloheximide chase experiment confirms that leptin and resistin cause the stabilization of FASN and Cav-1 protein levels respectively in melanoma cells. Considering our previous study on HFD mice [7], normalized serum levels of these adipokines, via reduced

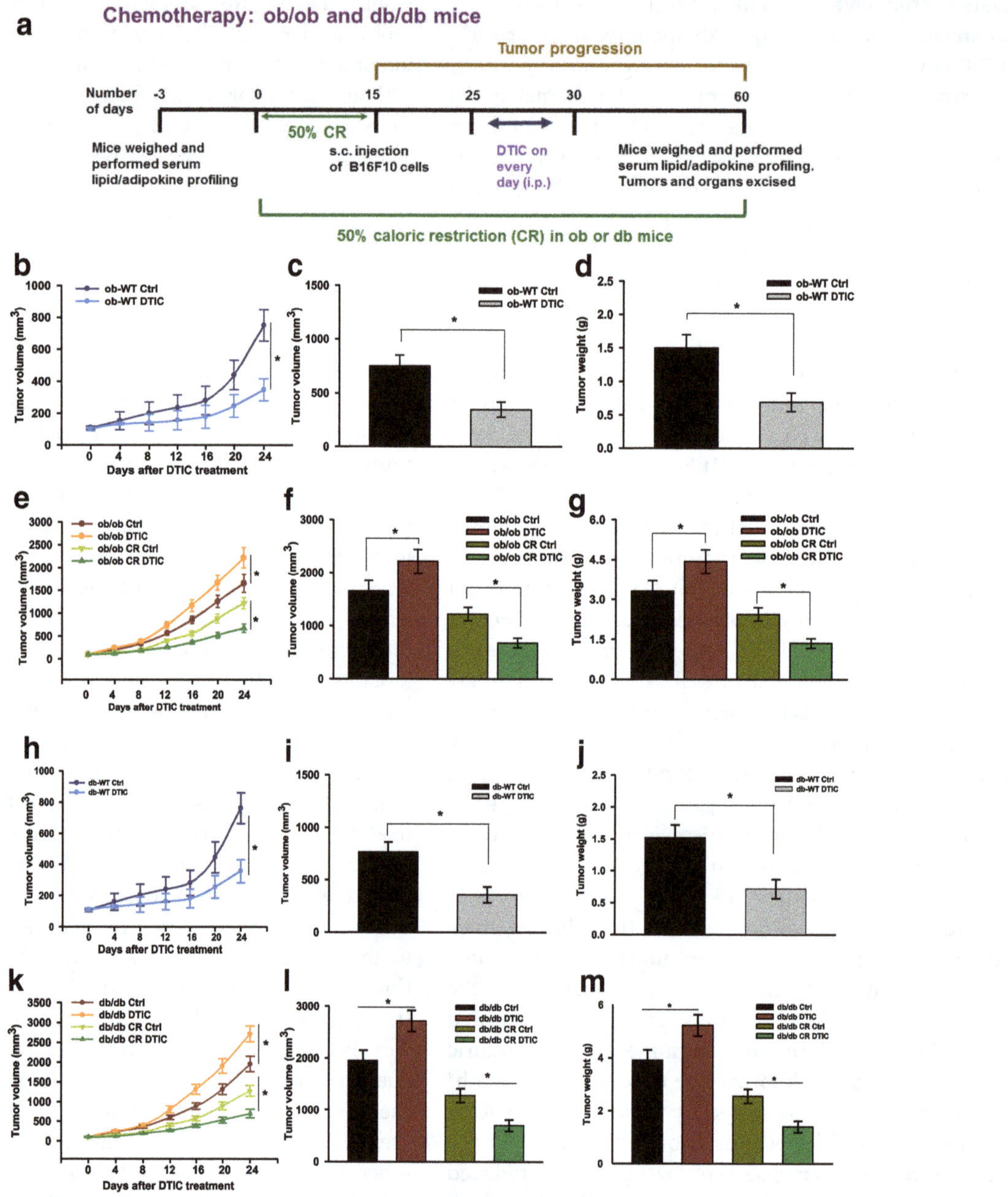

Fig. 4 Impact of leptin on melanoma progression and on the outcome of DTIC therapy in ob/ob and db/db mice. **a** Layout of the in vivo experiments. **b**–**d** ob-WT mice were injected with B16F10 cells (2×10^5 cells/mouse in 100 μl PBS). After the tumor formation, vehicle or DTIC treatment ($N = 6$ per each group) was given as per the experimental layout shown in **a**. **b** Tumor progression, **c** tumor volume, and **d** tumor weight. **e**–**g** ob/ob mice were divided into two major groups. One group was fed *ad libitum* on normal diet. In the second group, caloric intake was restricted to 50% by providing half the quantity of feed in normal before inoculating B16F10 cells. After 15 days, mice of all groups were injected subcutaneously with B16F10 cells (2×10^5 cells/mouse in 100 μl PBS). After tumor formation, vehicle or DTIC treatment ($N = 6$ per each group) was given as per the experimental layout shown in **a**. **e** Trend of tumor progression, **f** tumor volume, and **g** tumor weight. **h**–**j** db-WT mice were injected with B16F10 cells (2×10^5 cells/mouse in 100 μl PBS). After tumor formation, vehicle or DTIC treatment ($N = 6$ per each group) was given as per the experimental layout shown in **a**. **h** Trend of tumor progression, **i** tumor volume, and **j** tumor weight. **k**–**m** db/db mice were divided into two major groups. One group was fed *ad libitum* on normal diet. In the second group, caloric intake was restricted to 50% by providing half the quantity of feed in normal before inoculating B16F10 cells. After 15 days, mice of all groups were injected subcutaneously with B16F10 cells (2×10^5 cells/mouse in 100 μl PBS). After tumor formation, vehicle or DTIC treatment ($N = 6$ per each group) was given as per the experimental layout shown in **a**. At the end of the experiment, mice were sacrificed and tumors were collected. **k** Trend of tumor progression, **l** tumor volume, and **m** tumor weight. The results are given as means ± standard error of the mean. Statistical analysis was performed using two-tailed unpaired Student's *t* test (**b**, **h**), whereas one-way ANOVA, followed by the Tukey multiple comparison test was used for **e** and **k**. $^{*}p < 0.05$, when compared to respective controls

adiposity, could be associated with a reduction in FASN and Cav-1 protein levels and decrease in Akt activation, leading to reduced progression of melanoma in the experimental HFD mice.

Fatty acid metabolism plays a pivotal role in various aspects of cancer progression. It has been recently shown that adipocyte-derived fatty acids drive breast cancer cell proliferation and migration by promoting adipocyte lipolysis [37]. In the present study, we observed that leptin and resistin cause impairment in the effect of DTIC on melanoma cells in vitro. In addition to tumor promoting effect on cancer cells [38–41], FASN and Cav-1 have been reported to protect cancer cells from chemotherapy by inducing drug resistance [17]. Since FASN and Cav-1 were modulated by leptin and resistin respectively, the impairment in chemotherapeutic outcome of DTIC could be partly due to the involvement of FASN and Cav-1 proteins. Another protein with critical role in tumor growth and cancer drug resistance is Hsp90 [42, 43]. Hsp90 is also involved in the stabilization of various molecules required for tumor growth [44–47]. In this study, we show that leptin, in addition to stabilizing FASN protein, enhanced the protein and mRNA level of Hsp90. Thus, the mutual involvement of FASN and Hsp90 could contribute to the unresponsiveness of melanoma cells to DTIC in the presence of leptin. To confirm this proposition, we show that simultaneous inhibition of FASN and Hsp90 together, in the leptin-treated A375 cells, indeed immensely enhanced the cytotoxic effect of DTIC. Another mechanism that stimulates drug-resistant phenotype is overexpression of P-gp in order to prevent cytotoxic effects of anticancer drugs [48]. In this study, resistin was found to increase P-gp mRNA and protein levels. Therefore, resistin-mediated impairment of DTIC treatment in melanoma cells could be due to collective involvement of Cav-1 and P-gp, both being integral component of plasma membrane of cancer cells. Similar to FASN and Hsp90 inhibition together in leptin-stimulated cells, simultaneous inhibition of Cav-1 and P-gp in resistin-treated A375 cells prominently reduced survival upon exposure to DTIC. Consistent with these findings, improvement in the effect of DTIC was observed upon culturing B16F10 and B16F1 cells in mice serum immuno-depleted of leptin and resistin.

As observed in our in vivo studies, irrespective of the presence of leptin, we noticed the impairment of DTIC therapy in ob/ob and db/db mice. Nevertheless, our in vitro data clearly demonstrate the growth promoting and chemotherapy-impairment effect of leptin. This implies that leptin, in part, likely plays an important role in tumor growth as well as in the outcome of DTIC therapy. In addition, since we observed a trend of tumor progression and impaired therapeutic outcome in ob/ob mice (which lack functional leptin) as compared to their wild-type counterparts, obesity-associated factors (other than leptin) could also influence tumor progression and the impairment of chemotherapy. As serum level of resistin is very high in ob/ob mice, and we observed in vitro that resistin is equally partly responsible for causing impairment in the efficacy of DTIC, it is conceivable that even in the absence of leptin, resistin could be involved in impairing the efficacy of DTIC in ob/ob mice, as resistin is very well known to induce drug-resistant phenotype in various cancers [14, 15, 49, 50]. Although, our in vitro results established the fact that both leptin and resistin are involved in impairing the response of melanoma cells to DTIC, it is difficult to validate their role in vivo due to lack of resistin knockout animals as well as resistin neutralizing antibody. Moreover, CR in both ob/ob and db/db mice significantly reduced tumor growth and improved the efficacy of DTIC which correlated with normalization of the serum levels of obesity-associated factors. As per observations from our laboratory and other research groups [51–53], ob/ob and db/db mice consume ~ 6 g diet per day, while their WT counterpart mice eat ~ 3 g diet per day (which is essentially 50% of the diet consumed by ob/ob and db/db mice). Therefore, to mimic the diet consumption similar to their WT counterparts, ob/ob and db/db mice were restricted to 50% food intake. The culture of B16F10 and B16F1 cells in the presence of serum from the experimental ob/ob and db/db mice confirms that obesity-associated circulating factors are important for melanoma progression. Culturing melanoma cells in medium containing serum of calorically restricted (CR) ob/ob and db/db mice reveals that normalization in the levels of obesity-associated factors has a profound impact on tumor growth and outcome of chemotherapy. Thus, obesity-associated factors including leptin and resistin are crucial for cancer cell growth as well as for outcome of therapeutic response. However, the possibility of the involvement of other obesity-associated factors (including adipokines and nutritional factors) in cancer progression and chemotherapeutic outcome cannot be ruled out. Our results clearly indicated that leptin and resistin partly contribute to melanoma progression and in impairing the outcome of dacarbazine therapy. Host factors other than leptin and resistin (including insulin, other adipokines and nutritional factors) could also play a pivotal role. Nonetheless, our in vitro studies (especially treatment of melanoma cells with leptin and resistin, as well as their immune-depletion) demonstrate that these adipokines critically affect melanoma growth, and the chemotherapeutic outcome, by modulating melanoma promoting proteins. Moreover, our data show that depletion of leptin and resistin from the serum collected from obese mice resulted in the improved response of melanoma cells as compared to the undepleted serum suggestive of their role in modulating the response of melanoma cells to DTIC. Currently, our laboratory is actively pursuing to understand the role

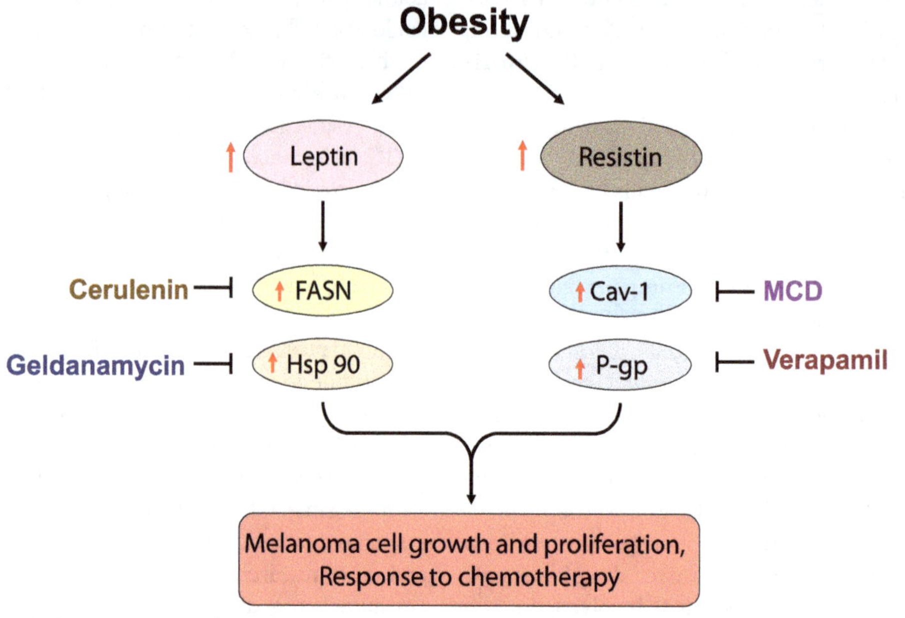

Fig. 5 Proposed model of study on impact of leptin on melanoma growth and the outcome of dacarbazine therapy. Leptin modulates FASN and Hsp90 levels while resistin modulates Cav-1 and P-gp, thereby enhancing melanoma growth. Collectively, these events are responsible in part for impaired outcome of DTIC therapy. Inhibition of these molecules restricts melanoma growth and improves the outcome of chemotherapy

of other obesity-associated factors (including both adipokines and nutritional factors) on cancer progression. Collectively, these data suggest that both leptin and resistin partly play a crucial role in melanoma growth and adversely affect the chemotherapeutic outcome by modulating the molecules which are involved in tumor growth and drug resistance. In a nutshell, this study highlights the role of leptin and resistin in melanoma growth, and impairment in the chemotherapeutic outcome.

Conclusions

To conclude, this study investigates the role of increased levels of obesity-associated important adipokines leptin and resistin in melanoma growth and the outcome of DTIC-based therapy. Both of these adipokines activate Akt in melanoma cells. Leptin modulates FASN and Hsp90, while resistin increases Cav-1 and P-gp levels, thereby enhancing melanoma growth, and impairing the chemotherapeutic outcome (see the schematic overview in Fig. 5). Thus, this study provides a mechanistic link between these two adipokines and melanoma progression, as well as outcome of chemotherapy. Overall, our study suggests that controlling the circulating levels of these adipokines by life style interventions or inhibition of their molecular effectors is critical for better management of obesity-promoted cancer progression, and in improving the outcome of chemotherapy.

Additional file

Additional file 1: Figure S1. Validation of immunodepletion of leptin form serum collected from HFD C57BL/6J mice. **Figure S2.** A375 cells were cultured in the presence of leptin or resistin along with inhibitors for 48 h. **Table S1.** Evaluation of obesity-associated factors in WT and db/db mice. **Table S2.** Evaluation of obesity-associated factors in WT and db/db mice. (DOC 319 kb)

Acknowledgements

Authors thank Dr. S.C. Mande, Director, NCCS, Pune, India, and Dr. G.C. Mishra, former Director, NCCS, Pune, India, for being very supportive and giving all the encouragement to carry out this work. P.M., S.V.S., and S.S. thank University Grants Commission (UGC), New Delhi, India; B.C., N.M., and S.C. thank Council for Scientific and Industrial Research (CSIR), India, for a research fellowship. The support from Experimental Animal Facility (EAF), Confocal Microscopy Facility, Fluorescence Activated Cell Sorter (FACS) Facility, Central Instrumental Facilities, technical staff of NCCS, and other group members is also duly acknowledged. We also acknowledge Radoslav Janostiak (Yale University School of Medicine, New Haven, USA) for reading and editing the manuscript.

Note

This work was carried out for the partial fulfillment of a Ph.D. thesis (of P.M.) submitted to Savitribai Phule Pune University, Pune, India.

Funding

This work was supported in part by an intramural grant from the National Centre for Cell Science (NCCS) funded by the Department of Biotechnology (DBT), Government of India, and an extramural grant from the Department of Science and Technology (DST), Government of India (Grant No. SR/SO/HS-0136/2012). The funding agencies had no involvement in the study design, data collection, interpretation, and analysis; decision to publish; or writing of the manuscript.

Authors' contributions

MKB and PM conceived and designed the experiments. PM, BC, and MKB wrote the manuscript; PM, BC, SVS, NM, MVV, SS, and SC performed the experiments and analyzed the data. All the authors read, reviewed, and edited the manuscript.

Competing interests

The authors declare that they have no competing interests.

References

1. Tremblay A, Doucet E. Obesity: a disease or a biological adaptation? Obes Rev. 2000;1:27–35.
2. Khandekar MJ, Cohen P, Spiegelman BM. Molecular mechanisms of cancer development in obesity. Nat Rev Cancer. 2011;11:886–95.
3. Gregor MF, Hotamisligil GS. Inflammatory mechanisms in obesity. Annu Rev Immunol. 2011;29:415–45.
4. Lumeng CN, Saltiel AR. Inflammatory links between obesity and metabolic disease. J Clin Invest. 2011;121:2111–7.
5. van Kruijsdijk RC, van der Wall E, Visseren FL. Obesity and cancer: the role of dysfunctional adipose tissue. Cancer Epidemiol Biomark Prev. 2009;18:2569–78.
6. Lashinger LM, Rossi EL, Hursting SD. Obesity and resistance to cancer chemotherapy: interacting roles of inflammation and metabolic dysregulation. Clin Pharmacol Ther. 2014;96:458–63.
7. Malvi P, Chaube B, Singh SV, Mohammad N, Pandey V, Vijayakumar MV, et al. Weight control interventions improve therapeutic efficacy of dacarbazine in melanoma by reversing obesity-induced drug resistance. Cancer Metab. 2016;4:21. eCollection 2016
8. Chi M, Chen J, Ye Y, Tseng HY, Lai F, Tay KH, et al. Adipocytes contribute to resistance of human melanoma cells to chemotherapy and targeted therapy. Curr Med Chem. 2014;10:1255–67.
9. Duong MN, Cleret A, Matera EL, Chettab K, Mathé D, Valsesia-Wittmann S, et al. Adipose cells promote resistance of breast cancer cells to trastuzumab-mediated antibody-dependent cellular cytotoxicity. Breast Cancer Res. 2015;17:57.
10. Liu Z, Xu J, He J, Liu H, Lin P, Wan X, et al. Mature adipocytes in bone marrow protects myeloma cells against chemotherapy through autophagy activation. Oncotarget. 2015;6:34329–41.
11. Vendrell J, Broch M, Vilarrasa N, Molina A, Gómez JM, Gutiérrez C, et al. Resistin, adiponectin, ghrelin, leptin, and proinflammatory cytokines: relationships in obesity. Obes Res. 2004;12:962–71.
12. Andò S, Catalano S. The multifactorial role of leptin in driving the breast cancer microenvironment. Nat Rev Endocrinol. 2011;8:263–75.
13. Kim HJ, Lee YS, Won EH, Chang IH, Kim TH, Park ES, et al. Expression of resistin in the prostate and its stimulatory effect on prostate cancer cell proliferation. BJU Int. 2011;108:E77–83.
14. Feng Z, Zhang H. Resistin and cancer risk: a mini-review. Endocrinol Metabol Syndrome. 2011;S4:003.
15. Lee JO, Kim N, Lee HJ, Lee YW, Kim SJ, Park SH, et al. Resistin, a fat-derived secretory factor, promotes metastasis of MDA-MB-231 human breast cancer cells through ERM activation. Sci Rep. 2016;6:18923.
16. Pandey V, Vijayakumar MV, Ajay AK, Malvi P, Bhat MK. Diet-induced obesity increases melanoma progression: involvement of Cav-1 and FASN. Int J Cancer. 2012;130:497–508.
17. Meena AS, Sharma A, Kumari R, Mohammad N, Singh SV, Bhat MK. Inherent and acquired resistance to paclitaxel in hepatocellular carcinoma: molecular events involved. PLoS One. 2013;8:e61524.
18. Malvi P, Chaube B, Pandey V, Vijayakumar MV, Boreddy PR, Mohammad N, et al. Obesity induced rapid melanoma progression is reversed by orlistat treatment and dietary intervention: role of adipokines. Mol Oncol. 2015;9:89–703.
19. Bradley G, Ling V. P-glycoprotein, multidrug resistance and tumor progression. Cancer Metastasis Rev. 1994;13:223–33.
20. Giordano C, Vizza D, Panza S, Barone I, Bonofiglio D, Lanzino M, et al. Leptin increases HER2 protein levels through a STAT3-mediated up-regulation of Hsp90 in breast cancer cells. Mol Oncol. 2013;7:379–91.
21. Kleinridders A, Lauritzen HP, Ussar S, Christensen JH, Mori MA, Bross P, et al. Leptin regulation of Hsp60 impacts hypothalamic insulin signaling. J Clin Invest. 2013;123:4667–80.
22. Xiao L, Lu X, Ruden DM. Effectiveness of hsp90 inhibitors as anti-cancer drugs. Mini Rev Med Chem. 2006;6:1137–43.
23. Xiao L, Rasouli P, Ruden DM. Possible effects of early treatments of hsp90 inhibitors on preventing the evolution of drug resistance to other anti-cancer drugs. Curr Med Chem. 2007;14:223–32.
24. Lin WW, Karin M. A cytokine-mediated link between innate immunity, inflammation, and cancer. J Clin Invest. 2007;117:1175–83.
25. Kushiro K, Nunez NP. Ob/ob serum promotes a mesenchymal cell phenotype in B16BL6 melanoma cells. Clin Exp Metastasis. 2011;28:877–86.
26. Honma S, Shimodaira K, Shimizu Y, Tsuchiya N, Saito H, Yanaihara T, et al. The influence of inflammatory cytokines on estrogen production and cell proliferation in human breast cancer cells. Endocr J. 2002;49:371–7.
27. Balkwill F. Cancer and the chemokine network. Nat Rev Cancer. 2004;4:540–50.
28. Yoshimura A. Signal transduction of inflammatory cytokines and tumor development. Cancer Sci. 2006;97:439–47.
29. Sirin O, Kolonin MG. Treatment of obesity as a potential complementary approach to cancer therapy. Drug Discov Today. 2013;18:567–73.
30. Yan D, Avtanski D, Saxena NK, Sharma D. Leptin-induced epithelial-mesenchymal transition in breast cancer cells requires β-catenin activation via Akt/GSK3- and MTA1/Wnt1 protein-dependent pathways. J Biol Chem. 2012;287:8598–612.
31. Uddin S, Bu R, Ahmed M, Hussain AR, Ajarim D, Al-Dayel F, et al. Leptin receptor expression and its association with PI3K/AKT signaling pathway in diffuse large B-cell lymphoma. Leuk Lymphoma. 2010;51:1305–14.
32. Brandon EL, Gu JW, Cantwell L, He Z, Wallace G, Hall JE. Obesity promotes melanoma tumor growth: role of leptin. Cancer Biol Ther. 2009;8:1871–9.
33. Moon HS, Chamberland JP, Diakopoulos KN, Fiorenza CG, Ziemke F, Schneider B, et al. Leptin and amylin act in an additive manner to activate overlapping signaling pathways in peripheral tissues: in vitro and ex vivo studies in humans. Diabetes Care. 2011;34:132–8.
34. Hu X, Juneja SC, Maihle NJ, Cleary MP. Leptin: growth factor in normal and malignant breast cells and for normal mammary gland development. J Natl Cancer Inst. 2002;94:1704–11.
35. Calabro P, Samudio I, Willerson JT, Yeh ET. Resistin promotes smooth muscle cell proliferation through activation of extracellular signal-regulated kinase 1/2 and phosphatidylinositol 3-kinase pathways. Circulation. 2004;110:3335–40.
36. Cao H, Huang Y, Wang L, Wang H, Pang X, Li K, et al. Leptin promotes migration and invasion of breast cancer cells by stimulating IL-8 production in M2 macrophages. Oncotarget. 2016;7(40):65441-65453.
37. Balaban S, Shearer RF, Lee LS, van Geldermalsen M, Schreuder M, Shtein HC, et al. Adipocyte lipolysis links obesity to breast cancer growth: adipocyte-derived fatty acids drive breast cancer cell proliferation and migration. Cancer Metab. 2017;5:1.
38. Di Vizio D, Adam RM, Kim J, Kim R, Sotgia F, Williams T, et al. Caveolin-1 interacts with a lipid raft-associated population of fatty acid synthase. Cell Cycle. 2008;7:2257–67.
39. Flavin R, Peluso S, Nguyen PL, Loda M. Fatty acid synthase as a potential therapeutic target in cancer. Future Oncol. 2010;6:551–62.
40. Bauerschlag DO, Maass N, Leonhardt P, Verburg FA, Pecks U, Zeppernick F, et al. Fatty acid synthase overexpression: target for therapy and reversal of chemoresistance in ovarian cancer. J Transl Med. 2015;13:146.
41. Chatterjee M, Ben-Josef E, Thomas DG, Morgan MA, Zalupski MM, Khan G, et al. Caveolin-1 is associated with tumor progression and confers a multi-modality resistance phenotype in pancreatic cancer. Sci Rep. 2015;5:10867.
42. Goetz MP, Toft DO, Ames MM, Erlichman C. The Hsp90 chaperone complex as a novel target for cancer therapy. Ann Oncol. 2003;14:1169–76.
43. Jhaveri K, Taldone T, Modi S, Chiosis G. Advances in the clinical development of heat shock protein 90 (Hsp90) inhibitors in cancers. Biochim Biophys Acta. 2012;1823:742–55.
44. Tsutsumi S, Beebe K, Neckers L. Impact of heat-shock protein 90 on cancer metastasis. Future Oncol. 2009;5:679–88.
45. Trepel J, Mollapour M, Giaccone G, Neckers L. Targeting the dynamic HSP90 complex in cancer. Nat Rev Cancer. 2010;10:537–49.
46. Teng Y, Ngoka L, Mei Y, Lesoon L, Cowell JK. HSP90 and HSP70 proteins are essential for stabilization and activation of WASF3 metastasis-promoting protein. J Biol Chem. 2012;287:10051–9.
47. Azoitei N, Diepold K, Brunner C, Rouhi A, Genze F, Becher A, et al. HSP90 supports tumor growth and angiogenesis through PRKD2 protein stabilization. Cancer Res. 2014;74:7125–36.
48. Goldman B. Multidrug resistance: can new drugs help chemotherapy score against cancer? J Natl Cancer Inst. 2003;95(4):255–7.

50. Pang J, Shi Q, Liu Z, He J, Liu H, Lin P, et al. Resistin induces multidrug resistance in myeloma by inhibiting cell death and upregulating ABC transporter expression. Haematologica. 2017;2016:154062.
51. Hedbacker BK, Wysocki RW, Asilmaz E, Ahima RS, Farooqi IS, et al. Antidiabetic effects of IGFBP2, a leptin-regulated gene. Cell Metab. 2010;11:11–22.
52. Xia Z, Sniderman AD, Cianflone K. Acylation-stimulating protein (ASP) deficiency induces obesity resistance and increased energy expenditure in ob/ob mice. J Biol Chem. 2002;277:45874–9.
53. de Luca C, Kowalski TJ, Zhang Y, Elmquist JK, Lee C, Kilimann MW, et al. Complete rescue of obesity, diabetes, and infertility in db/db mice by neuron-specific LEPR-B transgenes. J Clin Invest. 2005;115:3484–93.

4

Beta-hydroxybutyrate (3-OHB) can influence the energetic phenotype of breast cancer cells, but does not impact their proliferation and the response to chemotherapy or radiation

Catharina Bartmann[1], Sudha R. Janaki Raman[2], Jessica Flöter[2], Almut Schulze[2], Katrin Bahlke[1], Jana Willingstorfer[1], Maria Strunz[1], Achim Wöckel[1], Rainer J. Klement[3], Michaela Kapp[1], Cholpon S. Djuzenova[4], Christoph Otto[5] and Ulrike Kämmerer[1*]

Abstract

Background: Ketogenic diets (KDs) or short-term fasting are popular trends amongst supportive approaches for cancer patients. Beta-hydroxybutyrate (3-OHB) is the main physiological ketone body, whose concentration can reach plasma levels of 2–6 mM during KDs or fasting. The impact of 3-OHB on the biology of tumor cells described so far is contradictory. Therefore, we investigated the effect of a physiological concentration of 3 mM 3-OHB on metabolism, proliferation, and viability of breast cancer (BC) cells in vitro.

Methods: Seven different human BC cell lines (BT20, BT474, HBL100, MCF-7, MDA-MB 231, MDA-MB 468, and T47D) were cultured in medium with 5 mM glucose in the presence of 3 mM 3-OHB at mild hypoxia (5% oxygen) or normoxia (21% oxygen). Metabolic profiling was performed by quantification of the turnover of glucose, lactate, and 3-OHB and by Seahorse metabolic flux analysis. Expression of key enzymes of ketolysis as well as the main monocarboxylic acid transporter MCT2 and the glucose-transporter GLUT1 was analyzed by RT-qPCR and Western blotting. The effect of 3-OHB on short- and long-term cell proliferation as well as chemo- and radiosensitivity were also analyzed.

Results: 3-OHB significantly changed the oxygen consumption rate (OCR) and extracellular acidification rate (ECAR) in BT20 cells resulting in a more oxidative energetic phenotype. MCF-7 and MDA-MB 468 cells had increased ECAR only in response to 3-OHB, while the other three cell types remained uninfluenced. All cells expressed MCT2 and GLUT1, thus being able to uptake the metabolites. The consumption of 3-OHB was not strongly linked to mRNA overexpression of key enzymes of ketolysis and did not correlate with lactate production and glucose consumption. Neither 3-OHB nor acetoacetate did interfere with proliferation. Further, 3-OHB incubation did not modify the response of the tested BC cell lines to chemotherapy or radiation.

(Continued on next page)

* Correspondence: frak057@mail.uni-wuerzburg.de
[1]Department of Obstetrics and Gynaecology, University Hospital of Würzburg, Josef-Schneider-Str. 4, 97080 Würzburg, Germany

(Continued from previous page)

Conclusions: We found that a physiological level of 3-OHB can change the energetic profile of some BC cell lines. However, 3-OHB failed to influence different biologic processes in these cells, e.g., cell proliferation and the response to common breast cancer chemotherapy and radiotherapy. Thus, we have no evidence that 3-OHB generally influences the biology of breast cancer cells in vitro.

Keywords: Ketogenic diet, β-Hydroxybutyrate, Ketone bodies, Breast cancer, Seahorse, Metabolic profile, Chemotherapy, Ionizing radiation

Background

Breast cancer (BC) is one of the most common cancers and affects about one in eight women during their lifetime [1]. In general, modern BC therapy includes different therapeutic approaches, such as surgical removal of the tumor, chemotherapy, radiation, and hormone therapy [2]. In addition to these conventional therapies, a large number of patients seek supportive therapies like specific diets to improve their outcome. The correlation between different types of diet and the incidence and progression of cancer is increasingly becoming the focus of research [3–7]. In this respect, avoiding carbohydrates to specifically "starve cancer cells" is the most popular trend amongst "cancer diets." The rationale for this dietary regime is often based on the "Warburg effect," which describes the preferential fermentation of glucose to lactate even under availability of sufficient oxygen [8, 9]. Therefore, reducing carbohydrate intake and thus lowering blood glucose seems to be a promising strategy for cutting cancer off from glucose supply [10–12].

Besides fasting, the strictest form of such a "very low carb" diet is called the ketogenic diet (KD). The KD is characterized by consuming the predominant proportion of calories from fat, balancing those derived from protein and thus consuming very few calories from glucose or other carbohydrates. Different KD regimens were shown to be safe and well tolerated in a variety of malignancies [13–19] and lead to the metabolic state of a physiological ketosis [20]. During ketosis, the "ketone bodies" acetoacetate (AcAc) and D-β-hydroxybutyrate (R-3-hydroxybutyrate: 3-OHB) are predominantly produced in the liver and can be detected in the peripheral blood and urine above normal levels [21]. 3-OHB is found at similar or higher concentrations than AcAc and therefore, considered the principal "ketone body." In humans, the median concentration of 3-OHB in plasma reaches approximately 3 mM under short-term fasting conditions [22], up to 6 mM during long-term starvation [23] and regularly at least 2 mM under a ketogenic diet [24].

3-OHB is transported into cells via monocarboxylic acid transporters (MCT). The isoforms MCT1, MCT2, and MCT4 can transport lactate and ketone bodies across the cell membrane [25, 26]. Here, MCT2 has the highest affinity for 3-OHB, whereas MCT1 and 4 have a higher affinity for lactate [27, 28]. In mitochondria, 3-OHB is degraded via ketolysis into acetyl-CoA, which then is metabolized within the Krebs cycle and the respiratory chain to generate energy [29–32]. Since the oxidation of 3-OHB generates more energy per mol oxygen used compared to glucose, it is sometimes labeled a "superfuel" [33]. However, cells need functioning mitochondria as well as sufficient oxygen supply to generate energy from 3-OHB. The latter is hampered in the hypoxic microenvironment of larger tumors, which has already been shown in vivo for breast cancer tissue in patients [34].

There are somewhat contradicting results regarding the effect of 3-OHB on growth and biology of tumor cells cultured in vitro and in experimental tumors in mice. In some studies, ketone bodies seem to be associated with cancer progression, metastasis, and poor clinical outcome [35, 36]. In contrast, it was shown that a ketogenic diet significantly reduces tumor growth in mice [37, 38]. Further, an antiproliferative effect of 3-OHB was already shown for different cancer cells, such as glioblastoma and tumor stem cells [37], melanoma, cervical carcinoma, or neuroblastoma [39–41]. Several studies also described a significant delay of tumor growth in mice and humans in a systemic ketosis [16, 18, 37, 38, 40, 42–49]. In this respect, Rodrigues and coworkers reported evidence for a "β-hydroxybutyrate paradox" [50]. They postulated that the effect of 3-OHB on cancer growth would depend on the tumor's energetic phenotype. Thus, "oxidative cells" would use 3-OHB as an additional energy source so that tumors with predominantly "oxidative cells" increase their growth when this metabolite is available. Other cells with a more "glycolytic, Warburg-like phenotype" would be unable to metabolize 3-OHB in which case it could accumulate intracellularly and inhibit tumor growth via signaling and epigenetic mechanisms [50].

In view of this preclinical pro- and contra evidence and the fact that increasing numbers of patients are adopting a ketogenic diet or short-term fasting during oncological therapy, we studied the impact of 3-OHB on seven different BC cell lines in vitro. Here, we initially analyzed the energetic profile of these cells and correlated this to the effect of 3-OHB on cell proliferation.

Further, we investigated the possibility of synergism between ketosis and radio- or chemotherapy [51]. To mimic a physiological state of metabolites found in the circulation of patients performing a KD, we performed experiments with 3 mM 3-OHB, representing pronounced ketosis, and 5 mM glucose, typical for the blood glucose level found in persons on a KD (range 4.9–5.2 mM) [19, 52–57]. Furthermore, we investigated cells at both an oxygen supply of 5% oxygen (= 5 kPA), a typical mean concentration between well-vascularized benign breast tissue (6.5 kPA) and non-hypoxic tumor regions (3.2–4.7 kPA) in vivo [58] and 21% oxygen (21 kPA), as a common condition used in cell culture.

Methods

Breast cancer cell lines and culture

The BC cell lines BT20, BT474, HBL100, MCF-7, MDA-MB 231, MDA-MB 468, and T47D were obtained from Cell Lines Service GmbH (CLS; Eppelheim, Germany), and their receptor status, subtype, and mutation status are summarized in Table 1 [59–65]. The BT474 and the MDA-MB 231 cell lines were purchased directly from CLS for the experiments and used at low passage. All other cell lines were authenticated via genetic profiling of SRT loci by CLS before running the experiments. Aliquots of the cell lines were freshly cultured from frozen samples in 75-cm^2 cell culture flasks (TPP, Trasadingen, Switzerland) in Dulbecco's modified Eagle's medium (DMEM)/Hams F12 (1:1) medium (Gibco, ThermoFisher Scientific, Darmstadt, Germany) supplemented with 10% fetal calf serum (FCS; Biochrom, Berlin, Germany) and 50 ng/ml Gentamycin (Sigma-Aldrich, Munich, Germany) in the presence of 5% CO_2 and 21% oxygen, respectively.

Turnover of metabolites

For quantification of glucose, lactate, and 3-OHB metabolism, cells were seeded and cultured at conditions described in the cell proliferation assay. After 5 days, supernatants were collected and the levels of 3-OHB were analyzed by the PrecisionXceed® instrument with the corresponding test strips FreeStyle Precision® β-Ketone (Abbott, Wiesbaden, Germany). The concentrations of glucose and lactate were measured with the Cobas 8000 modular analyzer series (Roche Diagnostics; Mannheim, Germany) at the central laboratory of the University Hospital of Würzburg. Concentrations of metabolites were expressed in millimolar per optical density (OD) of crystal violet dye extracts in each well at day 3 or 5 of culture. The amount of solubilized dye in OD is directly proportional to the cell number. Therefore, after removing the supernatant carefully for metabolite quantification, adherent cells were fixed with 100 μl methanol

Table 1 Subtype of the breast cancer cell lines used in the experiments

Cell line	Receptor			Subtype	Ref.	Mutations*
	ER	PR	Her2			
BT20	–	(–)	np	Basal A	[60]	ATM; BRCA2; CBLB; CDKN2A; COL1A1; RAP1GDS1; RB1; PIK3CA TP53
	0	0	0–1	Basal	[61]	
BT474	+	(+)	+	Luminal	[60]	EPS15; HIST1H3B; NSD1; PIK3CA; PPP2R1A; RHOA; TP53
	0	8	3+	Luminal B	[61]	
	+	+/–	+	Luminal B	[59]	
HBL100	–	(–)	np	Basal B	[60]	np
MCF-7	+	(+)	np	Luminal	[60]	ATP2B3; CDKN2A; EP300; ERBB4; MAP3K13; PIK3CA
	6	6	0–1	Luminal A	[61]	
	+	+/–	–	Luminal A	[59]	
MDA-MB 231	–	(–)	np	Basal B	[60]	BRAF; CD79A; KRAS; CNKN2A; NF2; PBRM1; PDGFRA; TP53
	0	0	0–1+	Basal	[61]	
MDA-MB 468	(–)	(–)	np	Basal A	[60]	CACNA1D; INPP4B; PTEN; RB1; TP53
	0	0	0	Basal	[61]	
	–	–	–	Basal	[59]	
T47D	+	(+)	np	Luminal	[60]	ACVR1; ARID1A; PIK3CA; TP53
	+	+	–	Luminal A	[59]	

The subtype of the breast cancer cell lines used was classified before by gene expression profile and the expression of the estrogen (ER), progesterone (PR), and human epidermal growth factor receptor 2 (Her2) receptor. The abbreviations of receptors and breast cancer subtype classification shown here are published [59–61]. Semiquantified receptor status: results with "–", "(–)", "0", and "0–1+" are classified as negative and results with "+", "(+)", "+/–", 6, and 8 are classified as positive for receptor expression (also summarized by [62])

np not published

*Mutations shown here are described by [63–65]

(Sigma-Aldrich) for 10 min at room temperature (RT) and then dried. Cells were stained by incubation in 100 μl crystal violet solution per well (0.4% crystal violet [Merck, Darmstadt, Germany] in 1:3 methanol: phosphate-buffered saline) for 10 min at RT and then washed several times with distilled water. Crystal violet was extracted from cells with 100 μl of 10% acetic acid per well on a plate shaker for 30 min, and OD was determined at 570 nm by using a standard ELISA-Plate reader.

Energetic profiling by Seahorse technique

The oxygen consumption rate (OCR) and extracellular acidification rate (ECAR) were analyzed with the Seahorse XF Cell Mito Stress Test (Part #103015-100; Agilent Technologies, Santa Clara, CA, USA) in a Seahorse XFe96 Analyzer (Agilent Technologies). The day before the experiment, 40,000 cells per well were plated in a 96-well Seahorse plate in 100 μl DMEM/10% FCS/Gentamycin/5 mM glucose medium with or without 3 mM 3-OHB (sodium-hydroxybutyrate, Sigma-Aldrich). The Agilent Seahorse XFe96 Sensor Cartridge was hydrated with 200 μl/well of XF calibrant solution overnight in a non-CO_2 incubator at 37 °C. On the day of the experiment, 100 ml of Seahorse assay medium containing 1 mM pyruvate, 2 mM glutamine, and 5 mM glucose was prepared. The pH of the pre-warmed (37 °C) medium was adjusted to 7.4 with 0.1 N NaOH. Twenty milliliters of the assay medium was used to prepare 3 mM 3-OHB, and the pH was readjusted to 7.4 with 0.1 N HCl. Cells were washed twice with 200 μl of the corresponding Seahorse medium and incubated in 175 μl of the respective Seahorse medium per well in a non-CO_2 incubator at 37 °C for 1 h. Meanwhile, the Seahorse sensor cartridge ports were loaded with 25 μl of inhibitors to have a final concentration of 2 μM oligomycin (port A, Calbiochem), 1 μM FCCP (port B, Sigma-Aldrich), and 0.5 μM rotenone/antimycin A (port C, Sigma-Aldrich). The experimental design was setup using the WAVE software program, and measurements were performed in the Seahorse XFe96 Analyzer. After the measurement, supernatant from the cells was removed and the cells were fixed by addition of 100 μl methanol (Sigma-Aldrich) for 10 min at RT and air dried. Subsequently, the cells were stained using crystal violet solution as described for the colony formation assay (see below). For quantification, stained plates were incubated with 200 μl of 10% acetic acid per well with shaking for 15 min and the resulting solution was analyzed in a plate reader (Tecan GENios plus, Tecan Deutschland GmbH, Crailsheim, Germany) at 630 nm.

Cell proliferation assay

Adherent growing cells were seeded in 96-well flat bottom plates (TPP) at cell numbers determined for each cell line to reach semiconfluency after 3 days under the respective oxygen and low glucose conditions and to reach confluency after 5 days via preliminary testing. Thus, 250–350 cells per well, depending on the cell line, were seeded in 200 μl DMEM/10%FCS/Gentamycin/5 mM glucose. Cell plates were cultured for 5 days at 5% CO_2 and 37 °C in humidified chambers at oxygen concentrations of 21 or 5% in hypoxia-incubators (Coy Laboratories Products Inc., Grass Lake, MI, USA) respectively. At least 3 independent wells per cell line were tested either with or without 3 mM 3-OHB or 1.5 mM acetoacetate (lithium salt) and LiCl (both Sigma-Aldrich) as control in parallel. Four independent experiments were performed with fresh cultured cell aliquots. At day 5, supernatants were removed for metabolite testing, 100 μl of fresh medium containing 5-bromo-2′-deoxyuridine (BrdU) were added for another 24 h, and cell proliferation rate was then analyzed by the BrdU test (Roche; Cell Proliferation ELISA) according to the manufacturer's instructions.

Colony formation assay

For the colony formation assay, cells were cultured at 100 cells/well in 48 well plates (TTP) with 500 μl medium (DMEM/10% FCS/Gentamycin/5 mM glucose) with or without 3 mM 3-OHB at oxygen concentrations of 5 or 21% for 14 to 18 days, depending on the cell line. Half of the medium was replenished every 4 days. Crystal violet staining was performed for evaluation of the adherent colonies. Therefore, supernatant was carefully removed; adherent cells were fixed with 250 μl methanol (Sigma-Aldrich) for 10 min at RT and then dried. Colonies were stained by incubation in crystal violet solution (same as above) for 10 min and then washed several times with distilled water. Stained colonies were documented by using the ImmunoCapture 6.2 in the ImmunoSpot Analyzer® (Cellular Technology, Shaker Heights, OH, USA). Two independent experiments were performed with 8 replicate wells per condition (5 and 21% oxygen with and without 3-OHB) for each cell line.

Reverse transcriptase quantitative polymerase chain reaction (RT-qPCR) and Western blotting

For RT-qPCR and Western blot analyses, aliquots of cells were cultured under the same medium (DMEM/10% FCS/Gentamycin/5 mM glucose; with or without 3 mM 3-OHB) and oxygen (21 or 5%) conditions to reach subconfluency after 5 days in 75-cm^2 cell culture flasks.

RNA extraction, cDNA synthesis (iScript, Bio-Rad), and qPCR (Mesa Green containing Meteor Taq hotstart polymerase, Eurogentic) as well as Western blotting were performed as described previously [66]. The primers and conditions of the qPCR are described in Table 2. In brief, qPCR reactions were performed on a

Table 2 Details of the primer pairs used in this study

Gene	Forward primer/reverse primer	cDNA size (bp)	PubMed access no.
β-Actin	5'-CCT TGC CAT CCT AAA AGC C-3' 5'-CAC GAA AGC AAT GCT ATC AC-3'	96	NM_001101
PPIA	5'-TGT CCA TGG CAA ATG CTG GAC CC-3' 5'-GCG CTC CAT GGC CTC CAC AA-3'	140	NM_021130.3
BDH1	5'-CGC CGG GTG AAG GCG-3' 5'-GAA TGG CCC AGT TCC TCC C-3'	92	NM_004051.4
SCOT	5'-GCC ATT GCC AGT AAG CCA AG-3' 5'-CCA GGC TTT CAC CAA AGC AA-3'	99	NM_000436.3
ACAT1	5'-CGG CAG ATG CAG CGA AGA GG-3' 5'-AGG TTC TAC AGC AGC GTC AGC A-3'	77	NM_000019.3

DNA sequences and PubMed accession numbers for each gene are indicated. qPCR reactions were performed on a CFX96 real-time PCR system (Bio-Rad) operated by CFX Manager Software (version 3.0). The two-step cycler protocol was 5 min at 95 °C, 40 cycles of 15 s at 95 °C, 60 s at 60 °C, followed by 5 min at 72 °C and used for all primer pairs
PPIA peptidylprolyl isomerase A, *BDH* 3-hydroxybutyrate dehydrogenase, *SCOT* succinyl-CoA transferase (3-oxoacid CoA transferase), *ACAT* acetyl-CoA-acetyltransferase

CFX96 real-time PCR system (Bio-Rad) operated by CFX Manager Software (version 3.0). The cycler protocol was 5 min at 95 °C (initial denaturation), 40 cycles of 15 s at 95 °C, 60 s at 60 °C (two-step protocol), and 5 min at 72 °C (final extension) for all primer pairs used. Fold expression of genes of interest (Table 2) expression relative to reference genes PPIA and β-actin was calculated with the ΔΔCq method [67]. Post-amplification melting curves were controlled to exclude primer-dimer artifacts and contaminations (not shown). Data from two independent cell culture experiments in triplicate reactions for each primer pair were summarized (Fig. 3b).

For Western blotting, pellets of 1×10^6 tumor cells were lysed and protein concentrations were determined using the Bradford method [68] and Coomassie Brilliant Blue (Roti-Quant; Roth, Karlsruhe, Germany) reagent. Afterwards, samples were mixed with 5× loading buffer (Fermentas GmbH, St. Leon-Roth, Germany), denatured at 95 °C for 5 min, chilled on ice, and stored at − 20 °C for further analysis. Equal amounts of proteins (20 μg) were separated on a 10% polyacrylamide gel. The antibodies used are listed in Table 3.

Chemosensitivity and radiosensitivity

For both sensitivity tests, the cells were seeded as in the prior tests in 96-well plates in standard medium with 5 mM glucose and incubated for 48 h at oxygen concentrations of 5 or 21% respectively.

For chemosensitivity testing, the test drug concentration (TDC) of epirubicin was defined as 0.5 μg/ml, of paclitaxel as 13.6 μg/ml, and of carboplatin as 15.8 μg/ml, as described in the literature [69–72]. The cell culture medium (see above) with or without 3 mM 3-OHB and eight different dilutions of the chemotherapeutic drugs (epirubicin: highest concentration: 25% TDC and twofold dilution series; paclitaxel highest concentration: 50% TDC and tenfold dilution series or carboplatin highest concentration: 400% TDC and twofold dilution series) were added. TDC concentrations for the experiments were selected by cell viability assays performed in preliminary tests with all cell lines (not shown). After 3 days of cell culture, BrdU was added for the final 24 h of culture and the BrdU test performed as described above.

For radiosensitivity testing, subconfluent monolayers of cells were irradiated in the culture plates filled with 200 μl/well with the corresponding growth medium with graded single doses (0–8 Gy) and then cultivated for 10 days at either 5 or 21% oxygen concentration. Irradiation was performed using a 6 MV Siemens linear accelerator (Siemens, Concord, CA, USA) at a dose rate of 2 Gy/min. Half of the medium was changed every 4 days. At the end of the incubation period, BrdU was added and cell proliferation was measured by the BrdU test 24 h thereafter.

Statistics

Data are presented as means (± standard error of mean [SEM]). p values lower than 0.05 in the non-parametric Mann-Whitney U test were considered significant. The software GraphPad Prism 6 (La Jolla, CA 92037 USA) was used to create the figures and to perform statistical analysis. IC50 was determined via the nonlinear regression dose-response curve (inhibition) function of the Prism software.

Results

Glucose consumption and lactate production is not influenced by 3-OHB

Glucose consumption and production of lactate were normalized to the optical density (OD) of crystal violet dye extracts, which is directly proportional to the cell

Table 3 Antibodies for Western blot

Antibody	Gen/name	Company	Clone	Species	Dilution	MW of antigen
Primary	Beta-actin	Abcam	mAbcam 8226	Mouse	1:10000	42 kDa
	Monocarboxylic acid transporter 2 (MCT-2)	Abcam	Polyclonal	Rabbit	1:2000	52 kDa
	Glucose transporter 1 (GLUT1)	USBiological	Polyclonal	Rabbit	1:1000	55 kDa
Secondary	HRP-labeled goat-anti-mouse	KPL	Polyclonal	Goat	1:10000	
	HRP-labeled goat-anti-rabbit	Abcam	Polyclonal	Goat	1:20000	

MW molecular weight

number, as readout for the rate of aerobic glycolysis (Warburg effect) or respiration, respectively. With these measurements, we were able to categorize the metabolic characteristics of the seven tested cell lines as follows: BT20 and MDA-MB 231 exhibit high glucose consumption (with an average of more than 5.0 mM) normalized to cell number as reflected by OD readout of the crystal violet assay) and high lactate production (with an average of more than 15 mM/OD). HBL100, MCF-7, MDA-MB 468, and T47D consume relatively low amounts of glucose (< 3.5 mM/OD) and show low lactate production (< 10 mM/OD), while BT474 show very low levels of glucose consumption (< 1 mM/OD) and lactate production (< 5 mM/OD). Interestingly, independent of the respective metabolic characteristics, 3 mM 3-OHB failed to significantly influence the consumption of glucose or production of lactate in the presence of either 5 or 21% oxygen (Fig. 1).

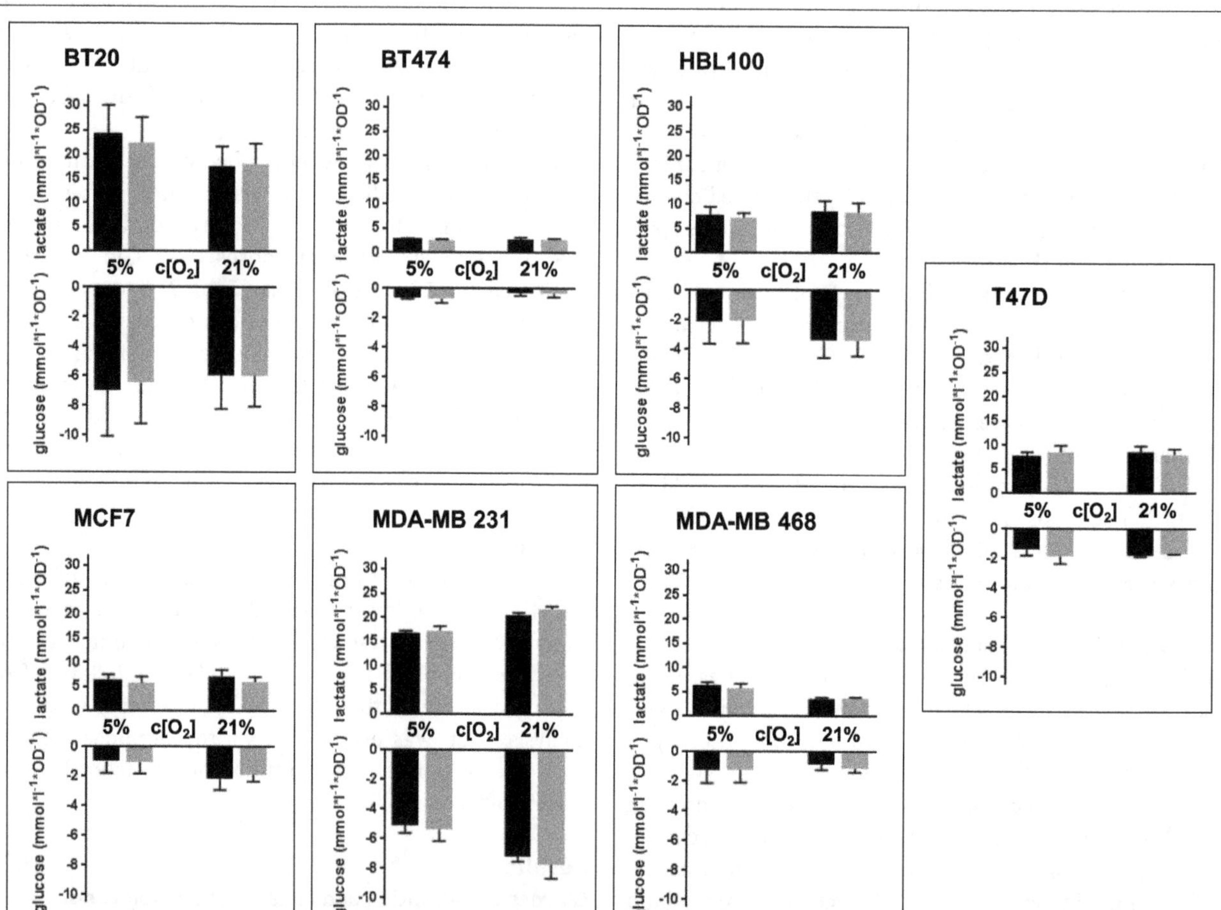

Fig. 1 The graphs represent the rate of lactate production (mmol × l^{-1} × optical density $(OD)^{-1}$; upper panel) and glucose consumption (mmol × l^{-1} × OD^{-1}; lower panel) normalized to total cell content (OD) after 5 days of culture in 5 or 21% oxygen (gray column = 3 mM 3-OHB; black column = control). Each column represents mean ± SEM of four independent experiments

3-OHB changes oxygen consumption rate and extracellular acidification rate in BT20 cells

Seahorse analysis confirmed the metabolic phenotype found in the glucose consumption/lactate production rate analysis. All cell lines except T47D exhibited a more aerobic/energetic cell type, corresponding to cells that divide but generate their energy predominantly from oxidative phosphorylation (OXPHOS) (Fig. 2a).

This basal metabolic phenotype did not correlate with the reaction of these cells to 3-OHB, since 3-OHB significantly influenced the oxygen consumption rate (OCR) in BT20 cells only. Here, OCR increased from 77.8 ± 5.8 to 124.0 ± 10.0 pmol/min (mean ± SEM; $p < 0.001$), when cells were cultured in the presence of 3-OHB (Fig. 2b, c). For all other cell lines, we found no evidence that 3-OHB influenced oxygen consumption (Fig. 2c, left graph). In addition, the effect of 3-OHB on extracellular acidification rate (ECAR) was analyzed. In the case of BT20 cells, ECAR significantly increased from 61.2 ± 4.3 mpH (milli pH)/min to 80.3 ± 7.7 mpH/min ($p < 0.05$) with 3-OHB. An increase from 83.6 ± 3.1 mpH/min to 99.5 ± 5.2 mpH/min ($p < 0.05$) and from 54.2 ± 1.8 mpH/min to 62.5 ± 2.3 mpH/min ($p < 0.01$) was observed in MCF7 and MDA-MB 468 cells under the influence of 3-OHB, respectively (Fig. 2c, right side).

Thus in general, no direct correlation between the metabolic reaction to 3-OHB and the basal energetic phenotype of the cell lines was seen.

Consumption of 3-OHB is not strongly linked to overexpression of ketolytic enzymes and does not correlate with the observed effects on metabolic phenotype

To investigate whether BC cells were able to use 3-OHB as a substrate for intermediate metabolism, we next determined uptake rates thereof in the panel of breast cancer cell lines. All cell lines depleted 3-OHB from the culture medium but the magnitude of depletion differed substantially between them (Fig. 3a). Interestingly, we detected variable levels of mRNA expression for key enzymes of ketolysis, namely 3-hydroxybutyrate dehydrogenase 1 (BDH1), succinyl-CoA transferase (SCOT), and acetyl-CoA-acetyltransferase (ACAT), in the seven human breast cancer cell lines (Fig. 3b). In BT474 cells, which showed a relevant consumption of 3-OHB (Fig. 3a), we detected high levels of mRNA for all three key enzymes. SCOT and ACAT, but not BDH1, were overexpressed in HBL100 cells, which showed reduced 3-OHB consumption compared to BT474 cells. All other cell lines revealed low levels of mRNA expression for ketolytic enzymes with a moderate ACAT mRNA expression in MDA-MB 231 and T47D cells. However, changes in mRNA expression levels of ketolytic enzymes in response to 3-OHB and reduced oxygen conditions varied between the tested BC cell lines. We observed an overall decrease in expression of all three enzymes in MCF7 and MDA-MB 231 cells with further decrease (MCF7) or a moderate increase of BDH1 and ACAT in the presence of 3-OHB. All enzymes were downregulated in HBL100 and MCF7 cells, but and only BDH1 and ACAT in MDA-MB 231 cells in response to low oxygen (5% oxygen). This regulation was not observed in BT20, BT474, MDA-MB 468, and T47D. In summary, the data show no strong correlation between mRNA overexpression and consumption of 3-OHB or oxygen concentration.

Moreover, the extent of 3-OHB uptake was not linked with the extent of the Warburg effect in each cell line as shown in Fig. 2a. There was also no significant difference in the concentration of 3-OHB remaining in the medium after incubation with cells at 5 or 21% oxygen (Fig. 3a). By Western blot analysis (Fig. 3c), we showed that MCT2, the key transporter for 3-OHB into cells [27], was expressed highly by all seven cell lines. In particular, MCT2 expression was higher at mild hypoxia in the majority of cell lines. Therefore, the transport of 3-OHB across the plasma membrane seems not to be a limiting factor for 3-OHB consumption by BC cells. GLUT1 as a key transporter for glucose into tumor cells was detected in all cell lines, and its expression was not influenced by 3-OHB (Fig. 3c). Together, our results demonstrate that 3-OHB does not significantly change the expression of ketolytic enzymes or of the transporter molecules MCT2 and GLUT1. Nevertheless, BC cell lines show marked differences in their ability to deplete 3-OHB from the medium indicating that mRNA expression patterns of ketolytic enzymes were not associated with consumption rate of 3-OHB.

Short-term and long-term cell proliferation of breast cancer cells is not affected by incubation with 3-OHB

To analyze whether 3-OHB can affect cancer cell proliferation independent of their metabolic phenotype, we incubated the BC cell lines with 5 mM glucose, with and without addition of 3 mM 3-OHB in the presence of 5 or 21% oxygen, respectively. Here, we found a slight reduction (< 10%) in short-term (5 days) proliferation following 3-OHB treatment in BT20, MCF-7, MDA-MB 231, MDA-MB 468, and T47D cells at either oxygen concentration, while BT474 and HBL100 cells were not affected (Fig. 4a). Since AcAc, the second ketone body which rises in circulation upon a ketogenic diet, was described to increase proliferation in BRAF V600E melanoma cells [73], we performed cell proliferation assays in the presence of this metabolite over 5 days in parallel to the 3-OHB experiments. As shown in the Additional file 1, there was no significant effect of AcAc

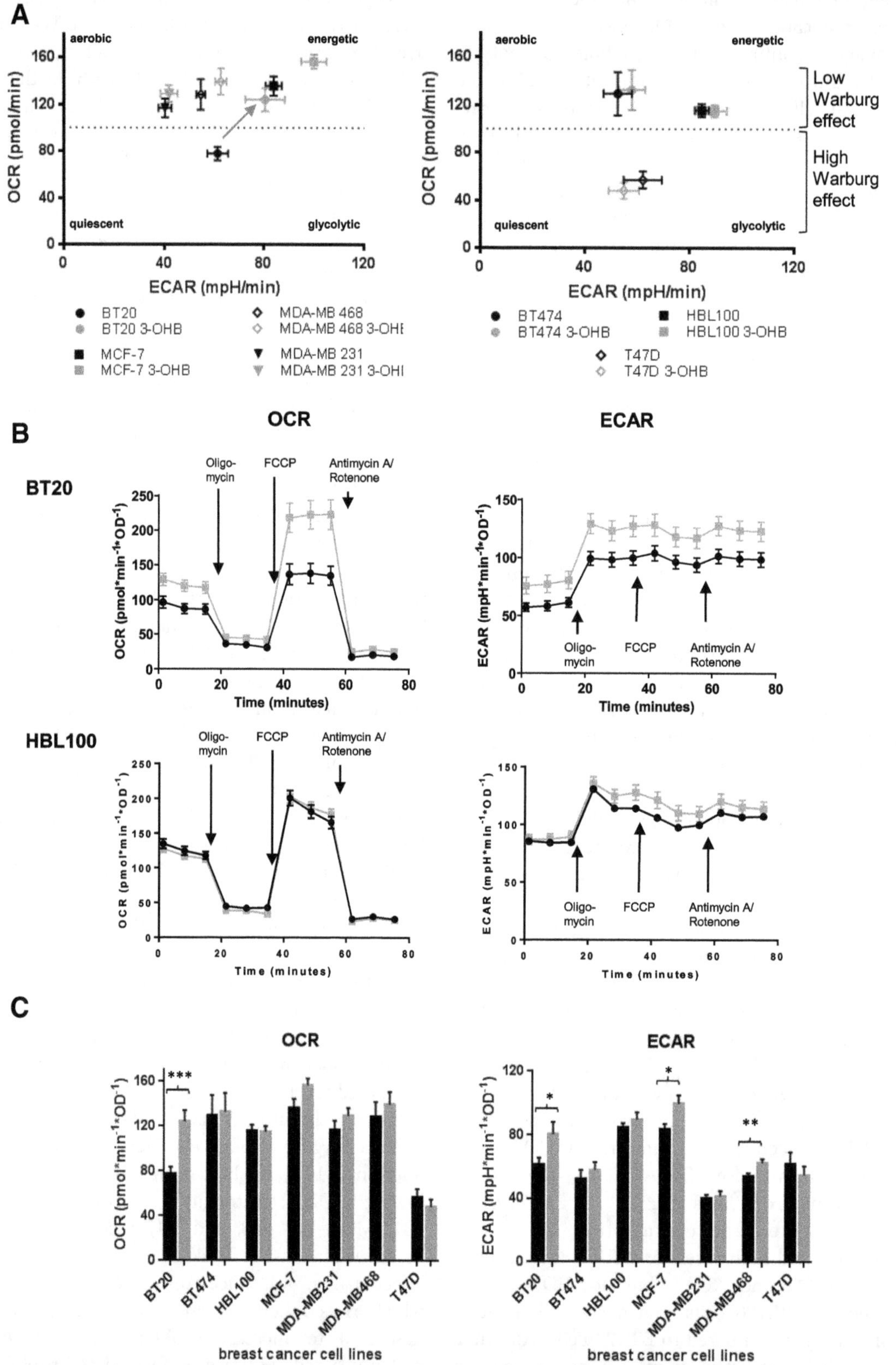

Fig. 2 (See legend on next page.)

(See figure on previous page.)
Fig. 2 a Energetic phenotype as revealed by Seahorse flux analysis in cultures without 3-OHB (black symbols) and with 3 mM 3-OHB (gray symbols). Arrow indicates the significant ($p < 0.05$) shift in energetic phenotype observed with the BT20 cell line. Graph summarizes the results of four independent seahorse experiments with four replicate wells for each cell line. **b** The curves of OCR and ECAR for the BC cell lines with the most prominent changes (BT20) and without any changes (HBL100) depending on the addition of 3-OHB are shown here. The graph represents the three measuring points of basal levels of respiration/acidification, and changes after addition of oligomycin, FCCP, and antimycin A/rotenone (black line and dots = control, gray line and boxes = 3-OHB). **c** Column statistics of the baseline OCR and ECAR of BC cell lines with 3-OHB (gray column) compared to control (black column) (***$p < 0.001$; **$p < 0.01$; *$p < 0.05$). Each column summarizes mean ± SEM of four independent seahorse experiments with four replicate wells per experiment for each cell line

on the proliferation rate of the BC cell lines tested. A slight increase in proliferation of BT20 cells at 5% oxygen concentration did not reach statistical significance. Since AcAc was used as lithium salt, control experiments with LiCl at corresponding Li concentration were performed, but did not differ from the proliferation rates seen with Li-free cell culture medium (not shown).

To test the effect of 3 mM 3-OHB on long-term proliferation, we performed a colony formation assay for at least 14 days of culture. Similar to the results of the short-term proliferation assay, we found no significant differences in number and size of cell colonies between cultures treated with 3-OHB and control cultures. Of note, oxygen concentration influenced size and number of cell colonies of BT474, HBL100, and MDA-MB 231 cells (Fig. 4b).

3-OHB incubation does not influence the response of BC cells to chemotherapy or ionizing radiation

We next addressed the question whether exposure to 3-OHB may affect the sensitivity of BC cells to different treatment modalities. We therefore exposed the BC cell lines to epirubicin, paclitaxel, or carboplatin, three chemotherapeutic agents commonly used in breast cancer treatment. Here, we did not find any significant influence of 3-OHB on the effect of these drugs on cancer cell viability at either 5 or 21% oxygen (Fig. 5a and Additional file 2). The cumulative IC50 of paclitaxel was 4.0 ± 1.1 ng/ml (mean ± SEM) (control) versus 2.7 ± 0.8 ng/ml (3 mM 3-OHB) at 5% oxygen and 3.7 ± 1.3 ng/ml (control) versus 3.8 ± 1.2 ng/ml (3 mM 3-OHB) at 21% oxygen. The mean cumulative IC50 of epirubicin was 28.3 ± 6.1 ng/ml in control cells versus 28.5 ± 7.8 ng/ml (3 mM 3-OHB) at 5% oxygen concentration and 18.9 ± 3.6 ng/ml (control) versus 18.0 ± 2.7 ng/ml (3 mM 3-OHB) at 21% oxygen concentration. In the case of carboplatin, the mean cumulative IC50 was 6.6 ± 1.4 μg/ml (control) versus 6.0 ± 1.4 μg/ml (3-OHB) at 5% oxygen and 5.0 ± 2.4 μg/ml (control) versus 4.8 ± 2.3 μg/ml (3-OHB) at 21% oxygen concentration. Representative results of the sensitivity tests are shown in Fig. 5b, c.

Further, we found that 3-OHB did not significantly sensitize BC cells to radiation at either 21 or 5% oxygen. Hypoxia per se, however, showed a tendency to confer a higher radio-resistance to the tumor cells (Fig. 6a + b) consistent with the known action of oxygen as a radiosensitizer. Two representative examples of dose-response curves are shown for the highest responders to radiation at both oxygen conditions in Fig. 6c–f. In analyzing the cell lines individually, however, a tendency to confer a higher radiosensitivity is seen for those tumor cells grown in 3-OHB at 5% oxygen in all but the MDA-MB 321 cell lines (Additional file 3).

Discussion

In this study, we have shown that beta-hydroxybutyrate (3-OHB), the main ketone body found in the circulation after fasting or ketogenic diets (KDs), was able to change the energetic phenotype of BT20 breast cancer cells when applied at physiological concentrations of 3 mM. However, this effect of 3-OHB on energy metabolism was not observed in any of the other BC cell lines investigated herein. Moreover, 3-OHB did not interfere with turnover of glucose and lactate and neither significantly affected short- and long-term cancer cell proliferation, or their sensitivity to chemotherapy or ionizing radiation in any of the cell lines tested. This implies that 3-OHB at a physiological concentration of 3 mM seems to be inert in affecting energetic processes essential for proliferation or cell survival in the tested BC cell lines in vitro. In addition, we found that AcAc, the second ketone body elevated under a KD, also did not significantly influence proliferation of any BC cell line measured over 5 days. While preclinical data have shown that AcAc promotes proliferation of BRAF-V600-positive melanoma cells [73], it is interesting that in a pilot study [13] it was a patient with BRAF V600E-positive/BRAF-inhibitor-resistant melanoma who responded favorably to a KD; this highlights the limitations of translating preclinical study results to humans.

This research was performed, since a possible influence of 3-OHB on cancer growth has gained substantial interest over the past years. In particular, different regimes for KDs are currently investigated in several

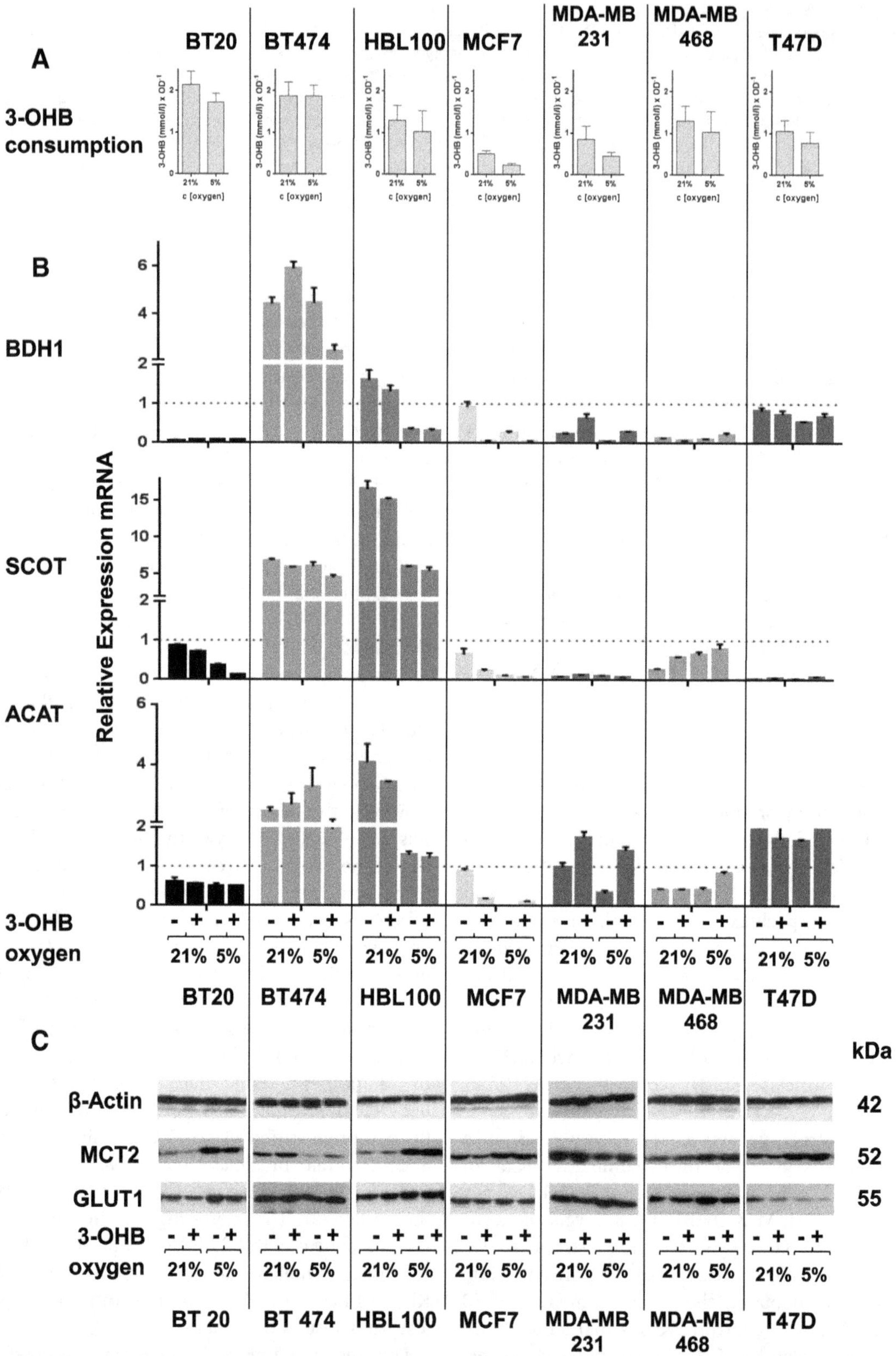

Fig. 3 (See legend on next page.)

(See figure on previous page.)

Fig. 3 a The columns show the amount of 3-OHB (in mM) consumed by the cells normalized to their cell number as given by optical density (OD) measured with the crystal violet assay. Columns represent mean ± SEM of two independent experiments with three replicate wells per experiment. There was no significant difference in the consumption of 3-OHB between cultivation at 21 and 5% oxygen. A tendency to reduced 3-OHB consumption was observed at 5% oxygen. **b** Relative expression of mRNA for the ketolytic enzymes BDH1 (β-hydroxybutyrate dehydrogenase), SCOT (succinyl-CoA:3-ketoacid coenzyme A transferase), and ACAT (acetyl-CoA acetyltransferases) in the tested BC cell lines. Each column represents mean ± SEM of data from two independent cell culture experiments in triplicate reactions for each primer pair. **c** All cell lines express the most important transporter for 3-OHB, the monocarboxylate transporter 2 (MCT2), and the glucose transporter 1 (GLUT1) on protein level. Beta-actin served as loading control. Representative Western blot images of the four test conditions (21 and 5% oxygen with and without 3-OHB) for each cell line are shown

clinical trials to improve the outcome for cancer patients [74]. Several reports indicate a significant benefit of ketosis and especially 3-OHB on slowing cancer progression in different preclinical cancer models and patients [13, 37, 42, 44, 49, 75–77], amongst them one recent case study successfully applying a KD as part of a multimodal pro-oxidative therapy in a stage IV triple-negative breast cancer patient [78]. On the other hand, there are other publications describing a negative impact of ketosis/3-OHB on tumor cell growth in vitro and in mouse models [35, 36, 79, 80].

Therefore, we initially analyzed the energetic profile of seven different BC cell lines using substrate turnover quantification and energetic flux analysis. The basic energetic

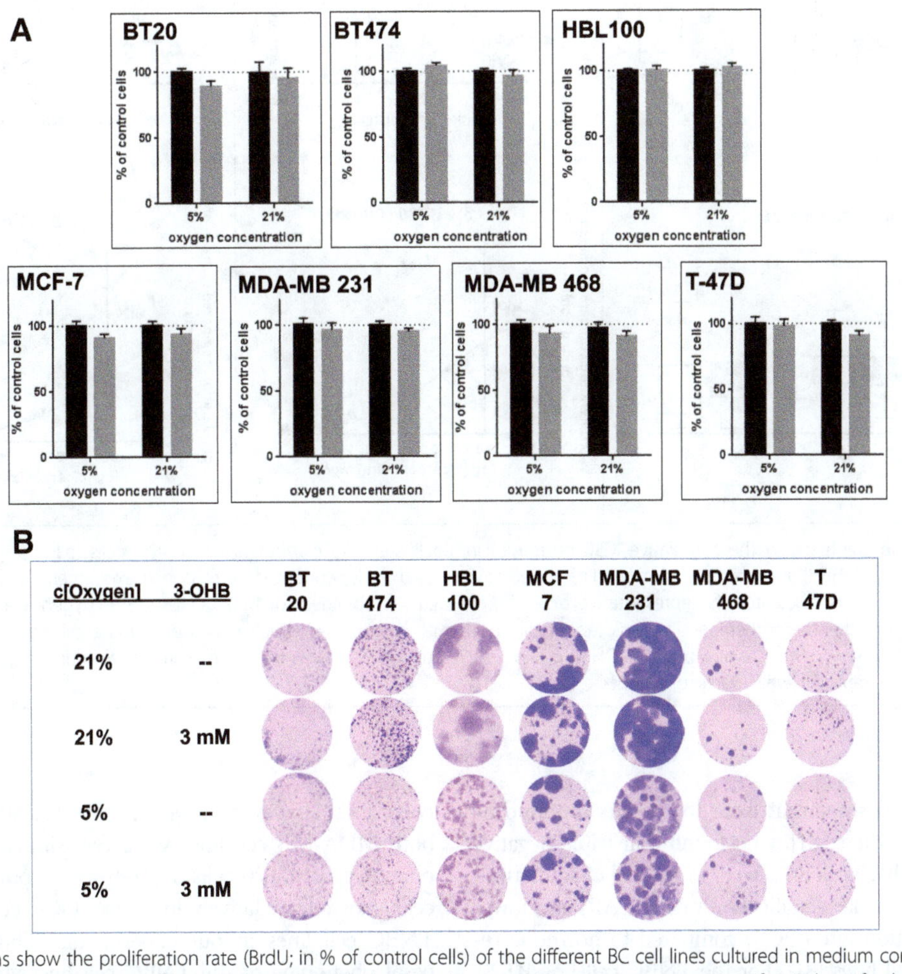

Fig. 4 a The graphs show the proliferation rate (BrdU; in % of control cells) of the different BC cell lines cultured in medium containing 3 mM 3-OHB (gray column) compared to control without 3-OHB (black column) at 5 or 21% oxygen concentration after 5 days of culture (differences are not statistically significant). The columns summarize mean ± SEM of data of four independent experiments with three replicate wells per experiment for each cell line. **b** The figure shows representative results (one out of eight replicates for each cell line) of the colony formation assay for the tested BC cell lines after 14 days of culture. The cell lines show no significant alteration in number and size of colonies upon addition of 3-OHB. BT474, HBL-100, and MDA-MB 231 showed an overall reduced colony size at 5% oxygen concentration compared to 21% oxygen concentration

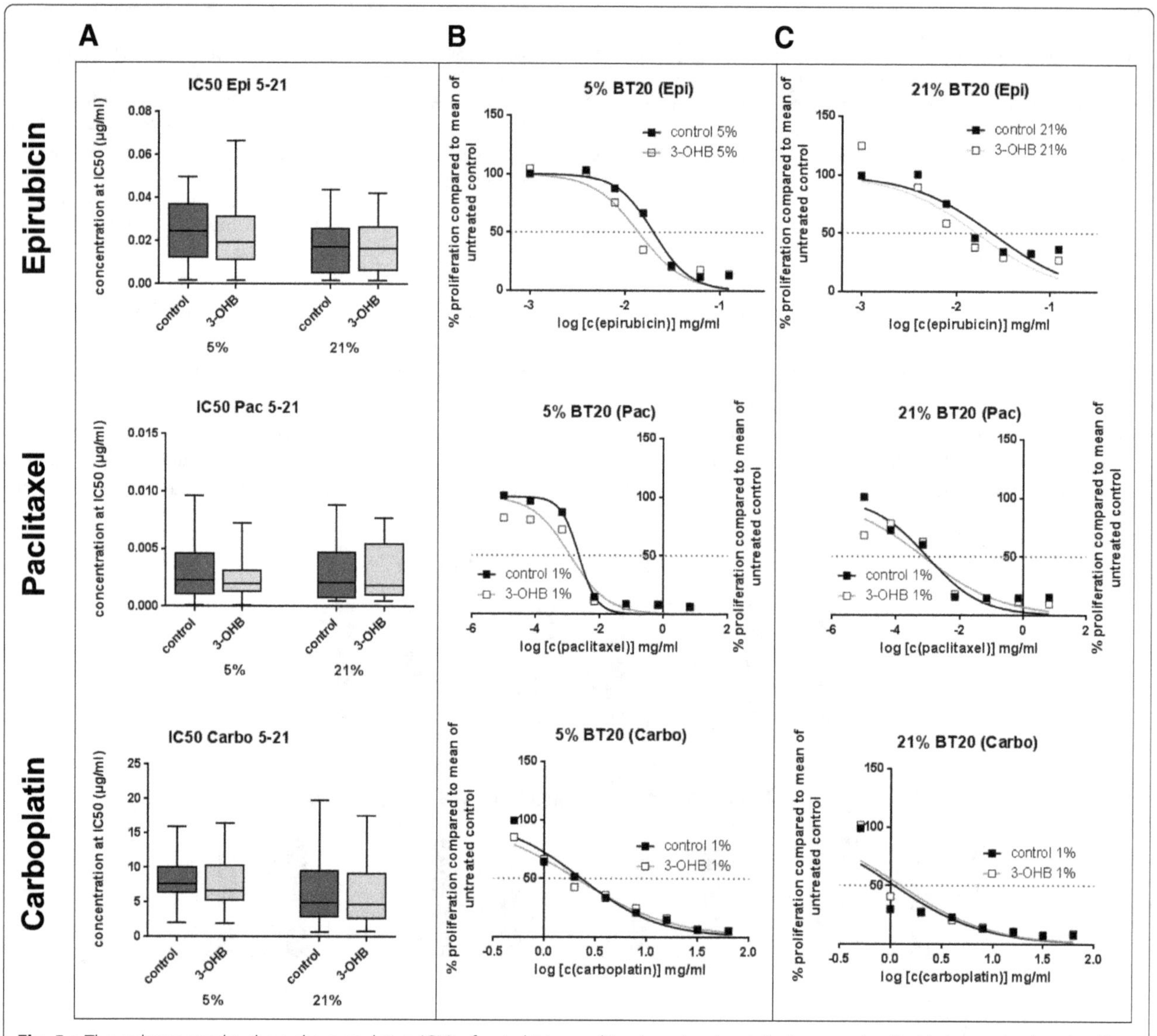

Fig. 5 a The column-graphs show the cumulative IC50 of epirubicin, paclitaxel, and carboplatin in control cells (dark gray box) and cells cultured with 3 mM 3-OHB (light gray box). Per cell line, three to four each independent dose-response experiments with six replicate wells per experiment were calculated. **b** Representative dose-response curves obtained for BT-20 cells at 5% oxygen in chemotherapy sensitivity testing with the chemotherapeutic drugs (epirubicin, paclitaxel, carboplatin) which was used for the calculation of the IC50 (dashed line) (black box = control, white box = 3-OHB). **c** Same as **b** but for 21% oxygen. Curves summarize four independent experiments with six replicate wells per experiment

phenotypes differed somewhat from the results reported by Pelicano and coworkers [81], who found that triple-negative breast cancer (TNBC) cell lines were in general characterized by a higher extracellular acidification rate (ECAR) and lower oxygen consumption rate (OCR) compared to hormone receptor positive cell lines [81]. For the TNBC cell line BT20, we found an energetic profile that was low in OCR and ECAR and was comparable to the hormone receptor positive T47D cell line. Furthermore, the TNBC cell lines MDA-MB 231 and MDA-MB 468 showed very similar energetic profiles in our experiments and those of Pelicano and colleagues. However, in the study of Pelicano and colleagues, both MDA-MB cell lines were very similar to the energetic phenotype of BT20 cells. In contrast, in our study, the BT20 cells showed a relatively low basal OCR compared to other TNBC cell lines in our experiments. This more oxidative basal phenotype of the TNBC cell line MDA-MB 468 was recently also shown by Lanning and colleagues, even at high glucose conditions of 10 mM [82]. However, this study also described a low oxidative phenotype for the MDA-MB 231 cell line which was remarkably lower than that of MDA-MB 468, while in our investigation, both cell lines showed

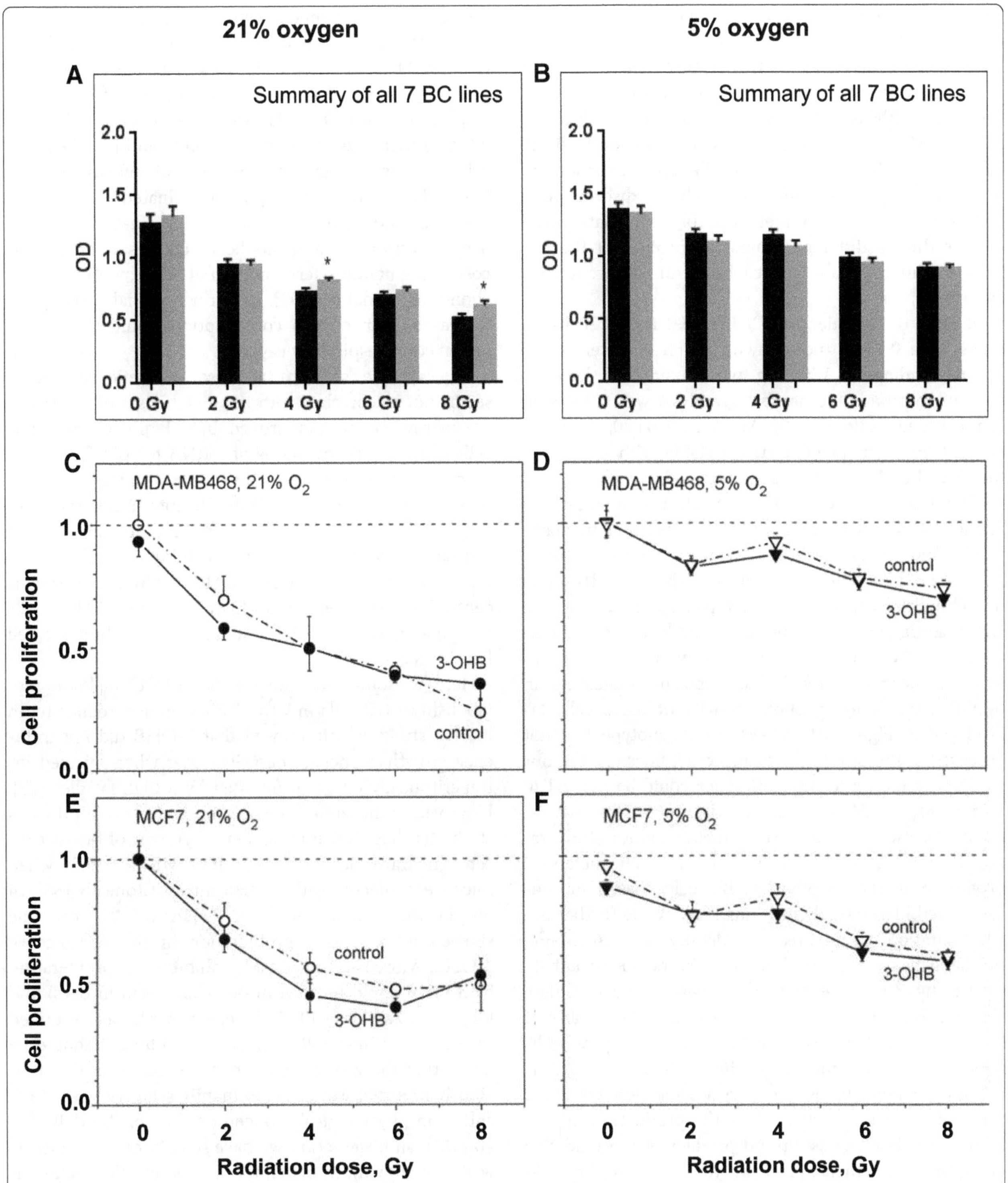

Fig. 6 Cell proliferation after irradiation measured by BrdU, summarized for all BC cell lines at 21% (**a**) and 5% (**b**) oxygen concentration (black column = control; gray column = 3 mM 3-OHB). No significant influence of 3-OHB was seen. Columns represent mean ± SEM of three independent experiments with six replicate wells per experiment. Two representative dose-response curves for MCF7 and MDA-MB 468 are shown (**c**–**f**). MDA-MB 468 cells were sensitive to radiation (**c**, **d**), while MCF7 cells were relatively insensitive even to high doses (**e**, **f**). Open and filled symbols represent mean (± SD) of S-phase cell counts in 3-OHB-untreated control and 3-OHB-treated cells, respectively. The data were normalized to the corresponding values of non-irradiated cells at 21 or 5% oxygen, respectively

comparable values of OCR. It is likely that these discrepancies between metabolic profiling data can arise from small differences in the culture conditions, for example different metabolite concentrations in fetal calf serum. Nevertheless, we can conclude that under the experimental conditions used here, only BT20 cells shifted their metabolic profile upon exposure to reduced oxygen concentration. Those discrepancies between our and other metabolic profiling data could also be due to different expression profiles of the cell lines in different laboratories based on different subclones [83, 84].

Of note, our quotient of OCR/ECAR for BT20 had a range from 0.9–2.4 (not shown), which is closer to the original findings of Warburg, who found that the quotient of respiration to aerobic glycolysis was 0.3–0.9 in tumor tissue sections [8, 9]. Apart from BT20, the other BC cell lines remained relatively stable with respect to the OCR/ECAR ratio in the presence of 3-OHB.

We found that 3-OHB increases both basic OCR and maximal OCR after inhibition of ATP synthesis by oligomycin and in the presence of the uncoupling agent FCCP in BT20 cells. This indicates that 3-OHB alters mitochondrial capacity, for example, by increasing the expression/activity of respiratory complexes or by inducing mitochondrial biogenesis. In addition, glycolysis was also increased after 3-OHB exposure, indicating an overall increase in metabolic activity of these cells (as displayed in Fig. 2a). However, this phenotype was not observed in the other breast cancer cell lines used in our study. One reason for this difference could be that BT20 is the only TNBC cell line that is mutant for BRCA2 (Table 1). Indeed, a large-scale metabolomics study recently found that BT20 cells differ in their metabolic profile compared to other TNBC cells, based on unsupervised hierarchical clustering [85]. While further experimentation is required to identify the underlying mechanisms for the overall increase in metabolic activity caused by 3-OHB exposure in these cells, our data clearly show that 3-OHB does not affect the viability of BT20 cells or their response to chemotherapy or radiation, despite this metabolic effect. Notably, ECAR is not only dependent on medium acidification via lactic acid but can also be affected by the production of carbonic acid (H_2CO_3) as an end product of the oxidative degradation of metabolites in the tricarboxylic acid (TCA) cycle [86, 87]. Here, a very important aspect is the observation that breast cancer cell lines, and especially the TNBC cell lines, often use glutamine as a relevant nutrient to support their metabolic demands [88, 89]. Moreover, glutamine can also be converted to pyruvate and lactate by malic enzyme [90]. Since glutamine is not a limiting factor in our cell culture medium, we cannot exclude that the observed increase in ECAR is due to glutamine metabolism in the cell lines investigated. Therefore, the increase in ECAR in parallel to elevated OCR in BT20 cells is likely to correspond to a generally more "energetic phenotype" of enhanced respiration and CO_2 or lactate-induced acidification [86, 87]. Another possible interpretation would be mitochondrial uncoupling via overexpression of uncoupling protein 2 (UCP2) that, although not evaluated in our study, has been shown to occur in BC cell lines [91]. UCP2 overexpression has a metabolic action by supporting glucose and glutamine fermentation at the expense of mitochondrial oxidation [92]. If mitochondrial uncoupling increased, then oxygen consumption would not strictly be linked to respiratory capacity.

Anyway, the shift to a more energetic phenotype seems not to correlate with the metabolism of 3-OHB as an energy source. As proven by RT-qPCR, the BT20 cells express very low levels of mRNA for BDH1, the key entry enzyme of ketolysis, and in line with this, consume only small amounts of 3-OHB. Of note, BT20 cells also displayed the highest basal rate of glucose consumption and lactic acid production of all cell lines tested and this rate was not influenced by 3-OHB at physiological concentrations. Further, the proliferation rate of BT20 cells was unaffected by 3-OHB, similar to the other six cell lines tested.

Here, we found no evidence that 3-OHB fuels the metabolism of BC cells in vitro. This is in accordance to an in vivo study, which showed that 3-OHB did not influence growth of melanoma cells either when injected intraperitoneally or when elevated by a high-fat diet [73]. However, at the same time, it is in contrast to a previous study that has shown an increased growth of breast cancer xenografts derived from MDA-MB 231 cells when mice were injected with 3-OHB intraperitoneally [36]. In our in vitro experiments, the MDA-MB 231 cell line showed no increased proliferation in the presence of 3-OHB. Moreover, no notable inhibition of proliferation by 3-OHB could be seen in our short-term (5 days) and long-term (at least 14 days) experiments, as described for other cell lines [39–41]. In this context, it should be noted that the growth inhibitory effects for 3-OHB previously reported were predominantly seen with very high and non-physiological concentrations of 3-OHB (5–40 mM), an observation we have seen in our cell lines as well (not shown). In detail, the first description of an antiproliferative effect of 3-OHB on different cancer cell lines was published by Magee et al. in 1979. The authors tested concentrations of 3-OHB between 10 and 40 mM [39]. In 2009, Skinner et al. described an effect of 3-OHB on the viability of human neuroblastoma cells. Again, the authors used very high concentrations of 3-OHB between 24 and 43 mM [41]. Interestingly, an antiproliferative effect of 3-OHB was also described for a physiological concentration of 5 mM 3-OHB in brain tumor cells, but at a very high glucose concentration of 25 mM that represents a more pathophysiological ketoacidotic situation [40]. Our intent was to investigate the effect of 3-OHB in vitro under conditions more likely to be found in cancer patients on KDs. That is why we used physiological concentration of 3-OHB (3 mM) and glucose (5 mM) [22–24]. Using cell culture conditions comparable to our experiments, Martuscelli described an antiproliferative effect of 3-OHB in glioblastoma cell lines and tumor stem cells with half maximal inhibitory concentration (IC50) of 2 mM 3-OHB in the presence of low (4 mM) and physiological (5–6 mM) glucose concentrations [37]. These contrary results described for the effect of 3-OHB on BC cells and glioma cells may reflect differences in their ability to consume 3-OHB.

Previous studies have shown variable gene expression levels of key enzymes involved in ketolytic metabolism in cancer cell lines of different entities [41, 93–97]. In line with these data, we found different mRNA expression patterns of ketolytic enzymes in BC cell lines. In BT474 and HBL100, mRNA transcripts for all ketolytic enzymes were detectable. This was associated with the highest relative consumption rate of 3-OHB by these cells. In contrast, the other BC cell lines failed to express increased levels of at least one of these key enzymes. This mRNA expression pattern was independent from the subtype of BC [59–61] (Table 1) and not influenced by 3-OHB. In accordance to the results of Antalis and colleagues [98], we found very low mRNA transcripts for ACAT1 for BDH1 in MCF-7 cells, which was linked to their inability to consume 3-OHB. Altogether, the expression of ketolytic enzymes on mRNA level seems not to be associated with the rate of 3-OHB consumption and unrelated to levels of glucose consumption and lactate production; however, we are aware, that mRNA expression did not allow to judge about enzymatic activity.

Cells take up ketone bodies by monocarboxylate transporters (MCTs), a family of proton-linked plasma membrane transporters that carry ketone bodies across biological membranes. The most important transporter for 3-OHB into cancer cells is MCT2 [25, 99–101], and previous studies describe an overexpression of MCT2 in BC cells [102]. Here, we found a strong expression of MCT2 in all seven BC cell lines, so that the absence of 3-OHB effects in the cells cannot be explained by defective MCT expression. Since the expression of GLUT1 was found to be related to poor prognosis in breast cancer [103, 104], we analyzed if its expression could be reduced by 3-OHB. However, as for MCT2, we could not detect any modulation of the GLUT1 receptor expression in dependency of 3-OHB, an observation also described in cardiomyocytes [105].

The KD is increasing in popularity, and an increasing number of cancer patients are trying the KD simultaneously with chemotherapy and radiation therapy. Recent clinical trials, e.g., NCT01419483, investigate safety and tolerance of a KD during combined chemotherapy and radiation. We analyzed the response of 3-OHB-treated BC cells to chemotherapy and radiation in vitro. No significant changes in the dose-response to three chemotherapeutical drugs most commonly used in BC treatment [106–110] were observed. Thus, the sensitizing effect of a ketogenic diet on radiochemotherapy in vivo [111] might be mediated by effects other than direct influences on cancer cells. In this context, the clinical study published by Klement and Sweeney [112] is of interest. The authors described an adequate tumor regression for a small cohort of cancer patients undergoing a KD and radiation therapy. Further, two mouse studies with glioma and lung cancer confirm the radio-sensitizing effect of a ketogenic diet [111, 113]. To date, no information is available on a possible radio-sensitizing effect of 3-OHB. Our in vitro results with 3 mM 3-OHB indicate a non-significant tendency of this ketone body to sensitize most BC cells to ionizing radiation.

Conclusions

The intent of the study was to investigate the effect of 3-OHB on seven BC cell lines in vitro under conditions likely to be found in patients on a KD or short-term starvation. We have found strong evidence that a physiological concentration of 3 mM 3-OHB and AcAc did not impact cell proliferation and the response to standard BC chemotherapy and ionizing radiation is not changed by 3-OHB. These findings were independent from the diverse genetic background of the cell lines and differences in mRNA expression of ketolytic enzymes and 3-OHB uptake. Taken together, we found that 3-OHB at physiological concentrations has no major impact on BC cell proliferative behavior and the metabolic activity in vitro and especially does not fuel tumor cell growth. These results support clinical observations that physiologically increased 3-OHB serum concentrations induced either by a ketogenic diet or by short-term starvation do neither support nor inhibit breast cancer cell proliferation. Thus, a ketogenic diet should be safe for breast cancer patients as already described for patients with diverse cancer types (for review, see [114]).

Additional files

Additional file 1: The graphs show the proliferation rate (BrdU; in % of control cells) for the seven different breast cancer cell lines cultured in medium containing 1.5 mM AcAc (white column) compared to control without AcAc (black column) at 5% or 21% oxygen concentration after 5 days of culture (differences are not statistically significant). The columns represent mean ± SEM of data of 4 independent experiments with 3 replicate wells per experiment for each cell line. (PPTX 104 kb)

Additional file 2: Graphs present the IC50 with the 95% confidence intervals for the seven tested cell lines obtained for the three cytostatic drugs epirubicin, paclitaxel and carboplatin comparing the IC50 obtained for cells cultured with 3 mM 3-OHB (gray blots) with the control cells grown in medium free of 3-OHB (black boxes). Each blot represents 3–4 independent dose-response experiments with 6 replicate wells per experiment. None of the differences are statistically significant; however a strong tendency to a reduction in IC50 of paclitaxel is seen for T47D grown in 3-OHB medium compared to the control. (PPTX 104 kb)

Additional file 3: Columns represent mean ± SEM of cell proliferation after irradiation shown for the seven cell lines at 21% and 5% oxygen concentration (gray column = with 3-OHB; black column without 3-OHB) (summarized in Fig. 6). The BT20, BT474 and T47D cell lines cultured in the presence of 3-OHB showed a trend towards increased radio-resistance at 21% oxygen (with some significant results at single doses). In contrast, in MCF-7 and MDA-MB 468, 3-OHB cultured cells showed a trend towards impaired cell proliferation following radiation at the same oxygen concentration. At 5% oxygen concentration, 3-OHB seemed to have a sensitizing effect to radiation in some cell lines. Columns represent mean ± SEM of 3 independent experiments with 6 replicate wells per experiment. *< 0.05, ***p* < 0.01, ****p* < 0.001. (PPTX 152 kb)

Abbreviations

3-OHB: Beta-hydroxybutyrate; AcAc: Acetoacetate; ACAT: *Homo sapiens* acetyl-CoA-acetyltransferase; BDH: 3-Hydroxybutyrate dehydrogenase; BrdU: 5-Bromo-2′-deoxyuridine; CLS: Cell Lines Service GmbH; DMEM: Dulbecco's modified Eagle's medium; ECAR: Extracellular acidification rate; FCS: Fetal calf serum; GLUT1: Glucose transporter 1; KD: Ketogenic diet; MCT: Monocarboxylic acid transporter; mpH: Milli pH; MW: Molecular weight; OCR: Oxygen consumption rate; OD: Optical density; OXPHOS: Oxidative phosphorylation; PPIA: Peptidylprolyl isomerase A; SCOT: Succinyl-CoA transferase; SEM: Standard error of mean; TDC: Test drug concentration; TNBC: Triple-negative breast cancer

Acknowledgements

We thank Monika Koospal and Susanne Kolb for the support of the RT-qPCR experiments and Astrid Katzer for the assistance with the radiation.

Funding

Part of this work was supported by a grant of the Interdisciplinary Centre for Clinical Research (IZKF) University Hospital of Würzburg (Z-2/66 to C.B.).

Authors' contributions

CB and UK originated the study and were responsible for the data collection, analysis, interpretation, and drafting the manuscript. SRJR, JF, AS, CSD, and CO performed the experiments, analyzed the data, and participated in writing the manuscript. RJK and AW helped with editing the manuscript and discussing the data. KB, JW, MS, and MK performed the experiments. All authors read and approved the final manuscript.

Competing interests

The authors declare that they have no competing interests.

Author details

[1]Department of Obstetrics and Gynaecology, University Hospital of Würzburg, Josef-Schneider-Str. 4, 97080 Würzburg, Germany. [2]Department of Biochemistry and Molecular Biology, Theodor-Boveri-Institute, Biocenter, University of Würzburg, 97070 Würzburg, Germany. [3]Department of Radiotherapy and Radiation Oncology, Leopoldina Hospital, 97422 Schweinfurt, Germany. [4]Department of Radiotherapy, University Hospital of Würzburg, 97080 Würzburg, Germany. [5]Experimental Surgery, Department of General, Visceral, Vascular, and Pediatric Surgery, University Hospital of Würzburg, 97080 Würzburg, Germany.

References

1. DeSantis CE, Fedewa SA, Goding Sauer A, Kramer JL, Smith RA, Jemal A. Breast cancer statistics, 2015: convergence of incidence rates between black and white women. CA Cancer J Clin. 2016;66:31–42.
2. Gnant M, Thomssen C, Harbeck N. St. Gallen/Vienna 2015: a brief summary of the consensus discussion. Breast Care (Basel). 2015;10:124–30.
3. Huang J, Pan G, Jiang H, Li W, Dong J, Zhang H, Ji X, Zhu Z. A meta-analysis between dietary carbohydrate intake and colorectal cancer risk: evidence from 17 observational studies. Biosci Rep. 2017;37
4. Ye Y, Wu Y, Xu J, Ding K, Shan X, Xia D. Association between dietary carbohydrate intake, glycemic index and glycemic load, and risk of gastric cancer. Eur J Nutr. 2017;56:1169–77.
5. van den Brandt PA, Schulpen M. Mediterranean diet adherence and risk of postmenopausal breast cancer: results of a cohort study and meta-analysis. Int J Cancer. 2017;140:2220–31.
6. Palacios C, Daniel CR, Tirado-Gomez M, Gonzalez-Mercado V, Vallejo L, Lozada J, Ortiz A, Hughes DC, Basen-Engquist K. Dietary patterns in Puerto Rican and Mexican-American breast cancer survivors: a pilot study. J Immigr Minor Health. 2017;19:341–8.
7. Augustin LS, Libra M, Crispo A, Grimaldi M, De Laurentiis M, Rinaldo M, D'Aiuto M, Catalano F, Banna G, Ferrau F, et al. Low glycemic index diet, exercise and vitamin D to reduce breast cancer recurrence (DEDiCa): design of a clinical trial. BMC Cancer. 2017;17:69.
8. Warburg O. On respiratory impairment in cancer cells. Science. 1956;124: 269–70.
9. Warburg OP, Karl, Negelein E. Über den Stoffwechsel der Carcinomzelle. In: Biochemische Zeitschrift, vol 152; 1924. p. 115–47.
10. Klement RJ, Kammerer U. Is there a role for carbohydrate restriction in the treatment and prevention of cancer? Nutr Metab (Lond). 2011;8:75.
11. Ryu TY, Park J, Scherer PE. Hyperglycemia as a risk factor for cancer progression. Diabetes Metab J. 2014;38:330–6.
12. Monzavi-Karbassi B, Gentry R, Kaur V, Siegel ER, Jousheghany F, Medarametla S, Fuhrman BJ, Safar AM, Hutchins LF, Kieber-Emmons T. Pre-diagnosis blood glucose and prognosis in women with breast cancer. Cancer Metab. 2016;4:7.
13. Tan-Shalaby JL, Carrick J, Edinger K, Genovese D, Liman AD, Passero VA, Shah RB. Modified Atkins diet in advanced malignancies—final results of a safety and feasibility trial within the Veterans Affairs Pittsburgh Healthcare System. Nutr Metab (Lond). 2016;13:52.
14. Klement RF, Richard D, Gross EC, Champ CE, D'Agostino DP, Fine EJ, Kämmerer U, Poff A, Rho JM, Seyfried TN, Scheck AC. Need for new review of article on ketogenic dietary regimes for cancer patients. Med Oncol. 2017;34:1–4.
15. Schwartz K, Chang HT, Nikolai M, Pernicone J, Rhee S, Olson K, Kurniali PC, Hord NG, Noel M. Treatment of glioma patients with ketogenic diets: report of two cases treated with an IRB-approved energy-restricted ketogenic diet protocol and review of the literature. Cancer Metab. 2015;3:3.
16. Rieger J, Bahr O, Maurer GD, Hattingen E, Franz K, Brucker D, Walenta S, Kammerer U, Coy JF, Weller M, Steinbach JP. ERGO: a pilot study of ketogenic diet in recurrent glioblastoma. Int J Oncol. 2014;44:1843–52.
17. Champ CE, Palmer JD, Volek JS, Werner-Wasik M, Andrews DW, Evans JJ, Glass J, Kim L, Shi W. Targeting metabolism with a ketogenic diet during the treatment of glioblastoma multiforme. J Neuro-Oncol. 2014;117:125–31.
18. Fine EJ, Segal-Isaacson CJ, Feinman RD, Herszkopf S, Romano MC, Tomuta N, Bontempo AF, Negassa A, Sparano JA. Targeting insulin inhibition as a metabolic therapy in advanced cancer: a pilot safety and feasibility dietary trial in 10 patients. Nutrition. 2012;28:1028–35.
19. Schmidt M, Pfetzer N, Schwab M, Strauss I, Kammerer U. Effects of a ketogenic diet on the quality of life in 16 patients with advanced cancer: a pilot trial. Nutr Metab (Lond). 2011;8:54.
20. Wheless JW. History of the ketogenic diet. Epilepsia. 2008;49(Suppl 8):3–5.

21. Laffel L. Ketone bodies: a review of physiology, pathophysiology and application of monitoring to diabetes. Diabetes Metab Res Rev. 1999;15:412–26.
22. Pan JW, Rothman TL, Behar KL, Stein DT, Hetherington HP. Human brain beta-hydroxybutyrate and lactate increase in fasting-induced ketosis. J Cereb Blood Flow Metab. 2000;20:1502–7.
23. Cahill GF Jr. Fuel metabolism in starvation. Annu Rev Nutr. 2006;26:1–22.
24. Kim DY, Rho JM. The ketogenic diet and epilepsy. Curr Opin Clin Nutr Metab Care. 2008;11:113–20.
25. Perez-Escuredo J, Van Hee VF, Sboarina M, Falces J, Payen VL, Pellerin L, Sonveaux P: Monocarboxylate transporters in the brain and in cancer. Biochim Biophys Acta 2016, 1863:2481–2497.
26. Halestrap AP. The monocarboxylate transporter family—structure and functional characterization. IUBMB Life. 2012;64:1–9.
27. Broer S, Broer A, Schneider HP, Stegen C, Halestrap AP, Deitmer JW. Characterization of the high-affinity monocarboxylate transporter MCT2 in Xenopus laevis oocytes. Biochem J. 1999;341(Pt 3):529–35.
28. Dimmer KS, Friedrich B, Lang F, Deitmer JW, Broer S. The low-affinity monocarboxylate transporter MCT4 is adapted to the export of lactate in highly glycolytic cells. Biochem J. 2000;350(Pt 1):219–27.
29. Newman JC, Verdin E. Beta-hydroxybutyrate: much more than a metabolite. Diabetes Res Clin Pract. 2014;106:173–81.
30. Hashim SA, VanItallie TB. Ketone body therapy: from the ketogenic diet to the oral administration of ketone ester. J Lipid Res. 2014;55:1818–26.
31. Veech RL, Chance B, Kashiwaya Y, Lardy HA, Cahill GF Jr. Ketone bodies, potential therapeutic uses. IUBMB Life. 2001;51:241–7.
32. Vidali S, Aminzadeh S, Lambert B, Rutherford T, Sperl W, Kofler B, Feichtinger RG. Mitochondria: the ketogenic diet—a metabolism-based therapy. Int J Biochem Cell Biol. 2015;63:55–9.
33. Cahill GF Jr, Veech RL. Ketoacids? Good medicine? Trans Am Clin Climatol Assoc. 2003;114:149–61. discussion 162-143
34. Vaupel P, Kelleher DK, Hockel M. Oxygen status of malignant tumors: pathogenesis of hypoxia and significance for tumor therapy. Semin Oncol. 2001;28:29–35.
35. Martinez-Outschoorn UE, Prisco M, Ertel A, Tsirigos A, Lin Z, Pavlides S, Wang C, Flomenberg N, Knudsen ES, Howell A, et al. Ketones and lactate increase cancer cell "stemness," driving recurrence, metastasis and poor clinical outcome in breast cancer: achieving personalized medicine via Metabolo-Genomics. Cell Cycle. 2011;10:1271–86.
36. Bonuccelli G, Tsirigos A, Whitaker-Menezes D, Pavlides S, Pestell RG, Chiavarina B, Frank PG, Flomenberg N, Howell A, Martinez-Outschoorn UE, et al. Ketones and lactate "fuel" tumor growth and metastasis: evidence that epithelial cancer cells use oxidative mitochondrial metabolism. Cell Cycle. 2010;9:3506–14.
37. Martuscello RT, Vedam-Mai V, McCarthy DJ, Schmoll ME, Jundi MA, Louviere CD, Griffith BG, Skinner CL, Suslov O, Deleyrolle LP, Reynolds BA. A supplemented high-fat low-carbohydrate diet for the treatment of glioblastoma. Clin Cancer Res. 2016;22:2482–95.
38. Shukla SK, Gebregiworgis T, Purohit V, Chaika NV, Gunda V, Radhakrishnan P, Mehla K, Pipinos II, Powers R, Yu F, Singh PK. Metabolic reprogramming induced by ketone bodies diminishes pancreatic cancer cachexia. Cancer Metab. 2014;2:18.
39. Magee BA, Potezny N, Rofe AM, Conyers RA. The inhibition of malignant cell growth by ketone bodies. Aust J Exp Biol Med Sci. 1979;57:529–39.
40. Poff AM, Ari C, Arnold P, Seyfried TN, D'Agostino DP. Ketone supplementation decreases tumor cell viability and prolongs survival of mice with metastatic cancer. Int J Cancer. 2014;135:1711–20.
41. Skinner R, Trujillo A, Ma X, Beierle EA. Ketone bodies inhibit the viability of human neuroblastoma cells. J Pediatr Surg. 2009;44:212–6. discussion 216
42. Klement RJ, Champ CE, Otto C, Kammerer U. Anti-tumor effects of ketogenic diets in mice: a meta-analysis. PLoS One. 2016;11:e0155050.
43. Mavropoulos JC, Buschemeyer WC 3rd, Tewari AK, Rokhfeld D, Pollak M, Zhao Y, Febbo PG, Cohen P, Hwang D, Devi G, et al. The effects of varying dietary carbohydrate and fat content on survival in a murine LNCaP prostate cancer xenograft model. Cancer Prev Res (Phila). 2009;2:557–65.
44. Nebeling LC, Miraldi F, Shurin SB, Lerner E. Effects of a ketogenic diet on tumor metabolism and nutritional status in pediatric oncology patients: two case reports. J Am Coll Nutr. 1995;14:202–8.
45. Otto C, Kaemmerer U, Illert B, Muehling B, Pfetzer N, Wittig R, Voelker HU, Thiede A, Coy JF. Growth of human gastric cancer cells in nude mice is delayed by a ketogenic diet supplemented with omega-3 fatty acids and medium-chain triglycerides. BMC Cancer. 2008;8:122.
46. Poff AM, Ari C, Seyfried TN, D'Agostino DP. The ketogenic diet and hyperbaric oxygen therapy prolong survival in mice with systemic metastatic cancer. PLoS One. 2013;8:e65522.
47. Seyfried TN, Sanderson TM, El-Abbadi MM, McGowan R, Mukherjee P. Role of glucose and ketone bodies in the metabolic control of experimental brain cancer. Br J Cancer. 2003;89:1375–82.
48. Zuccoli G, Marcello N, Pisanello A, Servadei F, Vaccaro S, Mukherjee P, Seyfried TN. Metabolic management of glioblastoma multiforme using standard therapy together with a restricted ketogenic diet: case report. Nutr Metab (Lond). 2010;7:33.
49. Csaba Toth ZC. Halted progression of soft palate cancer in a patient treated with the paleolithic ketogenic diet alone: a 20-months follow-up. Am J Med Case Rep. 2016;4:288–92.
50. Rodrigues LM, Uribe-Lewis S, Madhu B, Honess DJ, Stubbs M, Griffiths JR. The action of beta-hydroxybutyrate on the growth, metabolism and global histone H3 acetylation of spontaneous mouse mammary tumours: evidence of a beta-hydroxybutyrate paradox. Cancer Metab. 2017;5:4.
51. Klement RJ. The influence of ketogenic therapy on the 5 R's of radiobiology. Int J Radiat Biol. 2017:1–13.
52. Paoli A, Bianco A, Grimaldi KA, Lodi A, Bosco G. Long term successful weight loss with a combination biphasic ketogenic Mediterranean diet and Mediterranean diet maintenance protocol. Nutrients. 2013;5:5205–17.
53. Paoli A, Cenci L, Grimaldi KA. Effect of ketogenic Mediterranean diet with phytoextracts and low carbohydrates/high-protein meals on weight, cardiovascular risk factors, body composition and diet compliance in Italian council employees. Nutr J. 2011;10:112.
54. Zajac A, Poprzecki S, Maszczyk A, Czuba M, Michalczyk M, Zydek G. The effects of a ketogenic diet on exercise metabolism and physical performance in off-road cyclists. Nutrients. 2014;6:2493–508.
55. Urbain P, Strom L, Morawski L, Wehrle A, Deibert P, Bertz H. Impact of a 6-week non-energy-restricted ketogenic diet on physical fitness, body composition and biochemical parameters in healthy adults. Nutr Metab (Lond). 2017;14:17.
56. Dashti HM, Mathew TC, Hussein T, Asfar SK, Behbahani A, Khoursheed MA, Al-Sayer HM, Bo-Abbas YY, Al-Zaid NS. Long-term effects of a ketogenic diet in obese patients. Exp Clin Cardiol. 2004;9:200–5.
57. Perez-Guisado J, Munoz-Serrano A, Alonso-Moraga A. Spanish ketogenic Mediterranean diet: a healthy cardiovascular diet for weight loss. Nutr J. 2008;7:30.
58. Vaupel P, Schlenger K, Knoop C, Hockel M. Oxygenation of human tumors: evaluation of tissue oxygen distribution in breast cancers by computerized O2 tension measurements. Cancer Res. 1991;51:3316–22.
59. Holliday DL, Speirs V. Choosing the right cell line for breast cancer research. Breast Cancer Res. 2011;13:215.
60. Neve RM, Chin K, Fridlyand J, Yeh J, Baehner FL, Fevr T, Clark L, Bayani N, Coppe JP, Tong F, et al. A collection of breast cancer cell lines for the study of functionally distinct cancer subtypes. Cancer Cell. 2006;10:515–27.
61. Subik K, Lee JF, Baxter L, Strzepek T, Costello D, Crowley P, Xing L, Hung MC, Bonfiglio T, Hicks DG, Tang P. The expression patterns of ER, PR, HER2, CK5/6, EGFR, Ki-67 and AR by immunohistochemical analysis in breast cancer cell lines. Breast Cancer (Auckl). 2010;4:35–41.
62. Dai X, Cheng H, Bai Z, Li J. Breast cancer cell line classification and its relevance with breast tumor subtyping. J Cancer. 2017;8:3131–41.
63. Baenke F, Dubuis S, Brault C, Weigelt B, Dankworth B, Griffiths B, Jiang M, Mackay A, Saunders B, Spencer-Dene B, et al. Functional screening identifies MCT4 as a key regulator of breast cancer cell metabolism and survival. J Pathol. 2015;237:152–65.
64. Smith SE, Mellor P, Ward AK, Kendall S, McDonald M, Vizeacoumar FS, Vizeacoumar FJ, Napper S, Anderson DH. Molecular characterization of breast cancer cell lines through multiple omic approaches. Breast Cancer Res. 2017;19:65.
65. Catalogue of somatic mutations in cancer. (https://cancer.sanger.ac.uk/cosmic).
66. Kammerer U, Gires O, Pfetzer N, Wiegering A, Klement RJ, Otto C. TKTL1 expression in human malign and benign cell lines. BMC Cancer. 2015;15:2.
67. Pfaffl MW. A new mathematical model for relative quantification in real-time RT-PCR. Nucleic Acids Res. 2001;29:e45.
68. Bradford MM. A rapid and sensitive method for the quantitation of microgram quantities of protein utilizing the principle of protein-dye binding. Anal Biochem. 1976;72:248–54.

69. Chang J, Lee A, Lee J, Lim W, Sung SH, Moon BI. Correlation between the molecular subtype of breast cancer and the in vitro adenosine triphosphate-based chemosensitivity assay. J Korean Surg Soc. 2013;84:313–20.
70. Lin Y, Lv F, Liu F, Guo X, Fan Y, Gu F, Gu J, Fu L. High expression of pyruvate kinase M2 is associated with chemosensitivity to epirubicin and 5-fluorouracil in breast cancer. J Cancer. 2015;6:1130–9.
71. Kurbacher CM, Mallmann P, Kurbacher JA, Hübner H, Krebs D. Chemosensibilitätstestungen in der gynäkologischen Onkologie: Erfahrungen mit einem ATP-Biolumineszenzassay. Geburtshilfe Frauenheilkd. 1996;56:70–8.
72. Gwe Ahn S, Ah Lee S, Woo Lee H, Min Lee H, Jeong J. In vitro chemoresponse assay based on the intrinsic subtypes in breast cancer. Jpn J Clin Oncol. 2014;44:624–31.
73. Xia S, Lin R, Jin L, Zhao L, Kang HB, Pan Y, Liu S, Qian G, Qian Z, Konstantakou E, et al. Prevention of dietary-fat-fueled ketogenesis attenuates BRAF V600E tumor growth. Cell Metab. 2017;25:358–73.
74. NCT01865162 N, NCT02983942, NCT02939378, NCT03160599, NCT01754350, NCT02516501, NCT03075514, NCT01535911 (www.clinicaltrials.gov).
75. Branca JJ, Pacini S, Ruggiero M. Effects of pre-surgical vitamin D supplementation and ketogenic diet in a patient with recurrent breast cancer. Anticancer Res. 2015;35:5525–32.
76. Jansen N, Walach H. The development of tumours under a ketogenic diet in association with the novel tumour marker TKTL1: a case series in general practice. Oncol Lett. 2016;11:584–92.
77. Schwalb MTM, Hines S, Reinwald H, Ruggiero M. Clinical observation of a novel, complementary, immunotherapeutic approach based on ketogenic diet, chondroitin sulfate, vitamin D 3, oleic acid and a fermented milk and colostrum product. Am J Immunol. 2016;12:91–8.
78. Iyikesici MS, Slocum AK, Slocum A, Berkarda FB, Kalamian M, Seyfried TN. Efficacy of metabolically supported chemotherapy combined with ketogenic diet, hyperthermia, and hyperbaric oxygen therapy for stage IV triple-negative breast cancer. Cureus. 2017;9:e1445.
79. Martinez-Outschoorn UE, Lin Z, Whitaker-Menezes D, Howell A, Lisanti MP, Sotgia F. Ketone bodies and two-compartment tumor metabolism: stromal ketone production fuels mitochondrial biogenesis in epithelial cancer cells. Cell Cycle. 2012;11:3956–63.
80. Martinez-Outschoorn UE, Lin Z, Whitaker-Menezes D, Howell A, Sotgia F, Lisanti MP. Ketone body utilization drives tumor growth and metastasis. Cell Cycle. 2012;11:3964–71.
81. Pelicano H, Zhang W, Liu J, Hammoudi N, Dai J, Xu RH, Pusztai L, Huang P. Mitochondrial dysfunction in some triple-negative breast cancer cell lines: role of mTOR pathway and therapeutic potential. Breast Cancer Res. 2014;16:434.
82. Lanning NJ, Castle JP, Singh SJ, Leon AN, Tovar EA, Sanghera A, MacKeigan JP, Filipp FV, Graveel CR. Metabolic profiling of triple-negative breast cancer cells reveals metabolic vulnerabilities. Cancer Metab. 2017;5:6.
83. Chatterjee R. Cell biology. Cases of mistaken identity. Science. 2007;315:928–31.
84. Chatterjee R. Cell biology. When 60 lines don't add up. Science. 2007;315:929.
85. Dubuis S, Baenke F, Scherbichler N, Alexander LT, Schulze A, Zamboni N. Metabotypes of breast cancer cell lines revealed by non-targeted metabolomics. Metab Eng. 2017;43:173–86.
86. Mookerjee SA, Brand MD. Measurement and analysis of extracellular acid production to determine glycolytic rate. J Vis Exp. 2015:e53464.
87. Mookerjee SA, Goncalves RL, Gerencser AA, Nicholls DG, Brand MD. The contributions of respiration and glycolysis to extracellular acid production. Biochim Biophys Acta. 2015;1847:171–81.
88. Wise DR, Thompson CB. Glutamine addiction: a new therapeutic target in cancer. Trends Biochem Sci. 2010;35:427–33.
89. Lampa M, Arlt H, He T, Ospina B, Reeves J, Zhang B, Murtie J, Deng G, Barberis C, Hoffmann D, et al. Glutaminase is essential for the growth of triple-negative breast cancer cells with a deregulated glutamine metabolism pathway and its suppression synergizes with mTOR inhibition. PLoS One. 2017;12:e0185092.
90. DeBerardinis RJ, Mancuso A, Daikhin E, Nissim I, Yudkoff M, Wehrli S, Thompson CB. Beyond aerobic glycolysis: transformed cells can engage in glutamine metabolism that exceeds the requirement for protein and nucleotide synthesis. Proc Natl Acad Sci U S A. 2007;104:19345–50.
91. Fine EJ, Miller A, Quadros EV, Sequeira JM, Feinman RD. Acetoacetate reduces growth and ATP concentration in cancer cell lines which over-express uncoupling protein 2. Cancer Cell Int. 2009;9:14.
92. Vozza A, Parisi G, De Leonardis F, Lasorsa FM, Castegna A, Amorese D, Marmo R, Calcagnile VM, Palmieri L, Ricquier D, et al. UCP2 transports C4 metabolites out of mitochondria, regulating glucose and glutamine oxidation. Proc Natl Acad Sci U S A. 2014;111:960–5.
93. Chang HT, Olson LK, Schwartz KA. Ketolytic and glycolytic enzymatic expression profiles in malignant gliomas: implication for ketogenic diet therapy. Nutr Metab (Lond). 2013;10:47.
94. Matsumoto K, Fujiwara Y, Nagai R, Yoshida M, Ueda S. Expression of two isozymes of acyl-coenzyme A: cholesterol acyltransferase-1 and -2 in clear cell type renal cell carcinoma. Int J Urol. 2008;15:166–70.
95. Maurer GD, Brucker DP, Bahr O, Harter PN, Hattingen E, Walenta S, Mueller-Klieser W, Steinbach JP, Rieger J. Differential utilization of ketone bodies by neurons and glioma cell lines: a rationale for ketogenic diet as experimental glioma therapy. BMC Cancer. 2011;11:315.
96. Patel MS, Russell JJ, Gershman H. Ketone-body metabolism in glioma and neuroblastoma cells. Proc Natl Acad Sci U S A. 1981;78:7214–8.
97. Sawai M, Yashiro M, Nishiguchi Y, Ohira M, Hirakawa K. Growth-inhibitory effects of the ketone body, monoacetoacetin, on human gastric cancer cells with succinyl-CoA: 3-oxoacid CoA-transferase (SCOT) deficiency. Anticancer Res. 2004;24:2213–7.
98. Antalis CJ, Arnold T, Rasool T, Lee B, Buhman KK, Siddiqui RA. High ACAT1 expression in estrogen receptor negative basal-like breast cancer cells is associated with LDL-induced proliferation. Breast Cancer Res Treat. 2010;122:661–70.
99. Benton CR, Campbell SE, Tonouchi M, Hatta H, Bonen A. Monocarboxylate transporters in subsarcolemmal and intermyofibrillar mitochondria. Biochem Biophys Res Commun. 2004;323:249–53.
100. Pinheiro C, Reis RM, Ricardo S, Longatto-Filho A, Schmitt F, Baltazar F. Expression of monocarboxylate transporters 1, 2, and 4 in human tumours and their association with CD147 and CD44. J Biomed Biotechnol. 2010; 2010:427694.
101. Valenca I, Pertega-Gomes N, Vizcaino JR, Henrique RM, Lopes C, Baltazar F, Ribeiro D. Localization of MCT2 at peroxisomes is associated with malignant transformation in prostate cancer. J Cell Mol Med. 2015;19:723–33.
102. Cheng C, Edin NF, Lauritzen KH, Aspmodal I, Christoffersen S, Jian L, Rasmussen LJ, Pettersen EO, Xiaoqun G, Bergersen LH. Alterations of monocarboxylate transporter densities during hypoxia in brain and breast tumour cells. Cell Oncol (Dordr). 2012;35:217–27.
103. Eilertsen M, Andersen S, Al-Saad S, Kiselev Y, Donnem T, Stenvold H, Pettersen I, Al-Shibli K, Richardsen E, Busund LT, Bremnes RM. Monocarboxylate transporters 1-4 in NSCLC: MCT1 is an independent prognostic marker for survival. PLoS One. 2014;9:e105038.
104. Macheda ML, Rogers S, Best JD. Molecular and cellular regulation of glucose transporter (GLUT) proteins in cancer. J Cell Physiol. 2005;202:654–62.
105. Tardif A, Julien N, Pelletier A, Thibault G, Srivastava AK, Chiasson JL, Coderre L. Chronic exposure to beta-hydroxybutyrate impairs insulin action in primary cultures of adult cardiomyocytes. Am J Physiol Endocrinol Metab. 2001;281:E1205–12.
106. Bria E, Nistico C, Cuppone F, Carlini P, Ciccarese M, Milella M, Natoli G, Terzoli E, Cognetti F, Giannarelli D. Benefit of taxanes as adjuvant chemotherapy for early breast cancer: pooled analysis of 15,500 patients. Cancer. 2006;106:2337–44.
107. Kern P, Kalisch A, von Minckwitz G, Putter C, Kolberg HC, Pott D, Kurbacher C, Rezai M, Kimmig R. Neoadjuvant, anthracycline-free chemotherapy with carboplatin and docetaxel in triple-negative, early-stage breast cancer: a multicentric analysis of rates of pathologic complete response and survival. J Chemother. 2016;28:210–7.
108. Shao N, Wang S, Yao C, Xu X, Zhang Y, Zhang Y, Lin Y. Sequential versus concurrent anthracyclines and taxanes as adjuvant chemotherapy of early breast cancer: a meta-analysis of phase III randomized control trials. Breast. 2012;21:389–93.
109. Sharma P, Lopez-Tarruella S, Garcia-Saenz JA, Ward C, Connor CS, Gomez HL, Prat A, Moreno F, Jerez-Gilarranz Y, Barnadas A, et al. Efficacy of neoadjuvant carboplatin plus docetaxel in triple-negative breast cancer: combined analysis of two cohorts. Clin Cancer Res. 2017;23:649–57.
110. Turner N, Biganzoli L, Di Leo A. Continued value of adjuvant anthracyclines as treatment for early breast cancer. Lancet Oncol. 2015;16:e362–9.
111. Allen BG, Bhatia SK, Buatti JM, Brandt KE, Lindholm KE, Button AM, Szweda LI, Smith BJ, Spitz DR, Fath MA. Ketogenic diets enhance oxidative stress and radio-chemo-therapy responses in lung cancer xenografts. Clin Cancer Res. 2013;19:3905–13.

112. Klement RJ, Sweeney RA. Impact of a ketogenic diet intervention during radiotherapy on body composition: I. Initial clinical experience with six prospectively studied patients. BMC Res Notes. 2016;9:143.
113. Abdelwahab MG, Fenton KE, Preul MC, Rho JM, Lynch A, Stafford P, Scheck AC. The ketogenic diet is an effective adjuvant to radiation therapy for the treatment of malignant glioma. PLoS One. 2012;7:e36197.
114. Klement RJ. Beneficial effects of ketogenic diets for cancer patients: a realist review with focus on evidence and confirmation. Med Oncol. 2017;34:132.

5

Inflammation-induced DNA methylation of DNA polymerase gamma alters the metabolic profile of colon tumors

Ashley R. Maiuri[1], Hongde Li[2], Barry D. Stein[2], Jason M. Tennessen[2] and Heather M. O'Hagan[1,3*]

Abstract

Background: Inflammation, metabolism, and epigenetic modulation are highly interconnected processes that can be altered during tumorigenesis. However, because of the complexity of these interactions, direct cause and effect during tumorigenesis have been difficult to prove. Previously, using a murine model of inflammation-induced colon tumorigenesis, we determined that the promoter of the catalytic subunit of DNA polymerase gamma (*Polg*) is DNA hypermethylated and silenced in inflammation-induced tumors, but not in non-inflammation-induced (mock) tumors, suggesting that inflammation can induce silencing of *Polg* through promoting DNA methylation during tumorigenesis. *Polg* is the only mitochondrial DNA polymerase and mutations in *Polg* cause mitochondrial diseases in humans. Because of the role of mitochondria in metabolism, we hypothesized that silencing of *Polg* in inflammation-induced tumors would result in these tumors having altered metabolism in comparison to mock tumors.

Methods: Inflammation-induced and mock colon tumors and colon epithelium from a mouse model of inflammation-induced colon tumorigenesis were assayed for alterations in *Polg* expression, mitochondria, and metabolism. Organoids derived from these tissues were used to study the direct effect of loss of *Polg* on mitochondria and metabolism.

Results: We demonstrate that inflammation-induced tumors with reduced *Polg* expression have decreased mitochondrial DNA content and numbers of mitochondria compared to normal epithelium or mock tumors. Tumoroids derived from mock and inflammation-induced tumors retained key characteristics of the original tumors. Inflammation-induced tumoroids had increased glucose uptake and lactate secretion relative to mock tumoroids. shRNA-mediated knockdown of *Polg* in mock tumoroids reduced mtDNA content, increased glucose uptake and lactate secretion, and made the tumoroids more resistant to oxidative stress.

Conclusions: These results suggest that inflammation-induced DNA methylation and silencing of *Polg* plays an important role in the tumorigenesis process by resulting in reduced mitochondria levels and altered metabolism. An enhanced understanding of how metabolism is altered in and drives inflammation-induced tumorigenesis will provide potential therapeutic targets.

Keywords: Inflammation, DNA methylation, DNA polymerase gamma, Mitochondria, Glucose uptake, Glycolysis

* Correspondence: hmohagan@indiana.edu
[1]Medical Sciences, Indiana University School of Medicine, Bloomington, Indiana, USA
[3]Indiana University Melvin and Bren Simon Cancer Center, Indianapolis, Indiana, USA

Background

Inflammation is known to directly contribute to epigenetic and metabolic alterations as well as tumor formation [1]. Furthermore, epigenetics and metabolism affect each other [2, 3]. For example, epigenetic alterations, including DNA methylation and histone modification, can result in heritable changes in expression of genes involved in metabolism without altering the DNA sequence of these genes. Additionally, alterations in metabolism can affect the availability of metabolites that act as cofactors or inhibitors of epigenetic enzymes.

Metabolism differs in cancer cells compared to normal cells with one of these changes being an increase in glycolysis [4]. This change in metabolism in cancer cells supports their higher proliferative rate and increased need to generate macromolecules for accelerated mitosis. One hallmark of increased glycolysis is an increase in glycolytic flux, which allows cancer cells to take up high levels of glucose even in the presence of physiological levels of ATP [5].

Mitochondria produce ATP through oxidative phosphorylation (OXPHOS) and in the process generate reactive oxygen species (ROS), redox molecules, and metabolites. They can sense cellular stress and assist cells in adapting to the environment making them important to the function of both normal and cancer cells. Because of their multiple cellular functions, the role of mitochondria in carcinogenesis is complex and can vary between cancers. While some cancers depend on mitochondrial respiration, other cancers have dysregulated mitochondria resulting in less efficient OXPHOS [6]. DNA polymerase γ (POLG) is the only mitochondrial DNA polymerase and is involved in the replication and repair of mitochondrial DNA (mtDNA). Furthermore, POLG is the only DNA polymerase capable of maintaining mitochondrial numbers [7]. POLG is a heterodimeric enzyme consisting of the catalytic core encoded by the *POLG* gene and an accessory subunit encoded by *POLG2*. Mutations in *POLG* result in reduced mitochondria and mitochondrial disorders in humans [8]. Experimentally reducing *POLG* expression levels results in decreased mtDNA levels [9]. Each mitochondrion contains multiple copies of mtDNA, and the copy number changes in response to energy demands. Expression of *POLG* and mtDNA copy number are controlled during development with high energy-consuming cells having a higher mtDNA copy number than lower energy cells [10]. DNA methylation of the promoter CpG island of *POLG* has been associated with reduced gene expression and decreased mtDNA copy number in highly proliferative versus terminally differentiated cells and several cancer cell lines [10, 11]. While DNA hypermethylation of *Polg* in human colorectal cancer has not been specifically studied, data from The Cancer Genome Atlas (TCGA) suggests that some colorectal cancers have increased levels of *Polg* promoter DNA methylation [12]. Furthermore, mutations in *POLG* have been found in human breast cancers and are associated with decreased mtDNA levels and decreased mitochondrial activity [13].

We use a mouse model of inflammation-induced tumorigenesis to study the initiation of DNA methylation by inflammation. In this model, mice are infected with a human commensal bacterium, enterotoxigenic *Bacteroides fragilis* (ETBF). ETBF infection induces acute followed by chronic inflammation in the distal colon [14]. Infection of multiple intestinal neoplasia (Min) mice, which are heterozygous for loss of the tumor suppressor gene *adenomatous polyposis* (*Apc*), results in Th17 inflammation-driven tumorigenesis in the distal colon [15]. ETBF-infected Min mice develop on average 13 distal colon tumors (ETBF Min tumors) as compared to mock-infected mice that only occasionally develop colon tumors (Mock Min tumors--0.3 tumors per mouse) [16]. Using this model, we have demonstrated that inflammation-induced tumors have DNA hypermethylated regions relative to epithelium from mock-infected mice (mock Min epithelium) that are not present in non-inflammation-induced tumors from mock-infected mice (mock Min tumors) [16]. Inflamed epithelium isolated from ETBF-infected mice after the removal of tumors (ETBF Min epithelium) has an intermediate level of DNA hypermethylation at regions altered in ETBF Min tumors. Importantly, we demonstrated that the initiation of epigenetic changes is dependent on the mismatch repair protein MSH2 (MutS homolog 2) recruiting epigenetic proteins to sites of inflammation-induced oxidative damage. Mice lacking MSH2 in their intestinal epithelial cells (*Msh2*$^{l/l}$*VC*Min) are deficient in mismatch repair, and ETBF infection of these mice results in an increase in tumorigenesis that is localized to the same region of the colon as in Min mice (a mean of 30 distal colon tumors per mouse) [16]. Interestingly, these tumors (ETBF *Msh2*$^{l/l}$*VC*Min tumors) have very few regions with DNA hypermethylation and their genome-wide methylation profiles are more similar to mock Min tumors than ETBF Min tumors. *Polg* was one of the genes found to be specifically silenced through promoter CpG-island DNA hypermethylation in inflammation-induced tumors with wildtype MSH2, and a lack of MSH2 in intestinal epithelial cells prevented *Polg* methylation and loss of expression in inflammation-induced tumors [16].

Because of POLG's role in mitochondrial function, we hypothesized that reduced expression of *Polg* would result in reduced mtDNA and altered metabolism in inflammation-induced tumors as compared to non-inflammation-induced tumors. This study reports a novel functional role for *Polg* methylation during inflammation-driven tumorigenesis, specifically a reduction in mitochondria that is correlated with an increase in glucose uptake and resistance to oxidative stress.

Methods

Animal model

Min$^{Apc\Delta716\pm}$ and *Msh2*$^{l/l}$*VC*Min mice were handled and inoculated with ETBF as described previously [15, 16]. For all experiments, both males and females were used, mice were randomized between mock and ETBF groups, and mice of different genotypes were cohoused. Individual tumors were removed from dissected colons at 4 or 8 weeks post-infection with the aid of a dissecting microscope and stored at − 80 °C until further analysis. Distal (0–2 cm measured from the rectum) epithelium was collected by scraping the mucosal surface of the dissected colon (after removal of any tumors), washed three times in PBS, and then subjected to the indicated protocol. Such scraping has been shown to be an effective method to obtain samples of intestinal epithelial cells [17].

Quantitative methylation-specific PCR (qMSP) and mtDNA content

Isolated DNA (QIAamp DNA Micro Kit, Qiagen) was bisulfite-treated (EZ DNA methylation-Gold kit, Zymo Research), and qMSP assays were performed as described previously [16]. Quantification of mtDNA levels relative to nuclear DNA (ApoB– Apolipoprotein B) was performed using qPCR and the delta Ct method [18, 19]. See Additional file 1: Table S1 for primers used.

Gene expression

RNA was prepared from epithelium, tumors, or organoids using Trizol followed by cleanup with a RNeasy kit (Qiagen). cDNA was prepared, and qPCR was done using TaqMan assays (see Additional file 1: Table S1 for assays used). Expression of candidate genes was normalized to expression of a housekeeping gene (*PPIA*).

Transmission electron microscopy

Four weeks post-infection colons were dissected, opened, and rinsed with PBS. A 1-mm section was cut from the most distal 0–0.5 cm region and fixed on ice in 2.5% glutaraldehyde, 4% paraformaldehyde, 0.1 M sodium cacodylate, and pH 7.2 for 16 h. While on ice, the samples were processed further by being put into four changes of buffer to remove fixative, followed by 2% osmium tetroxide in 0.1 M sodium cacodylate buffer, pH 7.2 for 2 h, two changes of buffer to remove residual osmium tetroxide, and through a graded ethanol dehydration series to 100% ethanol. At room temperature, the samples were placed in three changes of 100% ethanol, 2:1, 1:1, 1:2 of ethanol/propylene oxide, 100% propylene oxide, infiltrated first with 1:1, 1:3, 1:6 propylene oxide/Embed 812 resin (Electron Microscopy Sciences, Hatfield, PA), and then with three changes of 100% resin before polymerization at 65 °C for 18 h. The polymerized blocks were sectioned at 70 nm thickness using a Leica Ultracut UCT ultramicrotome. Sections were placed on 300-mesh copper grids. The grids were stained first with saturated uranyl acetate, washed with water, and then with lead citrate. The grids were viewed with a JEOL company JEM-1010 transmission electron microscope and photographed using a Gatan 1 k × 1 k model 794 MultiScan camera. A single tumor was imaged per condition with five images taken per sample by a blinded investigator.

Metabolomic analysis

Metabolomic analysis was performed using gas chromatography-mass spectrometry (GC-MS) as previously described with slight modifications [20]. Namely, ~ 5–10 mg of distal colon epithelium or tumors were washed twice in ice-cold PBS; then, metabolites were extracted with 800 µL of 90% cold methanol containing 2 µg/mL of succinic acid-2,2,3,3-d4 as an internal standard using the Omni Bead Ruptor 24 homogenizer (Omni International), and dried with a Speed-Vac. Dried extracts were derivatized with O-methoxylamine hydrochloride and *N*-methyl-*N*-trimethylsilyltrifluoracetamide containing 1% trimethylchlorosilane, respectively. Derivatized samples were analyzed in an Agilent 6890 GC-5973iMS equipment with a 30-m Phenomex ZB5-5 MSi column with a 5-m long guard column. Raw data were normalized with the internal standard and tissue mass.

Organoids

Organoids were derived from mock distal colon epithelium (colonoids) or mock or inflammation-induced Min colon tumors (tumoroids) as demonstrated previously and grown in basal growth media containing EGF (epidermal growth factor), Noggin, R-Spondin1, and Wnt3a (colonoids) or EGF and Noggin (tumoroids) [21, 22]. shRNA-mediated *Polg* knockdown was performed by dissociating tumoroids into single cells using TrypLE, plating in Matrigel and incubating in media containing polybrene plus nontarget (NT) or *Polg*-concentrated lentivirus for 2 h. Then, the media were changed to normal tumoroid medium supplemented with 10 µM Y27632. Forty-eight hours later, media were replaced with fresh media containing 4 µg/ml puromycin. Knockdown organoids were passaged at least one time before performing downstream assays.

Proliferation assay

Tumoroids were disassociated into single cells and 4000 cells in 25 μL Matrigel were plated per well of a 48-well plate. On the indicated day, tumoroids were lysed by homogenization in 200 μL Lactate Assay Buffer (BioVision). The DNA concentration of the lysate was then determined using the Qubit dsDNA HS assay (Invitrogen), which is highly selective for DNA over RNA. Readings were found to be proportional to but more sensitive than cell numbers (data not shown). A similarly treated well without any cells added was used as a blank for the readings. Total DNA content was calculated by multiplying the concentration of DNA by the total volume of buffer.

Glucose uptake, glucose depletion, and lactate secretion

Glucose uptake assays were performed using the Glucose Uptake Colorimetric Assay Kit (BioVision) with some modifications. After 5 days of growth, tumoroids were incubated in 250 μL KRPH buffer (20 mM HEPES, 5 mM KH_2PO_4, 1 mM $MgSO_4$, 1 mM $CaCl_2$, 136 mM NaCl, 4.7 mM KCl, pH 7.4) for 40 min followed by the addition of 25 μL of 10 mM 2-DG (2-deoxy-D-glucose) and an additional 20-min incubation. Washed tumoroids were then removed from the Matrigel by pipetting up and down in cold PBS and lysed in extraction buffer. A 2-DG6P standard curve was performed during each experiment and used to calculate 2-DG uptake. As per the manufacturer's recommendation, protein concentration (BCA) assays were performed on the same cell lysate from each sample that was used for the glucose uptake assay to determine the protein concentration, which was then used to normalize the 2-DG uptake.

The same wells of tumoroids were used for glucose depletion and lactate secretion assays. Media were collected from each tumoroid well at the indicated day post-plating and used immediately for the assays. Glucose levels were measured using 2 μL media and the Glucose (HK) Assay Kit (Sigma-Aldrich) following the manufacturer's directions. Media from a similarly treated well without any cells added were used to determine the starting glucose levels. The glucose standard provided with the kit was used during each experiment to calculate glucose levels. Glucose depletion was calculated by subtracting the glucose levels in the media of a given well from the media from the no cells well. The concentration of DNA in each well was determined as in the "Proliferation assay" section and used to normalize the depleted glucose levels. To determine lactate levels, media were diluted 1:10 or 1:20 in lactate assay buffer and 2 μL was assayed with the Lactate Colorimetric/Fluorometric Assay Kit (BioVision) following the manufacture's protocol. A L(+)-Lactate standard was assayed during each experiment and used to calculate lactate levels. Lactate levels were normalized to DNA concentration as above. For NT and Polg KD tumoroids, lactate levels in media of wells containing tumoroids were determined as above at day 5 post-plating.

Tumoroid viability

Seventy-two hours after the addition of PBS or 0.5 mM H_2O_2 to the media of tumoroid cultures, the media were removed and 250 μL of KRPH buffer was added plus MTT (3-(4,5-dimethylthiazol-2-yl)-2,5-diphenyltetrazolium bromide) to a final concentration of 500 μg/ml and incubated at 37 °C for 1 h. Matrigel and MTT were solubilized as previously described [23].

Statistical analysis

Expression data, qMSP, mtDNA content, metabolite levels, glucose uptake, and cell viability are presented as the mean ± standard error (SEM). Data are evaluated by Mann-Whitney *U* test and considered statistically significant with a p value < 0.05. Sample sizes are indicated in associated figure legends for assays using tumor tissue. For all assays performed with organoid experiments were performed three times with two to three biological replicates per experiment. The mean ± SEM is computed using all biological replicates from all experiments.

Results

DNA methylation of *Polg* is associated with reduced mtDNA content in inflammation-induced colon tumors

Using methyl CpG-binding domain sequencing (MBD-seq), we previously found that inflammation-induced tumors (ETBF Min tumors) collected from Min mice 8 weeks post-ETBF infection have unique DNA hypermethylated regions that are mostly not hypermethylated in non-inflammation-induced tumors (mock Min tumors) [16]. Additionally, we demonstrated that in mice lacking expression of the mismatch repair protein MSH2 in their intestinal epithelium, the inflammation-induced DNA hypermethylation and expression alterations in tumors were reduced as compared to ETBF Min tumors [16]. The CpG-island containing promoter of *Polg* is one of regions specifically DNA hypermethylated in ETBF Min tumors. As POLG is the only mitochondrial DNA polymerase involved in the replication and repair of mitochondrial DNA, and mitochondria play a critical role in tumorigenesis, tumor progression, and metabolic regulation, we decided to explore the association between the DNA methylation of *Polg* and tumor metabolism. Tumors can be macrodissected as early as 4 weeks post-infection in our mouse model. Therefore, we assayed *Polg* DNA methylation in early tumors and epithelium from Min and $Msh2^{l/l}$*VC*Min mice as well as 8-week tumors and epithelium for comparison. Four- and 8-week ETBF Min tumors had significantly higher levels of *Polg* DNA methylation than epithelium from mock-infected mice (mock Min epithelium) (Fig. 1a). In contrast, ETBF Min epithelium and mock Min and ETBF *Msh2*$^{l/l}$*VC*Min tumors had increased *Polg* DNA methylation compared to mock Min epithelium 8 weeks post-mock infection, but not at 4 weeks, and this increase in DNA methylation was still significantly less than the *Polg* methylation in ETBF Min tumors. No significant changes in *Polg* promoter methylation were detected in inflamed epithelium from *Msh2*$^{l/l}$*VC*Min mice (Fig. 1a). Lack of DNA methylation in the CpG island containing promoter of *Gapdh* in all samples serves as a negative control.

Promoter CpG-island DNA hypermethylation is known to be associated with reduced gene expression. *Polg* expression was decreased in 4- and 8-week ETBF Min tumors relative to mock and ETBF Min epithelium and mock Min and ETBF *Msh2*$^{l/l}$*VC*Min tumors (Fig. 1b). Confirming the relationship between DNA methylation and expression, *Polg* expression in 8-week ETBF Min tumors was less than 4-week ETBF Min tumors. Additionally, *Polg* expression was only decreased in ETBF epithelium and mock Min and ETBF *Msh2*$^{l/l}$*VC*Min tumors versus mock epithelium 8 weeks post-infection when there is a corresponding increase in DNA methylation. There was a trend towards reduced expression of *Polg* in ETBF *Msh2*$^{l/l}$*VC*Min epithelium 8 weeks post-ETBF, but the change was not statistically significant (Fig. 1b).

Because reduced expression of *Polg* has been associated with reduced mtDNA content [9], we assayed mtDNA content relative to genomic DNA content in the various tissue types. At 4 and 8 weeks post-infection, ETBF Min tumors had significantly less mtDNA content than mock or ETBF Min epithelium or mock Min or ETBF *Msh2*$^{l/l}$*VC*Min tumors (Fig. 1c, d). mtDNA content in mock Min tumors was not significantly different from the mock epithelium at either time point. At 4 weeks post-ETBF mtDNA content in ETBF *Msh2*$^{l/l}$*VC*Min tumors was slightly reduced depending on the locus examined, but was unchanged or increased at the 8-week time point (Fig. 1d). mtDNA content in ETBF epithelium was also partially reduced at 4 weeks, but returned to normal levels at 8 weeks post-ETBF. Altogether, these data demonstrate that inflammation-induced tumors with *Polg* promoter CpG-island DNA hypermethylation have reduced *Polg* gene expression and mtDNA content.

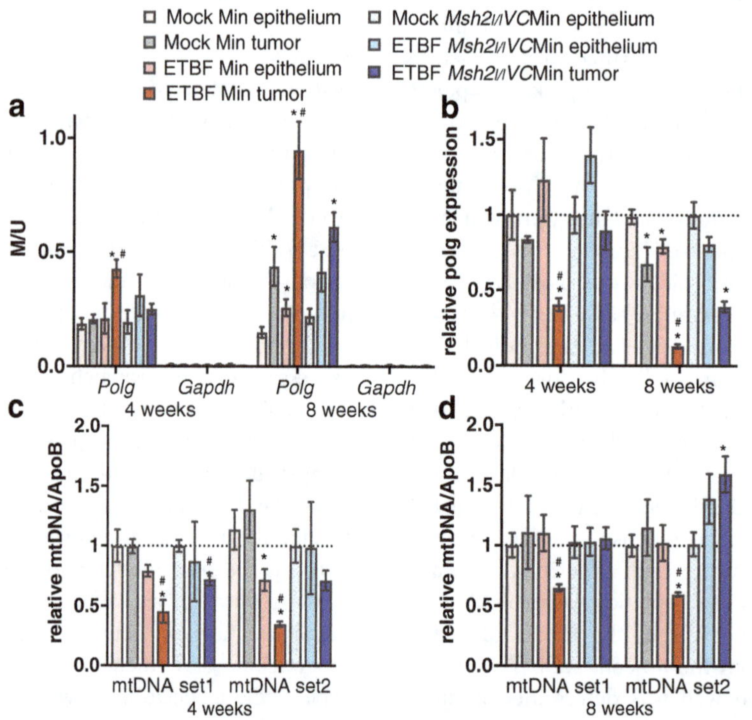

Fig. 1 Tumors with promoter DNA methylation and reduced expression of *Polg* have reduced mitochondrial DNA content. **a** qMSP of bisulfite-treated DNA from indicated tissue 4 or 8 weeks post-infection using methylation-specific primers in promoter CpG islands of indicated genes. Mean ± SEM. $N = 4$–5 for epithelium, $N = 5$–9 for tumors. *$P < 0.05$ compared with mock epithelium. #$P < 0.05$ compared to ETBF Min epithelium and mock Min and ETBF *Msh2*$^{l/l}$*VC*Min tumors. **b** *Polg* gene expression by qPCR relative to mock epithelium. Mean ± SEM. $N = 4$–8 for epithelium, $N = 6$–12 for tumors, asterisk and number sign as in **a**. DNA from tissue (**c**) 4 weeks or (**d**) 8 weeks post-infection was used in qPCR assays with primer sets specific for two different regions of mitochondrial DNA or the genomic ApoB. Mean ± SEM. $N = 4$–5 for epithelium, $N = 5$–9 for tumors, asterisk and number sign as in **a**

Inflammation-induced tumors with wildtype MSH2 have fewer mitochondria

Mitochondria have multiple copies of mtDNA, and the number can vary between cell types [10], suggesting that the decrease in mtDNA content in the ETBF tumors could be from decreased number of mtDNA copies per mitochondria or decreased numbers of total mitochondria in the tumors. Therefore, we used transmission electron microscopy (TEM) to image mitochondria in tumors from our mouse model. Because of size limitations of TEM, we used tissues from mice 4 weeks post-infection when tumors are still relatively small. Since mitochondria can be relocalized inside cells in response to stress, it was important to use control tissue that was undergoing similar inflammation-induced stress [24]. Therefore, ETBF *Msh2*$^{l/l}$*VC*Min tumors are the best comparison tissue for ETBF Min tumors. TEM images of ETBF Min tumors had fewer mitochondria than ETBF *Msh2*$^{l/l}$*VC*Min tumors (2.0 versus 9.6 mitochondria per image, respectively) (Fig. 2). There were no obvious structural differences in the mitochondria that were present between the two different tumor types. This finding suggests that reduced expression of *Polg* by inflammation-induced DNA hypermethylation results in fewer mitochondria in tumors although some are still present and likely necessary for cell survival.

Altered expression of metabolic genes and metabolite levels in inflammation-induced tumors

Altered mitochondrial function has been associated with increased aerobic glycolysis [6]. To determine the alterations in metabolic gene expression in ETBF Min tumors versus mock Min epithelium, we first used a PCR array for detecting expression of genes involved in glucose metabolism as well as screened additional candidates by qPCR. Using a two-fold cutoff, three genes on the array had increased expression in inflammation-induced tumors (*Phosphoribosyl pyrophosphate synthetase 1-Like 1 Prps1l1*; *Hexokinase 3 - Hk3*; *Glycogen phosphorylase, muscle associated - Pygm*) and 17 genes had decreased expression on the PCR array (Additional file 1: Table S2). We verified expression alterations of genes with the greatest fold change (*Glucokinase –Gck*; *Aldolase, fructose-bisphosphate B – Aldob*; *Prps1l1*; *Hk3*) by qRT-PCR, and all expression changes were validated (Fig. 3a and Additional file 1: Figure S1A). To determine which gene expression changes may be associated with reduced expression of *Polg* and reduced mitochondria, we also performed qRT-PCR using mock Min tumors and ETBF-induced *Msh2*$^{l/l}$*VC*Min tumors, which have higher levels of *Polg* expression and mtDNA content than ETBF Min tumors. *Hif1a* (*Hypoxia inducible factor 1 alpha*), *Glut1* (*glucose transporter 1*), and *Hk2* had increased expression in ETBF Min tumors relative to mock Min epithelium as well as relative to mock Min and ETBF *Msh2*$^{l/l}$*VC*Min tumors (Fig. 3a). None of these genes had significant increases in expression in the other tumor types relative to mock Min epithelium. *Hif1a* expression was also increased in mock *Msh2*$^{l/l}$*VC*Min epithelium and ETBF epithelium from Min and *Msh2*$^{l/l}$*VC*Min mice relative to mock Min epithelium. Expression of *6-phophofructose-2-kinas/fructose2,6-biphosphatase 3* (*Pfkfb3*), the only isoform of *Pfkb* that is induced by inflammatory stimuli and hypoxia, was significantly increased in all tumors assayed relative to mock Min epithelium and was significantly higher in ETBF Min tumors than mock Min or ETBF *Msh2*$^{l/l}$*VC*Min tumors (Fig. 3a). *Pfkfb3* expression was not altered in ETBF epithelium from either genotype. *Gck* expression was reduced in all tumor types, but was significantly lower in ETBF Min tumors compared to the other tumor types (Fig. 3a). *Gck* expression was also decreased in ETBF *Msh2*$^{l/l}$*VC*Min epithelium. Interestingly, all of the expression changes in ETBF Min tumors are associated with increased glycolytic flux [5, 25]. Stabilization

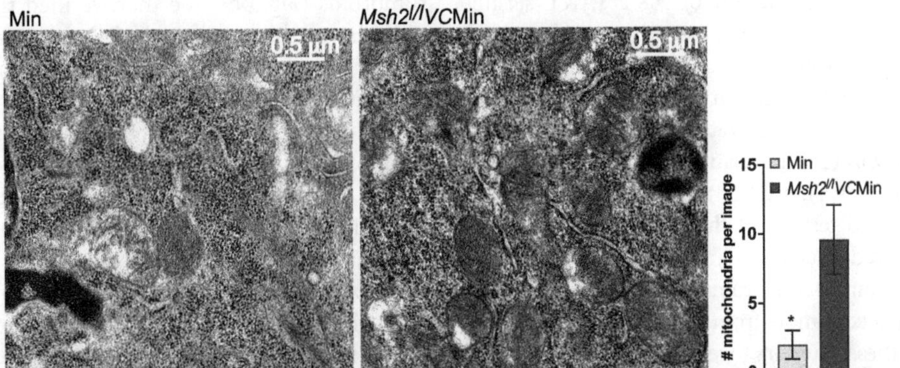

Fig. 2 Inflammation-induced tumors with wildtype MSH2 have fewer mitochondria. One tumor each from mice of the indicated genotypes 4 weeks post-ETBF infection was imaged by transmission electron microscopy. Red asterisk indicates mitochondria. Five images at the same magnification were taken per sample in a blinded fashion, and the numbers of mitochondria per image were counted. Mean ± SEM. $^*P < 0.05$

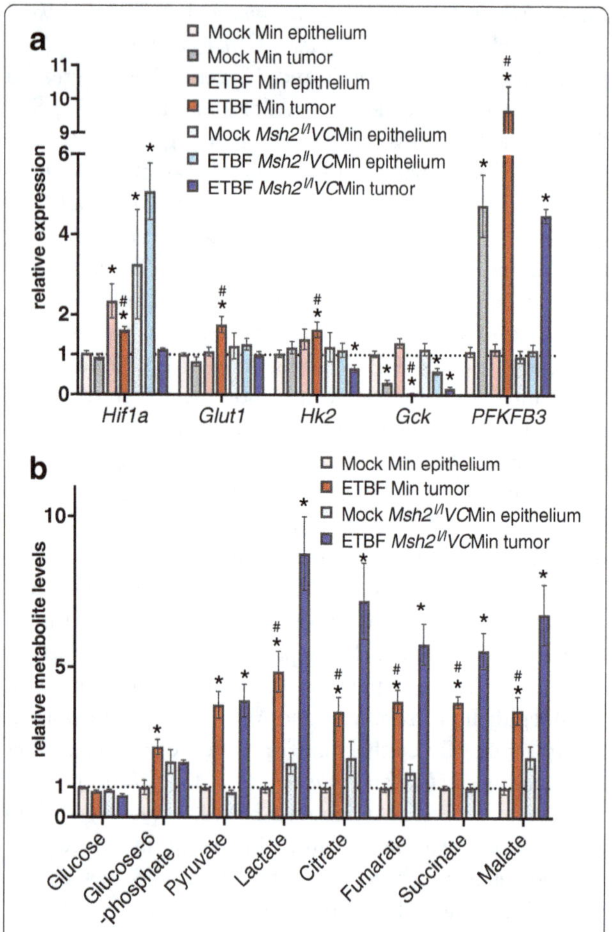

Fig. 3 Inflammation-induced tumors have altered metabolism. **a** Gene expression by qPCR relative to mock Min epithelium from indicated tissue 8 weeks post-infection. Mean ± SEM. *N* = 4–8 for epithelium, *N* = 6–12 for tumors. **P* < 0.05 compared with mock Min epithelium. #*P* < 0.05 compared to mock Min and ETBF $Msh2^{l/l}$VCMin tumors. **b** Metabolites in tissues as in **a**. Mean ± SEM. *N* = 4 tissue, six tumors. **P* < 0.05 compared with mock epithelium. #*P* < 0.05 compared to ETBF $Msh2^{l/l}$VCMin tumors

of HIF1α protein and activation of AKT (AKT serine/threonine kinase 1) are common occurrences in tumors and both of them can alter the expression of metabolic genes [26]. However, by western blot, total HIF1α and phosphorylated AKT were elevated to similar levels in ETBF and mock Min tumors relative to mock Min epithelium (Additional file 1: Figure S1B).

To more directly determine if the inflammation-induced tumors have altered metabolism, we assayed metabolite levels in epithelium and tumors. We focused on inflammation-induced tumors from Min and *$Msh2^{l/l}$VC*Min mice because these tumors were undergoing similar inflammation-induced stress but had different *Polg* and mtDNA levels. While there was no change in glucose levels, the levels of glucose-6-phosphate (G-6P) were higher in ETBF Min tumors than mock Min epithelium (Fig. 3b). G-6P levels in ETBF *$Msh2^{l/l}$VC*Min tumors were unaltered relative to mock *$Msh2^{l/l}$VC*Min epithelium. Pyruvate levels were increased similarly in ETBF Min and *$Msh2^{l/l}$VC*Min tumors relative to their respective epithelium (Fig. 3b). Lactate and the tricarboxylic acid (TCA) metabolites (citrate, fumarate, succinate, malate) were elevated in both tumor types relative to their respective epithelium (Fig. 3b). However, levels of these metabolites were significantly higher in ETBF *$Msh2^{l/l}$VC*Min tumors relative to ETBF Min tumors. Altogether, these data suggest that both types of tumors have altered metabolite levels relative to their respective mock epithelium, but that ETBF Min tumors have increased G-6P and lower mitochondrial metabolites than ETBF *$Msh2^{l/l}$VC*Min tumors.

Tumoroids derived from inflammation-induced tumors have increased glucose uptake

The increased expression of genes related to glycolytic flux as well as increased G-6P metabolite levels suggest that inflammation-induced tumors have increased glucose uptake. To be able to directly assay glucose uptake in tumor cells, we derived organoids from tumors from mock or ETBF-infected Min mice (tumoroids) as well as organoids from mock colon epithelium (colonoids). Since tumoroids and colonoids only consist of tumor or epithelial cells, respectively, they provide a reductionist approach to examining cellular changes without other cells that are normally present in the mucosal layer of the colon [27]. Colonoids formed characteristic budding structures, whereas mock and ETBF tumoroids formed cystic structures that were similar in appearance to each other (Fig. 4a). ETBF tumoroids proliferated significantly faster than mock tumoroids as demonstrated by increased DNA content per well of tumoroids at days 4, 5, and 6 post-plating for ETBF relative to mock tumoroids (Fig. 4b). We verified that ETBF tumoroids maintain reduced *Polg* expression relative to colonoids and mock tumoroids (Fig. 4c). We then verified that ETBF tumoroids have the increased *Polg* promoter CpG-island methylation present in ETBF Min tumors by performing qMSP on isolated DNA. ETBF tumoroids did have higher levels of DNA methylation at the *Polg* promoter than colonoids and mock tumoroids, but not at the *Gapdh* promoter, which does not undergo inflammation-induced DNA hypermethylation (Fig. 4d). Furthermore, ETBF tumoroids had lower levels of mtDNA than colonoids and mock tumoroids consistent with our previous data (Fig. 4e). Interestingly, ETBF tumoroids had increased glucose uptake relative to mock tumoroids (Fig. 4f; measured 5 days after plating). To confirm these results by a different assay, glucose levels in the media that the tumoroids were growing in were measured and normalized to the

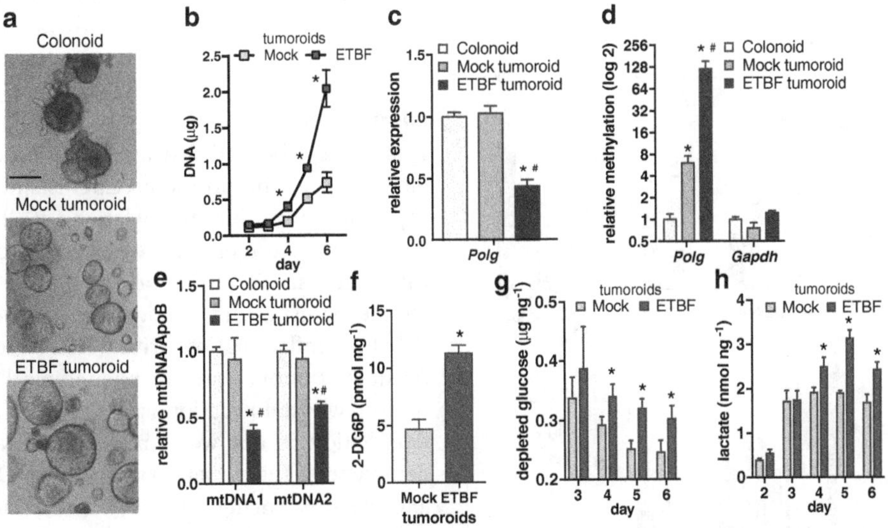

Fig. 4 Tumoroids derived from inflammation-induced tumors have increased glucose uptake. **a** Representative images of colonoids derived from mock Min epithelium and tumoroids derived from mock or ETBF Min tumors 8 weeks post-infection. Scale bar, 100 μm. **b** Total DNA content in wells of mock and ETBF tumoroids as in **a** collected at the indicated days post-plating. Mean ± SEM. The data is from three independent experiments each with two biological replicates. $^*P < 0.05$. **c** *Polg* gene expression in organoids as in **a** by qPCR relative to epithelium organoids. Mean ± SEM. The data is from three independent experiments each with two biological replicates. $^*P < 0.05$ compared to epithelium. $^\#P < 0.05$ compared to mock tumoroid. **d** qMSP of bisulfite-treated DNA from organoids as in **a** using methylation-specific primers in promoter CpG islands of indicated genes. Bar indicates mean ± SEM. The data is from three independent experiments each with two biological replicates, asterisk and number sign as in **c**. **e** DNA from organoids as in **a** was used in qPCR assays with primer sets specific for two different regions of mitochondrial DNA or the genomic ApoB. Mean ± SEM. The data is from three independent experiments each with two biological replicates, asterisk and number sign as in **c**. **f** Glucose uptake by tumoroids derived as in **a**. 2-DG6P levels were normalized to protein concentrations of the samples to account for differences in cell number. Mean ± SEM. The data is from three independent experiments each with three biological replicates. $^*P < 0.05$. **g** At the indicated day post-plating, glucose levels in media from wells with tumoroids were subtracted from glucose levels in media from a well with Matrigel, but without cells, and then normalized to DNA concentration of the tumoroids. Mean ± SEM. The data is from three independent experiments each with two biological replicates. $^*P < 0.05$. **h** Lactate levels in media from wells with tumoroids at the indicated day post-plating normalized to DNA concentration. Mean ± SEM. The data is from three independent experiments each with two biological replicates. $^*P < 0.05$

DNA content of the tumoroids. ETBF tumoroids depleted the media of more glucose than mock tumoroids at days 4, 5, and 6 post-plating (Fig. 4g). Since aerobic glycolysis results in increased production and secretion of lactate, we measured lactate levels in the media and normalized these values to DNA content. Lactate secretion by ETBF tumoroids was more than mock tumoroids at days 4, 5, and 6 post-plating (Fig. 4h). Changes in glucose levels in the media were undetectable at 2 days post-plating, and glucose and lactate levels were not different between the tumoroid types at 3 days post-plating. These findings demonstrate that epigenetic changes persist in tumoroids and that tumoroids derived from inflammation-induced tumors with reduced *Polg* expression have increased proliferation, glucose uptake, and lactate secretion than mock tumoroids.

Reduction of Polg expression increases glucose uptake and resistance to oxidative stress in mock tumoroids

Tumors have many epigenetic and other types of alterations compared to normal epithelium. To determine if reduced *Polg* expression directly affects glucose uptake, we first knocked down *Polg* in colonoids derived from the epithelium of WT-uninfected mice. shRNA knockdown of *Polg* resulted in decreased *Polg* expression and reduced mtDNA (Additional file 1: Figure S2A&B). However, glucose uptake was similar in nontarget (NT) and *Polg* knockdown (KD) colonoids suggesting that reduced expression of *Polg* in WT colonoids is not sufficient to alter glucose uptake (Additional file 1: Figure S2C).

To determine if reduced *Polg* expression is sufficient to alter metabolism in tumor cells, we knocked down *Polg* in mock tumoroids. *Polg* KD tumoroids had less *Polg* expression than NT KD tumoroids (Fig. 5a). The *Polg* KD tumoroids also had less mtDNA content than NT tumoroids and similar mtDNA content as ETBF tumoroids (Fig. 5b). *Polg* KD tumoroids had significantly increased glucose uptake and lactate secretion relative to NT tumoroids, but less than ETBF tumoroids suggesting that, at least in part, the increased glucose uptake and lactate secretion in ETBF tumoroids is due to the promoter DNA methylation and reduced expression of *Polg* (Fig. 5c, d).

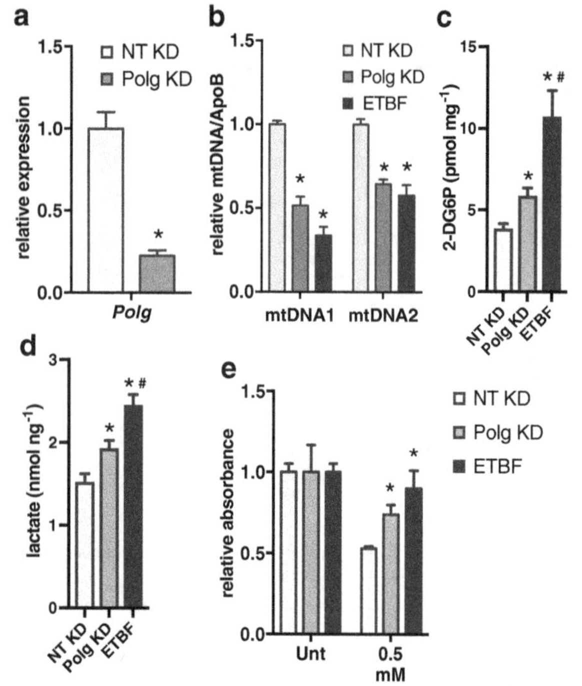

Fig. 5 Reduced *Polg* expression increases glucose uptake and resistance to oxidative stress. **a** *Polg* gene expression in nontarget (NT) or *Polg* knockdown (KD) mock tumoroids by qPCR relative to NT organoids. Mean ± SEM. The data is from three independent experiments each with two biological replicates. $^*P < 0.05$. **b** DNA from tumoroids as in **a** was used in qPCR assays with primer sets specific for two different regions of mitochondrial DNA or the genomic ApoB. Mean ± SEM. The data is from three independent experiments each with two biological replicates. $^*P < 0.05$ compared to NT. **c** Glucose uptake by tumoroids derived as in **a** normalized to protein concentration. Mean ± SEM. The data is from three independent experiments each with three biological replicates. $^*P < 0.05$ compared to NT. $^\#P < 0.05$ compared to Polg KD. **d** Lactate levels in media from wells with tumoroids as in **a** normalized to DNA concentration. Mean ± SEM. The data is from three independent experiments each with two biological replicates, asterisk and number sign as in **c**. **e** Cell viability relative to untreated assayed by MTT in tumoroids derived as in **a** 72 h after mock treatment (Unt) or 0.5 mM H_2O_2. Mean ± SEM. The data is from three independent experiments each with two biological replicates. $^*P < 0.05$ compared to NT

Mitochondria are major intracellular producers of reactive oxygen species (ROS) and are susceptible to oxidative damage [28]. They also play a key role in initiation and execution of apoptosis. Therefore, we hypothesized that tumoroids with fewer mitochondria would be more resistant to oxidative stress than those with normal levels. We determined that ETBF and *Polg* KD tumoroids are more resistant to oxidative stress than NT KD tumoroids by measuring cell viability 72 h after mock or 0.5 mM hydrogen peroxide (H_2O_2) treatment (Fig. 5d). Altogether, these findings demonstrate that KD of *Polg* reduces mtDNA content in both colonoids and tumoroids and increases glucose uptake, lactate secretion, and resistance to oxidative stress specifically in tumoroids.

Discussion

It is well established that inflammation can induce silencing of genes by promoter CpG-island DNA hypermethylation, and this methylation, if it occurs in the promoters of tumor suppressor genes, can participate in tumorigenesis [29]. Tumorigenesis can also be initiated by mechanisms independent of chronic inflammation. Whether inflammation-driven DNA methylation events result in tumors that are phenotypically different from tumors whose formation is not directly from chronic inflammation is not well understood. Here, we uniquely demonstrate that inflammation-driven DNA methylation and gene silencing of *Polg* in murine colon tumors results in tumors with fewer mitochondria and altered metabolism in comparison to non-inflammation-induced tumors. Furthermore, tumoroids derived from these two types of tumors retain their DNA methylation, mitochondria, and metabolic differences. Using the tumoroids as a manipulatable system, we demonstrate that increased glucose uptake, lactate secretion, and resistance to oxidative stress in inflammation-induced colon tumors are, at least in part, due to decreased *Polg* expression.

Human colorectal cancer tissue has lower mtDNA copy number than surrounding normal tissue, and the copy number negatively correlates with disease progression [30–32]. There is also evidence of alterations in mitochondrial function in the epithelium of patients with inflammatory bowel disease, a condition that increases risk for developing colon cancer [33]. However, in these studies, which use human primary samples, it is unclear if decreased mtDNA is directly involved in disease progression or is a consequence of the disease itself. Here, we demonstrate that, in the setting of inflammation-induced tumors, decreases in mtDNA copy and in numbers of mitochondria are directly associated with increased glucose uptake, lactate secretion, and resistance to oxidative stress.

The cause-effect relationship between glycolysis and cancer is controversial. Mitochondria produce ATP through OXPHOS and synthesize key molecules needed for cellular proliferation. Some level of functional mitochondria and mtDNA is necessary for the survival of cancers cells [26]. However, dysfunction of mitochondria in tumor cells through mtDNA mutations and/or reduction in mtDNA copy number alters OXPHOS resulting in increased reliance on aerobic glycolysis [6]. Upregulation of glycolysis produces ATP to compensate for decreased ATP production by mitochondria. Glycolysis also provides intermediates for macromolecular biosynthesis and redox homeostasis [34]. These connections suggest that alterations in mitochondrial functions have a role in initiating or sustaining some tumors [6]. The loss of *Polg* expression in our system directly results in reduced mitochondria and a shift towards increased glycolysis. Importantly, the DNA methylation, reduced *Polg* expression, and decrease in number of mitochondria occur early in the tumorigenesis process (at the earliest time point when we can macroscopically detect tumors) and occur to some extent in all inflammation-induced wildtype MSH2 tumors, we have tested in our model. The strong selective pressure for this process suggests that it results in a survival benefit for cells that harbor DNA hypermethylation of the promoter of *Polg*.

Mitochondria are the major producer of intracellular ROS and reactive nitrogen species (RNS). Damage of mitochondria and impairment of mitochondrial respiratory function enhances ROS release into the cytoplasm [28]. Mitochondria also play a significant role in the induction of apoptosis [35]. While ROS can play a positive role in tumorigenesis, ROS levels above the antioxidant capability of the tumor cells are detrimental [36]. Having fewer mitochondria present in cells at sites of chronic inflammation would result in less mitochondrial damage and therefore potentially less intracellular ROS production and reduced induction of apoptosis. On the other hand, increased redox potential of ETBF Min tumors could account for the increased resistance to ROS. Even though glucose uptake is higher in ETBF than mock tumoroids, the levels of glucose in tumor tissues are not changed significantly suggesting that the additional glucose is rapidly metabolized. Only the upstream metabolite, G-6P, is higher in ETBF Min tumors. The levels of the TCA cycle intermediates and lactate are lower in ETBF Min tumors, and the levels of pyruvate are not changed. The glucose could be metabolized through the pentose phosphate pathway rather than glycolysis, which would result in production of the reducing agent NADPH (nicotinamide adenine dinucleotide phosphate) [34]. However, we found no differences in NADPH or reduced glutathione (GSH) levels between different tumor or tumoroid types (data not shown). While the exact mechanism of increased resistance to ROS needs to be further elucidated, we demonstrate that tumoroids with reduced expression of *Polg* (and consequently fewer mitochondria) are more resistant to oxidative stress suggesting a possible mechanism for the selective advantage for epigenetic silencing of *Polg* during chronic inflammation-induced tumorigenesis.

Conclusions

Polg DNA methylation changes in inflammation-induced colon tumors make them metabolically different from non-inflammation-induced tumors and more resistant to oxidative stress. Understanding the metabolic differences and the role epigenetics plays in establishing and maintaining these differences is important for developing strategies to best treat cancers in patients that are caused by different etiologies. For example, pursuing differences in metabolism by using glycolytic inhibitors against cancer cells with mitochondrial defects may allow for targeted oncology therapeutics.

Additional file

Additional file 1: Figure S1. Additional gene and protein expression in mock and ETBF-induced tumors. A) Gene expression by qPCR relative to mock epithelium from indicated tissue 8 weeks post-infection. Mean ± SEM. $N = 6$. $^*P < 0.05$ compared with mock Min epithelium. $^{\#}P < 0.05$ compared to *Msh2$^{l/l}$VCMin* ETBF tumors. B) Western blots were run using protein isolated from indicated tissue 8 weeks post-infection. Blots are representative of two independent sets of biological replicates. **Figure S2.** *Polg* knockdown in colonoids derived from normal epithelium does not alter glucose uptake. A) *Polg* gene expression by qRT-PCR relative to nontarget (NT) knockdown colonoids derived from wt epithelium. Bar represents mean ± SEM. $^*P < 0.05$. B) DNA from organoids as in A was used in qPCR assays with primer sets specific for a region of mitochondrial DNA or the genomic ApoB. Bars indicate mean ± SEM. $^*P < 0.05$. C) Glucose uptake by tumoroids derived as in A. Mean ± SEM. NS not significant. **Table S1.** Primer sequences for qMSP and mtDNA content and assays used for TaqMan gene expression. **Table S2.** Fold change in expression by RT2 Profiler Glucose Metabolism PCR Array. (DOCX 3724 kb)

Abbreviations

2-DG: 2-Deoxy-D-glucose; AKT: AKT serine/threonine kinase 1; Aldob: Aldolase, fructose-bisphosphate B; Apc: Adenomatous polyposis; EGF: Epidermal growth factor; ETBF: Enterotoxigenic *Bacteroides fragilis*; F2,6BP: Fructose-2,6-biphosphate; G-6P: Glucose-6-phosphate; Gck: Glucokinase; GC-MS: Gas chromatography-mass spectrometry; Glut-1: Glucose transporter 1; GSH: Reduced glutathione; H_2O_2: Hydrogen peroxide; HIF1α: *Hypoxia inducible factor 1 alpha*; HK: Hexokinase; KD: Knockdown; MBD-seq: Methyl CpG-binding domain sequencing; Min: Multiple intestinal neoplasia; MSH2: MutS Homolog 2; *Msh2$^{l/l}$VCMin*: *Msh2$^{lox/lox}$VillinCreMin*; mtDNA: Mitochondrial DNA; MTT: 3-(4,5-Dimethylthiazol-2-yl)-2,5-diphenyltetrazolium bromide); NADPH: Nicotinamide adenine dinucleotide phosphate; NT: Nontarget; OXPHOS: Oxidative phosphorylation; PFK1: Phosphofructokinase 1; PFKFB: 6-Phophofructose-2-kinas/fructose2,6-biphosphatase; Polg: DNA polymerase gamma; Prps1l1: Phosphoribosyl pyrophosphate synthetase 1-Like 1; Pygm: Glycogen phosphorylase, muscle associated; qMSP: Quantitative methylation-specific PCR; RNS: Reactive nitrogen species; ROS: Reactive oxygen species; SEM: Standard error of the mean; TCA: Tricarboxylic acid; TCGA: The Cancer Genome Atlas; TEM: Transmission electron microscopy

Funding

This work was supported by a grant from the NIEHS (R01ES023183 to H.M. O'Hagan). J.M.T. is supported by a NIH R35 Maximizing Investigators' Research Award (MIRA; 1R35GM119557) from NIGMS. The granting agencies had no role in the study or the writing of the manuscript.

Authors' contributions

ARM and HMOH performed the mouse and organoid experiments and analyzed and interpreted the data for them. HL performed the metabolomic analysis and assisted with study design and writing of the manuscript. BDS performed the TEM in a blinded fashion. JMT assisted with the study design and direction and writing of the manuscript. HMOH wrote the majority of the manuscript. All authors read and approved the final manuscript.

Competing interests
The authors declare that they have no competing interests.

Author details
[1]Medical Sciences, Indiana University School of Medicine, Bloomington, Indiana, USA. [2]Department of Biology, Indiana University, Bloomington, Indiana, USA. [3]Indiana University Melvin and Bren Simon Cancer Center, Indianapolis, Indiana, USA.

References
1. Raghuraman S, Donkin I, Versteyhe S, Barrès R, Simar D. The emerging role of epigenetics in inflammation and immunometabolism. Trends Endocrinol Metab. 2016;27:782–95.
2. Johnson C, Warmoes MO, Shen X, Locasale JW. Epigenetics and cancer metabolism. Cancer Lett. 2015;356:309–14.
3. Kinnaird A, Zhao S, Wellen KE, Michelakis ED. Metabolic control of epigenetics in cancer. Nat Rev Cancer. 2016;16:694–707.
4. Pavlova Natalya N, Thompson Craig B. The emerging hallmarks of cancer metabolism. Cell Metab. 2016;23:27–47.
5. Marie SK, Shinjo SM. Metabolism and brain cancer. Clinics (Sao Paulo). 2011;66(Suppl 1):33–43.
6. Wallace DC. Mitochondria and cancer. Nat Rev Cancer. 2012;12:685–98.
7. Hance N, Ekstrand MI, Trifunovic A. Mitochondrial DNA polymerase gamma is essential for mammalian embryogenesis. Hum Mol Genet. 2005;14:1775–83.
8. Stumpf JD, Saneto RP, Copeland WC. Clinical and molecular features of polg-related mitochondrial disease. Cold Spring Harb Perspect Biol. 2013;5:a011395.
9. Chandel NS, Schumacker PT. Cells depleted of mitochondrial DNA (ρ0) yield insight into physiological mechanisms. FEBS Lett. 1999;454:173–6.
10. Lee W, Johnson J, Gough DJ, Donoghue J, Cagnone GLM, Vaghjiani V, et al. Mitochondrial DNA copy number is regulated by DNA methylation and demethylation of polga in stem and cancer cells and their differentiated progeny. Cell Death Dis. 2015;6:e1664.
11. Kelly RD, Mahmud A, McKenzie M, Trounce IA, St John JC. Mitochondrial DNA copy number is regulated in a tissue specific manner by DNA methylation of the nuclear-encoded DNA polymerase gamma A. Nucleic Acids Res. 2012;40:10124–38.
12. TCGA. Comprehensive molecular characterization of human colon and rectal cancer. Nature. 2012;487:330–7.
13. Singh KK, Ayyasamy V, Owens KM, Koul MS, Vujcic M. Mutations in mitochondrial DNA polymerase-gamma promote breast tumorigenesis. J Hum Genet. 2009;54:516–24.
14. Rhee KJ, Wu S, Wu X, Huso DL, Karim B, Franco AA, et al. Induction of persistent colitis by a human commensal, enterotoxigenic bacteroides fragilis, in wild-type c57bl/6 mice. Infect Immun. 2009;77:1708–18. PMCID: PMC2663167
15. Wu S, Rhee KJ, Albesiano E, Rabizadeh S, Wu X, Yen HR, et al. A human colonic commensal promotes colon tumorigenesis via activation of T helper type 17 T cell responses. Nat Med. 2009;15:1016–22. PMCID: PMC3034219
16. Maiuri AR, Peng M, Sriramkumar S, Kamplain CM, DeStefano Shields CE, Sears CL, et al. Mismatch repair proteins initiate epigenetic alterations during inflammation-driven tumorigenesis. Cancer Res. 2017;77:3467–78.
17. Ortega-Cava CF, Ishihara S, Rumi MA, Aziz MM, Kazumori H, Yuki T, et al. Epithelial toll-like receptor 5 is constitutively localized in the mouse cecum and exhibits distinctive down-regulation during experimental colitis. Clin Vaccine Immunol. 2006;13:132–8.
18. Machado TS, Macabelli CH, Sangalli JR, Rodrigues TB, Smith LC, Meirelles FV, et al. Real-time pcr quantification of heteroplasmy in a mouse model with mitochondrial DNA of c57bl/6 and nzb/binj strains. PLoS One. 2015;10:e0133650.
19. Li R, Jia Y, Pan S, Li X, Song H, Zhao R. Glucocorticoid receptor mediates the effect of high-fat diet on mitochondrial oxidative phosphorylation in mouse liver. DNA Cell Biol. 2016;35:51–8.
20. Tennessen JM, Barry WE, Cox J, Thummel CS. Methods for studying metabolism in drosophila. Methods. 2014;68:105–15.
21. Mahe MM, Aihara E, Schumacher MA, Zavros Y, Montrose MH, Helmrath MA, et al. Establishment of gastrointestinal epithelial organoids. Curr Protoc Mouse Biol. 2013;3:217–40.
22. Xue X, Shah YM. In vitro organoid culture of primary mouse colon tumors. J Vis Exp. 2013:e50210.
23. Grabinger T, Luks L, Kostadinova F, Zimberlin C, Medema JP, Leist M, et al. Ex vivo culture of intestinal crypt organoids as a model system for assessing cell death induction in intestinal epithelial cells and enteropathy. Cell Death Dis. 2014;5:e1228.
24. Desai Salil P, Bhatia Sangeeta N, Toner M, Irimia D. Mitochondrial localization and the persistent migration of epithelial cancer cells. Biophys J. 2013;104:2077–88.
25. Clem B, Telang S, Clem A, Yalcin A, Meier J, Simmons A, Rasku MA, et al. Small-molecule inhibition of 6-phosphofructo-2-kinase activity suppresses glycolytic flux and tumor growth. Mol Cancer Ther. 2008;7:110–20.
26. Bensinger SJ, Christofk HR. New aspects of the Warburg effect in cancer cell biology. Semin Cell Dev Biol. 2012;23:352–61.
27. Sato T, Stange DE, Ferrante M, Vries RG, Van Es JH, Van den Brink S, et al. Long-term expansion of epithelial organoids from human colon, adenoma, adenocarcinoma, and Barrett's epithelium. Gastroenterology. 2011;141:1762–72.
28. Boland ML, Chourasia AH, Macleod KF. Mitochondrial dysfunction in cancer. Front Oncol. 2013;3:292.
29. Niwa T, Tsukamoto T, Toyoda T, Mori A, Tanaka H, Maekita T, et al. Inflammatory processes triggered by helicobacter pylori infection cause aberrant DNA methylation in gastric epithelial cells. Cancer Res. 2010;70:1430–40.
30. Cui H, Huang P, Wang Z, Zhang Y, Zhang Z, Xu W, et al. Association of decreased mitochondrial DNA content with the progression of colorectal cancer. BMC Cancer. 2013;13:110.
31. Larman TC, DePalma SR, Hadjipanayis AG, Protopopov A, Zhang J, Gabriel SB, et al. Spectrum of somatic mitochondrial mutations in five cancers. Proc Natl Acad Sci U S A. 2012;109:14087–91.
32. Skonieczna K, Malyarchuk BA, Grzybowski T. The landscape of mitochondrial DNA variation in human colorectal cancer on the background of phylogenetic knowledge. Biochim Biophys Acta. 2012;1825:153–9.
33. Novak EA, Mollen KP. Mitochondrial dysfunction in inflammatory bowel disease. Front Cell Dev Biol. 2015;3:62.
34. DeBerardinis RJ, Chandel NS. Fundamentals of cancer metabolism. Sci Adv. 2016;2:e1600200.
35. Galluzzi L, Kepp O, Kroemer G. Mitochondria: master regulators of danger signalling. Nat Rev Mol Cell Biol. 2012;13:780–8.
36. Jeschke J, O'Hagan HM, Zhang W, Vatapalli R, Calmon MF, Danilova L, et al. Frequent inactivation of cysteine dioxygenase type 1 contributes to survival of breast cancer cells and resistance to anthracyclines. Clin Cancer Res. 2013;19:3201–11.

6

Molecular features that predict the response to antimetabolite chemotherapies

Mahya Mehrmohamadi[1,2,3,4], Seong Ho Jeong[4] and Jason W. Locasale[1,2,3*]

Abstract

Background: Antimetabolite chemotherapeutic agents that target cellular metabolism are widely used in the clinic and are thought to exert their anti-cancer effects mainly through non-specific cytotoxic effects. However, patients vary dramatically with respect to treatment outcome, and the sources of heterogeneity remain largely unknown.

Methods: Here, we introduce a computational method for identifying gene expression signatures of response to chemotherapies and apply it to human tumors and cancer cell lines. Furthermore, we characterize a set of 17 antimetabolite agents in various contexts to investigate determinants of sensitivity to these agents.

Results: We identify distinct favorable and unfavorable metabolic expression signatures for 5-FU and Gemcitabine. Importantly, we find that metabolic pathways targeted by each of these antimetabolites are specifically enriched in its expression signatures. We provide evidence against the common notion about non-specific cytotoxic functions of antimetabolite drugs.

Conclusions: This study demonstrates through unbiased analyses that the activities of metabolic pathways likely contribute to therapeutic response.

Keywords: Antimetabolite chemotherapies, Molecular determinants of response to chemotherapy, Gemcitabine, 5-fluorouracil

Background

Cancer cells adapt their metabolism to meet the requirements of inappropriate growth, survival, and proliferation [1–3]. Since these demands are often not present in normal cells to the same extent, there is considerable interest in exploiting metabolic alterations for therapeutic advances [4, 5]. Antimetabolite chemotherapies are one of the most commonly used therapeutic strategies for the treatment of neoplastic disease [6]. Historically, some of the first successful chemotherapeutic agents were derived from intermediates in the synthesis of folates [7, 8]. Subsequently, there are now at least 17 agents approved in the USA that target a specific metabolic enzyme [9]. These agents can often be tolerated and can achieve remarkable responses in advanced-stage cancers leading to complete remission in many cases. However, the clinical responses to these agents are heterogeneous with patients exhibiting varying degrees of sensitivity or resistance.

To date, there is little molecular information that is used clinically for prognostication for these agents. For instance, 5-fluorouracil (5-FU) is a widely used antimetabolite chemotherapy that interferes with pyrimidine biosynthesis by targeting the enzyme thymidylate synthetase (TYMS). Previous studies that have associated the expression levels of *TYMS* and tumor response to 5-FU have been controversial, and currently, *TYMS* expression is not used as a biomarker in clinical decision-making [10]. Other studies have found *TP53* mutational status a predictor of 5-FU therapy [11, 12]. However, it remains unclear whether the activities of specific pathways that are targeted by 5-FU associate with anti-tumor responses. Notably, a recent metabolomics study provided evidence that pyrimidine homeostasis is disrupted in response to 5-FU suggesting metabolic specificity in determinants of response to this drug [13]. A recent study used a large panel of cell lines from the catalog of somatic mutations

* Correspondence: jason.locasale@duke.edu
[1]Duke Cancer Institute, Duke University School of Medicine, Durham, NC 27710, USA
[2]Duke Molecular Physiology Institute, Duke University School of Medicine, Durham, NC 27710, USA

in cancer (COSMIC) collection and characterized molecular markers of response to hundreds of different drugs [11]. This drug panel included a number of antimetabolite chemotherapies together with a number of other agents grouped as "cytotoxic drugs." This study comprehensively evaluated thousands of molecular features in their ability to act as predictive markers of sensitivity and found the *TP53* mutational status as the most dominant marker for antimetabolite agents such as 5-FU and Gemcitabine. For 5-FU, a handful of copy number variants (CNVs) was also found to be predictive of cell line resistance [11]. However, this study did not explore gene expression beyond only 11 common pathways, which found no significant predictors. It remains to be investigated whether any differences among antimetabolite agents can be captured in gene expression signatures of response and whether such gene expression signatures can add to our power of distinguishing subtypes with heterogeneous therapeutic outcome.

Previous assessments of molecular markers of response to chemotherapy have mostly been carried out in cancer cell lines. The wealth of genomic information on annotated human tumors now publically available through the cancer genome atlas (TCGA) allows for these questions to be addressed in patients in a more systematic way than previously possible. We and others have successfully utilized the TCGA to decipher novel aspects of cancer metabolism using computational approaches that integrate genomic information on thousands of human tumors [14–18]. A previous study applied an unbiased investigation of genomic data on ovarian cancer tumors from the TCGA and specifically looked for prognostic markers of response to Cisplatin using progression-free survival of recipients [19]. Despite difficulties in studying drug response in human patients in the presence of numerous confounding factors and heterogeneity in therapeutic regimens, the unbiased framework introduced in that study provided useful insights on novel genetic and epigenetic subgroups with variable outcome [19]. This motivated us to apply a similar approach to identify gene expression subgroups of response to antimetabolite chemotherapies.

Here, we carry out an investigation of a set of antimetabolite chemotherapies that target metabolic enzymes. These agents target different pathways including folate synthesis, nucleotide metabolism, and glutathione biosynthesis. Instead of analyzing target enzyme expressions, we develop an unbiased approach to identify gene expression signatures of response. Subsequently, we assess specificity and heterogeneity in cell line sensitivities to various antimetabolite agents. Together, our results introduce specific metabolic determinants of response to these agents.

Methods

Discretizing gene expressions and defining favorability scores

We considered TCGA's COAD and PAAD cohorts. Level-3 RNA-seq RSEM gene-normalized counts were downloaded for each tumor through the GDC portal (https://gdc.cancer.gov/). The values were log2 normalized, and in each data set, genes with a count of 2 or smaller in over 80% of the samples were removed as low-count genes. We used the following criteria to discretize the signature gene expression matrix and label expressions "favorable" or "unfavorable" based on their relationship with progression-free survival (PFS; time-zero is date of diagnosis in the corresponding plots). A gene was assigned a value of 1 and was considered favorable if its high expression (higher than median plus half of the standard deviation for that gene) co-occurred with better prognosis (i.e., patient exhibited both high expression and good prognosis based on Cox survival test on the values of expression of a given gene), and a value of − 1 (unfavorable) if its high expression co-occurred with poor prognosis in univariate Cox regression:

$$F\begin{cases} = 1, \text{if Eij} \geq \text{med} + \text{s}/2 \textbf{ and } \text{j} \in \text{good survival} \\ = -1, \text{if Eij} \geq \text{med} + \text{s}/2 \textbf{ and } \text{j} \in \text{poor survival} \\ = 0, \text{otherwise} \end{cases}$$

where Eij represents expression of gene "i" in individual tumor "j."

For discretizing cell line expression data, the following modified scheme was used where cell lines were labeled either "sensitive" or "resistant" to a drug if their IC-50 value was at either extreme of the distribution of IC-50 values for that given drug across all cell lines.

$$F\begin{cases} = 1, \text{if Eij} \geq \text{med} + \text{s}/2 \textbf{ and } \text{j} \in \text{sensitive} \\ = -1, \text{if Eij} \geq \text{med} + \text{s}/2 \textbf{ and } \text{j} \in \text{resistant} \\ = 0, \text{otherwise} \end{cases}$$

where Eij represents expression of gene "i" in cell line "j."

Genome-wide identification of survival-associated expression

Progression-free survival times for TCGA's COAD and PAAD cohorts were obtained through the cBioPortal for cancer genomics. We used cancer progression or patient death as "events" in Cox models and used the last day of follow-up to right censor the data in cases where no event was documented. R packages "survival" was used for univariate survival analyses independently for all genes (Fig. 1a and Fig. 3a).

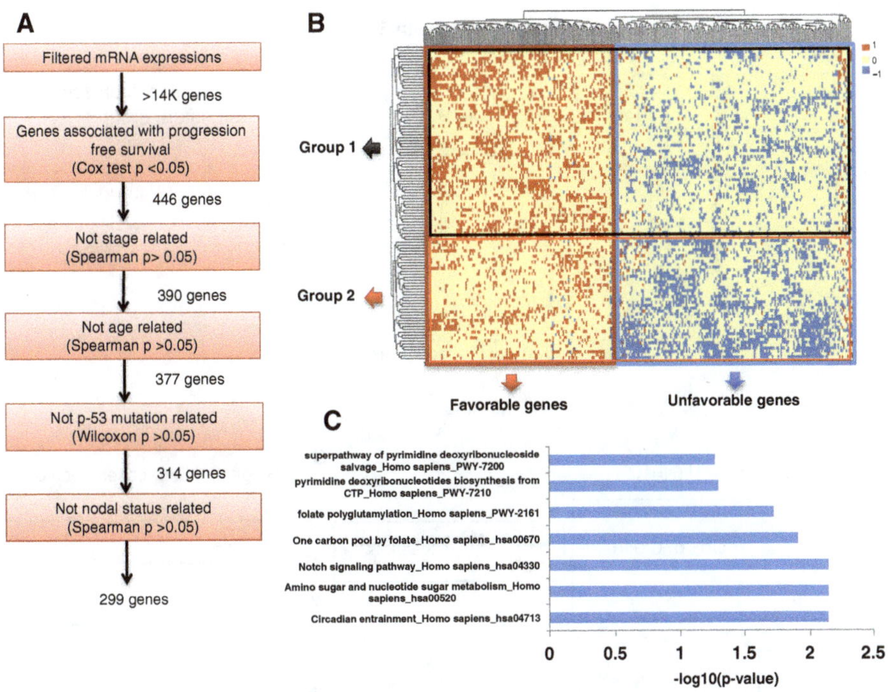

Fig. 1 Combined gene expression signatures of response to 5-FU in colon cancer identify novel subgroups. **a** Schematic of the step-wise filtering used for gene selection in colon cancer (TCGA COAD). **b** Hierarchical clustering of heatmap of the discretized gene favorability scores. Columns represent genes and rows represent individuals. Favorable scores are shown by the color red ($F = 1$), unfavorable by blue ($F = -1$), and neutral by yellow ($F = 0$) (see the "Methods" section). **c** Pathways enriched in the unfavorable gene set. Enrichment p values are calculated using Fisher's exact test (see the "Methods" section)

Survival analysis using gene signatures

When considering survival analysis for subgroups identified by our favorability scoring method (described in the following), we used the subgroup assignments based on the k-means clustering of favorability matrix in each case to label samples as "favorable signature group" and "unfavorable signature group." Subsequently, Cox regression was performed to assess the significance of the difference between PFS of the two groups as shown in Fig. 2a and Fig. 3d.

Cross validation

To assess potential over-fitting of our approach for stratifying response subsets, we repeated the favorability scoring and the subsequent clustering using 5-fold cross validation as follows: we divided the cohort of COAD tumors into five independent test subsets. For each round of cross validation, we left one of the test subsets out and performed the survival analysis as described above only on the remaining four subsets (the training set). We next performed the survival analysis on the test subset using the training set gene expression data to determine "high" and "low" expression thresholds for each gene. The median log likelihood test p value for the significance of the difference between survival rates of the two subsets was $p = 5.706671\text{e-}06$ (with standard deviation of 0.003) on the training and $p = 0.019$ (with standard deviation of 0.017) on the test sets.

Cell line sensitivity analyses

For the COSMIC cell lines, RMA-normalized gene expressions were obtained through the Sanger Institute (http://cancer.sanger.ac.uk/cosmic). Genes with a coefficient of variation of 0.05 or smaller were removed. To test association with drug response, inhibitory concentration (IC-50) values were correlated with gene expression values and a Kendal tau was calculated. Genes with a correlation of over 0.2 and an associated p value of 0.01 or less were selected for subsequent discretization step (Fig. 4a and Additional file 1: Figure S2A).

Gene selection approach

Genes that passed our first filter, i.e., showed a significant association with PFS (Cox p value < 0.05), were subsequently evaluated by additional clinical and genetic attributes. To eliminate genes whose expression levels were significantly affected by *TP53* mutational status, we compared expression levels in *TP53* mutant with *TP53* wild-type samples, and a Wilcoxon non-parametric test was used to assess statistical difference. This test allowed filtering out genes significantly associated with *TP53* mutation. For other clinical attributes, such as cancer

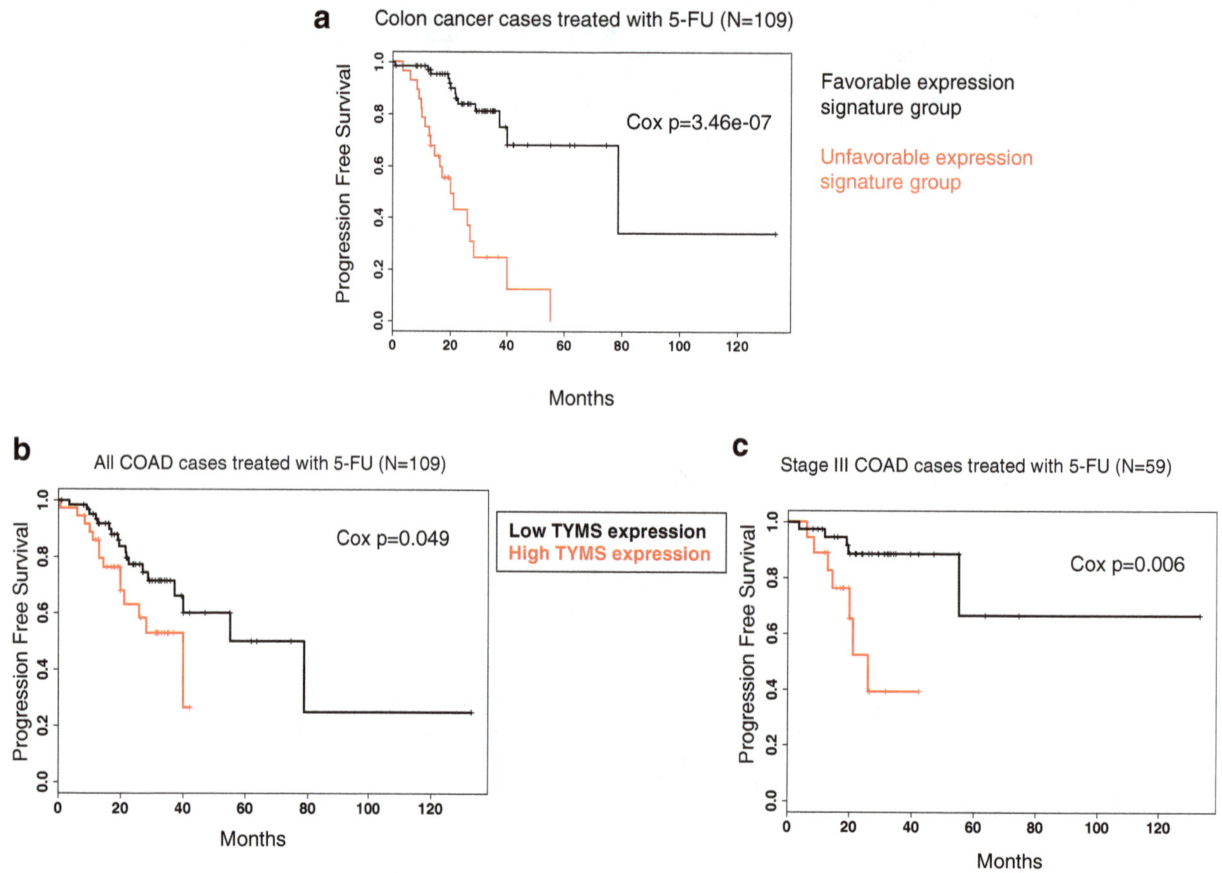

Fig. 2 Relationship between target enzyme expression and response to 5-FU in colon cancer. **a** Kaplan-Meier plot showing progression free survival in the two tumor subgroups identified in Fig. 1b. **b** Kaplan-Meier plot compares progression free survival in high-TYMS expression vs. low-TYMS expression subgroups of TCGA COAD patients. **c** Kaplan-Meier plot compares progression free survival in high-TYMS expression vs. low-TYMS expression subgroups of stage III TCGA COAD patients

stage, patient age, tumor grade, and nodal status, the Spearman correlation was used to test associations between gene expression and these clinical factors across samples. Finally, genes that passed all of the above filters were used for subsequent discretization analyses.

Survival analysis using expression of target enzymes

To assess the strength of direct target enzymes of 5-FU and Gemcitabine as markers of PFS, we considered expression levels of *TYMS* and *RRM1* (*RRM2*), respectively. We first used the function "cutp" in the R package "survMisc" to find the best cutting point in the continuous gene expression. We then used this cutting point as a threshold to divide the samples into two groups of "low" and "high" expression for samples below and above the cut point, respectively.

Independent cross validation for pancreatic cancer

To validate the clinical significance of the gene signatures comprised of 665 genes in pancreatic cancer, we looked at publicly available datasets (Accession: **GSE17891**) of a pancreas cohort comprised of 27 patients. First, we clustered the patients based on their 665 gene signatures by Spearman Rank Correlation Clustering, and there were two distinct clusters. We performed Kaplan-Meier survival analysis based on the clustering, and we found that the gene signature was able to stratify the cohort into two groups with distinct survival outcomes despite the small cohort size ($n = 27$). To compare this result to those of using single gene expression levels, we performed Kaplan-Meier analysis for RRM1 and RRM2. We divided the cohort into half according to RRM1 and RRM2 gene expression levels ($n = 14$ for high gene expression and $n = 13$ for low gene expression).

Pathway enrichment analyses

Pathway enrichment analysis was performed on the resulting gene list for each cancer type using Enrichr [20]. *P* values from the Fisher's exact test are reported for significant ($p < 0.05$) KEGG pathways (and HumanCyc (https://humancyc.org/) pathways for potential metabolic signatures not defined by KEGG pathways in detail).

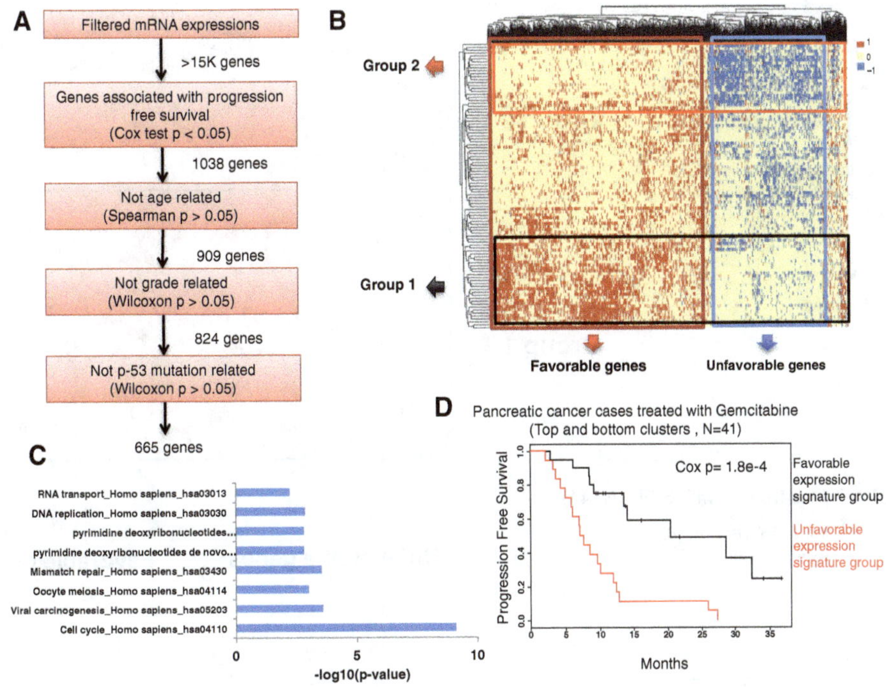

Fig. 3 Combined gene expression signatures of response to Gemcitabine in pancreatic cancer identify novel subgroups. **a** Schematic of the step-wise filtering used for gene selection in pancreatic cancer (TCGA PAAD). **b** Hierarchical clustering of heatmap of the discretized gene favorability scores. Columns represent genes and rows represent individuals. Favorable scores are shown by the color red ($F = 1$), unfavorable by blue ($F = -1$), and neutral by yellow ($F = 0$) (see the "Methods" section). **c** Pathways enriched in the unfavorable gene set. Enrichment p values are calculated using Fisher's exact test. **d** Kaplan-Meier plot showing the progression free survival in the two tumor subgroups identified in part (**b**)

Analyses of non-gene expression cell attributes

We obtained IC-50 values for the 17 antimetabolite compounds across a panel of 60 cell lines from the National Cancer Institute (NCI-60) [21]. To complement our gene expression analyses, we took advantage of the NCI-60 cell line panel where in addition to the comprehensive annotation of cell lines, a previous study has quantified the consumption and release rates (CORE) of hundreds of metabolites by each of these cell lines. We obtained cell volumes, proliferation rates, CORE values, and dose-response sensitivity information (IC-50 values) for 17 antimetabolite drugs across this cell line panel (https://dtp.cancer.gov/discovery_development/nci-60/). CORE values are positive if a metabolite is released into the media by cancer cells and is negative if the metabolite is consumed. The list of these antimetabolic agents is as follows: Gemcitabine, Methotrexate, Pemetrexed, Thioguanine, Thiopurine, Fluorouracil, 5-Fluorouracil deoxyriboside, Hydroxyurea, Ara-C, Azacytidine, Cladribine, Decitabine, Pentostatin, Cytarabine, Fludarabine phosphate, Clofarabine, and Capecitabine.

Growth rate calculations

We obtained growth rate by correcting proliferation rates for volumes. At time zero—right after the cell division, the cell volume (V_0) is the minimum. At time T_1, the cell gets bigger to V_1. If we define growth rate (k_g) as the increase of cell volume per time it takes, we can come up with the equation below:

$$V_1 = V_0 + T_1 k_g$$

At doubling time (T_d), the cell will divide into two, and we assume two divided cells will have the same volume as the initial volume, V_0.

$$V_2 = 2V_0 = V_0 + T_d k_g$$

$$V_0 = T_d k_g \tag{1}$$

$$T_d = \frac{\ln 2}{k_p} \tag{2}$$

$$V_0 = \left(\frac{\ln 2}{k_p}\right) k_g \tag{1,2}$$

We then solved the above equation to obtain the following equation for growth rate:

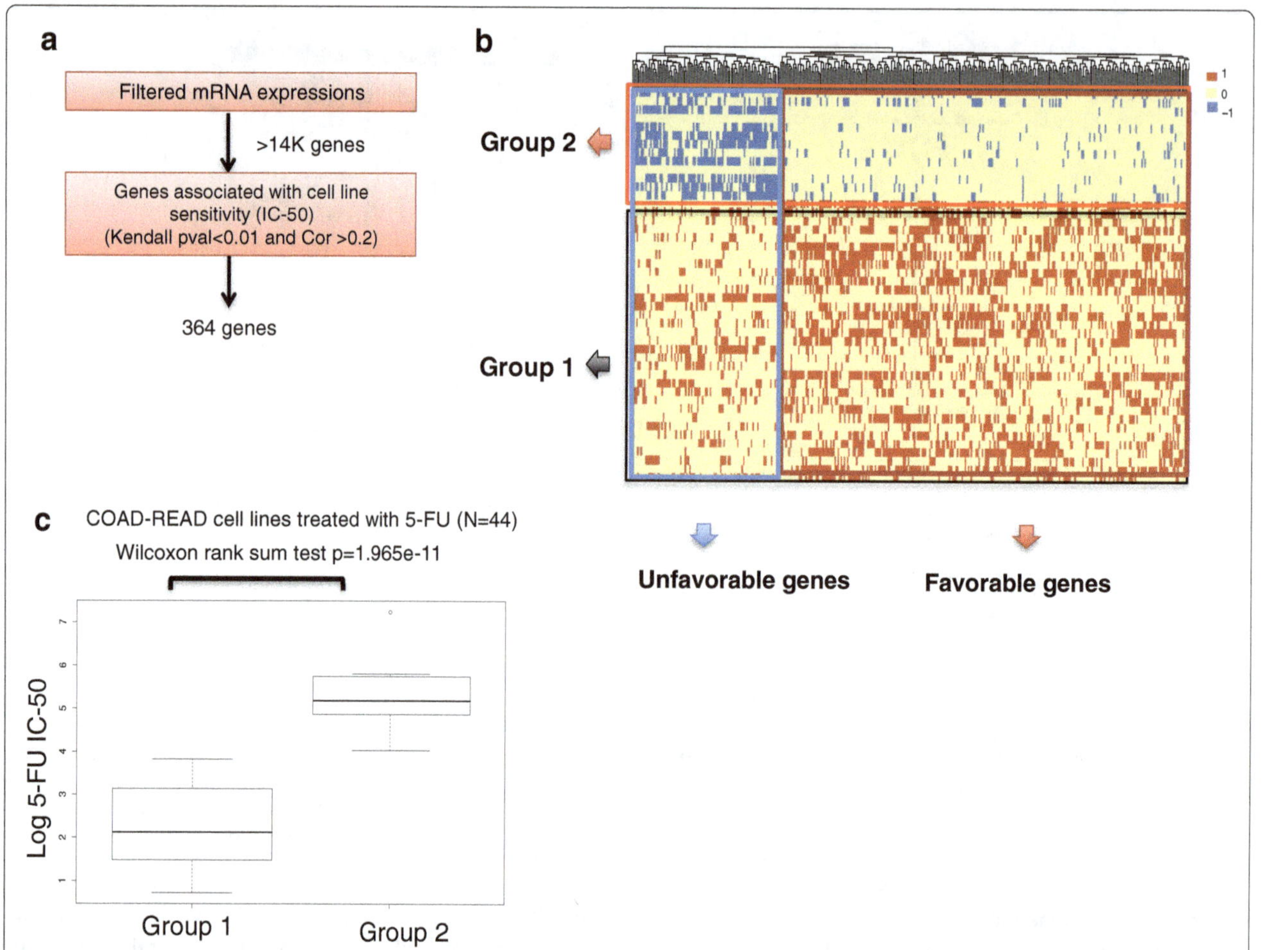

Fig. 4 Combined gene expression signatures of response to 5-FU across colon cancer cell lines identify novel subgroups. **a** Schematic of the step-wise filtering used for gene selection in colon cancer (COSMIC COAD-READ). **b** Hierarchical clustering of heatmap of the discretized gene favorability scores. Columns represent genes and rows represent individuals. Favorable scores are shown by the color red ($F = 1$), unfavorable by blue ($F = -1$), and neutral by yellow ($F = 0$) (see the "Methods" section). **c** Box-plots comparing the resistance to 5-FU (log IC-50 values) between the two cell line subgroups identified in part (**b**) (error bars show the range of the data points in each group)

$$k_g = \frac{V_0 k_p}{\ln 2}$$

Results

Gene expression signatures of patient response to antimetabolite chemotherapies are enriched for metabolic pathways

To identify gene expression signatures associated with patients' response to chemotherapies, we undertook an unbiased genome-wide selection approach adapted and modified from a previous framework [19] (Fig. 1a). We used the TCGA as the source of our clinically annotated genomic data on human tumors [22]. Progression-free survival (PFS), a readily available metric of clinical outcome, was used as a measure of patient response to chemotherapy. TCGA cancer types in which patients were treated with a common antimetabolite agent were considered if both RNA-seq gene expression and follow-up data were available for a large enough cohort of patients ($N > 50$) that would allow quantitative analysis. Since our goal was to identify subtypes of cancer patients with "good response" and "poor response," we considered each cancer type separately. These criteria limited our analyses of human data to 5-FU treatment in colorectal cancers and Gemcitabine treatment in pancreatic cancers (see the "Methods" section). Both of these agents target one-carbon metabolism, a metabolic pathway that has previously been shown to play diverse critical roles in cancer initiation, progression, and pathogenesis [4, 14–16, 23, 24].

A total of 109 colon cancer patients were considered who received adjuvant 5-FU therapy as part of their chemotherapy regimen [22]. For this genome-wide study, we considered all of the genes in the genome after filtering out low-count mRNA expressions (see the

"Methods" section). We first calculated association between expression of each gene with PFS using univariate Cox regression (see the "Methods" section) and excluded genes that did not show a significant ($p < 0.05$) association (Fig. 1a). Next, we considered the remaining 446 genes and further filtered out stage-, age-, *TP53* mutation-, and nodal status-associated genes to eliminate confounding factors that might affect the association of genes with 5-FU response (see the "Methods" section). This filtering leads to a set of 299 genes that were each individually significantly associated with patient response to 5-FU in colon cancer, and their relationship to PFS was independent of stage, age, *TP53* mutation, and nodal status of the tumors (Fig. 1a). Notably, this set included TYMS—the direct target enzyme of 5-FU.

We next set out to assess the combined power of the 299 genes in separating response subgroups. For this, we used a scheme previously proposed by Hsu et al. for DNA methylation [19] and modified the method to apply to gene expression analysis (see the "Methods" section). First, we converted the gene expression matrix into a discretized matrix of "favorability scores," where a gene with high expression in a patient in the better prognosis subgroup was assigned a score of 1 ("favorable"), and a gene with high expression co-occurring with poorer prognosis subgroup was assigned a score of − 1 ("unfavorable"), and all other cases were assigned a score of 0 ("neutral") (see the "Methods" section). The clustered heatmap of the favorability scores discovered distinct subsets of genes (favorable vs. unfavorable) as well as distinct subgroups of patients (Fig. 1b). To assess the functional relevance of the favorable and unfavorable gene signatures, we performed gene set enrichment analysis based on the Kyoto Encyclopedia of Genes and Genomes (KEGG) pathways. The unfavorable gene set was enriched for the following KEGG pathways: circadian entrainment ($p = 7e\text{-}03$); nucleotide sugar metabolism ($p = 7e\text{-}03$); Notch signaling ($p = 7e\text{-}03$); and one-carbon metabolism ($p = 1e\text{-}02$) (Fig. 1c). *TYMS, SHMT2, GALT, RENBP,* and *AMDHD2* were among the metabolic genes that had an unfavorable expression in colon cancer, meaning that their high expression in patients treated with 5-FU was associated with poorer prognosis. Consistent with our results, one-carbon metabolic fluxes have previously been shown to correlate with sensitivity to 5-FU in vitro and in mice [13]. These observations illustrate the importance of specific metabolic target pathways of 5-FU in explaining part of the variability in patient response to this drug. Enrichment analysis on the favorable gene cluster showed enrichment of lipid metabolic KEGG pathways (synthesis of unsaturated fatty acids ($p = 4e\text{-}04$) and fatty acid metabolism ($p = 2e\text{-}03$)), with SCD and ACOX1 fatty acid de-saturases being among the metabolic genes in this group. Lipid synthesis has long been known to increase upon carcinogenesis, producing cellular membrane subunits for rapidly proliferating cells [25]. However, lipidome analyses have shown that the role of fatty acids in cancers are more complex, with an enrichment of saturated fatty acids causing the loss of membrane fluidity, increase in drug resistance, and increase in malignancy of cancer cells [26]. Our results confirm previous studies by identifying fatty acid oxidases and de-saturases SCD and ACOX1 as favorable enzymes, suggesting a role for fatty acid metabolism.

To compare the two patient subgroups identified by our approach, we performed *k*-means clustering on the matrix of favorability scores and identified a distinct subgroup enriched with favorable genes (group 1 in Fig. 1b) and a second subgroup enriched with unfavorable gene expression (group 2 in Fig. 1b) (see "Methods" section). When PFS was compared between these two subgroups, we found a highly significant difference (Cox $p = 3.46e\text{-}07$, hazard ratio (HR) = 6.7; Fig. 2a). Interestingly, when limiting the gene expression signatures to 17 metabolic genes among the 299, we could still see a significant separation (Cox $p = 1.3e\text{-}03$) suggesting that the metabolic genes alone are predictive of outcome. To control for potential bias, we repeated this procedure using 5-fold cross validation. We found the difference between the two subgroups to be significant in all five testing subsets (see "Methods" section). Next, we assessed the power of *TYMS* expression alone in distinguishing response subgroups. For this, we divided tumors into two groups based on their *TYMS* expression level: "low-TYMS" and "high-TYMS" (see "Methods" section). We then compared PFS between the two groups using Cox regression and found a modestly significant difference in response between the low-TYMS and high-TYMS groups ($p = 4.9e\text{-}02$; Fig. 2b). Given that adjuvant 5-FU therapy is usually administered in stage III colon cancer, we repeated this analysis in stage III tumors only ($N = 59$) and found a slightly stronger association ($p = 6e\text{-}03$; Fig. 2c). In both analyses, we found that higher expression of *TYMS* is associated with poorer response to 5-FU therapy, consistent with previous reports [27, 28], possibly explained by larger doses of the drug needed to achieve *TYMS* inhibition in high-expressing tumors. These results show that our scheme of discretizing combined gene expression signatures followed by favorability scoring and clustering is able to identify prognosis subgroups that are significantly more distinct than the subgroups identified based on *TYMS* expression alone, despite *TYMS* being the direct target of 5-FU and gene strongly correlated with drug response. Importantly, our gene expression signatures are not associated with other prominent clinical predictors of prognosis (e.g., age, stage, nodal status, and *TP53* mutation), as we controlled for these confounding factors in the gene selection step (see the "Methods" section; Fig. 1a). This suggests that the gene expression signatures identified here offer additional information about prognosis beyond what is already captured by commonly used clinical metrics. Since metabolism is an interconnected network of reactions that work in concert; thus, the combined activity of multiple connected genes and pathways results in a better reflection of the biological state of a tumor than the activity of individual enzymes.

We next set out to apply our gene expression analysis method to an independent TCGA cohort consisting of pancreatic cancer patients ($N = 100$) who were treated with adjuvant Gemcitabine chemotherapy as part of their chemotherapy regimen. Gemcitabine is another chemotherapeutic agent that targets nucleotide and glutathione metabolism. Gene selection and filtering steps resulted in a set of 665 genes associated with PFS in this cohort after controlling for patient age, tumor grade, and *TP53* mutational status (Fig. 3a). Visualization of a discretized expression heatmap made apparent subsets of favorable and unfavorable genes (Fig. 3b). Pathway analysis of the favorable gene set showed Glycerophospholipid metabolism (p = 1e-04) pathway being enriched, while the following KEGG pathways were enriched in the unfavorable expression signature: mitotic cell cycle and nuclear division (p < 10e-9), viral carcinogenesis (p = 2e-04), mismatch repair (p = 2e-04), apoptosis (p = 8e-03), and Pyrimidine metabolism (p = 1e-02) (Fig. 3c). Notably, the unfavorable gene set included ribunucleotide reductases *RRM1* and *RRM2*—direct targets of Gemcitabine— as well as *DTYMK* and *TK1* in thymidine metabolism and *NT5E* in purine degradation pathways, demonstrating a role for specific target pathways of Gemcitabine in explaining the response to this agent. The favorable gene signature included the following metabolic genes: *PLA2G2D, PLA2G4A, PLA2G4C,* and *PLD2* phospholipases, *LPGAT1, PNPLA6, AGPAT1,* and *AGPAT4.* This observation further supports previous cancer profiling studies that have established important structural and signaling roles for phospholipids in the pathogenesis and malignancy of cancer cells [25].

We next performed *k*-means clustering on the matrix of favorability scores across these 665 genes and identified clear subgroups of patients. Comparison of the subgroup enriched with unfavorable gene expression with that of the favorable subgroup showed a significant difference in PFS (Cox p = 1.8e-04, HR = 3.5; Fig. 3d). When limited to 39 metabolic genes among the 665, we still observed a significant separation of response subgroups (Cox p = 1.3e-04). Notably, when considered individually, *RRM1* and *RRM2* each had far less distinctive power (Cox p = 6e-03 for *RRM1* and p = 5e-03 for *RRM2*; Additional file 1: Figure S1A, B) than the combined gene sets, further confirming the advantage of our approach by considering pathways rather than individual genes. Together, these results show the relevance of metabolic states of tumors in predicting drug response and also confirm the generalizability of this approach in identifying clinically distinct subgroups of cancer patients using gene expression signatures. Finally, our signature of 665 genes was used in a cross validation test from an independent study on 27 pancreatic cancer patients (see "Methods" section) [29]. In this cohort as well, while RRM1 and RRM2 expression were not capable of subdividing patients with respect to survival on Gemcitabine (Additional file 1: Figure S1A, B), our gene signature identified two survival subgroups significantly different in response (Likelihood ratio test = 4.57 on 1 df, p = 0.0326 Additional file 1: Figure S1C; see the "Methods" section).

Analysis of gene expression signatures of response to antimetabolites in cell lines confirms metabolic specificity

Due to limitations in the availability of sufficiently annotated human data with gene expression and follow-up information, we next turned to cancer cell line collections to further test the applicability of our method. We used the catalog of somatic mutations in cancer (COSMIC) cell line set as the largest collection of annotated cancer cell lines and obtained microarray gene expression data as well as drug sensitivity information in the form of 50% of maximal inhibition of cell proliferation (IC-50) for the same agents we had previously tested in human samples (i.e., 5-FU and Gemcitabine). In the case of cell lines, we considered a gene favorable if its high expression co-occurred with higher sensitivity to drug treatment (lower IC-50) and unfavorable if its high expression co-occurred with lower sensitivity (higher IC-50) (see the "Methods" section).

A set of 44 cell lines from colorectal origin was considered. For the gene selection step, we calculated the correlation between expression of every gene in the genome with IC-50 value for 5-FU and selected genes with a Kendall's tau value of 0.2 or larger and a corresponding p value of 0.01 or smaller. A total of 364 genes passed this filter (Fig. 4a). Subsequently, the discretization and favorability scoring approach as described in the previous section was applied to this matrix and the clustering heatmap was visualized (Fig. 4b). Distinct subsets were immediately obvious, with favorable genes enriched in protein processing (p = 4e-05), arginine and proline metabolism (p = 7e-03), and glutathionie metabolism (p = 8e-03), while the unfavorable genes were not significantly enriched in any of the KEGG pathways. Notably, Dihydropyrimidine dehydrogenase (*DPYD*) was the only metabolic gene identified in the unfavorable set, consistent with its biological function [23] and previous reports of its predictive power in 5-FU treated rectal cancers [30].

Next, we compared response to 5-FU between the two subgroups of cell lines identified by *k*-means clustering of the favorability matrix. The subgroup of cells enriched with the unfavorable gene expression signature had a significantly higher IC-50 for 5-FU (higher resistance) than the subgroup enriched with the favorable signature (Wilcoxon test $p = 1.96e\text{-}11$; Fig. 4c). Together, these results confirm the generalizability of this method for identification of novel subgroups with distinct response to 5-FU and also find a specific metabolic target (*DPYD*) as a marker of cell line sensitivity.

We next considered all COSMIC cell lines derived from pancreatic origins regarding their sensitivity to Gemcitabine. This set included only 17 cell lines, limiting the statistical power of this analysis. Only 201 genes passed our initial filtering (Additional file 1: Figure S3A). A visualization of the favorability heatmap illustrated two distinct clusters of genes, one with a mostly favorable expression score, but the second one with heterogeneous scores across the cell lines (Additional file 1: Figure S3B). Pathway analysis of the favorable set identified chemical carcinogenesis ($p = 7e\text{-}03$), glutathionie metabolism ($p = 2e\text{-}02$), and drug metabolism ($p = 4e\text{-}02$) KEGG pathways significantly enriched, while the unfavorable set was enriched in adherens junctions ($p = 5e\text{-}03$), cacterial invasion ($p = 6e\text{-}03$), and glycophospholipid synthesis ($p = 7e\text{-}03$). Finally, comparison of sensitivity to Gemcitabine between two of the cell line subgroups with distinct signatures revealed a significant difference in IC-50 (Wilcoxon p value = 8e-04; Additional file 1: Figure S3C), showing the power of this approach even when applied to very small data sets. Overall, our analyses of response to 5-FU and Gemcitabine in cell lines also confirmed relevance of metabolic determinants of response; however, we did not observe a perfect correspondence between the markers identified in human studies and those identified in cell lines. This result is important given that the majority of experiments aimed at drug response are typically performed in cell line settings. Our results suggest that cell line IC-50 values do not perfectly mimic cancer outcome in response to chemotherapies in patients. This is perhaps partly due to culture conditions and other limitations with using cell lines as models for cancer and partly explained by the fact that unlike the controlled experimental settings, the majority of patients underwent combination chemotherapies that could partially confound statistical analyses.

Signatures of response to antimetabolite agents exhibit specificity and variability

So far, our results have shown considerable contribution from the metabolic gene expression network in distinguishing drug response subsets within human tumors as well as cancer cell lines. Careful consideration of two nucleotide metabolism inhibitors—5-FU in colon and Gemcitabine in pancreatic cancers—revealed subtle differences in gene expression signatures associated with favorable and unfavorable response in each case, suggesting antimetabolite agents exert their function through different cellular pathways in these tissues and therefore be associated with different clinical markers.

Our approach utilized gene expression levels of metabolic enzymes as surrogates for metabolic fluxes or enzyme activities in tumors. Next, we attempted to complement our results by taking advantage of direct metabolite measurements across a panel of 60 cancer cell lines (NCI-60). We calculated correlation between the metabolic activities in the form of consumption or release rates (CORE) as previously reported [31], and IC-50 values of 17 antimetabolite compounds (see the "Methods" section; Fig. 5a). Interestingly, the release rate of phosphocholine showed a strong negative correlation with sensitivity to six of the antimetabolite agents tested (Fig. 5a). This result suggests that cells that have a higher rate of phosphocholine production are less sensitive to drug treatments, consistent with our gene expression results showing the enrichment of phospholipid metabolic genes in response signatures. Previous studies have shown that an increase in phosphatidylcholine affects cancer cell membrane dynamics and correlates with higher tumor malignancy and poorer overall survival [25]. Our results agree with previous reports suggesting high activity of enzymes that degrade phosphatidylcholine renders cells more sensitive to drug treatments, potentially contributing to a more favorable outcome for chemotherapy [25]. An example of a specific interaction that was detected at the level of metabolite consumption and release was the case of Fludarabine—a purine analog—that was significantly associated with CORE of 2-deoxycytidine (Fig. 5a). Together, these results identify relationships between directly measured metabolic signatures of cancer cells and their sensitivity to antimetabolite chemotherapies, and also demonstrate variability among the 17 antimetabolites tested regarding their interaction with cellular metabolism.

The gene expression results suggest that despite common cytotoxic effects of antimetabolite agents, they might have distinct biological markers in cells that are specific to their functions. Furthermore, the analysis of metabolic CORE profiles in cell lines suggested that markers of sensitivity to antimetabolite agents might be more variable than previously appreciated. This motivated us to further assess specificity of determinants of response across a large set of antimetabolite agents. We

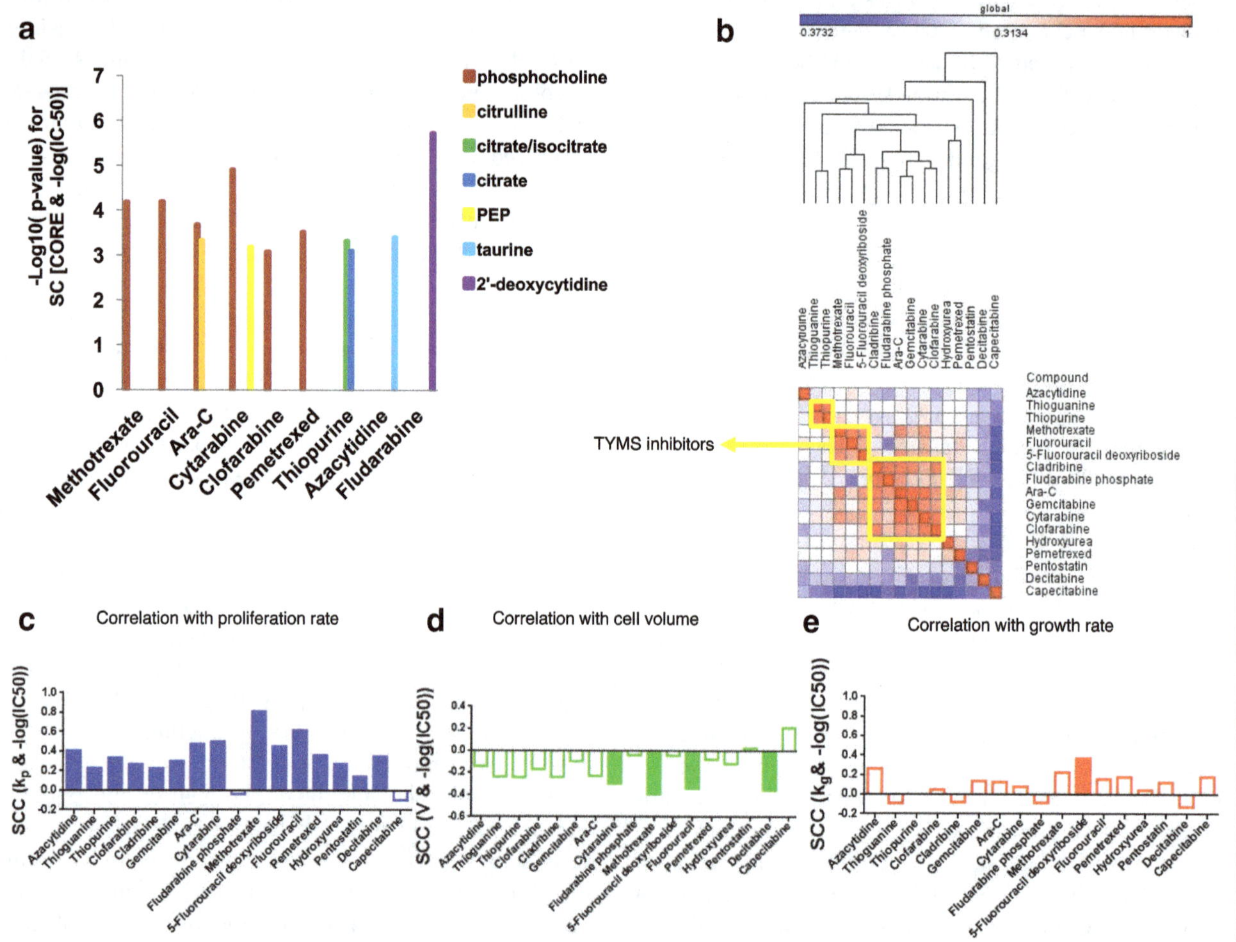

Fig. 5 Analysis of additional determinants of sensitivity to antimetabolite agents demonstrates variability among these agents. **a** The significance of association between metabolic profiles (consumption and release rates (CORE)) and sensitivity to drugs (– log (IC-50)) was assessed using Spearman correlations (SC) across the NCI-60 cell line panel. The *y*-axis shows negative log-10 of the corresponding correlation *p* values for only the significant associations found (*q* value < 0.05). **b** Hierarchical clustering of the Pearson similarity matrix between the IC-50 values of 17 antimetabolite agents across the NCI-60 panel. The diagonal shows correlation of each drug with itself (= 1). The *yellow boxes* show three distinct clusters of drugs. **c** Spearman correlation coefficient (SCC) between proliferation rate (kp) and sensitivity to each drug (– log (IC-50)) is shown. *Solid bars* show significant correlations (FDR-corrected *q* value < 0.05). **d** Spearman correlation coefficient (SCC) between cell volume (V) and sensitivity to each drug (– log (IC-50)) is shown. Solid bars show significant correlations (FDR-corrected *q* value < 0.05). **e** Spearman correlation coefficient (SCC) between growth rate (kg) and sensitivity to each drug (– log (IC-50)) is shown. *Solid bars* show significant correlations (FDR-corrected q-value < 0.05)

considered a set of 17 antimetabolite chemotherapeutic compounds (see the "Methods" section). These agents target enzymes involved in a number of metabolic pathways including de novo nucleotide metabolism, amino acid metabolism, and glutathione metabolism. To assess the extent of correlation in the sensitivities of cell lines to these compounds, we computed a similarity matrix of pairwise Pearson correlations between the IC-50 values for antimetabolite. Three distinct clusters were identified by hierarchical clustering: a cluster including Thiopurine and Thioguanine, a cluster for an anti-folate Methotrexate (MTX) and pyrimidine analogs (5-FU and 5-FUDR), and a cluster for other purine analogs (Fig. 5b). The antimetabolite compounds in the second cluster shared TYMS as a target enzyme. This analysis suggests that in general, compounds with common mechanisms of action tend to have similar sensitivity profiles across cell lines, suggesting some degree of specificity in response to antimetabolites.

A common notion is that cytotoxicity of antimetabolite chemotherapies occurs in all rapidly dividing cells and thus lacks specificity. It has also been proposed that cell size, cell proliferation, and cellular metabolism are invariably coupled [21]. Given that data on proliferation rate, cell size, and metabolic profiles are readily available for the NCI-60 cell lines, we sought to re-investigate these relationships in the context of association with cell line sensitivities to antimetabolite agents. Spearman rank correlations between IC-50 and proliferation rate were computed and revealed significant positive correlations

(q values < 0.05 in all cases except Capecitabine and Fluodarabine phosphase; Fig. 5c). When the cell volumes were correlated with responses to antimetabolites, all compounds except for Capecitabine showed a negative correlation (four compounds had q value < 0.05) (Fig. 5d). Together, these results confirm that cytotoxicity, as defined as the concentration of drug needed to achieve toxic dosages, is lower with smaller cells that also tend to divide more rapidly due to their size [21]. The significant negative correlation between proliferation rate and cell volume suggested that to obtain an overall growth rate corresponding to the rate of synthesis of macromolecules, the proliferation rate should be corrected for cell volume (see the "Methods" section). We next correlated dose responses with the volume-corrected proliferation rate, referred to hereinafter as the "growth rate" (Fig. 5e). The strong correlations that were observed between IC-50 values and proliferation rate were absent when considering the growth rates (Fig. 5e). This suggests that although cytotoxicity of antimetabolite agents appears highly nonspecific with selectivity pertaining only to proliferation rate, these effects are completely removed when considering an overall growth rate. Importantly, a recent study independently demonstrated that growth rate inhibition normalizations correct for confounders in measuring cell line sensitivity to cancer drugs [32]. Together, our results provide evidence that unlike the common notion, variation in response to antimetabolite agents is not explained solely by differences in the rates of production of macromolecules in cells (i.e., growth rate), but is also explained by specific factors related to the functions of these agents in cells.

Discussion

The specificity of antimetabolite chemotherapeutic agents has unclear, and previous reports have been controversial around prognostic values for expression levels of target enzymes for most of these agents. Given that the metabolic network is composed of complex interactions between multiple enzymes and pathways, we hypothesized that perhaps by defining gene signatures instead of individual enzyme markers, we would gain power in distinguishing subgroups of tumors with differential response to therapy.

Here, we introduced an unbiased approach for the assessment of combined prognostic power of expression of multiple genes and used this platform to define favorable and unfavorable signatures. Notably, we showed that these signatures allow for distinguishing novel "poor prognosis" (high progression rate) from "good prognosis" (low progression rate) subgroups far more robustly than individual target genes. Importantly, since the gene selection steps control for expression differences related to other important clinical and genetic attributes of response, we are assured that the gene signature analysis captures information about response subgroups beyond the already established markers.

In both studied cases of 5-FU in colon cancer and Gemcitabine in pancreatic cancer, we found that expression of metabolic pathways related to direct targets of the drugs is enriched in the unfavorable gene set. This confirmed that tumors with higher activity of target pathways require higher doses of drug to elicit the inhibitory response and are therefore more resistant to treatment. However, our results discovered that metabolic state of cells are not fully reflected in the expression levels of individual target enzymes but rather captured more robustly in the collection of functionally and chemically linked enzymes in pathways. Although we were only able to illustrate the applicability of our method in two independent cohorts of human tumors due to data limitations, results suggest generalizability of this method to other antimetabolite agents as well.

Gene signatures associated with favorable and unfavorable response to 5-FU and Gemcitabine exhibited functional similarities overall, but distinct markers for each drug were also discovered. In both cases of 5-FU and Gemcitabine, high expressions of the target metabolic pathways (i.e., nucleotide metabolism) were associated with unfavorable outcome, while high expression of lipid metabolizing pathways was associated with favorable outcome. These results point to common general mechanisms of cellular response to these drugs. However, a deeper look into specific genes and pathway within the signatures for 5-FU and Gemcitabine identified some differences. For instance, while "One-carbon metabolism" and "Nucleotide sugar metabolism" were identified as the unfavorable signature for 5-FU, "Pyrimidine metabolism" was discovered in the case of Gemcitabine. Furthermore, *TYMS* was among the unfavorable genes for 5-FU, while *RRM1* and *RRM2* were among the unfavorable genes for Gemcitabine. Together, these results suggest that despite similarities in overall mechanisms of action, antimetabolite agents have specific biological markers that have not been very well characterized and appreciated in the past.

Our complementary analyses of cancer cell line sensitivities to the same chemotherapeutic agents also proved useful in identifying distinct subgroups using the gene signature approach. Other than lipid metabolic genes, the gene sets identified as favorable and unfavorable signatures in cell lines did not completely match those identified from the analysis of response in patients. The main sensitivity predictor in vitro seemed to be "Glutathione metabolism" and "Drug metabolism" that were found in cases of 5-FU and Gemcitabine to be associated with favorable outcome (i.e., higher sensitivity of cells to drug treatment). This observation is consistent with previous reports showing a critical role for glutathione metabolism in detoxification and protection against drugs in vitro [33]. These results illustrated that despite the availability and convenience of using cell lines as models of human tumors for drug response studies, analysis of patient tumors is advantageous in that it provides insights that are not fully reflected in cancer cell lines, potentially due to unwanted effects of culture media. This lack of concordance between in vitro and in vivo gene signatures can be interpreted as either differences in resistance mechanisms or differences in the gene expression correlates of resistance in vivo and in vitro.

Together, our analyses of human tumors and cancer cell lines elucidated considerable variability among different antimetabolite agents, as well as specificity in metabolic markers of sensitivity to them. These demonstrate that despite the common notion, different classes of antimetabolite agents vary according to their distinct cellular functions. Our results suggest that potentially important biological markers of response to antimetabolite compounds exist, and a better understanding of these factors will provide useful insights for clinical decision-making. Notably, we showed that gene expression signatures have significant power to capture part of the previously unexplained variation in patients' responses to 5-FU and Gemcitabine in colon and pancreatic cancers, respectively. Future studies using larger cohorts of human tumors with well-annotated patient follow-up information can provide valuable additional insights about antimetabolite response signatures. Importantly, metabolism can not only be targeted with new drugs, but also by repurposing approved metabolic drugs for cancer therapy [34]. In general, drugs that target cellular metabolism are of new clinical interest [35], and future studies similar to this work are needed to shed light on identification of patient subgroups that are likely to benefit from antimetabolite therapies.

Conclusions

This study demonstrates through unbiased analyses of multiple independent datasets that the activity of metabolic pathways likely contributes to the therapeutic response to antimetabolite chemotherapeutic agents that target these pathways. Importantly, we show that information captured by the metabolic network has the potential of stratifying patients beyond the ability of common markers currently used in the clinic such as tumor grade and cancer stage. Areas of translational relevance of these findings include novel biomarker design based on the metabolic network, and also identification of patients who are likely to benefit from antimetabolite chemotherapies. Together, results presented in this manuscript are of significant interest to the cancer and metabolism research communities and have important and immediate clinical implications for treatment decision-making.

Additional file

Additional file 1: Supplementary Figures. **Figure S1.** Relationship between target enzyme expression and response to Gemcitabine in TCGA pancreatic cancer. A) Kaplan-Meier plot compares progression free survival in high-RRM1 expression vs. low-RRM1 expression subgroups of TCGA PAAD patients. B) Kaplan-Meier plot compares progression free survival in high-RRM2 expression vs. low-RRM2 expression subgroups TCGA PAAD patients. **Figure S2.** Relationship between target enzyme expression and survival in an independent pancreatic cancer cohort. A) Kaplan-Meier plot compares overall survival in high-RRM1 expression vs. low-RRM1 expression subgroups of patients. B) Kaplan-Meier plot compares overall survival in high-RRM2 expression vs. low-RRM2 expression subgroups of patients. C) Kaplan-Meier plot compares overall survival in subgroups of patients divided based on our gene signature (see Methods). **Figure S3.** Identifying gene expression signatures of sensitivity to Gemcitabine in pancreatic cancer cell lines. A) Schematic of the step-wise filtering used for gene selection in pancreatic cancer (COSMIC PAAD). B) Hierarchical clustering heatmap of the discretized gene favorability scores. Columns represent genes and rows represent individuals. Favorable scores are shown by the color red (F=1), unfavorable by blue (F= -1), and neutral by yellow (F=0) (see Methods). C) Box-plots comparing the resistance to Gemcitabine (log IC-50 values) between the two cell line subgroups identified in part B (error bars show the range of the data points in each group). (DOCX 225 kb)

Abbreviations

5-FU: 5-fluorouracil; CNVs: Copy number variants; CORE: Consumption and release rates; COSMIC: Catalog of somatic mutations in cancer; IC-50: Inhibitory concentration; MTX: Methotrexate; PFS: Progression-free survival; TCGA: The cancer genome atlas; TYMS: Thymidylate synthetase

Funding

This work was supported by grants R01CA193256 and P30CA014236 to J.W.L. from the National Institutes of Health (NIH). MM was supported by F99 CA212457 from the NCI and a Graduate Fellowship from the Duke University School of Medicine.

Authors' contributions

JWL and MM designed the study. MM performed all human analyses and wrote the manuscript. SJ performed the analyses of drug response in cell lines. JWL supervised the project and revised the manuscript. All authors read and approved the final manuscript.

Competing interests

The authors declare that they have no competing interests.

Author details

[1]Duke Cancer Institute, Duke University School of Medicine, Durham, NC 27710, USA. [2]Duke Molecular Physiology Institute, Duke University School of Medicine, Durham, NC 27710, USA. [3]Department of Pharmacology and Cancer Biology, Duke University School of Medicine, Durham, NC 27710, USA. [4]Department of Molecular Biology and Genetics, Field of Genetics, Genomics and Development, Cornell University, Ithaca, NY 14853, USA.

References

1. Pavlova NN, Thompson CB. The emerging hallmarks of cancer metabolism. Cell Metab. 2016;23:27–47.

2. Schulze A, Harris AL. How cancer metabolism is tuned for proliferation and vulnerable to disruption. Nature. 2012;491:364–73.
3. DeBerardinis RJ, Chandel NS. Fundamentals of cancer metabolism. Sci Adv. 2016;2:e1600200.
4. Locasale JW. Serine, glycine and one-carbon units: cancer metabolism in full circle. Nat Rev Cancer. 2013;13:572–83.
5. Hirschey MD, et al. Dysregulated metabolism contributes to oncogenesis. Semin Cancer Biol. 2015;35(Suppl):S129–50.
6. Chabner BA, Roberts TG Jr. Timeline: chemotherapy and the war on cancer. Nat Rev Cancer. 2005;5:65–72.
7. Farber S, Diamond LK. Temporary remissions in acute leukemia in children produced by folic acid antagonist, 4-aminopteroyl-glutamic acid. N Engl J Med. 1948;238:787–93.
8. Farber S. Some observations on the effect of folic acid antagonists on acute leukemia and other forms of incurable cancer. Blood. 1949;4:160–7.
9. Cheung-Ong K, Giaever G, Nislow C. DNA-damaging agents in cancer chemotherapy: serendipity and chemical biology. Chem Biol. 2013;20:648–59.
10. Showalter SL, et al. Evaluating the drug-target relationship between thymidylate synthase expression and tumor response to 5-fluorouracil. Is it time to move forward? Cancer Biol Ther. 2008;7:986–94.
11. Iorio F, et al. A landscape of pharmacogenomic interactions in cancer. Cell. 2016;166:740–54.
12. Kandioler D, et al. TP53 mutational status and prediction of benefit from adjuvant 5-fluorouracil in stage III colon cancer patients. EBioMedicine. 2015;2:825–30.
13. Ser Z, et al. Targeting one carbon metabolism with an antimetabolite disrupts pyrimidine homeostasis and induces nucleotide overflow. Cell Rep. 2016;15:2367–76.
14. Nilsson R, et al. Metabolic enzyme expression highlights a key role for MTHFD2 and the mitochondrial folate pathway in cancer. Nat Commun. 2014;5:3128.
15. Mehrmohamadi M, Mentch LK, Clark AG, Locasale JW. Integrative modelling of tumour DNA methylation quantifies the contribution of metabolism. Nat Commun. 2016;7:13666.
16. Mehrmohamadi M, Liu X, Shestov AA, Locasale JW. Characterization of the usage of the serine metabolic network in human cancer. Cell Rep. 2014;9:1507–19.
17. Madhukar NS, Warmoes MO, Locasale JW. Organization of enzyme concentration across the metabolic network in cancer cells. PLoS One. 2015;10:e0117131.
18. Hu J, et al. Heterogeneity of tumor-induced gene expression changes in the human metabolic network. Nat Biotechnol. 2013;31:522–9.
19. Hsu FH, et al. Reducing confounding and suppression effects in TCGA data: an integrated analysis of chemotherapy response in ovarian cancer. BMC Genomics. 2012;13(Suppl 6):S13.
20. Chen EY, et al. Enrichr: interactive and collaborative HTML5 gene list enrichment analysis tool. BMC Bioinformatics. 2013;14:128.
21. Dolfi SC, et al. The metabolic demands of cancer cells are coupled to their size and protein synthesis rates. Cancer Metab. 2013;1:20.
22. Cancer Genome Atlas, N. Comprehensive molecular characterization of human colon and rectal cancer. Nature. 2012;487:330–7.
23. Shaul YD, et al. Dihydropyrimidine accumulation is required for the epithelial-mesenchymal transition. Cell. 2014;158:1094–109.
24. Kottakis F, et al. LKB1 loss links serine metabolism to DNA methylation and tumorigenesis. Nature. 2016;539:390–5.
25. Beloribi-Djefaflia S, Vasseur S, Guillaumond F. Lipid metabolic reprogramming in cancer cells. Oncogene. 2016;5:e189.
26. Rysman E, et al. De novo lipogenesis protects cancer cells from free radicals and chemotherapeutics by promoting membrane lipid saturation. Cancer Res. 2010;70:8117–26.
27. Hu YC, et al. Thymidylate synthase expression predicts the response to 5-fluorouracil-based adjuvant therapy in pancreatic cancer. Clin Cancer Res. 2003;9:4165–71.
28. Wakasa K, et al. Dynamic modulation of thymidylate synthase gene expression and fluorouracil sensitivity in human colorectal cancer cells. PLoS One. 2015;10:e0123076.
29. Collisson EA, et al. Subtypes of pancreatic ductal adenocarcinoma and their differing responses to therapy. Nat Med. 2011;17:500–3.
30. Huang MY, et al. DPYD, TYMS, TYMP, TK1, and TK2 genetic expressions as response markers in locally advanced rectal cancer patients treated with fluoropyrimidine-based chemoradiotherapy. Biomed Res Int. 2013;2013:931028.
31. Jain M, et al. Metabolite profiling identifies a key role for glycine in rapid cancer cell proliferation. Science. 2012;336:1040–4.
32. Hafner M, Niepel M, Chung M, Sorger PK. Growth rate inhibition metrics correct for confounders in measuring sensitivity to cancer drugs. Nat Methods. 2016;13:521–7.
33. Traverso N, et al. Role of glutathione in cancer progression and chemoresistance. Oxidative Med Cell Longev. 2013;2013:972913.
34. Liu X, Romero IL, Litchfield LM, Lengyel E, Locasale JW. Metformin targets central carbon metabolism and reveals mitochondrial requirements in human cancers. Cell Metab. 2016;24:728–39.
35. Chan AT. Metformin for cancer prevention: a reason for optimism. Lancet Oncol. 2016;17:407–9.

7

Protein interaction and functional data indicate MTHFD2 involvement in RNA processing and translation

Costas Koufaris[1,2,3] and Roland Nilsson[1,2,3*]

Abstract

Background: The folate-coupled metabolic enzyme MTHFD2 is overexpressed in many tumor types and required for cancer cell proliferation, and is therefore of interest as a potential cancer therapeutic target. However, recent evidence suggests that MTHFD2 has a non-enzymatic function which may underlie the dependence of cancer cells on this protein. Understanding this non-enzymatic function is important for optimal targeting of MTHFD2 in cancer.

Methods: To identify potential non-enzymatic functions of MTHFD2, we defined its interacting proteins using co-immunoprecipitation and mass spectrometry and integrated this information with large-scale co-expression analysis, protein dynamics, and gene expression response to MTHFD2 knockdown.

Results: We found that MTHFD2 physically interacts with a set of nuclear proteins involved in RNA metabolism and translation, including components of the small ribosomal subunit and multiple members of the RNA-processing hnRNP family. Interacting proteins were also in general co-expressed with MTHFD2 in experiments that stimulate or repress proliferation, suggesting a close functional relationship. Also, unlike other folate one-carbon enzymes, the MTHFD2 protein has a short half-life and responds rapidly to serum. Finally, shRNA against MTHFD2 depletes several of its interactors and yields an overall transcriptional response similar to targeted inhibition of certain ribosomal subunits.

Conclusions: Taken together, our findings suggest a novel function of MTHFD2 in RNA metabolism and translation.

Keywords: Interactome, Moonlighting, Heat shock proteins, RNA, Non-metabolic

Background

Altered metabolism is a hallmark of cancer cells that facilitates their growth and survival [1]. In particular, metabolism of folate-coupled one-carbon groups is reprogrammed in a wide variety of cancers [2–4]. One-carbon metabolism is localized into cytosolic, mitochondrial, and nuclear compartments (Fig. 1) and is required for the synthesis of purines, dTMP, and remethylation of homocysteine to methionine. Extensive evidence now supports that proliferating cancer cells primarily rely on the mitochondrial catabolism of serine via SHMT2 as their main source of one-carbon groups [5–7], rather than the corresponding cytosolic enzymes. The reason for this preference is unclear, but may be due to the mitochondrial NADH/NAD ratio favoring flux in the oxidative direction [8], or related to the associated reduction of NAD and NADP [7]. In the nucleus, the formate produced by the mitochondrial pathway supports synthesis of dTMP during DNA replication.

Within mitochondrial folate one-carbon metabolism, the enzyme MTHFD2 has attracted considerable attention as a potential target for cancer therapeutics [4, 9, 10], motivated by a favorable expression profile with high expression in various human tumor types [4] but low or undetectable levels in most adult tissues. The normal function of MTHFD2 may be in embryogenesis, since the enzyme has long been known to be highly expressed and essential during embryonic development [11], and a paralogous mitochondrial enzyme, MTHFD2L, is expressed in normal adult tissues [12]. Expression of MTHFD2 in tumors also correlates with poor disease outcome in

* Correspondence: roland.nilsson@ki.se

[1]Cardiovascular Medicine Unit, Department of Medicine, Karolinska Institutet, SE-171 76 Stockholm, Sweden

[2]Division of Cardiovascular Medicine, Karolinska University Hospital, SE-171 76 Stockholm, Sweden

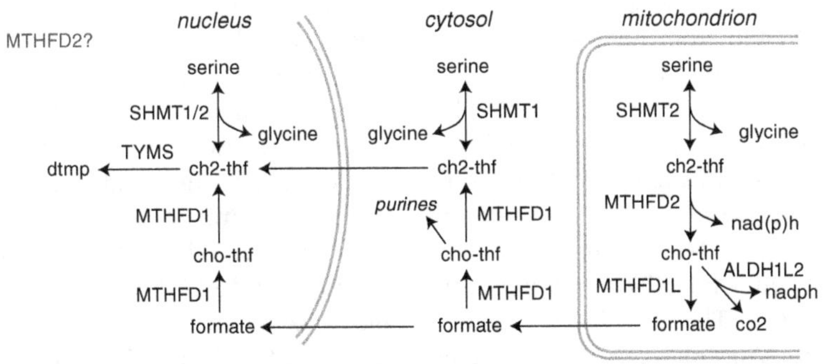

Fig. 1 Schematic diagram of enzymes, metabolites, and compartmentalization of folate one-carbon metabolism. One-carbon metabolism enzymes are now known to be present and active in three distinct compartments, the nucleus, mitochondria, and cytosol, linked by the flow of formate between them. The function of MTHFD2 in the mitochondria is well understood, although its function in the nucleus is not known

breast cancer [13], liver cancer [14], and acute myeloid leukemia (AML) [10]. Knockdown of MTHFD2 can inhibit cancer cell proliferation in vitro [4, 10, 15] and reduces (but does not abolish) tumor growth in vivo [7, 10]. This combination of specific expression in transformed cells and severe cell phenotypes upon knockdown render MTHFD2 a compelling potential drug target.

Nevertheless, several observations suggest that the known metabolic function of MTHFD2 may not be the sole explanation for its prominent role in cancer. First, supplementing cultures with formate, the primary product of the mitochondrial pathway (Fig. 1), fails to rescue MTHFD2 knockdown cancer cells [4, 10], indicating that another function of the MTHFD2 protein might be necessary for growth. Second, cells can rapidly adapt to loss of MTHFD2 by shifting to the cytosolic one-carbon pathway [7], suggesting a degree of redundancy where flux through the mitochondrial pathway is not strictly essential. Third, knockdown of the SHMT2 enzyme, which should also block the mitochondrial pathway, does not cause cell death unless glycine is removed [2, 16]. Moreover, the MTHFD2 protein was recently found to be present in the nucleus at sites of newly synthesized DNA, and over-expression of catalytically inactive MTHFD2 drives cell proliferation [17], suggestive of a role in signaling/regulation rather than metabolism. Knockdown of MTHFD2 also affects invasion and migration in vitro [14, 18], although no obvious mechanistic link exists between one-carbon metabolism and these phenotypes.

Given these observations, it is becoming clear that the effective targeting of the MTHFD2 protein requires a better understanding of its role in cancer cells beyond metabolism. Although chemical inhibitors of the MTHFD enzymatic activity have been reported [19, 20], different strategies may be required if a non-enzymatic function of the MTHFD2 enzyme is critical for cancer cells. For these reasons, we performed an initial investigation of the possible non-metabolic functions of MTHFD2 by mapping the protein's interacting partners, co-expression pattern and the transcriptional responses to knockdown. Taken together, our results suggest a previously unrecognized role for MTHFD2 in RNA metabolism and translation.

Methods

Cell culture

HCT-116 cell lines were obtained from the National Cancer Institute. The MTHFD2 CRISPR$^{-/-}$ knockout (D2-KO) and parental wildtype (WT) HCT-116 cells were obtained from the lab of Dr. Rabinowitz [7]. Cells were grown in RPMI-1640 medium supplemented with 5% FBS (Life technologies) and Penicillin/Streptomycin (Gibco) and maintained at 37 °C and 5% CO_2.

For serum starvation experiments, 200,000 cells were plated in six-well plates. The next day, the medium was removed, the cells were washed with PBS and then serum-free RPMI-1640 medium was added. Cyclohexamide was obtained from Sigma Aldrich (C4859). For the serum re-stimulation experiments, after 48 h of serum starvation, wells were washed with PBS and then fresh RPMI-1640 containing 20% FBS was added to the cells.

Real-time PCR

RNA was isolated from cells using the Qiagen RNeasy mini kit and quantified using a Nanodrop ND-1000 spectrophotometer. The RNA was reverse transcribed to cDNA using the VILO cDNA synthesis kit (Invitrogen). The qPCR reactions were performed in triplicate on a StepOne Real-Time PCR machine (Thermo Fisher Scientific) using the Fast SYBR Green master mix (Thermo Fisher Scientific). Oligos were ordered from Sigma Aldrich. Primer sequences are listed in Additional file 1. Relative amounts of mRNA were calculated using the $\Delta\Delta C_T$ method normalized to RPLPO mRNA as a reference.

Immunoblotting

Total protein was isolated from cells using RIPA buffer (Thermo Fisher Scientific), with the addition of × 100

Halt protease inhibitors (Thermo Fisher Scientific) just prior to the extraction. Protein from nuclear and cytosolic cellular compartments were fragmented as described previously [17]. Protein levels were quantified by the BCA assay (Pierce). Equal amounts of protein (10–20 μg) were loaded per lane of 10% SDS-PAGE gel. The following primary antibodies were incubated overnight: anti-MTHFD2 (Proteintech 12270-1-AP); anti-MTHFD1 (Proteintech 6113-1-AP); anti-MTHFD1L (Proteintech 10794-1-AP); Lamin A/C (Thermo Fisher Scientific MA3-1000); HSP60 (Abcam ab46798); Tubulin (Abcam ab6046); and COX IV (Abcam 33985). Quantification of protein bands was performed using the ImageJ software and values were normalized to tubulin for each sample.

Co-immunoprecipitation

WT and D2-KO HCT-116 cells were lysed using the moderate Pierce IP lysis buffer (Thermo Fisher Scientific) with addition of × 100 Halt protease inhibitors (Thermo Fisher Scientific). All steps were performed at 4 °C to reduce protein disassociation. The protein lysate was quantified using the BCA assay, and 1 or 2 mg of lysate was used for immunoprecipitation with no cross-linkage. Immunoprecipitation was performed using two separate anti-MTHFD2 antibodies (Proteintech 12270-1-AP (AP) and Genetex N1C3 (NC)) or an anti-rabbit immunoglobulin (IgG) (Santa Cruz). The immunoprecipitation was performed at 4 °C for 2 h using Dynabeads Protein A (Thermo Fisher Scientific) following the manufacturer's instructions.

In-gel digestion and mass spectrometry

Immunoprecipitated proteins were eluted from Dynabeads through a combination of elution buffer and heating and separated on a 10% SDS gel. In-gel staining of proteins was performed using the SilverQuest silver staining kit (Thermo Fisher Scientific). Protein lanes were excised manually and in-gel digested using a MassPREP robotic protein-handling system (Waters, Millford, MA, USA). Gel pieces were distained twice with 100 μL of 50 mM ammonium bicarbonate (AmBic) containing 50% acetonitrile at 40 °C for 10 min. Proteins were reduced with 10 mM DTT in 100 mM Ambic for 30 min at 40 °C and alkylated with 55 mM iodoacetamide in 100 mM AmBic at 40 °C for 20 min followed with in-gel digestion with 0.3 μg trypsin (sequence grade, Promega, Madison, WI, USA) in 50 mM at 40 °C AmBic for 5 h. The tryptic peptides were extracted with 1% formic acid in 2% acetonitrile, followed by 50% acetonitrile twice. The liquid was evaporated to dryness, and the peptides were reconstituted in 10 μL of 2% acetonitrile/0.1% formic acid. Five microliters of the samples was injected onto the LC-MS/MS system (Ultimate™ 3000 RSLCnano chromatography system and Q Exactive HF Orbitrap mass spectrometer, Thermo Scientific). The peptides were separated on an Easy-C18 column, 50 cm (Thermo Fisher Scientific) at 55 °C in a 120-min gradient at a flow rate of 300 nL/min. The linear gradient was from 5 to 26% of buffer B (98% acetonitrile/0.1% formic acid) in 115 min and to 95% of buffer B in 5 min.

We used data-dependent acquisition with a survey scan range of 300 to 1650 m/z, at a resolution of 120,000 m/z and selected up to 16 most abundant features with a charge state ≥2 for HCD fragmentation at a normalized collision energy of 26 and a resolution of 30,000 at m/z 200. To limit repeated sequencing, dynamic exclusion of sequenced peptides was set to 90 s. Thresholds for ion injection time and ion target values were set to 250 ms and 5 × 106 for the survey scans, and 120 ms and 2 × 105 for the MS/MS scans. Data were acquired using the Xcalibur software (Thermo Fisher Scientific). The spectra were analyzed using the Mascot search engine v. 2.4 (Matrix Science Ltd., UK) using carbamidomethylation (C) as fixed and deamidation (NQ), oxidation (M) as variable modification. The precursor mass tolerance was set to 10 ppm while MS/MS tolerance was 0.02 Da allowing 2 missed cleavages. The SwissProt database was used with taxonomy limited to *Homo sapiens*.

In total, we performed 12 Co-IP experiments (for HCT-116 WT, 4 using AP antibody, 2 using NC antibody, and 2 using IgG antibody; for HCT-116 D2-KO, 2 using AP antibody and 2 using NC antibody) followed by MS analysis. A protein was considered as high confidence if at least two unique peptides were detected in 50% of IP-MS samples for each of the MTHFD2 antibodies used and was not detected in any of the IP-MS samples from D2-KO cells, nor the IgG isotype control IP-MS samples.

Protein-protein interaction network

A protein-protein interaction network was extracted from the STRING database v10.5 [21] using the set of MTHFD2 interacting proteins identified here. Only experimental data (e.g., from co-purifications and yeast two hybrids) imported in STRING from primary sources were used for constructing the network. Threshold for connections between proteins was set at medium score (more than 0.400) as calculated in STRING, and gene ontology (GO) enrichment was calculated.

Half-life analysis

For half-life analysis, we used publicly available data on global protein half-life in NIH3T3 cells [22], HeLa, and C2C12 cells [23]. The list of 1652 proteins involved in metabolism were obtained from Recon2 [24] model of human metabolism, of which 596 were measured in HeLa, 575 in C2C12, and 605 in NIH3T3.

Co-expression analysis

Calculation of gene co-expression was performed using a clustering-based method, as described previously [17]. Briefly, we analyzed 25,485 genes represented on a variety of microarray platforms for co-expression with MTHFD2 across 8097 human, mouse and rat data sets obtained from the Gene Expression Omnibus (GEO). From the resulting matrix of coexpression scores x_{gd}, we computed the overall coexpression score w_g for each gene g by simply summing over all data sets d. We selected the 50 data sets showing highest coexpression for the D2PPI genes by scoring each data set by the weighted sum $\sum_g w_g x_{gd}$, where g ranges over the 29 genes in the D2PPI gene set; and similarly for the ATF4 gene set (Fig. 3b). Example data sets from GEO (Fig. 3c–f) were analyzed as deposited on GEO, with no further normalization. In cases where multiple probes against a single gene were present on the arrays, the probe with highest mean signal across all samples was used. Enrichment analysis was done using the GSEA-P statistic [25], and an enrichment p value was calculated by gene permutation (10,000 permutations). An independent analysis was made using the SEEK tool (http://seek.princeton.edu) with default settings [26].

Connectivity Map (CMap) analysis

Expression data from the Connectivity Map (CMap) project in Level 5 (signature) GCTX format was obtained from GEO (accession GSE92742), and data for 99 experiments with five distinct shRNA hairpins against MTHFD2 across 12,328 measured genes was extracted using R v.3.3.3 and the cmapR package (https://github.com/cmap/cmapR). Since the three hairpins TRCN0000036550, TRCN0000036551, and TRCN0000036553 exhibited strongest knockdown on MTHFD2 itself, these were used for subsequent analysis. Data from the ASC and NPC cell lines were discarded due to few replicates. The z-scores for the remaining 9 cell lines were averaged into a final z-score vector, which was used for enrichment analysis using the GSEA-P statistic [25]. The genesets examined were downloaded from ConsensusPathDB collection (http://cpdb.molgen.mpg.de/). An enrichment p value was calculated by gene permutation (10,000 permutations).

Connectivity scores between hairpins targeting three one-carbon enzymes included in CMap (MTHFD2, MTHFD1, and SHMT1) and hairpins targeting 3799 examined genes were analyzed using the CMap online tools (https://clue.io/cmap). Connectivity scores of more than 90 or less than −90 were considered as significantly enriched. Clustering analysis of connectivity scores was performed using ClustVis [27] with average linkage and correlation metric. Ribosomal genes were selected for analysis based on the KEGG ribosome gene set (entry hsa03010).

RNAi and CRISPR screening data analysis

Global RNAi and CRISPR screening data were performed as part of the Achilles project in 501 and 342 cell lines respectively [28, 29]. We also examined a second CRISPR study conducted in 14 AML cell lines [30]. To identify genes with similar dependencies across examined cell lines in the RNAi and CRISPR screens, we calculated Pearson's correlation for MTHFD2 against all examined genes in both datasets.

Results

Protein interaction partners of MTHFD2

Since a non-metabolic function of MTHFD2 would likely involve direct physical contact with other proteins, we decided to first perform co-immunoprecipitation (Co-IP) of MTHFD2-interacting proteins followed by mass spectrometry (MS) to identify its binding partners. To avoid potential artifacts due to unspecific antibody binding, we chose to perform Co-IP experiments in wildtype (WT) and CRISPR MTHFD2 knockout (D2-KO) HCT-116 cells [7], using two distinct MTHFD2 antibodies, 12270-1AP (AP; Proteintech) and N3C3 (NC; Genetex) as well as an isotype control (IgG) antibody (Fig. 2a). We first confirmed by immunoblotting and IP that the MTHFD2 protein was absent from D2-KO cells (Additional file 2). Next, we performed Co-IP followed by SDS-PAGE and silver-staining to verify the efficient immunoprecipitation of MTHFD2. This analysis revealed a strong band at the expected size of MTHFD2, as well as a large number of other immunoprecipitated protein bands (Fig. 2b). In D2-KO cells, the MTHFD2 band was not detected, but other protein bands were still observable, presumably due to non-specific binding of the antibodies used (Additional file 2). Detected peptide fragments in all examined Co-IP lysates are listed in Additional file 3. Reassuringly, MTHFD2 itself was reliably identified from WT cells using both antibodies and strongly decreased in the D2-KO lysates (Fig. 2c).

We defined high-confidence MTHFD2-interacting proteins as those that were reliably detected by Co-IP in WT but not D2-KO cells, using both the AP and NC antibodies, and were also absent from IgG lysates (Fig. 2a; Methods). With these criteria, we identified 29 MTHFD2-interacting proteins, from here on referred to as the D2PPI gene set (Table 1). The majority of these proteins have been reported to localize to the nucleus, consistent with previous evidence that MTHFD2 is also a nuclear protein [17]. While two mitochondrial RNA-binding proteins were present (LRPPRC; HSPA9), we found no other one-carbon enzymes among the

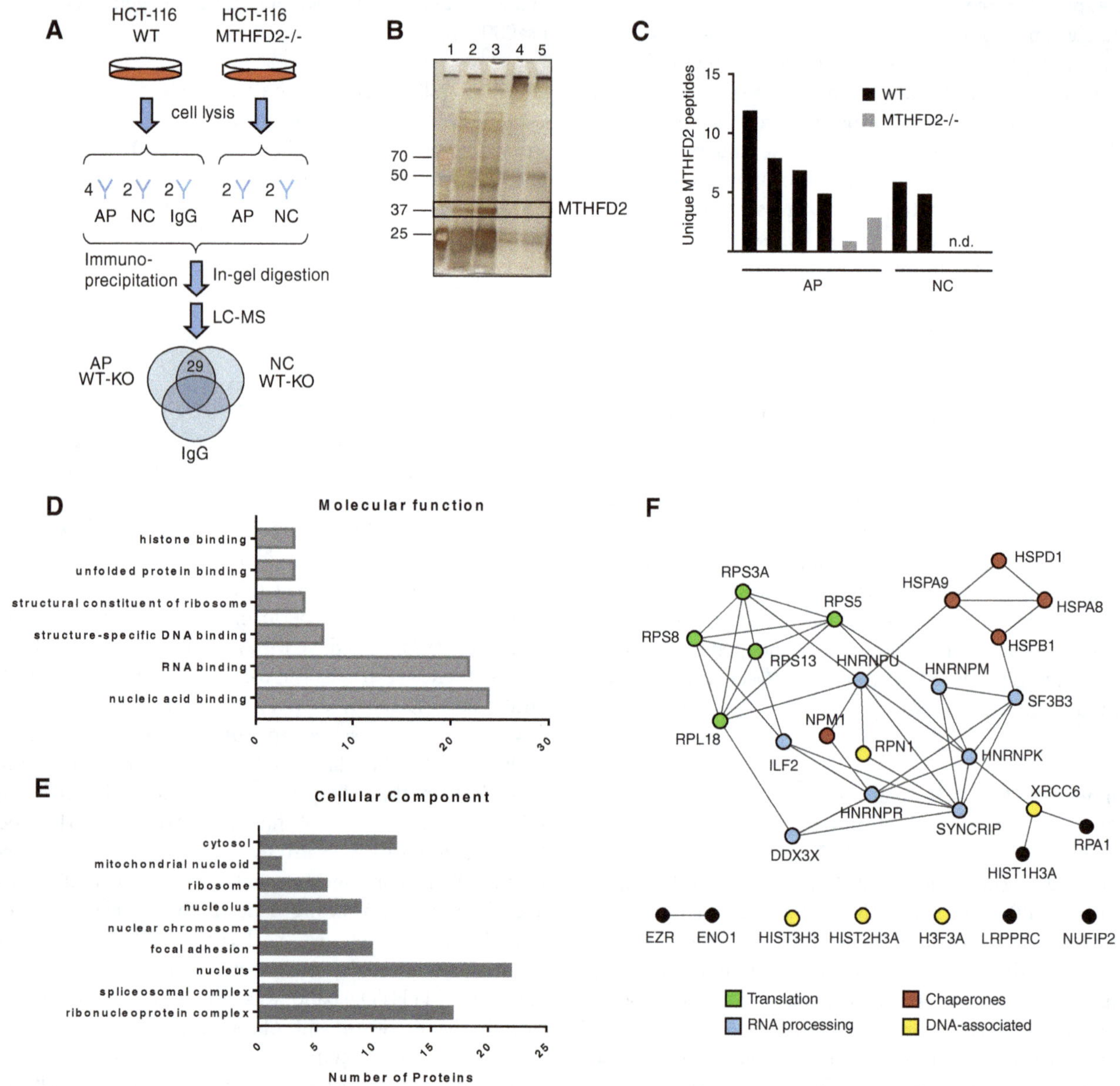

Fig. 2 Defining the MTHFD2 interactome. **a** Schematic of the strategy used for identifying MTHFD2 interactors. Immunoprecipitation was performed on parental HCT-116 cells (WT) and MTHFD2 knockout cells (D2-KO) using either one of two anti-MTHFD2 antibodies (AP and NC) or an anti-rabbit immunoglobulin (IgG) antibody. The numbers above antibody names indicate the number of replicate experiments performed for a given condition. After in-gel digestion and MS 29 proteins were found to be detected in IP from both anti-MTHFD2 antibodies in parental HCT-116 cells but not in IP performed in MTHFD2 knockout cells or using IgG antibody. **b** Representative silver-stained SDS-gel containing co-immunoprecipitated samples. Lane 1 contained a molecular weight ladder. Lane 2 and 3 lysates from wildtype HCT-116 cells after immunoprecipitation with anti-MTHFD2 antibody, lanes 4 and 5 lysates from same cells immunoprecipitated using anti-rabbit IgG antibody. **c** Number of unique peptides matching to MTHFD2 identified in replicate experiments with two anti-MTHFD2 antibodies in WT or knockout D2-KO cells. **d, e** Selected significantly enriched GO Molecular Function and Cellular Component respectively. **f** PPI network generated for 29 identified MTHFD2 interactors using experimental evidence in STRING database and medium confidence links (> 0.400). Nodes with no interaction are not shown. Thickness of edges represent strength of evidence supporting interaction. Members of protein functional groups are indicated according to color chart

D2PPI proteins. We did detect MTHFD1 using the AP antibody, but this protein was found in D2-KO cells as well, indicating that this interaction is due to unspecific binding. Hence, MTHFD2 does not appear to participate in the previously reported nuclear thymidylate synthesis complex [31].

Gene Ontology (GO) analysis of these proteins confirmed a highly significant enrichment of RNA binding proteins (24/29 proteins; $q < 10^{-20}$) (Fig. 2d; Additional file 4) and that a large fraction of these proteins were also nuclear (Fig. 2e). To determine if the D2PPI proteins

Table 1 MTHFD2 protein interactors identified by CoIP and MS

Symbol	Name	AP	NC	RNA binding	Unfolded protein binding	DNA Binding
HSPA8	Heat shock cognate 71 kDa protein	3/4	1/2	X	X	
HSPA9	Stress-70 protein, mitochondrial	3/4	1/2	X	X	
HSPB1	Heat shock protein beta-1	3/4	1/2	X		
HSPD1	60 kDa heat shock protein	3/4	1/2	X	X	X
NPM1	Nucleophosmin	2/4	1/2	X	X	
HIST1H3A	Histone H3.1	2/4	1/2			X
HIST2H3A	Histone H3.2	2/4	1/2			X
HIST3H3	Histone H3.1 t	2/4	1/2			X
H3F3A	Histone H3.3	2/4	1/2			X
XRCC6	X-ray repair cross-complementing protein 6	2/4	1/2	X		X
RPA1	Replication protein A 70 kDa DNA-binding subunit	2/4	1/2			X
HNRNPK	Heterogeneous nuclear ribonucleoprotein K	2/4	1/2	X		X
HNRNPM	Heterogeneous nuclear ribonucleoprotein M	3/4	1/2	X		
SYNCRIP	Heterogeneous nuclear ribonucleoprotein Q	2/4	1/2	X		
HNRNPR	Heterogeneous nuclear ribonucleoprotein R	2/4	1/2	X		
HNRNPU	Heterogeneous nuclear ribonucleoprotein U	2/4	2/2	X		X
SF3B3	Splicing factor 3B subunit 3	2/4	1/2	X		
LRPPRC	Leucine-rich PPR motif-containing protein, mitochondrial	3/4	1/2	X		X
ILF2	Interleukin enhancer-binding factor 2	2/4	1/2	X		X
NUFIP2	Nuclear fragile X mental retardation-interacting protein 2	2/4	1/2	X		
DDX3X	ATP-dependent RNA helicase DDX3X	2/4	1/2	X		X
RPL18	60S ribosomal protein L18a	2/4	1/2	X		
RPS13	40S ribosomal protein S13	2/4	1/2	X		
RPS3A	40S ribosomal protein S3a	2/4	1/2	X		
RPS5	40S ribosomal protein S5	2/4	1/2	X		
RPS8	40S ribosomal protein S8	2/4	1/2	X		
ENO1	Alpha-enolase	2/4	1/2	X		X
EZR	Ezrin	2/4	1/2	X		
RPN1	Dolichyl-diphosphooligosaccharide--protein glycosyltransferase subunit 1	2/4	1/2	X		

Numbers indicate the unique peptides mapped to protein in given CoIP replicate

belonged to any known complexes, we extracted a protein-protein interaction (PPI) network over these 29 proteins from the STRING database [21]. We obtained 47 physical interactions, which is two times more than expected by chance ($p < 10^{-7}$); hence, the D2PPI proteins are likely part of previously known protein complexes, including the small ribosomal subunit proteins (four RPS proteins), RNA processing proteins (several hnRNP family members; SF3B3; ILF2), protein chaperones (several heat shock proteins; NPM1), and histone/DNA repair proteins (three histone proteins; XRCC6; RPN1) (Fig. 2f). Hence, the proteins shown here to directly interact with MTHFD2 indicate a role for the protein in metabolism and translation of RNA.

Co-expression analysis of MTHFD2 and interacting proteins

To systematically assess if the D2PPI proteins indeed share a common function with MTHFD2, we next asked whether their mRNAs are also frequently co-expressed with MTHFD2. We have previously shown that frequent co-expression across diverse experimental conditions is highly predictive of closely related biological function [32, 33]. Using a previously described method [17], we scored 25,845 genes for co-expression with MTHFD2 in 8067 human, rat, and mouse microarray datasets (Additional file 5). Remarkably, D2PPI gene set was clearly enriched for coexpression with MTHFD2 ($p = 0.003$, permutation test), with 13 of 29 of genes within the 95th percentile of coexpression scores (Fig. 3a). An exception was the histone proteins H3F3A, HIST1H3A, HIST3H3,

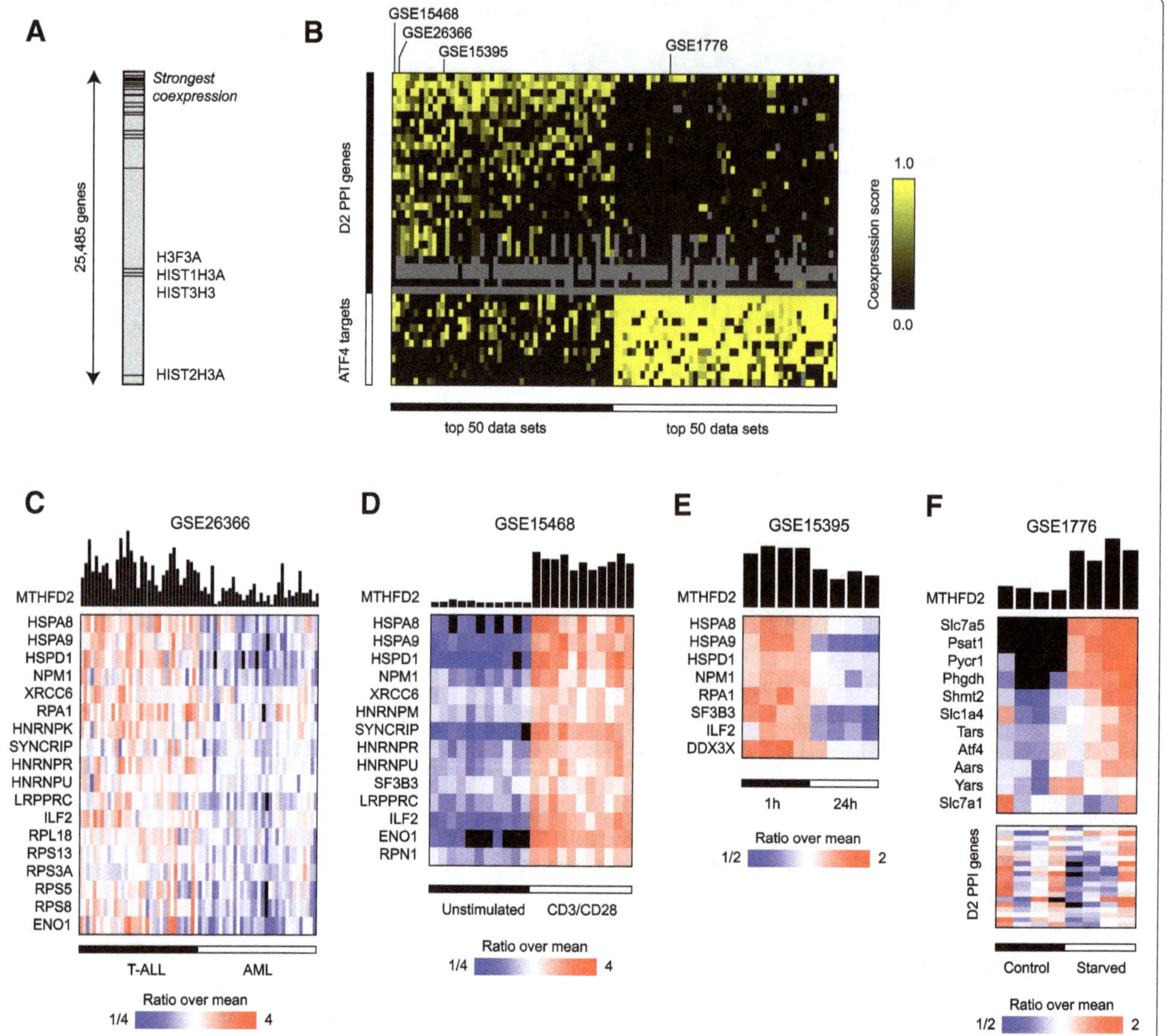

Fig. 3 MTHFD2-interacting proteins are coexpressed with MTHFD2 in response to stimuli. **a** Enrichment plot showing the ranks of MTHFD2-interacting (D2PPI) proteins ordered by overall coexpression with MTHFD2 across 8067 gene expression data sets (see Methods). **b** Heat map of coexpression score for the D2PPI and ATF4 gene sets, across the 50 data sets exhibiting with strongest coexpression for each set. Data sets selected for panels **c**–**f** are indicated by arrows. **c**–**f** Heat maps of expression level for selected data sets. For each gene, ratio over the overall mean is shown, according to scale bars. Only genes with nonzero coexpression scores are shown. MTHFD2 expression level is shown above in linear scale, with baseline equal to zero (arbitrary units)

and HIST2H3A that did not exhibit co-expression with MTHFD2; however, these proteins were not well-represented on the microarrays used, so this result may reflect low power to detect coexpression. An independent analysis of 3356 human gene expression datasets using the SEEK gene co-expression analysis tool [26] gave similar results (Additional file 5). To investigate factors that might drive the observed coexpression of the D2PPI gene set, we identified specific gene expression data sets where this set was coexpressed (Fig. 3b, Additional file 6). Among the top scoring data sets were several tumor gene expression studies, where expression varied between subtypes; for example, in one leukemia study, highest expression was found in T-ALL and lowest in AML subtypes, suggesting specific disease contexts where the D2PPI proteins may be relevant (Fig. 3c). We also noted a concerted induction of the D2PPI proteins in stimulated T cells (Fig. 3d), in line with previous observations of MTHFD2 induction in this setting [4], and also suppression of D2PPI genes in HCT-116 cancer cells in response to treatment with a CDK inhibitor (Fig. 3e). These data indicate that MTHFD2 and the D2PPI genes are frequently coexpressed and responsive to mitogenic stimuli and anti-proliferative drugs.

As previously shown [17], a set of ATF4-responsive mRNAs involved in amino acid metabolism and aminoacyl-tRNA synthesis, including the mitochondrial folate-coupled enzymes SHMT2 and MTHFD1L, was also strongly co-expressed with MTHFD2. However, we found that these genes co-express with MTHFD2 in different conditions than the MTHFD2-interacting proteins (Fig. 3b, Additional file 6), suggesting that the underlying mechanism is different. For example, the mitochondrial enzymes were induced in contexts of amino acid starvation, possibly reflecting the involvement of this pathway in amino acid synthesis, while the D2PPI genes were not (Fig. 3f). In summary, the D2PPI genes are co-regulated with MTHFD2 in specific biological conditions, providing independent evidence that they share a biological function with MTHFD2, which appears to be distinct from ATF4-driven induction of MTHFD2.

MTHFD2 is a rapidly regulated protein with a short half-life

Given the above finding that MTHFD2 and the D2PPI gene set is acutely regulated by pro- and anti-proliferative stimuli, we examined in more detail the dynamics of MTHFD2 regulation. Generally, metabolic enzymes are long-lived proteins, while proteins involved in RNA metabolism, cell cycle, and signaling have shorter half-lives [22]. In a reanalysis of global protein half-life data [22, 23], we noted that the half-life of the MTHFD2 protein was consistently within 17–22 h in HeLa, C2C12, and NIH3T3 cells, which was markedly lower than the other folate one-carbon enzymes (Fig. 4a) and within the 5–10th percentile of all detected enzymes (as defined by Recon2 [24]; 596–605 enzymes were detected across three cell lines) (Fig. 4b). We confirmed this short half-life of MTHFD2 by treatment with the cyclohexamide inhibitor of protein synthesis, which resulted in an approximate halving of protein levels after 24 h (Fig. 4c). Therefore, MTHFD2 is unusually short-lived for a metabolic enzyme in general, and one-carbon enzymes in particular.

Considering the short half-life of MTHFD2, we next examined the regulation of the MTHFD2 protein compared to other enzymes in the mitochondrial folate pathway. In HCT-116 cells, after 48 h serum starvation, MTHFD2 and SHMT2 mRNA was significantly decreased, while SHMT1, MTHFD1, and MTHFD1L was unaffected (Fig. 4d). At the protein level, MTHFD2 and MTHFD1L decreased noticeably at the 24 h time point, while MTHFD1 did not (Fig. 4e), consistent with the shorter half-life of MTHFD2. In serum restimulated HCT-116 cells, MTHFD2 protein was induced within 3 h (Fig. 4f), consistent with our previous report [17]. Moreover, induction of the protein was observed in both the nuclear and cytoplasmic compartments (Fig. 4h), and also on the mRNA level (Fig. 4g). Our data show therefore that enzymes of the one-carbon pathway differ in their response to serum depletion and stimulation, with MTHFD2 being particularly responsive.

Transcriptional response to MTHFD2 knockdown in cancer cells

To study the effects of loss of MTHFD2, and how these relate to its identified interacting proteins, we analyzed transcriptomics data from MTHFD2 shRNA knockdown cells generated by the Connectivity Map (CMap) project [34]. Interestingly, the D2PPI gene set was clearly decreased (ES -0.64, $p < 10^{-4}$) in MTHFD2 knockdown cells (Fig. 5a) and was among the most negatively enriched among examined collection of 3581 gene sets (Fig. 5b). Hence, loss of MTHFD2 affects expression of the D2PPI genes, consistent with a shared function.

The CMap data also allows assessing functional relationship between genes by scoring the similarity of transcriptional response of cancer cells to individual gene knockdown. In this regard, knockdown of MTHFD2 was highly similar (score > 90/100) to four out of the 14 D2PPI genes represented in CMap: HSPA8, HSPA9, HSPD1, and RPS3A. In contrast, with this criterion, other folate-metabolizing enzymes present in the CMap data set (MTHFD1, SHMT2, GLDC, AMT, TYMS, MTR, MTRR, FTCD, and DHFR) were not similar to MTHFD2, with the exception of MTHFD1 (score = 91.0, rank 414/3798), possibly reflecting the fact that loss of MTHFD1 also gives severe growth phenotypes [7]. In particular, SHMT2 was not closely related (score = 18.74 of 100, rank 2790/3798), consistent with the observations that loss of MTHFD2 is often detrimental to cells [4], while SHMT2 is not [2], and suggesting that at least some effects of MTHFD2 suppression are unrelated to mitochondrial folate metabolism.

Finally, we investigated the sets of genes that in CMap were highly similar to MTHFD2. We noted that, across all 3798 genes for which shRNA data was available in the CMap data set, MTHFD2 was highly similar (absolute score > 90) to 510 genes, compared to only 266 for SHMT2 and 169 for MTHFD1, indicating that loss MTHFD2 induces a response that more commonly occurs with gene knockdown. In addition, the set of 510 genes similar to MTHFD2 in this respect were clearly different from those of SHMT2 and MTHFD1 (Fig. 5c), again consistent with MTHFD2 having a distinct function. In particular, knockdown of MTHFD2, but not SHMT2 or MTHFD1, was highly similar to knockdown of a group of ribosomal proteins (Fig. 5d). Therefore, MTHFD2 is unique in that suppression of this protein causes cellular transcriptomic responses that are highly similar to those observed following the targeting of ribosomal proteins.

Comparison of RNAi and CRISPR suppression of MTHFD2

At first, the observation that MTHFD2 knockdown is similar to knockdown of ribosomal proteins, but not the

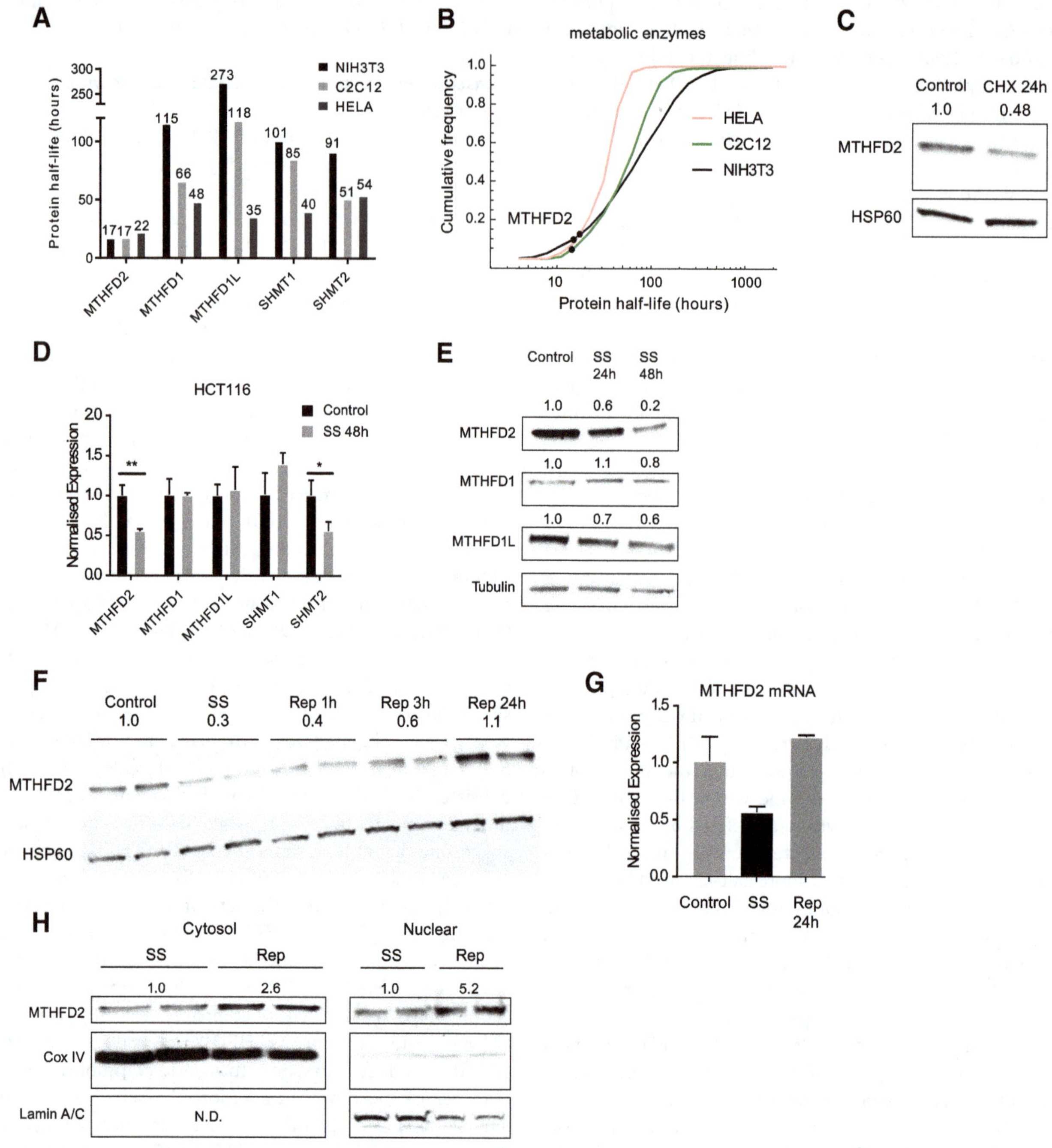

Fig. 4 MTHFD2 is a short-lived and dynamically regulated protein. **a** Half-life of enzymes of the one-carbon pathway in in HeLa, C2C12, and NIH3T3 cell lines. **b** Cumulative frequency of all quantified enzymes (596, 576, and 605 respectively) half-life in three cell lines. Dotted lines indicate relative half-life of MTHFD2 in each cell line. **c** Effect of treatment of HCT-116 cells for 24 h with 25 mg/ml protein translation inhibitor cyclohexamide on MTHFD2 protein levels. **d** qRT-PCR measurement of effect of 48 h serum starvation on mRNA of folate one-carbon enzymes. **e** Immunoblots of MTHFD1, MTHFD1L, MTHFD2, and beta-tubulin in HCT-116 grown in normal media or serum starved for 24 or 48 h. **f** Immunoblot showing time course of MTHFD2 protein response to serum replenishment in HCT-116 cells. SS, serum-starved; rep, serum replenishment (time point indicated). **g** Quantification of MTHFD2 mRNA in HCT-116 cells in control media, serum starved (SS) for 48 h, and serum starved followed by 24 h serum replenishment (rep). **h** Levels of MTHFD2 protein in nuclear and cytosolic compartments in HCT-116 cells that were serum starved for 48 h or in replenished media for 24 h after serum starvation. The COX IV and Lamin were used as cytosolic and nuclear markers respectively. Numbers in **f** and **g** indicate fold changes relative to control

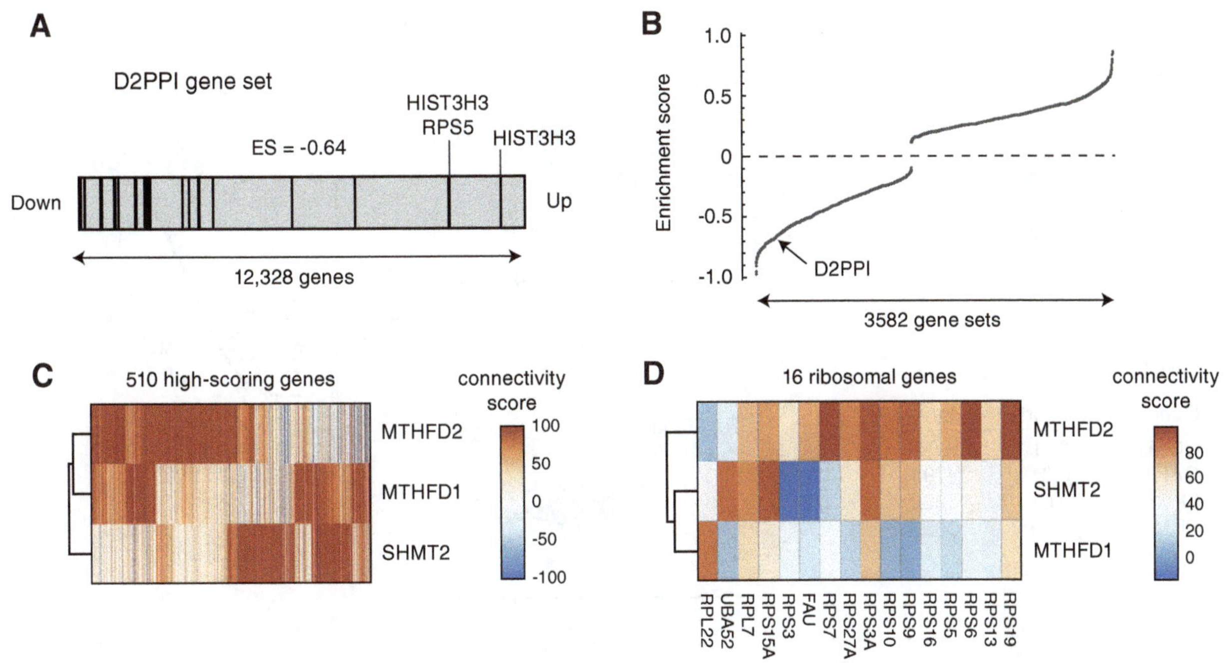

Fig. 5 Consequences of MTHFD2 knockdown. **a** Enrichment plot showing ranks of the D2PPI gene set among 12,328 genes responding to treatment with MTHFD2 shRNA in CMap study. Overall enrichment score was − 0.64. Genes with low enrichment scores (histones and RSP5) are indicated. **b** Distribution of enrichment scores for 3582 gene sets, with arrow indicating position of D2PPI gene set. **c** Heatmap showing connectivity scores for all 510 genes with significant associations (scores > 90 or < − 90) in CMap project with either of MTHFD2, MTHFD1 or SHMT2. Genes were clustered by average linkage and Pearson correlation distance. **d** Connectivity scores between MTHFD2, MTHFD1, and SHMT2 with ribosomal genes measured in the CMap project

upstream enzyme SHMT2, seemed counter-intuitive. A possible explanation is that shRNA knockdown cells still contain some residual protein, which may be sufficient to retain activity of a metabolic enzyme, but disrupts a more sensitive non-metabolic function such as control of translation. Indeed, there is evidence that a small amount of residual enzymatic activity can be sufficient to maintain necessary metabolic output, as seen for example with SHMT2 and formylmethionyl-tRNA pools [35]. To investigate this hypothesis, we compared the effects of shRNA knockdown to effects of CRISPR knockout, using genome-wide shRNA and CRISPR screening data from the Achilles project, measuring growth phenotypes across 501 and 341 cell lines, respectively. Here, genes with shared functions are expected to have similar dependency profiles across cell lines [30]. Overall, 977 genes were similar to MTHFD2 in the shRNA screening data, and 161 with CRISPR screening (Pearson's correlation, Bonferroni-corrected $p < 0.05$). Interestingly, genes involved in folate metabolism (SHMT2, GART, GCSH, FPGS) were similar to MTHFD2 in the CRISPR, but not in the shRNA screens (Fig. 6a, b, Additional file 7). Moreover, in a similar analysis of an independent CRISPR dataset comprising 14 AML cell lines, SHMT2, SLC25A32, and MTHFD1L were strongly correlated with MTHFD2, while cytosolic one-carbon enzymes showed weak correlations (Fig. 6c). However, in these data sets, the D2PPI proteins frequently showed strong growth phenotypes across all cell lines and were not significantly correlated with MTHFD2 (data not shown). This is consistent with the notion that in CRISPR MTHFD2 knockouts, the metabolic disruption dominates the effects on cell proliferation, while for shRNA knockdown, other functions of MTHFD2 may play a role.

Discussion

A common theme in cancer metabolism is that cancer-associated enzymes of interest as potential therapeutic targets [36–38] are frequently found to have non-metabolic "moonlighting" functions [39, 40]. In this study, we have demonstrated that MTHFD2 interacts with ribosomal and RNA processing proteins (Fig. 2, Table 1), which are also coexpressed with MTHFD2, and give similar transcriptional phenotypes upon shRNA knockdown. These distinct methods provide independent evidence suggesting that MTHFD2 has a previously unrecognized function in RNA metabolism and/or translation, although further experiments are required to confirm these findings, for example using ribosomal profiling, in-depth analysis of alternative splicing, and additional interaction data including reverse Co-IP experiments. The MTHFD2-interacting proteins clearly

A

CRISPR

Gene	Pearson R	Rank
GCSH	0.33	4
GART	0.29	38
FPGS	0.28	48
SHMT2	0.27	56

shRNA

Gene	Pearson R	Rank
GCSH	0.11	5004
GART	0.01	14794
FPGS	0.01	15822
SHMT2	-0.03	13686

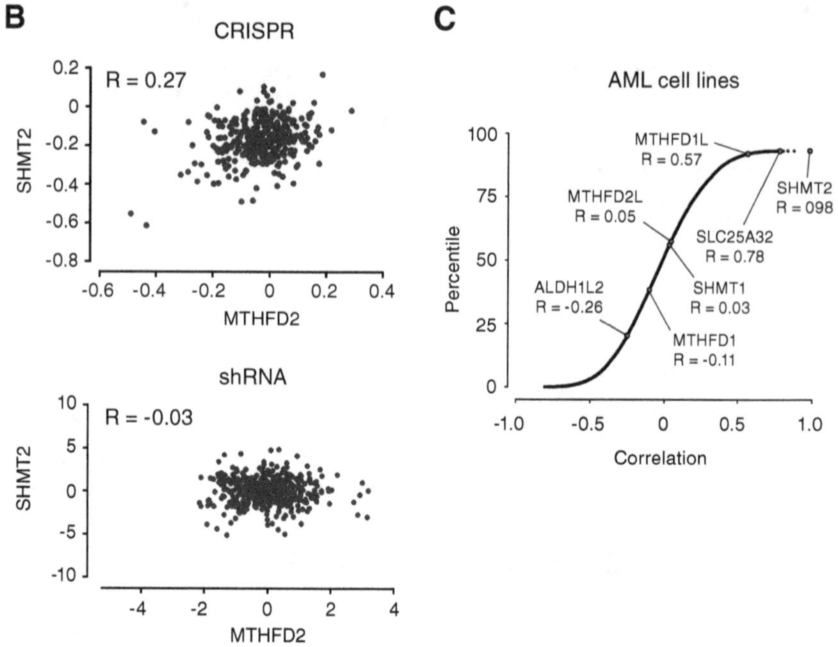

Fig. 6 Comparison of consequences of CRISPR knockout and RNAi knockdown of MTHFD2. **a** Pearson correlation and global rank between MTHFD2 and genes involved in folate metabolism in shRNA and CRISPR screens. **b** Comparison of growth effects caused by depletion of MTHFD2 and SHMT2 using shRNA and CRISPR in Achilles project. Each circle represents a tested cell line. Pearson's correlation is shown. **c** Distribution of correlations between growth phenotype effects of all examined genes and MTHFD2 across 14 AML cell lines. Selected genes involved in one-carbon metabolism are indicated by arrows

consist of previously known complexes of proteins with related, but also diverse, functions. We found multiple members of the heterogeneous ribonuclear protein (hnRNP) family of RNA binding proteins, which are of particular interest for several reasons. hnRNPs are known to interact with nascent RNA and control their stability, localization, splicing, and translation, and several family members have been implicated in regulation of cell proliferation and in the endothelial-mesenchymal transition (EMT) process [41, 42], which are also affected by RNAi against MTHFD2 [42–44]. While the consequences of interaction between MTHFD2 and hnRNPs are not yet clear, one possibility is that this interaction may allow nuclear MTHFD2 to exert some control over gene expression; indeed, there are many examples of hnRNP-interacting proteins influencing gene regulation via hnRNPs [45–47]. Moreover, hnRNPs may mediate signals on metabolic status: in particular, hnRNP-E1 has been reported to regulate gene transcription in response to folate starvation [48]. We also observed interactions with components of the small ribosomal subunit, and with several heat-shock proteins (HSPs) that assist with the folding and transportation of target proteins. While HSPs could interact with MTHFD2 simply to assist its own folding, it is also possible that MTHFD2 or other components of the observed complexes bind and that regulate the functions of the HSPs [49]. Interestingly, some of the observed hnRNPs are involved in heat shock responses as well [50], hinting at a common role. We also found interactions with proteins involved in DNA repair and replication (XRCC6 and RPN1), as well as histones (Fig. 2; Table 1, consistent with observations that the protein localize to regions of newly formed DNA [17]. Whether these findings represent more than one distinct function of the MTHFD2 protein, or rather are multiple aspects of a single mechanism, is not yet clear.

Although Co-IP coupled with MS is a powerful methodology for the unbiased detection of protein interactions, it is still a technique with false positives (due to off-target binding of antibodies) and false negatives (due to failure to capture protein-proteins interactions that are of transient nature, or due to other technical reasons). To reduce the impact of false positives, we utilized two antibodies and a CRISPR knockout control. Due to this stringent approach, it is more probable that we have missed some real protein interactors rather than identified false positives. Interestingly, we did not detect interactions between MTHFD2 and other one-carbon metabolism enzymes involved in nuclear dTMP synthesis (SHMT1, SHMT2, MTHFD1, TYMS or DHFR) [51], nor with nuclear lamin to which they are tethered [31]. Such interactions could of course have been missed in our experiments, since we used quite stringent criteria to obtain high-quality interactions and did not perform cross-linking during CoIP. Alternatively, MTHFD2 may reside in a different compartment. From a biochemical perspective, nuclear MTHFD2 would not be expected to contribute to dTMP synthesis, since this process requires CH_2-THF which MTHFD2 cannot generate on its own, as it lacks the formyl-THF synthase domain present in MTHFD1.

An open question is what drives the recruitment and association of MTHFD2 with cellular RNA-processing protein complexes. Because several of the D2PPI proteins are RNA-binding, one possibility is that MTHFD2 itself is an RNA-binding protein and encounters its partners while bound to specific RNAs. Indeed, a recent large-case study reported that RNA binding proteins tend to CoIP with a large number of other RNA binding proteins [52]. Additionally, MTHFD2 contains Rossman folds, NAD-binding domains that can also bind RNA, as in the example of GAPDH [53]. A number of enzymes have been shown to "moonlight" by binding RNA, including SHMT2 and MTHFD1 [54], and it has been suggested that this may allow metabolic status to influence gene regulation [55]. However, it is also possible that MTHFD2 is not a direct RNA-binding protein, but instead contacts one or more proteins around which the RNA-binding complex is organized. Further work is required to demonstrate whether MTHFD2 binds RNA species directly or indirectly, and understand how the observed protein-protein interactions are formed and function. Further experiments will also be important for validating and extending the findings of this study, such as Co-IP and transcriptomic studies of enzymatically inactive MTHFD2 in diverse nutritional and cell conditions. For example it will be of interest to determine whether the interaction partners of MTHFD2 are modified in response to availability of one-carbon units, growth factors or DNA damage.

Conclusions

Our study suggests a role for nuclear MTHFD2 in RNA metabolism and translation, besides its established function in mitochondrial folate metabolism. An intriguing possibility is that the MTHFD2-interacting proteins could provide a mechanism whereby MTHFD2 can affect gene expression and cell behaviour, perhaps serving to integrate information on folate metabolism. While the precise mechanism remains to be investigated, such a function would explain the observation that catalytically inactive MTHFD2 protein is sufficient to promote cell proliferation [17]. Future investigation of this non-enzymatic function will be important for pharmaceutically targeting MTHFD2; for example, inhibitors of MTHFD2 dehydrogenase activity may not be effective, and instead drugs that disrupt protein-protein interactions might be required.

Additional files

Additional file 1: Table S1. List of primers used for qRT-PCR in this study. (DOCX 12 kb)

Additional file 2: Figure S1. Validation of MTHFD2 knockout cell model. (a) Immunoblot of MTHFD2 in WT and D2-KO clones. Tubulin is shown as loading control. (b) Immunoprecipitation of MTHFD2 using Anti-MTHFD2 antibody from D2-KO and WT cells followed by immunoblotting for MTHFD2. (c) Silver-stained SDS-PAGE of CoIP lysates from WT and D2-KO cells. As indicated the CoIP were performed using either of the anti-MTHFD2 NC or AP antibodies. MTHFD2 bands are indicated by blue squares. As can be seen MTHFD2 were detected in IP samples from WT but not D2-KO cells. (PDF 311 kb)

Additional file 3: Mapped peptides detected by Mass Spectrometry in each of 12 CoIP lysate samples. (XLSX 748 kb)

Additional file 4: Significantly enriched GO Molecular Function and Cellular Component gene sets for 29 identified MTHFD2 protein interactors. (XLSX 15 kb)

Additional file 5: Co-expression scores between MTHFD2 and the D2PPI genes. The gene co-expression were calculated across 8097 human, rat, and mouse datasets using in-house tools, or against ~ 3000 human datasets using SEEK. (XLSX 11 kb)

Additional file 6: List of top data sets exhibiting coexpression between MTHFD2 and the D2PPI and ATF4 gene sets, respectively. (XLSX 17 kb)

Additional file 7: Correlation scores of MTHFD2 against all other genes in Achilles Project. (XLSX 1006 kb)

Abbreviations

AP: Proteintech 12,270–1-AP anti-MTHFD2 antibody; CoIP: Co-immunoprecipitation; D2-KO: MTHFD2 CRISPR knockout cell line; D2PPI: Set of D2 protein-protein interactors, listed in Table 1.; HNRNP: Heterogeneous ribonucleoprotein; HSP: Heat-shock proteins; IgG: Immunoglubulin G; MS: Mass spectrometry; MTHFD2: Methylenetetrahydrofolate dehydrogenase (NADP+ dependent) 2; NC: Genetex N1C3 anti-MTHFD2 antibody; PPI: Protein-protein interaction

Acknowledgements

We would like to thank Dr. Rabinowitz for providing us with the MTHFD2 CRISPR knockout cells. In-gel digestion, peptide extraction, MS analysis, and database searches of protein identification were performed by the Proteomics Karolinska (PK/KI) core facility at Karolinska Institute, Stockholm.

Funding

The project was funded by Cancerfonden (CAN 2016/632) and the Swedish Foundation for Strategic Research (FFL12-0220).

Authors' contributions

RN and CK conceived the study, designed the experiments, wrote the manuscript, and approved for the publication of the final manuscript. CK performed the experiments. CK and RN performed the computational analysis presented here.

Competing interests

The authors declare that they have no competing interests.

Author details

[1]Cardiovascular Medicine Unit, Department of Medicine, Karolinska Institutet, SE-171 76 Stockholm, Sweden. [2]Division of Cardiovascular Medicine, Karolinska University Hospital, SE-171 76 Stockholm, Sweden. [3]Center for Molecular Medicine, Karolinska Institutet, SE-171 76 Stockholm, Sweden.

References

1. Pavlova NN, Thompson CB. The emerging hallmarks of cancer metabolism. Cell Metab. 2016;23:27–47.
2. Jain M, Nilsson R, Sharma S, Madhusudhan N, Kitami T, Souza AL, et al. Metabolite profiling identifies a key role for glycine in rapid cancer cell proliferation. Science. 2012;336:1040–4.
3. Locasale JW. Serine, glycine and one-carbon units: cancer metabolism in full circle. Nat Rev Cancer. 2013;13:572–83.
4. Nilsson R, Jain M, Madhusudhan N, Sheppard NG, Strittmatter L, Kampf C, et al. Metabolic enzyme expression highlights a key role for MTHFD2 and the mitochondrial folate pathway in cancer. Nat Commun. 2014;5:3128.
5. Pike ST, Rajendra R, Artzt K, Appling DR. Mitochondrial C1-tetrahydrofolate synthase (MTHFD1L) supports the flow of mitochondrial one-carbon units into the methyl cycle in embryos. J Biol Chem. 2010;285:4612–20.
6. Lewis CA, Parker SJ, Fiske BP, McCloskey D, Gui DY, Green CR, et al. Tracing compartmentalized NADPH metabolism in the cytosol and mitochondria of mammalian cells. Mol Cell. 2014;55:253–63. Elsevier Inc
7. Ducker GSSS, Chen L, Morscher RJJJ, Ghergurovich JMMM, Esposito M, Teng X, et al. Reversal of cytosolic one-carbon flux compensates for loss of the mitochondrial folate pathway. Cell Metab. Elsevier Inc. 2016;23:1140–53.
8. Mejia NR, MacKenzie RE. NAD-dependent methylenetetrahydrofolate dehydrogenase is expressed by immortal cells. J Biol Chem. 1985;260: 14616–20.
9. Tedeschi PM, Vazquez A, Kerrigan JE, Bertino JR. Mitochondrial methylenetetrahydrofolate dehydrogenase (MTHFD2) overexpression is associated with tumor cell proliferation and is a novel target for drug development. Mol Cancer Res. 2015;13:1361–6.
10. Pikman Y, Puissant A, Alexe G, Furman A, Chen LM, Frumm SM, et al. Targeting MTHFD2 in acute myeloid leukemia. J Exp Med. 2016;213:1285–306.
11. Di Pietro E, Sirois J, Tremblay ML, MacKenzie RE. Mitochondrial NAD-dependent methylenetetrahydrofolate dehydrogenase-methenyltetrahydrofolate cyclohydrolase is essential for embryonic development. Mol Cell Biol. 2002;22:4158–66.
12. Bolusani S, Young BA, Cole NA, Tibbetts AS, Momb J, Bryant JD, et al. Mammalian MTHFD2L encodes a mitochondrial methylenetetrahydrofolate dehydrogenase isozyme expressed in adult tissues. J Biol Chem. 2011; 286:5166–74.
13. Liu F, Liu Y, He C, Tao L, He X, Song H, et al. Increased MTHFD2 expression is associated with poor prognosis in breast cancer. Tumor Biol. 2014;35:8685–90.
14. Liu X, Huang Y, Jiang C, Ou H, Guo B, Liao H, et al. Methylenetetrahydrofolate dehydrogenase 2 overexpression is associated with tumor aggressiveness and poor prognosis in hepatocellular carcinoma. Dig Liver Dis. 2016;48:953–60.
15. Koufaris C, Gallage S, Yang T, Lau C-H, Valbuena GN, Keun HC. Suppression of MTHFD2 in MCF-7 breast cancer cells increases glycolysis, dependency on exogenous glycine, and sensitivity to folate depletion. J Proteome Res. 2016;15:2618–25.
16. Kim D, Fiske BP, Birsoy K, Freinkman E, Kami K, Possemato RL, et al. SHMT2 drives glioma cell survival in ischaemia but imposes a dependence on glycine clearance. Nature. 2015;520:363–7.
17. Gustafsson Sheppard N, Jarl L, Mahadessian D, Strittmatter L, Schmidt A, Madhusudan N, et al. The folate-coupled enzyme MTHFD2 is a nuclear protein and promotes cell proliferation. Sci Rep. 2015;5:15029.
18. Lehtinen L, Ketola K, Mäkelä R, Mpindi J-P, Viitala M, Kallioniemi O, et al. High-throughput RNAi screening for novel modulators of vimentin expression identifies MTHFD2 as a regulator of breast cancer cell migration and invasion. Oncotarget. 2013;4:48–63.
19. Schmidt A, Wu H, MacKenzie RE, Chen VJ, Bewly JR, Ray JE, et al. Structures of three inhibitor complexes provide insight into the reaction mechanism of the human methylenetetrahydrofolate dehydrogenase/cyclohydrolase. Biochemistry. 2000;39:6325–35.
20. Fu C, Sikandar A, Donner J, Zaburannyi N, Herrmann J, Reck M, et al. The natural product carolacton inhibits folate-dependent C1 metabolism by targeting FolD/MTHFD. Nat Commun. 2017;8:1529.
21. Szklarczyk D, Morris JH, Cook H, Kuhn M, Wyder S, Simonovic M, et al. The STRING database in 2017: quality-controlled protein–protein association networks, made broadly accessible. Nucleic Acids Res. 2017;45:D362–8.
22. Schwanhäusser B, Busse D, Li N, Dittmar G, Schuchhardt J, Wolf J, et al. Global quantification of mammalian gene expression control. Nature. 2011;473:337–42.
23. Cambridge SB, Gnad F, Nguyen C, Bermejo JL, Krüger M, Mann M. Systems-wide proteomic analysis in mammalian cells reveals conserved, functional protein turnover. J Proteome Res. 2011;10:5275–84.
24. Thiele I, Swainston N, Fleming RMT, Hoppe A, Sahoo S, Aurich MK, et al. A community-driven global reconstruction of human metabolism. Nat Biotechnol. 2013;31:419–25.
25. Subramanianan A, Tamayo P, Mootha VK, Mukherjeed S, Ebert BL, Gillette MA, et al. Gene set enrichment analysis: a knowledge-based approach for interpreting genome-wide expression profiles. Proc Natl Acad Sci U S A. 2005;102:15545–50.
26. Zhu Q, Wong AK, Krishnan A, Aure MR, Tadych A, Zhang R, et al. Targeted exploration and analysis of large cross-platform human transcriptomic compendia. Nat Methods. 2015;12:211–4.
27. Metsalu T, Vilo J. ClustVis: a web tool for visualizing clustering of multivariate data using principal component analysis and heatmap. Nucleic Acids Res. 2015;43:W566–70.
28. Meyers RM, Bryan JG, McFarland JM, Weir BA, Sizemore AE, Xu H, et al. Computational correction of copy number effect improves specificity of CRISPR–Cas9 essentiality screens in cancer cells. Nat Genet. 2017;49: 1779–84.
29. Tsherniak A, Vazquez F, Montgomery PG, Weir BA, Kryukov G, Cowley GS, et al. Defining a cancer dependency map. Cell. 2017;170:564–576.e16.
30. Wang T, Yu H, Hughes NW, Liu B, Kendirli A, Klein K, et al. Gene Essentiality Profiling Reveals Gene Networks and Synthetic Lethal Interactions with Oncogenic Ras. Cell. 2017;168:890–903.e15.
31. Anderson DD, Woeller CF, Chiang E-P, Shane B, Stover PJ. Serine Hydroxymethyltransferase anchors de novo thymidylate synthesis pathway to nuclear Lamina for DNA synthesis. J Biol Chem. 2012;287: 7051–62.
32. Baughman JM, Nilsson R, Gohil VM, Arlow DH, Gauhar Z, Mootha VK. A computational screen for regulators of oxidative phosphorylation implicates SLIRP in mitochondrial RNA homeostasis. PLoS Genet. 2009;5:e1000590.
33. Nilsson R, Schultz IJ, Pierce EL, Soltis KA, Naranuntarat A, Ward DM, et al. Discovery of genes essential for heme biosynthesis through large-scale gene expression analysis. Cell Metab. 2009;10:119–30.
34. Subramanian A, Narayan R, Corsello SM, Peck DD, Natoli TE, Lu X, et al. A Next Generation Connectivity Map: L1000 Platform and the First 1,000,000 Profiles. Cell. 2017;171:1437–1452.e17.
35. Minton DR, Nam M, McLaughlin DJ, Shin J, Bayraktar EC, Alvarez SW, et al. Serine Catabolism by SHMT2 Is Required for Proper Mitochondrial Translation Initiation and Maintenance of Formylmethionyl-tRNAs. Mol Cell. 2018;69:610–621.e5.
36. Christofk HR, Vander Heiden MG, Harris MH, Ramanathan A, Gerszten RE, Wei R, et al. The M2 splice isoform of pyruvate kinase is important for cancer metabolism and tumour growth. Nature. 2008;452:230–3.
37. Son J, Lyssiotis CA, Ying H, Wang X, Hua S, Ligorio M, et al. Glutamine supports pancreatic cancer growth through a KRAS-regulated metabolic pathway. Nature. 2013;496:101–5.
38. Dang L, White DW, Gross S, Bennett BD, Bittinger MA, Driggers EM, et al. Cancer-associated IDH1 mutations produce 2-hydroxyglutarate. Nature. Nature Publishing Group. 2009;462:739–44.
39. Yang W, Lu Z. Pyruvate kinase M2 at a glance. J Cell Sci. 2015;128:1655–60.
40. Yu X, Li S. Non-metabolic functions of glycolytic enzymes in tumorigenesis. Oncogene. 2017;36:2629–36.
41. Geuens T, Bouhy D, Timmerman V. The hnRNP family: insights into their role in health and disease. Hum Genet. 2016;135:851–67.
42. Xu Y, Gao XD, Lee J-H, Huang H, Tan H, Ahn J, et al. Cell type-restricted activity of hnRNPM promotes breast cancer metastasis via regulating alternative splicing. Genes Dev. 2014;28:1191–203.
43. Zhang Z, Zhou C, Chang Y, Zhang Z, Hu Y, Zhang F, et al. Long non-coding RNA CASC11 interacts with hnRNP-K and activates the WNT/ß-catenin pathway to promote growth and metastasis in colorectal cancer. Cancer Lett. 2016;376:62–73.
44. Lai C-H, Huang Y-C, Lee J-C, Tseng JT-C, Chang K-C, Chen Y-J, et al. Translational upregulation of aurora-a by hnRNP Q1 contributes to cell proliferation and tumorigenesis in colorectal cancer. Cell Death Dis. 2017;8:e2555.
45. Ji Y, Tulin AV. Poly (ADP-ribose) controls DE-cadherin-dependent stem cell maintenance and oocyte localization. Nat Commun. 2012;3:760.
46. Lee P-T, Liao P-C, Chang W-C, Tseng JT. Epidermal growth factor increases the interaction between nucleolin and heterogeneous nuclear ribonucleoprotein K/poly (C) binding protein 1 complex to regulate the gastrin mRNA turnover. Mol Biol Cell. 2007;18:5004–13.
47. Leal G, Comprido D, de Luca P, Morais E, Rodrigues L, Mele M, et al. The RNA-Binding Protein hnRNP K Mediates the Effect of BDNF on Dendritic

mRNA Metabolism and Regulates Synaptic NMDA Receptors in Hippocampal Neurons. eNeuro. 2017;4:ENEURO.0268-17.2017.
48. Tang Y-S, Khan RA, Xiao S, Hansen DK, Stabler SP, Kusumanchi P, et al. Evidence favoring a positive feedback loop for physiologic auto upregulation of hnRNP-E1 during prolonged folate deficiency in human placental cells. J Nutr. 2017;147:482–98.
49. Calderwood SK, Gong J. Heat shock proteins promote cancer: It's a protection racket. Trends Biochem Sci. 2016;41:311–23.
50. Weighardt F, Cobianchi F, Cartegni L, Chiodi I, Villa A, Riva S, et al. A novel hnRNP protein (HAP/SAF-B) enters a subset of hnRNP complexes and relocates in nuclear granules in response to heat shock. J Cell Sci. 1999; 112(Pt 10):1465–76.
51. Field MS, Kamynina E, Agunloye OC, Liebenthal RP, Lamarre SG, Brosnan ME, et al. Nuclear enrichment of folate cofactors and methylenetetrahydrofolate dehydrogenase 1 (MTHFD1) protect de novo thymidylate biosynthesis during folate deficiency. J Biol Chem. 2014;289:29642–50.
52. Brannan KW, Jin W, Huelga SC, Banks CAS, Gilmore JM, Florens L, et al. SONAR discovers RNA-binding proteins from analysis of large-scale protein-protein Interactomes. Mol Cell. 2016;64:282–93.
53. Nagy E, Rigby WF. Glyceraldehyde-3-phosphate dehydrogenase selectively binds AU-rich RNA in the NAD(+)-binding region (Rossmann fold). J Biol Chem. 1995;270:2755–63.
54. Castello A, Fischer B, Eichelbaum K, Horos R, Beckmann BM, Strein C, et al. Insights into RNA biology from an atlas of mammalian mRNA-binding proteins. Cell. 2012;149:1393–406.
55. Hentze MW, Preiss T. The REM phase of gene regulation. Trends Biochem Sci. 2010;35:423–6.
56. Boisvert F-M, Ahmad Y, Gierlinski M, Charrière F, Lamont D, Scott M, et al. A quantitative spatial proteomics analysis of proteome turnover in human cells. Mol Cell Proteomics. 2012;11:M111.011429.

8

A precision therapeutic strategy for hexokinase 1-null, hexokinase 2-positive cancers

Shili Xu[1], Arthur Catapang[1], Daniel Braas[1,3], Linsey Stiles[6], Hanna M. Doh[1], Jason T. Lee[1,4,5], Thomas G. Graeber[1,3,4,5], Robert Damoiseaux[1,7], Orian Shirihai[6] and Harvey R. Herschman[1,2,4,5,8*]

Abstract

Background: Precision medicine therapies require identification of unique molecular cancer characteristics. Hexokinase (HK) activity has been proposed as a therapeutic target; however, different hexokinase isoforms have not been well characterized as alternative targets. While HK2 is highly expressed in the majority of cancers, cancer subtypes with differential HK1 and HK2 expression have not been characterized for their sensitivities to HK2 silencing.

Methods: HK1 and HK2 expression in the Cancer Cell Line Encyclopedia dataset was analyzed. A doxycycline-inducible shRNA silencing system was used to examine the effect of HK2 knockdown in cultured cells and in xenograft models of $HK1^-HK2^+$ and $HK1^+HK2^+$ cancers. Glucose consumption and lactate production rates were measured to monitor HK activity in cell culture, and ^{18}F-FDG PET/CT was used to monitor HK activity in xenograft tumors. A high-throughput screen was performed to search for synthetically lethal compounds in combination with HK2 inhibition in $HK1^-HK2^+$ liver cancer cells, and a combination therapy for liver cancers with this phenotype was developed. A metabolomic analysis was performed to examine changes in cellular energy levels and key metabolites in $HK1^-HK2^+$ cells treated with this combination therapy. The CRISPR Cas9 method was used to establish isogenic $HK1^+HK2^+$ and $HK1^-HK2^+$ cell lines to evaluate $HK1^-HK2^+$ cancer cell sensitivity to the combination therapy.

Results: Most tumors express both HK1 and HK2, and subsets of cancers from a wide variety of tissues of origin express only HK2. Unlike $HK1^+HK2^+$ cancers, $HK1^-HK2^+$ cancers are sensitive to HK2 silencing-induced cytostasis. Synthetic lethality was achieved in $HK1^-HK2^+$ liver cancer cells, by the combination of DPI, a mitochondrial complex I inhibitor, and HK2 inhibition, in $HK1^-HK2^+$ liver cancer cells. Perhexiline, a fatty acid oxidation inhibitor, further sensitizes $HK1^-HK2^+$ liver cancer cells to the complex I/HK2-targeted therapeutic combination. Although $HK1^+HK2^+$ lung cancer H460 cells are resistant to this therapeutic combination, isogenic $HK1^{KO}HK2^+$ cells are sensitive to this therapy.

Conclusions: The $HK1^-HK2^+$ cancer subsets exist among a wide variety of cancer types. Selective inhibition of the $HK1^-HK2^+$ cancer cell-specific energy production pathways (HK2-driven glycolysis, oxidative phosphorylation and fatty acid oxidation), due to the unique presence of only the HK2 isoform, appears promising to treat $HK1^-HK2^+$ cancers. This therapeutic strategy will likely be tolerated by most normal tissues, where only HK1 is expressed.

Keywords: Precision medicine, Warburg effect, Liver cancer, Cancer, Glycolysis, Hexokinase 2, Diphenyleneiodonium, Perhexiline, Fatty acid oxidation, Oxidative phosphorylation, Mitochondria complex-I, Synthetic lethality

* Correspondence: hherschman@mednet.ucla.edu
[1]Department of Molecular and Medical Pharmacology, David Geffen School of Medicine, University of California, Los Angeles, Los Angeles, CA 90095, USA
[2]Department of Biological Chemistry, David Geffen School of Medicine, University of California, Los Angeles, Los Angeles, CA 90095, USA

Background

Precision medicine depends on the identification of a unique molecular cancer subtype that may exist across tumors with different origins. The recent Food and Drug Administration (FDA) approval of Keytruda for treatment of a wide range of advanced cancers with the common biomarkers microsatellite instability-high (MSI-H) or mismatch repair deficient (dMMR) illustrates this concept of phenotype/genotype commonality, rather than tissue of origin, for a common therapeutic approach to subclasses of cancers from tissues of varying origin [1]. Larotrectinib, which targets the rare tropomyosin receptor kinase (TRK) fusion mutation, is another example of precision cancer medicine; larotrectinib has demonstrated efficacy in cancers from different tissues that share TRK fusion mutations [2]. FDA approval is currently being sought for the larotrectinib treatment of adult and pediatric TRK fusion cancers, based on molecular makeup rather than the tissue of origin [3].

Most cancers increase glycolysis (the "Warburg effect"), a metabolic event postulated to ensure sufficient supplies of energy (ATP), reducing equivalents (NADPH), and/or biochemical building blocks for cell growth and proliferation [4]. However, because of the conserved nature of the glycolytic pathway in normal tissues, global systemic inhibition of glycolysis results in adverse effects that make this approach of limited value; selective inhibition of cancer-driven glycolysis will be required for clinical cancer therapy.

The hexokinase (HK) enzymes, encoded by four genes (HK1/2/3/4), catalyze glucose phosphorylation, the first enzymatic step in glycolysis [5]. Most adult tissues use HK1 for glycolysis. HK3 is inhibited by physiological concentrations of glucose. HK4, also known as glucokinase (GCK), is expressed in hepatocytes, pancreatic β-cells, and glucose-sensing neurons. HK2 is expressed primarily in embryonic tissues and in adult muscle and adipose tissues. In addition, HK2 is expressed in a wide range of cancers [6–9], from tissues that normally express only HK1. HK2 gene deletion in adult mice does not significantly affect normal tissues [6]. Consequently, selective HK2 inhibitors have recently been developed [10], under the assumption that targeted HK2 inhibition will reduce progression of HK2-positive cancers and have minimal adverse effects. However, most previous studies on HK2 in cancer did not examine the contribution of HK1 to cancer glycolysis [6–9, 11]. Cancer subtypes with differential HK1/HK2 expression have not been characterized.

In addition to enhanced glycolysis, other modes of energy generation are utilized to support biological processes in cancer cells; these alternative energy-generating sources include oxidative phosphorylation and fatty acid oxidation [12, 13]. The availability and use of multi-source energy generation alternatives suggests both the flexibility of cancer cells in reprogramming their required energy generation under metabolic stress and their abilities to escape from alternative modes of energy generation blockade using monotherapies. Combination therapies that target compensatory energy metabolism pathways in cancer cells, but are tolerated by normal tissues, have not yet achieved clinical success, due to the conserved nature of energy metabolism shared by most cancer and normal cells.

We have developed a combination therapy specifically effective in cancers with the $HK1^-HK2^+$ molecular signature, a subset of cancers which originate from a wide variety of tissues. Using an $HK1^-HK2^+$ subpopulation of liver cancers as an example, we developed a synergistic combination of HK2 inhibition and partial inhibition of mitochondrial complex I and fatty acid oxidation to achieve synthetic lethality of these $HK1^-HK2^+$ tumors. However, like $HK1^+$ cells/tissues, $HK1^+HK2^+$ cancers are not susceptible to this therapy, despite the reduction in their HK2-driven glycolytic activity. Our findings warrant optimization of the triple-combination therapy as a precision medicine for further clinical development to treat $HK1^-HK2^+$ cancers, regardless of their tissues of origin.

Methods

Cell lines and tissue samples

Hep3B, HepG2, H460, H1299, HT29, HCT116, SW620, and Caco2 cells were from the American Type Culture Collection (ATCC). Huh7, JHH7, JHH5, and MDAMB468 cells were provided by Drs. Dennis Slamon and Richard Finn (UCLA). SUM159, MDAMB231, and HCC1937 cells were provided by Dr. Heather Christofk (UCLA). A549, SKOV3, OVCAR5, and HEY cells were provided by Dr. Caius Radu (UCLA). Hs766T, MiaPaca2, and Panc1 were provided by Dr. Timothy Donahue (UCLA). LNCaP, DU145, and PC3 cells were provided by Dr. Hong Wu (UCLA). 786-0 cells were provided by Dr. Allan Pantuck (UCLA). All cells used for the experiments were between passages 3 and 20. Cell lines were routinely authenticated based on morphology, growth characteristics, and HK expression profiles according to the CCLE gene expression dataset. All cells were maintained in RPMI1640 + 10% FBS, at 37 °C in 5% CO_2/95% air. Cells were routinely checked for *Mycoplasma* contamination by using MycoAlert (Lonza). Frozen human liver and liver cancer samples were provided by the UCLA Translational Pathology Core Laboratory.

High-throughput screen (HTS) for compounds synergistic with HK2 knockdown in cell growth inhibition

In the primary HTS screening, libraries of 3205 drug-like small molecules and 119 FDA-approved oncology drugs were screened for their ability to inhibit the growth of Hep3B/shHK2^{DOX} cells in the presence of

DOX. Hep3B/shHK2^{DOX} cells were pretreated with DOX for 48 h, then seeded in 384-well plates with 700 cells per well, and treated with DOX and individual library members at 10 μM for 72 h. Relative numbers of viable cells in response to different treatments were determined by the CellTiter-Glo assay (Promega). Compounds with z score < – 3 were selected for subsequent secondary screening. In the secondary screening, Hep3B/shHK2^{DOX} cells with or without 48-h DOX pretreatment, were treated subsequently with the selected compounds in dose response curves (DRCs 10, 2.5, 0.625, 0.156, 0.039, 0.010, 0.0024, and 0.0006 μM) for 72 h. Relative numbers of viable cells were determined by the alamarBlue assay (Invitrogen).

Media metabolite measurement

Medium was collected from culture plates and analyzed for glucose, lactate, and glutamine concentrations using a Biomedical Bioprofile Analyzer (Nova Biomedical). Cells seeded in 6-well plates received treatments described in the "Results" section and the figure legends. Twenty-four hours before the analysis, the media were refreshed. Medium added to wells with no cells was used as a blank control. After 24-h incubation, 1 ml of medium was collected from each sample and the blank control, and media samples were analyzed in the Bioprofile Analyzer. Values were normalized to cell number and time intervals. DPI was purchased from Cayman Chemical (#81050). PER was purchased from Cayman Chemical (#16982). FDG was purchased from Omicron Biochemicals Inc. (#GLC-010).

In vivo assessment of treatment efficacy and safety

Nu/nu mice (Jackson Laboratory) were used for in vivo efficacy and safety studies. Mice were fed ad libitum and kept in air-conditioned rooms at 20 ± 2 °C with a 12-h light-dark period. Animal care and manipulation were in accordance with the Guidelines for the Care and Use of Laboratory Animals. Cells (Hep3B, 5×10^6; Huh7, 2×10^6; HepG2, 2×10^6; H460, 1×10^6) in 100 μl RPMI/matrigel (1:1) were implanted subcutaneously in nu/nu mice under aseptic conditions. Body weight was measured biweekly. The body condition score (BCS) was also used to evaluate animal health. Tumor growth was assessed by biweekly measurement of tumor diameters with a vernier caliper. Tumor volume (mm^3) = $D \times d^2/2$, where D and d are the longest and shortest diameters, respectively. After subcutaneous tumor cell inoculation, tumors were allowed to grow to a volume of 200 mm^3. We chose tumors of this size because, in our experience, tumor xenografts of smaller sizes may regress. Mice were then randomly assigned into groups as indicated in the "Results" section and the figure legends. DOX was given in the diet (625 mg DOX per kg diet, daily DOX 1.6–2.7 mg in 3–5 g diet per mouse). DPI (#D491550, Toronto Research Chemicals) and PER were dissolved in DMSO as stock solutions at 20 and 300 mg/ml, respectively, diluted in 5% (*w*/*v*) hydroxyl-propyl-beta-cyclodextrin (Sigma) as injection solutions, and given daily by intraperitoneal (i.p.) injection at 2 and 30 mg/kg, respectively.

Statistics

Student's t-test was used for statistical analysis. P values were determined by Prism 5 (GraphPad Software, Inc.). Differences were considered statistically significant at $P < 0.05$.

Study approval

All reported animal studies were approved by the UCLA Chancellor's Animal Research Committee (ARC).

Results

The conversion of liver to liver cancer is accompanied by extinction of HK4 expression and tumor expression of either HK2 alone or HK1 and HK2

Our initial goal was to identify a tumor population likely to be highly sensitive to HK2 inhibition or silencing, to optimize evaluation of targeting HK2 as a therapeutic modality. Unlike most adult tissues, which express HK1 to drive glycolysis, the liver expresses HK4 (also known as glucokinase) and does not express either HK1 or HK2 (Fig. 1a). Liver cancers, however, no longer express HK4; instead, analysis of datasets of liver cancer samples [14, 15] revealed that, like many other cancers, HK2 is expressed in many liver tumors (Fig. 1b). Moreover, analysis of HK1 and HK2 expression in the TCGA liver cancer dataset demonstrates that a substantial portion (83%) of HK2$^+$ (HK2 RSEM > 1000) liver cancers are deficient in HK1 expression (HK1 RSEM < 1000) (Fig. 1c).

Because tumor biopsies are likely to have normal tissue contamination, it is not possible to evaluate tumors in the TCGA collection from other tissues of origins for tumor HK1 and HK2 expression; the presence of HK1 derived from most normal tissues would distort the estimate of HK1 tumor-derived levels in tumor biopsies. In contrast, contamination with normal liver, which does not express either HK1 or HK2, would not affect the evaluation of HK1 and HK2 expression in liver tumor samples.

Tumors of multiple origin contain HK1$^-$HK2$^+$ and HK1$^+$HK2$^+$ subsets

To confirm and extend the observations regarding the presence of HK1$^-$HK2$^+$ liver cancers and to determine whether HK1$^-$HK2$^+$ subsets exist in cancers from other tissues of origin, we examined the frequencies of HK1$^-$HK2$^+$ and HK1$^+$HK2$^+$ subsets in established cancer cell lines of the Cancer Cell Line Encyclopedia (CCLE) collection [16]. Subsets of cancer cell lines

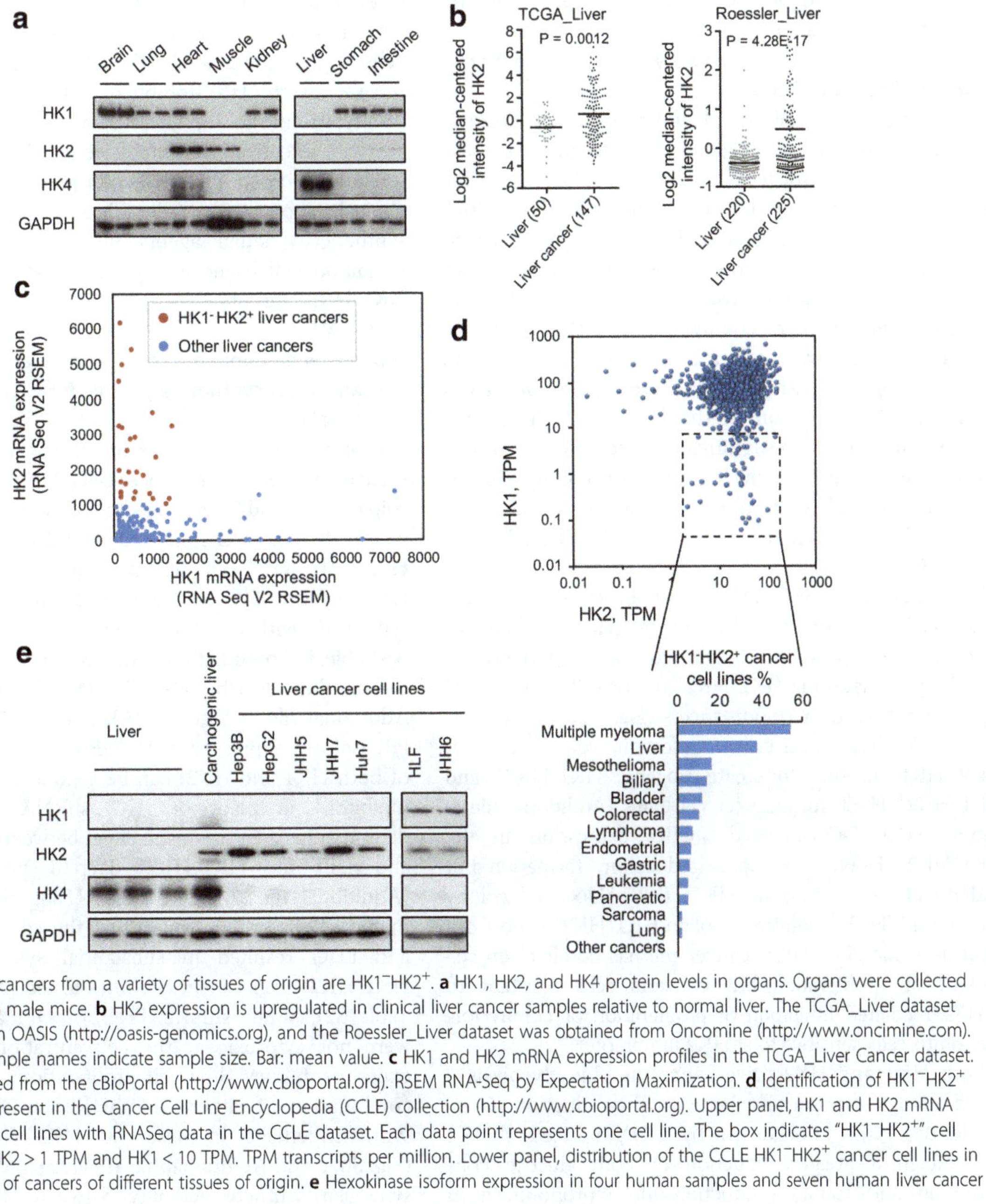

Fig. 1 Subsets of cancers from a variety of tissues of origin are HK1⁻HK2⁺. **a** HK1, HK2, and HK4 protein levels in organs. Organs were collected from two C57BL/6 male mice. **b** HK2 expression is upregulated in clinical liver cancer samples relative to normal liver. The TCGA_Liver dataset was obtained from OASIS (http://oasis-genomics.org), and the Roessler_Liver dataset was obtained from Oncomine (http://www.oncimine.com). Numbers after sample names indicate sample size. Bar: mean value. **c** HK1 and HK2 mRNA expression profiles in the TCGA_Liver Cancer dataset. Data were obtained from the cBioPortal (http://www.cbioportal.org). RSEM RNA-Seq by Expectation Maximization. **d** Identification of HK1⁻HK2⁺ cancer cell lines present in the Cancer Cell Line Encyclopedia (CCLE) collection (http://www.cbioportal.org). Upper panel, HK1 and HK2 mRNA expression of 935 cell lines with RNASeq data in the CCLE dataset. Each data point represents one cell line. The box indicates "HK1⁻HK2⁺" cell lines, defined as HK2 > 1 TPM and HK1 < 10 TPM. TPM transcripts per million. Lower panel, distribution of the CCLE HK1⁻HK2⁺ cancer cell lines in a broad spectrum of cancers of different tissues of origin. **e** Hexokinase isoform expression in four human samples and seven human liver cancer cell lines

exhibiting the $HK1^-HK2^+$ molecular characteristic are present, at varying frequencies, across a broad spectrum of cancer types from a wide variety of tissues of origin (Fig. 1d).

We chose to use liver cancer cell lines to investigate HK2 as a therapeutic target because of (i) the substantial contributions of both $HK1^-HK2^+$ and $HK1^+HK2^+$ tumor cell lines to the liver CCLE population, (ii) the lack of effective treatment for liver cancers, and (iii) the prediction of liver cancer as the third most lethal cancer in the USA in the next decade [17]. To confirm and extend these observations, we evaluated the expression of HK1 and HK2 in human liver samples and in a collection of liver cancer cell lines (Fig. 1e). At the protein level, all established human liver cancer cell lines we examined express HK2 and lack HK4. Moreover, as expected from the TCGA data, these liver cancer cell lines fall into two subpopulations: $HK1^-HK2^+$ (Hep3B, HepG2, JHH5, JHH7, Huh7) and $HK1^+HK2^+$ (HLF, JHH6) (Fig. 1e). We used these liver cancer cell lines to examine the therapeutic efficacy of the targeted inhibition of HK2.

HK2 shRNA-silencing mediated inhibition of proliferation and colony formation in $HK1^-HK2^+$ cancer cells, but not $HK1^+HK2^+$ cancer cells, is a property of cancer cells from a variety of tissues of origin

To examine tumor cell growth inhibition in response to HK2 knockdown, we investigated the consequences of expressing an HK2-targeted doxycycline (DOX)-inducible shRNA in our panel of $HK1^-HK2^+$ and $HK1^+HK2^+$ liver cancer cell lines. An inducible HK2 shRNA was used to avoid the potential selection for cells resistant to HK2 silencing. shHK2 expression suppressed both proliferation (Fig. 2a, lower panel) and colony formation (Fig. 2b) of the $HK1^-HK2^+$ liver cancer cell lines. However, in contrast to the results obtained with the $HK1^-HK2^+$ liver cancer cell lines, shHK2 expression in the $HK1^+HK2^+$ liver cancer cell lines had no significant effect on either cell proliferation (Fig. 2a, lower panel) or colony formation (Fig. 2b). These results were validated using two additional shRNA sequences for HK2 (Additional file 1: Figure S1A and S1B).

The lack of an shHK2 inhibitory response for $HK1^+HK2^+$ cancer cells is not unique to liver cancer cells; shHK2 inhibition of HK2 expression is unable to prevent proliferation or colony formation in $HK1^+HK2^+$ tumor cell lines derived from lung, breast, or colon cancers (Fig. 2c, d) as well as $HK1^+HK2^+$ liver cancer cells. In addition, we used CRISPR Cas9 HK1 deletion to create isogenic $HK1^-HK2^+$ and $HK1^+HK2^+$ H460 lung cancer cell lines (Additional file 1: Figure S1C). DOX-induced shHK2 expression in the $HK1^-HK2^+$ H460 cells suppressed colony formation but had no effect on isogenic $HK1^+HK2^+$ H460 cell colony formation (Fig. 2e); conversion of an $HK1^+HK2^+$ cancer cell to an isogenic $HK1^-HK2^+$ cancer cell has no effect on cell growth or proliferation but converts cells resistant to shHK2-mediated inhibition of proliferation or colony formation to cells sensitive to shHK2 inhibition.

Both HK1 and HK2 drive cancer aerobic glycolysis—glucose consumption and lactic acid production. Consequently, HK2 knockdown by DOX-induced shHK2 resulted in a greater reduction of both glucose consumption and lactate production more pronounced in $HK1^-HK2^+$ cancer cells (Hep3B, Huh7) compared to $HK1^+HK2^+$ cancer cells (SUM159) (Fig. 2f). However, before proceeding further with consideration of HK2-targeted therapy, we wanted to determine if reduction of HK2 activity in $HK1^-HK2^+$ cells would also reduce glucose consumption in vivo. In mouse subcutaneous Hep3B/shHK2^{DOX} tumor xenografts, HK2 knockdown by a 4-day DOX treatment in the diet reduced tumor glucose consumption as determined non-invasively by ^{18}F-fluorodeoxyglucose (FDG)/positron emission tomography (PET) imaging [18, 19] (Fig. 2g, h).

While HK2 knockdown in $HK1^-HK2^+$ liver cancer cells substantially reduced cell proliferation, the majority of the cells remained alive (Additional file 1: Figure S1D); after removing DOX from cultured Hep3B/shHK2^{DOX} cells, the DOX-treated $HK1^-HK2^+$ cells were able to recover from HK2-inhibited cytostasis and resumed proliferation (Fig. 2i). These data suggest that monotherapy with selective HK2 inhibitors in $HK1^-HK2^+$ tumors is unlikely to be curative, either in preclinical models or in clinical applications; identification of synergistic or synthetically lethal agents in combination with HK2 inhibition will be necessary for HK2-targeted therapy of $HK1^-HK2^+$ tumors.

Diphenyleneiodonium (DPI), in combination with HK2 knockdown, is synthetically lethal for $HK1^-HK2^+$ liver cancer cells

To search for partners synthetically lethal with HK2 silencing in $HK1^-HK2^+$ cancer cells, 119 FDA-approved oncology drugs and 3205 drug-like compounds were screened, with or without DOX-induced shHK2 HK2 knockdown, in Hep3B/shHK2^{dox} cells (Fig. 3a, Additional file 2: Table S1). None of the 119 FDA-approved oncology drugs were synergistic with HK2 knockdown. DPI was the molecule best able, in combination with HK2 knockdown, to reduce the number of viable Hep3B/shHK2^{dox} cells (Fig. 3a and Additional file 1: Figure S2A). Because HK2 is the only HK isoform expressed in Hep3B cells, FDG (an inhibitor of both HK1 and HK2) can be used as an "HK2-targeted inhibitor," in place of HK2 shRNA knockdown, to demonstrate the synergistic effect between HK2 inhibition and DPI for $HK1^-HK2^+$ Hep3B growth inhibition (Additional file 1: Figure S2B). Using the Chou-Talalay method [20], we confirmed that the combination of DPI and FDG resulted in substantial synergy in all five $HK1^-HK2^+$ liver cancer cell lines tested (Additional file 2: Table S2). While shHK2, FDG, or DPI as single agents were not cytotoxic at the concentrations used in this experiment, they slow cell proliferation; in contrast, the combination of either DPI/shHK2 or DPI/FDG caused synthetic lethality in these $HK1^-HK2^+$ liver cancer cells (Fig. 3b, c and Additional file 1: Figure S2C). However, the synergism/synthetic lethality between HK2 knockdown and DPI is restricted to $HK1^-HK2^+$ cancer cells and is not observed in $HK1^+HK2^+$ liver cancer cells or in $HK1^+HK2^+$ cancer cells from other tissues (Additional file 1: Figure S2D). It is important to note that we chose to use FDG instead of 2-deoxy-D-glucose (2DG, a commonly used reagent to study glycolysis) because 2DG inhibits both HK1/2-driven glycolysis and N-linked glycosylation, whereas FDG only inhibits HK1/2-driven glycolysis [21]. As a result, 2DG is toxic as a single agent but FDG is not [21].

DPI has been reported to inhibit NADPH oxidase (NOX) [22], nitric oxide synthase (NOS) [23], and mitochondrial complex I [24]. Tested in combination with

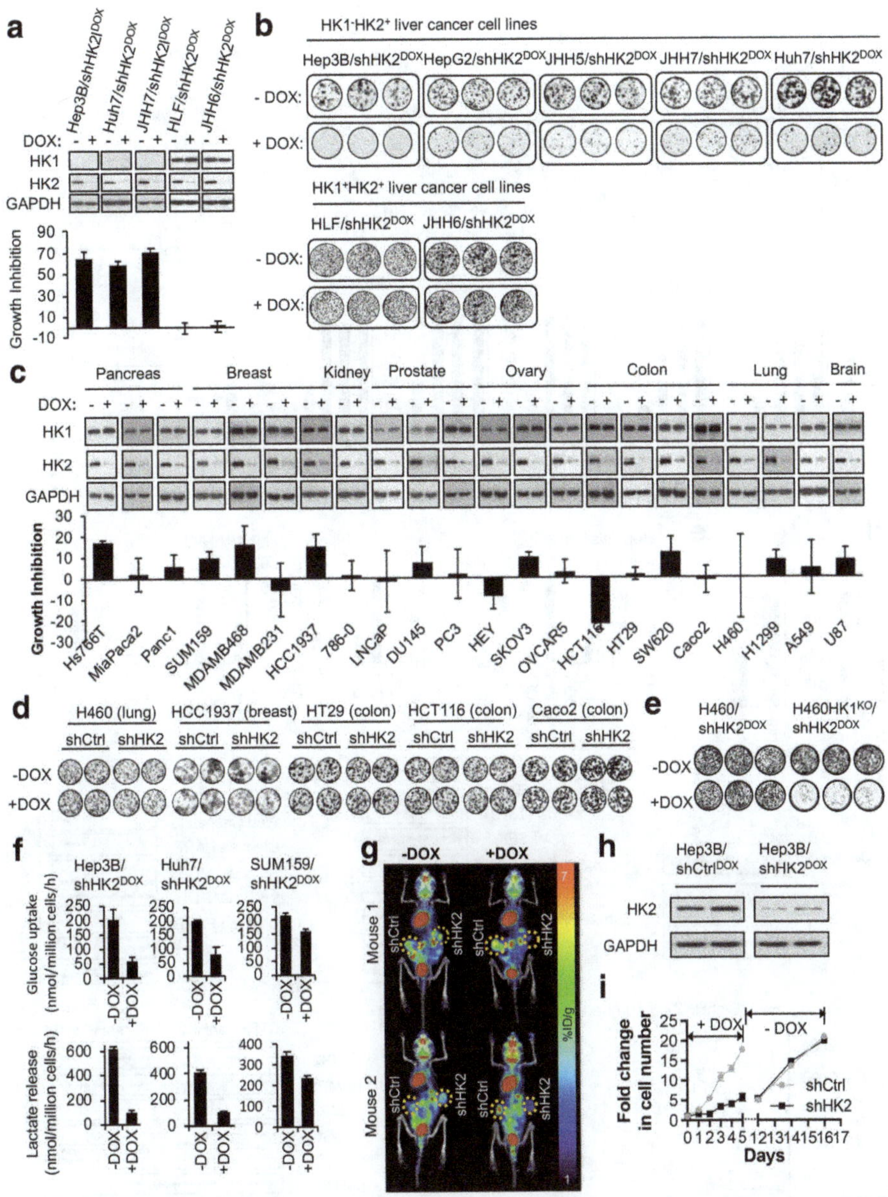

Fig. 2 HK1$^-$HK2$^+$ liver cancer cells are sensitive to HK2 knockdown-induced growth inhibition. **a** HK1$^-$HK2$^+$ liver cancer cells are sensitive to HK2 knockdown-induced growth inhibition. Top panel, HK2 knockdown by DOX-inducible shHK2^{DOX} after 72 h DOX (25 ng/ml) induction. Bottom panel, after a 7-day exposure to DOX to induce shRNA expression, relative cell numbers were measured using the MTT assay. Data are expressed as "growth inhibition" [100 × (1 − MTT assay values of DOX-treated cells/MTT assay values of untreated cells)]. **b** Effect of DOX-induced HK2 knockdown on colony formation by HK1$^-$HK2$^+$ and HK1$^+$HK2$^+$ liver cancer cells. Triplicate wells of each cell line are shown, stained at 15–20 days after plating. **c**, **d** DOX-induced HK2 silencing has limited or no effect on **c** cell proliferation or **d** colony formation in HK1$^+$HK2$^+$ cancer cells, regardless of tissue of origin. **e** DOX-induced shRNA HK2 knockdown inhibited colony formation by H460HK1^{KO}/shHK2^{DOX} isogenic cells but not by isogenic H460/shHK2^{DOX} cells. **f** HK2 knockdown inhibits glucose consumption (upper panels) and lactate production (lower panels) in Hep3B/shHK2^{DOX}, Huh7/shHK2^{DOX}, and SUM159/shHK2^{DOX} cells. Triplicate wells of cells were exposed to DOX or vehicle for 72 h. *Media* were then refreshed and, after 24 h, glucose consumption and lactate production were measured. **g** HK2 knockdown decreases ^{18}F-FDG/PET signal in a mouse subcutaneous Hep3B/shHK2^{DOX} xenograft model. Tumors on the left flank: Hep3B/shCtrl^{DOX}. Tumors on the right flank: Hep3B/shHK2^{DOX}. ^{18}F-FDG PET/CT scans were performed for each mouse before and after mice were switched to a DOX diet for 4 days. **h** Following the PET scans in panel **g**, HK2 knockdown was confirmed in tumor extracts by Western blotting. **i** Cytostasis induced in HK1$^-$HK2$^+$ liver cancer cells by HK2 knockdown is reversible. Hep3B/shHK2^{DOX} cells and Hep3B/shCtrl^{DOX} cells were treated with DOX for 2 days then re-plated in equal numbers in 96-well plates on day 0 in the continued presence of DOX. Cell proliferation during days 0–5 in the presence of DOX was measured (left panel). Cells from the two conditions (+DOX, −DOX) were pooled and cultured in DOX-free medium for 7 days (days 5–12) to allow the degradation of shRNAs in the cells and re-expression of HK2. The cells were then re-plated in 96-well plates and grown in the absence of DOX to generate the growth curves for days 12–16 (right panel). Relative cell proliferation was measured by the MTT assay and presented as fold change compared to the value on day 0. Each data point in panels **a**, **c**, and **f** represents mean ± SD of triplicate samples

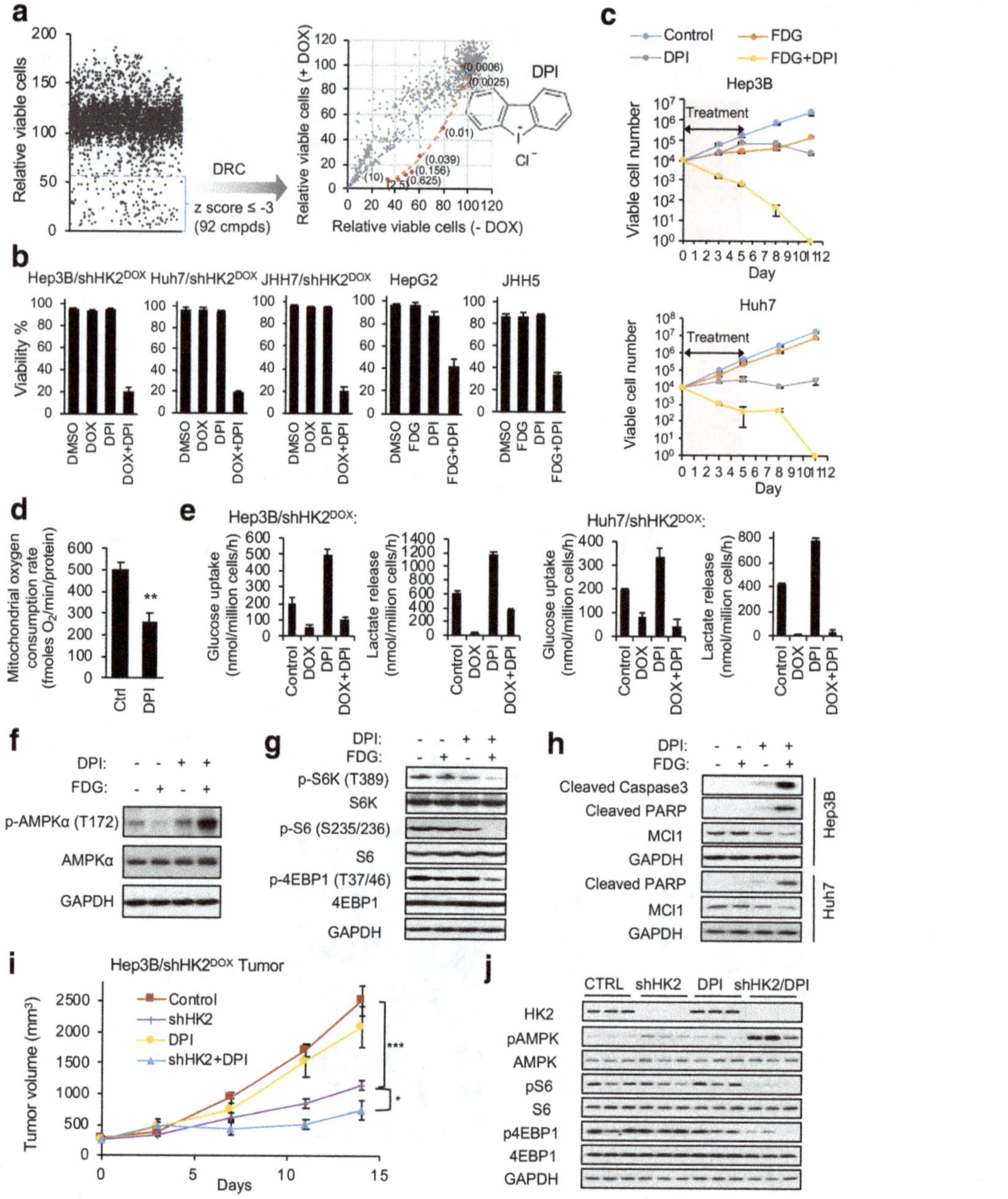

Fig. 3 (See legend on next page.)

(See figure on previous page.)

Fig. 3 DPI is a synthetically lethal partner in combination with HK2 knockdown or inhibition in $HK1^{-}HK2^{+}$ liver cancer cells. **a** A high-throughput screen of 3205 drug-like compounds and 119 FDA-approved oncology drugs identified DPI as the best synergistic agent with HK2 knockdown in $Hep3B/shHK2^{DOX}$ cells. Primary screening of all compounds at 10 μM was performed in combination with DOX-induced HK2 knockdown in $Hep3B/shHK2^{DOX}$ cells. Growth inhibition was measured by the CellTiter-Glo assay (left panel). Ninety-two compounds with *z* scores ≤ − 3 were tested in dose response curves (dose response concentrations 0, 0.0006, 0.0025, 0.01, 0.039, 0.156, 0.625, and 2.5 μM) in $Hep3B/shHK2^{DOX}$ cells cultured with or without DOX. Viable cells were normalized to DMSO-treated cells with or without DOX, respectively (right panel). The dots represent compounds at the tested concentrations. The red line connects the individual DPI concentration points. The chemical structure of DPI is shown. **b** DPI is synthetically lethal with HK2 knockdown or inhibition in $HK1^{-}HK2^{+}$ liver cancer cells. DOX/DPI 2-day DOX pretreatment prior to 72 h DPI (100 nM) treatment. FDG/DPI 72 h FDG (1 mM) and/or DPI (100 nM) treatments. Viability percentages were determined by trypan blue staining. **c** FDG/DPI combination irreversibly inhibits Hep3b and Huh7 $HK1^{-}HK2^{+}$ liver cancer cell proliferation. Viable cells were determined by trypan blue staining. **d** DPI decreases the oxygen consumption rate (OCR) of Hep3B cells. Cells were exposed to 100 nM DPI or vehicle for 2 h before OCR measurements. **e** DPI increases glycolysis of $HK1^{-}HK2^{+}$ liver cancer cells. Cells were pretreated with vehicle or DOX for 72 h prior to exposure to DPI (100 nM). Twenty-four hours later, culture media were analyzed for glucose and lactate. **f, g** FDG/DPI treatment activates AMPKα (**f**) and inactivates the mTOR pathway (**g**) in Hep3B cells. Cells were treated with 1 mM FDG and/or 100 nM DPI for 4 h. **h** FDG/DPI treatment triggers apoptosis. Hep3B $HK1^{-}HK2^{+}$ cells were treated with FDG (1 mM) and/or DPI (100 nM) for 24 h prior to apoptosis analyses. **i** DPI (2 mg/kg) enhances inhibition of tumor progression in response to HK2 silencing in $Hep3B/shHK2^{DOX}$ tumors. Mice-bearing tumor xenografts were treated when tumors reached 200 mm^3 (day 0). **j** Effects of HK2 knockdown and/or DPI (2 mg/kg) treatment on HK2 expression, AMPKα activation, and mTOR pathway inactivation in the xenograft $Hep3B/shHK2^{DOX}$ tumors described in panel **i**. Each data point in **a**–**c** and **e** represents mean ± SD of triplicate samples, and each data point in **d** and **i** represents mean ± SEM of five samples. $^{*}P < 0.05$, $^{***}P < 0.001$

HK2 knockdown, neither NOX inhibitors (GKT137831, apocynin; Additional file 1: Figure S3A) nor NOS inhibitors (L-NAME or L-NNA) (Additional file 1: Figure S3B) show synergy in $HK1^{-}HK2^{+}$ liver cancer cells. In contrast, the complex I inhibitor rotenone (ROT) is synthetically lethal in combination with HK2 knockdown (Additional file 1: Figure S3C). In addition, DPI treatment reduced, but did not eliminate, mitochondrial oxygen consumption (Fig. 3d), consistent with its inhibition of mitochondrial complex I, and increased cellular demand for glycolysis (Fig. 3e). These results indicate that DPI synergizes with HK2 silencing/inhibition in $HK1^{-}HK2^{+}$ liver cancer cells through the inhibition of mitochondrial complex I, reducing ATP production from the electron transport chain (ETC). The synergistic reduction in cellular energy levels by FDG/DPI or FDG/ROT triggered the activation of the cellular energy sensor AMPKα (Fig. 3f and Additional file 1: Figure S3D), suppressed the energy-dependent mTOR pathway (Fig. 3g and Additional file 1: Figure S3E) [25], and induced apoptosis (Fig. 3h and Additional file 1: Figure S3F).

In a mouse xenograft model of $HK1^{-}HK2^{+}$ $Hep3B/shHK2^{DOX}$ tumor progression, DOX-induced HK2 knockdown initiated when the tumors reached 200 mm^3 significantly reduced tumor growth (Fig. 3i). Although DPI alone had no significant effect on tumor growth, the DPI/shHK2 combination was significantly more effective in reducing tumor growth when compared to the effect of either shHK2 or DPI alone (Fig. 3i). The $Hep3B/shHK2^{DOX}$ tumors, in which HK2 was reduced to undetectable levels, did not express other active HK isoforms to compensate for glycolysis (Additional file 1: Figure S4). The combination shHK2/DPI treatment resulted in increased levels of phosphorylated AMPKα and dephosphorylation of S6 and 4EBP1 in xenograft $Hep3B/shHK2^{DOX}$ tumors (Fig. 3j), demonstrating the reduction in tumor energy production induced by the shHK2/DPI combination therapy.

Inhibition of fatty acid oxidation sensitizes $HK1^{-}HK2^{+}$ liver cancer cells to the FDG/DPI combination

Acetyl-CoA carboxylase (ACC), the first and rate-limiting enzyme in fatty acid biosynthesis, regulates fatty acid oxidation (FAO) [26]. Both the FDG/DPI and FDG/ROT combinations triggered ACC phosphorylation in Hep3B and Huh7 $HK1^{-}HK2^{+}$ liver cancer cells (Fig. 4a and Additional file 1: Figure S5A), an indicator of ACC inhibition. These data suggest the FDG/DPI combination treatment shifts the balance of cellular metabolism in $HK1^{-}HK2^{+}$ cancer cells from fatty acid elongation, which is used for membrane synthesis and cell proliferation, to FAO to provide additional fuel for energy generation through residual mitochondrial respiration (Fig. 3d) as a survival strategy. When compared to normal liver, liver cancers upregulate expression of genes involved in fatty acid elongation and downregulate expression of genes involved in FAO (Fig. 4b). These data also suggest FAO inhibitors might sensitize $HK1^{-}HK2^{+}$ cancer cells to the combination of DPI and HK2 inhibition but could be tolerated by HK4-expressing hepatocytes and by other normal tissues which express HK1.

Perhexiline (PER), a FAO inhibitor in clinical use as an anti-angina drug in Australia and Asia and currently in clinical trials in the USA [13], sensitized $HK1^{-}HK2^{+}$ Hep3B liver cancer cells to the FDG/DPI combination (Fig. 4c). In the presence of FDG and DPI, at sub-optimal concentrations (lower than the concentrations used in previous experiments) that did not cause

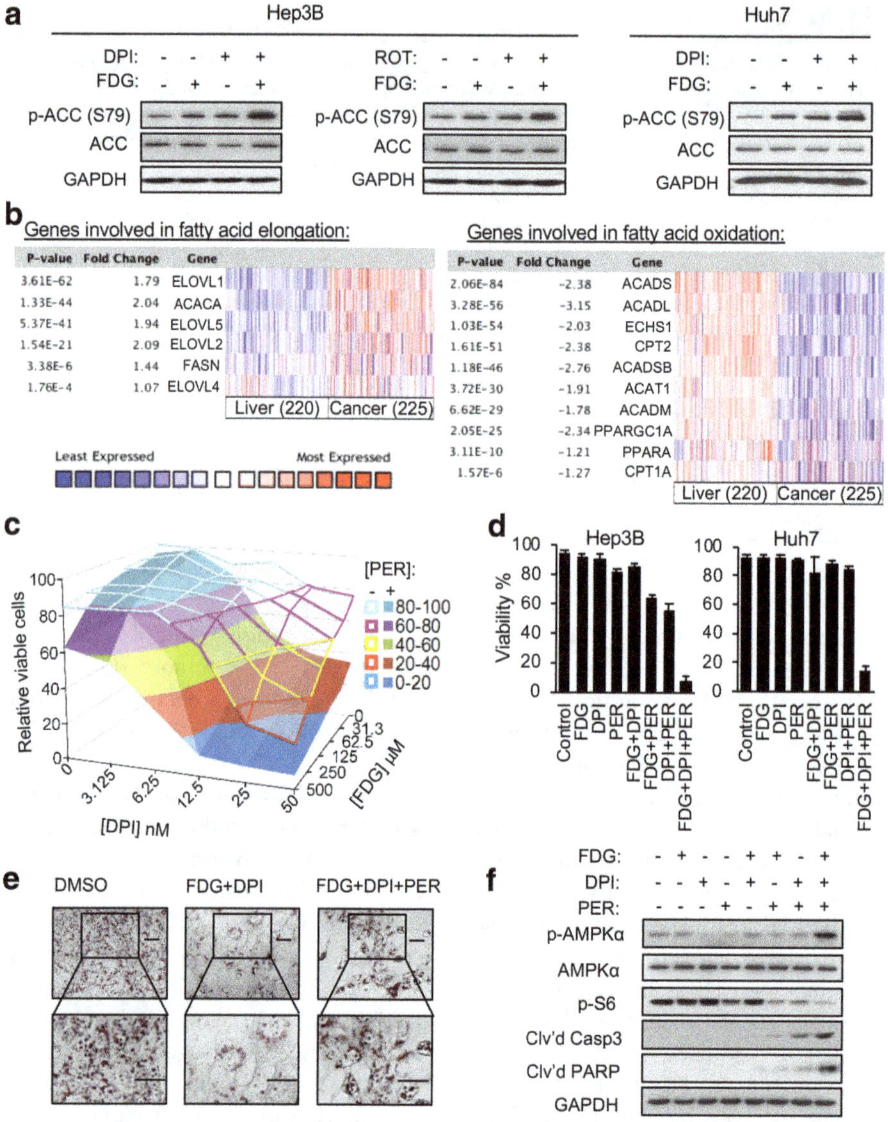

Fig. 4 Inhibition of fatty acid oxidation sensitizes HK1⁻HK2⁺ liver cancer cells to the cytotoxicity of the HK2 inhibition/DPI combination. **a** FDG/DPI or FDG/ROT combinations induce ACC phosphorylation. HK1⁻HK2⁺ liver cancer cells were treated with the indicated drug(s) for 24 h prior to analysis of ACC phosphorylation. FDG, 1 mM. DPI, 100 nM. ROT, 100 nM. **b** Clinical liver cancer samples show upregulated expression of genes involved in fatty acid elongation and downregulated expression of genes involved in FAO compared to normal liver tissues. Data were obtained from Oncomine (http://www.oncomine.com). **c** PER sensitizes Hep3B cells to FDG/DPI treatment. Cells were treated with FDG, plus or minus 5 μM PER, for 72 h and then assayed for viable cells by the MTT assay. Open surface, [DPI + FDG + vehicle] treatment. Filled surface, [DPI + FDG + PER] treatment. **d** PER sensitizes HK1⁻HK2⁺ liver cancer cells to the cytotoxicity of FDG/DPI treatment. Triplicate wells of (left) Hep3B or (right) Huh7 cells were treated with FDG (250 μM), DPI (15 nM), and/or PER (5 μM) for 72 h, followed by trypan blue staining to determine cell viability. Viability % = 100% × (trypan blue negative cells/total cells). Data are means ± SD. **e** PER rescues FDG/DPI-induced lipid droplet depletion in Hep3B cells. Hep3B cells were treated with DMSO, FDG (1 mM)/DPI (100 nM), or FDG (1 mM)/DPI (100 nM)/PER (5 μM) for 24 h, followed by Oil Red staining of intracellular lipid droplets. Representative images with indicated treatments are shown. Scale bars, 30 μM. **f** FDG, DPI, and/or PER modulation of AMPKα activation, mTOR pathway inactivation, and apoptosis induction in Hep3B/shHK2^{DOX} cells. Cells were treated with FDG (250 μM), DPI (15 nM), and/or PER (5 μM) for 24 h, and cell extracts were examined by Western blotting

significant cell death either alone or in combination, the addition of PER to HK1⁻HK2⁺ liver cancer cells resulted in substantial lethality (Fig. 4d). A similar sensitizing effect was observed with another FAO inhibitor, etomoxir (Additional file 1: Figure S5B). While the FDG/DPI combination significantly decreased lipid droplets (lipid droplets are an indicator of cellular fatty acid abundance) in HK1⁻HK2⁺ liver cancer cells, PER addition prevented the disappearance of lipid droplets (Fig. 4e). In addition, PER synergized with the FDG/DPI combination to activate AMPKα, suppress the mTOR pathway, and trigger apoptosis (Fig. 4f). In contrast, there was no significant synthetic lethality induced by the triple combination of shHK2/DPI/PER in $HK1^+HK2^+$ cancer cells (Additional file 1: Figure S5C), suggesting that our shHK2/DPI/PER triple-combination treatment is selectively cytotoxic for $HK1^-HK2^+$ cancer cells and is likely to be tolerated by normal tissues. Taken together, our results indicate that FAO inhibition further sensitizes $HK1^-HK2^+$ cells to the combined inhibition of glycolysis and the mitochondrial electron transport chain (ETC) and that the triple combination of HK2 inhibition, DPI, and PER simultaneously target the components of multiple energy generation sources (glycolysis, OXPHOS, FAO) in $HK1^-HK2^+$ liver cancer cells, resulting in synthetic lethality in cells that express HK2 but not HK1.

The HK2i/DPI/PER combination suppresses energy generation and alters cell metabolism in $HK1^-HK2^+$ liver cancer cells

Mitochondrial oxygen consumption rate (OCR) is an indicator of cellular energy production. To demonstrate a synergistic relationship among FDG, DPI, and PER, these inhibitors were used at sub-optimal concentrations (lower than the concentrations used in previous experiments), at which each individual agent did not substantially affect cell growth (Fig. 4c, d) or their OCR (Fig. 5a). The FDG/DPI/PER combination substantially reduced the basal OCR in $HK1^-HK2^+$ Hep3B cells within the first 2 h (Fig. 5a). PER enhanced the FDG/DPI combination-induced OCR reduction continued over a 24-h period (Fig. 5b). Decreased basal respiration in response to the triple combination suggests decreased ATP turnover in these cells, reflecting a state of reduced cellular energy generation [27].

Mass spectrometry was used to determine the levels of energy-related molecules extracted from $HK1^-HK2^+$ Hep3B cells after an 8-h treatment with FDG, DPI, and/or PER at sub-optimal concentrations, at which each individual agent did not substantially affect cell growth (Fig. 4c, d) or OCR (Fig. 5a). The increase in the ADP/ATP and AMP/ATP ratios in response to the triple treatment demonstrated the combined inhibition of ATP production from glycolysis, oxidative phosphorylation, and FAO (Fig. 5c). In addition, the combination of PER with FDG, DPI, or FDG/DPI substantially increased the creatine/P-creatine ratio (Fig. 5c), limiting the ability of $HK1^-HK2^+$ liver cancer cells to replenish ATP from P-creatine. These molecular energy changes, measured after an 8-h treatment, occurred before cell death as measured by trypan blue exclusion (Additional file 1: Figure S6A). The FDG/DPI/PER-induced reduction in ATP was also confirmed in living Hep3B cells expressing firefly luciferase, an ATP-dependent reporter enzyme (Additional file 1: Figure S6B). Metabolomic analysis also revealed that the pools of most metabolites of glycolysis and the TCA cycle, as well as nucleotide pools, were reduced in $HK1^-HK2^+$ liver cancer cells treated with FDG/DPI and were further decreased when PER was added into the combination (Fig. 5d). These data suggest that global changes in cell metabolism, in association with or caused by energy inhibition, may contribute to the HK2i/DPI/PER-induced synthetic lethality in $HK1^-HK2^+$ cancer cells.

The shHK2/DPI/PER combination suppresses established $HK1^-HK2^+$ liver tumor progression in vivo

We next compared the efficacy of the shHK2/DPI/PER triple combination to the efficacy of the shHK2/DPI double combination in xenograft $HK1^-HK2^+$ liver tumors. In each of the treatment groups, individual $HK1^-HK2^+$ Hep3B/shHK2^{DOX} mice were switched to the DOX-containing diet when their tumor reached 200 mm^3 (day 0) to induce HK2 knockdown. DPI and/or PER treatments were started 72 h later (day 3). While PER alone showed no significant effects on tumor growth (Additional file 1: Figure S7), PER significantly enhanced the potency of the shHK2/DPI combination in Hep3B/shHK2^{DOX} tumor progression (Fig. 6a, b). No significant change in body weight was detected among the different Hep3B/shHK2^{DOX} xenograft groups (Fig. 6c). While both the shHK2 + DPI and the shHK2 + DPI + PER treatments activated AMPKα and suppressed the mTOR signaling cascade, only the shHK2 + DPI + PER treatment induced the appearance in xenograft tumors of the apoptosis markers cleaved caspase-3 and cleaved caspase-7 (Fig. 6d). These data indicate that, with the reported maximum DPI tolerated dosage and schedule [28], the intratumor amount of DPI was not sufficient to achieve tumor synthetic lethality with HK2 knockdown. However, the addition of PER sensitized Hep3B tumors to the shHK2/DPI combination and induced tumor cell apoptosis.

The potency of the shHK2/DPI/PER combination was also examined with two additional $HK1^-HK2^+$ liver tumor xenografts, Huh7/shHK2^{DOX} and HepG2/shHK2^{DOX} (Fig. 6e–g). These results confirm the in vivo efficacy and safety of our triple-combination therapy in established $HK1^-HK2^+$ liver tumors.

The shHK2/DPI/PER combination is an effective precision therapy for treating $HK1^-HK2^+$ tumors, regardless of their tissues of origin

We used liver cancer cell lines to develop our $HK1^-HK2^+$ cancer cell-targeted combination therapy. As indicated earlier, analysis of the CCLE RNASeq dataset identified subsets of cancer cell lines, present in a broad spectrum of cancers from a wide variety of tissues of origin, that exhibit the $HK1^-HK2^+$ molecular signature (Fig. 1d). We suggest that this therapy will be effective in

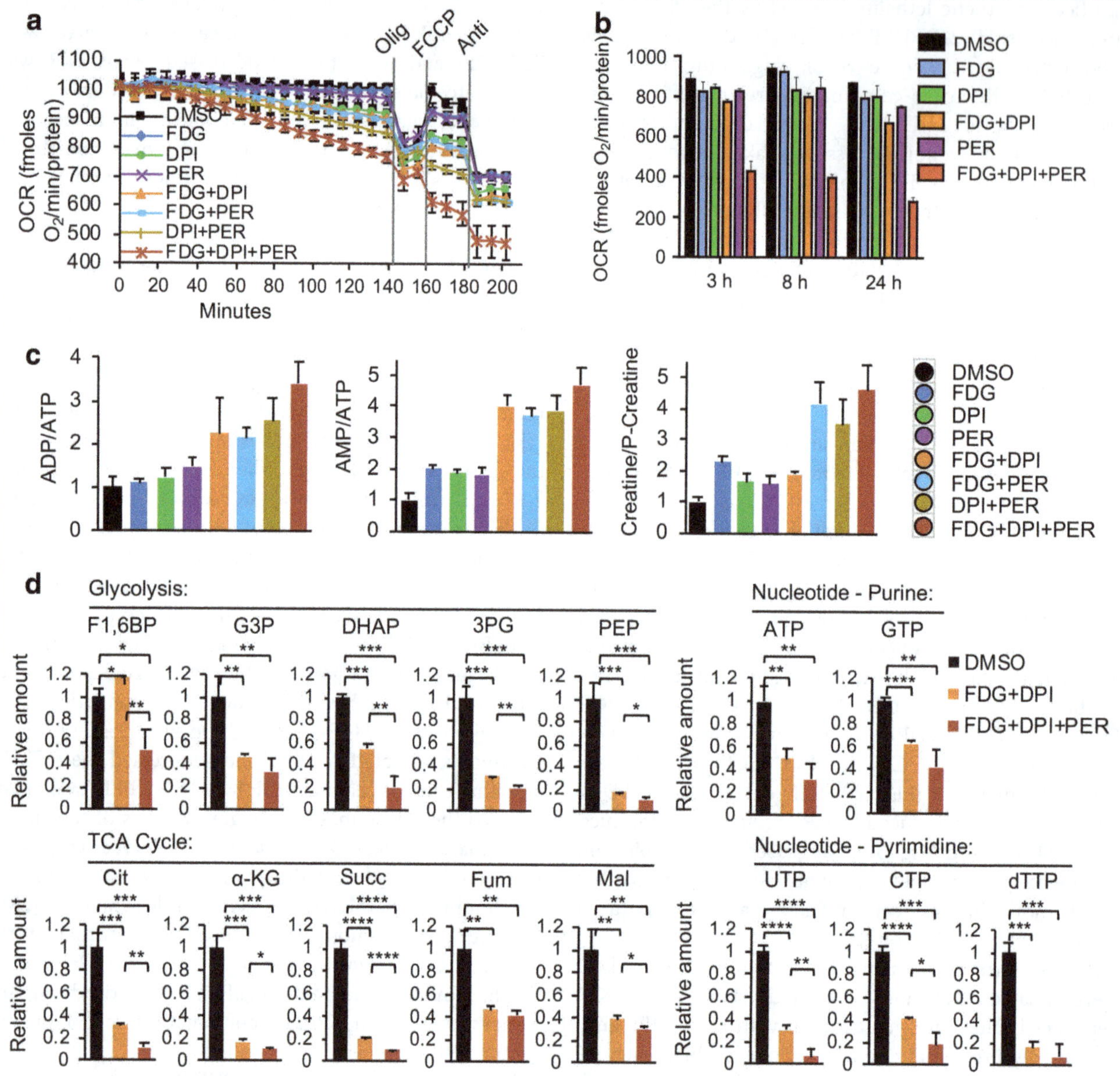

Fig. 5 Modulation of energy generation and metabolism in HK1⁻HK2⁺ Hep3B/shHK2^{DOX} cells in response to FDG/DPI/PER treatment. **a** FDG/DPI/PER combination treatment acutely decreases the OCR of Hep3B cells. FDG (250 μM), DPI (15 nM), and/or PER (5 μM) were added to cultured Hep3B cells, as single agents or in the combinations shown, at time 0. The OCR was measured by the Seahorse assay. Oligomycin (2 μM), FCCP (0.1 μM), and Antimycin (2 μM) were used to indicate the fraction of respiration coupled to oxidative ATP production, maximum mitochondrial respiration, and non-mitochondrial respiration, respectively. **b** OCR in Hep3B cells after 3, 8, and 24 h of drug exposure; concentrations are as in panel **a**. **c** The HK2i/DPI/PER triple combination decreases liver cancer cellular energy levels. After an 8-h drug treatment, AMP, ADP, ATP, creatine, and P-creatine amounts in Hep3B cells were determined by LC-MS. **d** Changes in pool sizes of glycolysis and TCA cycle metabolites, as well as purine and pyrimidine nucleotides, after vehicle, FDG/DPI, or FDG/DPI/PER treatment in Hep3B cells. F1,6BP fructose 1,6-biphosphate, G3P glyceraldehyde 3-phosphate, DHAP dihydroxyacetone phosphate, 3PG 3-phospho-glycerate, PEP phosphoenolpyruvate, Cit citrate, α-KG α-ketoglutarate, Succ succinate, Fum fumarate, Mal malate. Each data point in **a** and **b** represents mean ± SEM of five samples, and each data point in **c** and **d** represents mean ± SD of triplicate samples. *$P < 0.05$, **$P < 0.01$, ***$P < 0.001$, ****$P < 0.0001$

$HK1^-HK2^+$ cancer cells, regardless of their tissue of origin. However, $HK1^+HK2^+$ cancer cell lines from a variety of cancers (liver, breast, colon, prostate, ovary, lung), including the lung cancer H460 cell line, are resistant to HK2 silencing alone (Fig. 2a–d) or the synthetic lethality of the shHK2/DPI/PER (Additional file 1: Figure S5C). To test the potential generality of the efficacy of the shHK2/DPI/PER combination in cancers with the $HK1^-HK2^+$ molecular characteristic, regardless of their tissues of origin, we used the isogenic lung cancer cell

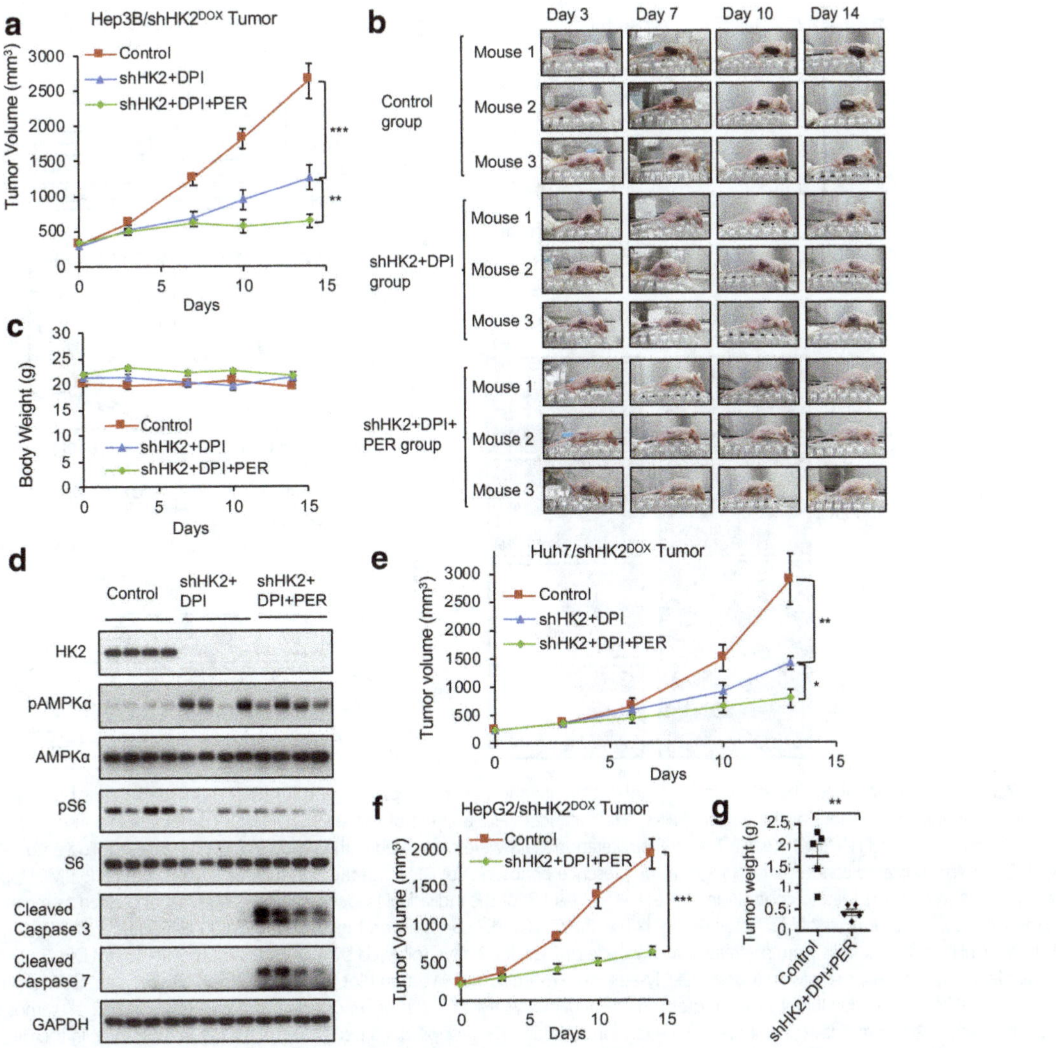

Fig. 6 PER sensitizes established xenograft HK1⁻HK2⁺ liver tumors to HK2 knockdown/DPI combination therapy. **a** PER enhances the ability of the HK2 knockdown/DPI combination to retard the progression of Hep3B/shHK2^{DOX} tumor xenografts. When tumors reached 200 mm^3 (day 0), xenografts were randomized into a control group and two treatment groups. The control mice (*n* = 7) were remained on the standard diet and were treated with vehicle. In the treatment groups, mice were placed on a DOX-supplemented diet (from day 0) and treated either with DPI (2 mg/kg, daily i.p. from day 3, *n* = 7) or with [DPI (2 mg/kg, daily i.p.) + PER (30 mg/kg, daily i.p), from day 3, *n* = 8]. **b** Representative images of tumor progression in three mice from each group in panel **a**. **c** Body weights of the mice in panel **a** bearing xenograft subcutaneous tumors, in response to the indicated treatments. **d** shHK2/DPI/PER treatment activates AMPKα and dephosphorylates S6 and elicits cleavage of caspase-3 and caspase-7. Hep3B/shHK2^{DOX} tumors from the indicated treatment groups were collected at day 15. Protein extracts from tissue homogenate supernatants were analyzed. **e** PER enhances the ability of the HK2 knockdown/DPI combination to retard the progression of HK1$^-$HK2$^+$ Huh7shHK2^{DOX} liver tumor xenografts. Experimental conditions are the same as those described in panel **a** (*n* = 6). **f** PER enhances the ability of the HK2 knockdown/DPI combination to retard the progression of HK1$^-$HK2$^+$ HepG2/shHK2^{DOX} liver tumor xenografts. Experimental conditions are the same as those described in panel **a** (*n* = 5). **g** HK2 knockdown/DPI/PER combination suppresses HepG2/shHK2^{DOX} tumor growth. Weights of HepG2/shHK2^{DOX} tumors after indicated treatments of the xenograft-bearing mice shown in panel **f** are shown. All data are expressed as means ± SEM. **P* < 0.05. ***P* < 0.01. ****P* < 0.001

line pair, HK1^{KO}HK2$^+$ H460 cells created by CRISPR Cas9 knockout, and their parental HK1$^+$HK2$^+$ H460 cells to establish HK1^{KO}HK2$^+$/shHK2^{DOX} H460 cells and HK1$^+$HK2$^+$/shHK2^{DOX} H460 cells (Additional file 1: Figure S1C). Unlike the HK1-expressing HK1$^+$HK2$^+$/shHK2^{DOX} H460 cells, the isogenic HK1^{KO}HK2$^+$/shHK2^{DOX} H460 cells are sensitive to the synthetic lethality of the shHK2/DPI/PER combination in cell culture (Fig. 7a). The shHK2/DPI/PER combination triggers the cleavage of caspase 3 in the isogenic HK1^{KO}HK2$^+$shHK2^{DOX} H460 cells but not in the HK1$^+$HK2$^+$shHK2^{DOX} H460 cells (Fig. 7b). While shHK2, DPI, or PER had no

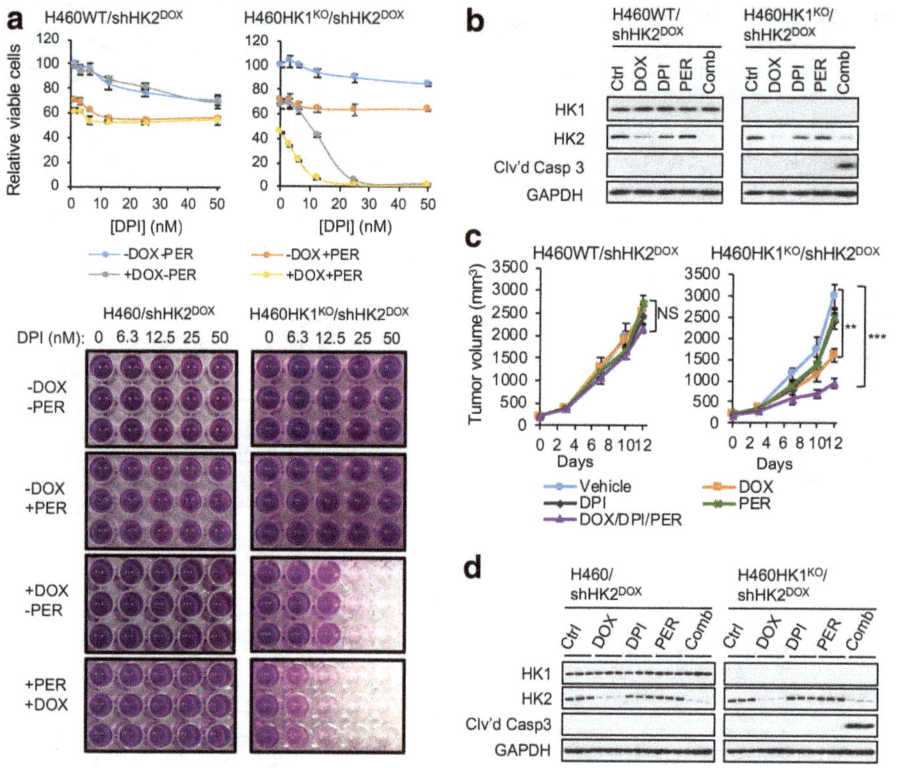

Fig. 7 The shHK2/DPI/PER combination does not inhibit proliferation or tumor progression for HK1$^+$HK2$^+$ cancer cells but is effective in inhibiting proliferation and progression for the isogenic HK1^{KO}HK2$^+$ cancer cells. **a** Effect of the shHK2/DPI/PER combination on isogenic HK1$^+$HK2$^+$ H460WT/shHK2^{DOX} and H460HK1^{KO}/shHK2^{DOX} cell proliferation. Cells were pretreated with vehicle or DOX for 2 days, followed by a 72-h treatment with DPI in the indicated concentration range, in the presence or absence of DOX and the presence or absence of PER (5 μM). Upper panels, MTT assay values were normalized to control samples (-DOX, -DPI, -PER) of the individual isogenic cell lines. Data are expressed as means ± SD. Lower panels, representative images of MTT assay results. **b** The shHK2/DPI/PER combination triggers apoptosis in H460HK1^{KO}/shHK2^{DOX} cells but not in H460WT/shHK2^{DOX} cells. Cells were pretreated with vehicle or DOX for 2 days, followed by a 24-h treatment with 15 nM DPI, 5 μM PER, and DOX, both as single agents and in combination (Comb). Cell lysates were examined by Western blot for HK1, HK2, and cleaved caspase 3 expression. **c** The shHK2/DPI/PER combination inhibits the progression of H460HK1^{KO}/shHK2^{DOX} tumor xenografts but not H460WT/shHK2^{DOX} tumor xenografts. When tumors reached 200 mm^3 (day 0), xenografts were randomized into five groups (*n* = 5 per group) receiving vehicle, DOX in the diet, DPI (2 mg/kg, daily i.p.), and PER (30 mg/kg, daily i.p.), both as single agents and in combination. Data are expressed as means ± SEM. $^{**}P < 0.01$. $^{***}P < 0.001$. NS not significant. **d** The shHK2/DPI/PER combination triggers apoptosis in H460HK1^{KO}/shHK2^{DOX} tumor xenografts but not H460WT/shHK2^{DOX} tumor xenografts. Three representative xenograft tumors in each group in panel **c** were homogenized for Western blotting analyses of indicated proteins

significant effect on xenograft HK1$^+$HK2$^+$ shHK2^{DOX} H460 tumor growth, shHK2 alone reduced tumor volume by 47%, and the shHK2/DPI/PER combination reduced tumor volume by 69% in HK1^{KO}HK2$^+$ shHK2^{DOX} H460 tumors (Fig. 7c). In addition to growth suppression in HK1^{KO}HK2$^+$ shHK2^{DOX} H460 tumors, the shHK2/DPI/PER combination also triggered tumor cell apoptosis (Fig. 7d). Taken together, our findings suggest that the HK2 inhibition/DPI/PER combination is a potential precision therapeutic approach to treatments for cancers with the HK1$^-$HK2$^+$ characteristic existing in a broad spectrum of cancer types, regardless of their tissues of origin.

Discussion

In this study, we describe a triple-combination therapy for treatment of HK1$^-$HK2$^+$ cancers that targets the HK1$^-$HK2$^+$ cancer-specific modes of energy generation, HK2-driven glycolysis, mitochondrial oxidative phosphorylation, and fatty acid oxidation. Using HK1$^-$HK2$^+$ liver cancer cells as an example, we illustrated that targeting each individual energy generation source is either cytostatic or has only a subtle effect on cell proliferation or tumor progression for HK1$^-$HK2$^+$ liver cancer cells. While the majority of cancers including liver cancer, from many tissues of origin, express both HK1 and HK2, in many types of cancers, there exist subsets of HK1$^-$HK2$^+$ tumors, i.e., tumors that express only HK2. The potential specificity of this therapy for this HK1$^-$HK2$^+$ subclass, and the extension of this therapy across cancers from a broad range of tissues of origin, results from this common phenotype that makes them vulnerable to this combination therapy.

We have studied HK2 knockdown in a large panel of naturally existing $HK1^+HK2^+$ and $HK1^-HK2^+$ cancer cells and found that only $HK1^-HK2^+$ cancer cells but not $HK1^+HK2^+$ cells as defined by mRNA and Western blot analyses are sensitive to HK2 knockdown. It is likely that there is a threshold effect for HK1 expression necessary to provide resistance to HK2 inhibition. Future studies in the titration of HK1 protein levels using genetic manipulation approaches, such as inducible knockdown of HK1 in $HK1^+HK2^+$ cancer cells with different concentrations of doxycycline or inducible expression of HK1 in $HK1^-HK2^+$ cancer cells with different concentrations of doxycycline, would quantify the threshold effect of HK1 required to provide resistance to HK2 inhibition in cancer cells. In addition, how the HK1 gene is silenced in the $HK1^-HK2^+$ subsets of cancers is unknown. Future studies in regulation of HK1 expression in cancers and in normal tissues may provide targets for combination therapies in conjunction with HK2 inhibition for cancer treatment.

It is important to note that, even at the highest DPI concentration (100 nM) we used in cell culture experiments, which is relevant to the tolerated plasma concentration previously determined in mice [28], DPI inhibits only 50% of OXPHOS activity (Fig. 3d). These data suggest that the residual OXPHOS system can still oxidize fuels provided by metabolic pathways such as pyruvate oxidation, glutamine catabolism, and FAO. When we partially inhibited HK2-driven glycolysis and OXPHOS in $HK1^-HK2^+$ cancer cells, we observed that FAO was upregulated as indicated by ACC phosphorylation (Fig. 4a) and disappearance of intracellular lipid droplets (Fig. 4e). Therefore, we targeted FAO with the clinical FAO inhibitor PER. The addition of PER sensitized $HK1^-HK2^+$ cancer cells to the combination of FDG and DPI, indicating that FAO plays an important role in providing fuels to the residual OXPHOS activity, among the different fuel-providing pathways.

Because cancer cells can flexibly reprogram their energy generation [29], loss of HK2 activity in $HK1^-HK2^+$ cancer cells is only cytostatic; however, the combined inhibition of these three critical pathways involved in ATP production leads to a profound decrease in energy generation and to synthetic lethality for $HK1^-HK2^+$ cancers. Identification/stratification of patients with an $HK1^-HK2^+$ cancer molecular characteristic will be essential for clinical translation of our combination therapy as a precision medicine for this tumor subtype in tumors of different origins.

While our manuscript was in preparation for submission, De Waal et al. [11] reported that cell proliferation and xenograft progression of HepG2 and Huh7 liver cancer cells, which are from the $HK1^-HK2^+$ liver cancer subset we studied (Fig. 1e), are restricted by $shHK2^{DOX}$ expression and that combination of $shHK2^{DOX}$ expression and OXPHOS inhibition with metformin further suppressed Huh7 xenograft progression. We also find $shHK2^{DOX}$ HK2 inhibition plus OXPHOS inhibition (in our case with DPI) reduces, but does not completely suppress, xenograft tumor progression for Huh7 (Fig. 6e) and Hep3B (Fig. 6a) $HK1^-HK2^+$ liver cancer xenografts. We suggest inhibition of the third major pathway driving ATP production, fatty acid oxidation, would enhance inhibition (by $shHK2^{DOX}$ + DPI/metformin) of $HK1^-HK2^+$ liver tumor xenograft growth and confirm this hypothesis for Hep3B, Huh7, and HepG2 liver tumor xenograft growth (Fig. 6a, e, and f).

De Waal et al. [11] emphasized that many liver cancers express HK2; however, a substantial proportion of liver cancers express both HK1 and HK2 or only HK1 (Fig. 1c). We find neither cell proliferation (Fig. 2a) nor colony formation (Fig. 2b) are affected by $shHK2^{DOX}$ HK2 inhibition for $HK1^+HK2^+$ HLF and JHH6 liver cancer cells, suggesting pharmacologic HK2 inhibition will not have therapeutic efficacy for $HK1^+HK2^+$ liver cancers.

CCLE cell gene expression profile analyses revealed cancers from tissues of multiple origins contain $HK1^-HK2^+$ subsets (Fig. 1d). To determine whether $HK1^-HK2^+$ cancers of other origins will be sensitive to HK2 inhibition, we created isogenic $HK1^-HK2^+$ cells from $HK1^+HK2^+$ H460 lung cancer cells. As expected, xenograft progression of $HK1^+HK2^+$ H460 cells was unaffected by $shHK2^{DOX}$ expression or the $shHK2^{DOX}$/DPI/PER combination (Fig. 7c). In contrast, $HK1^{KO}HK2^+$ H460 xenograft progression was inhibited by $shHK2^{DOX}$ expression or $shHK2^{DOX}$/DPI/PER (Fig. 7c). We conclude (i) that inhibition of HK2-driven glycolysis, OXPHOS, and FAO is likely to be a pan-tumor precision therapy approach to $HK1^-HK2^+$ tumors, regardless of their tissue of origin, and (ii) that cancer therapies that involve HK2 inhibition will be restricted to tumors that do not express HK1.

In addition to the hexokinases, several isoform switches in other metabolic enzymes occur during hepatocarcinogenesis, e.g., a splicing switch from ketohexokinase-C (KHK-C) to KHK-A involved in fructose metabolism [30], and a switch from 11β-HSD1 to 11β-HSD2 involved in glucocorticoid metabolism and gluconeogenesis [31]. Although the mechanisms of these metabolic isozyme switches and possible relationships among these switches during hepatocarcinogenesis are not currently understood, these additional cancer-specific isoforms may also be therapeutic targets for the development of effective cancer treatments.

Tumor progression for $HK1^-HK2^+$ liver cancer cells either by $shHK2^{DOX}$ + metformin [11] or by $shHK2^{DOX}$ + DPI (Fig. 3) is retarded but not completely suppressed. In vivo, DPI is maximally tolerated by mice at 2 mg/kg, with a plasma C_{max} value of 1 μM [28]. The combination of shRNA HK2 knockdown and daily DPI i.p. injection at 2 mg/kg did not cause $HK1^-HK2^+$ liver tumor cell apoptosis (Fig. 6d), suggesting that DPI at this dosage, in combination with HK2 knockdown, is not sufficient to cause lethality of $HK1^-HK2^+$ tumor cells in vivo. However, including PER in vivo to further sensitize $HK1^-HK2^+$ cancer cells to the shHK2/DPI combination improved the therapeutic effect on $HK1^-HK2^+$ tumors from growth inhibition to tumor cell death. Targeting fatty acid oxidation has recently been attracting additional attention for cancer therapy [13, 32, 33].

ATP is the principal energy currency in cell metabolism and is a versatile regulator of cellular activities [34, 35]. Maintenance of an adequate ATP supply is of crucial importance for cellular functions, for both normal tissues and for cancers. Targeting HK2-mediated glycolysis, mitochondrial respiration, and fatty acid oxidation in liver $HK1^-HK2^+$ cancer cells results in a synergistic decrease in cancer energy/ATP production. While a substantial drop in cellular energy levels causes $HK1^-HK2^+$ cancer cell death, the inhibition of different ATP generation sources may also have a profound impact on the distribution of compartmentalized intracellular ATP concentrations ("ATP inhomogeneity") [36]. For example, ATP produced from glycolysis is readily diffused in the cytosol, whereas transfer of respiration-derived ATP from mitochondrial to cytosol requires carrier proteins across mitochondrial membranes [37]. Nuclear ATP levels are compromised by inhibiting mitochondrial ATP production but not by inhibiting glycolysis [38]. The subcellular compartmentalization of ATP has important roles in multiple cellular activities, such as cell motility [36], muscle contraction [39], DNA repair [40], and chromatin remodeling [38]. Further study will be required to explore the impact of our combination therapy on the ATP inhomogeneity in $HK1^-HK2^+$ cancer cells derived from alternative tissues and the consequent effects on cell viability.

To translate our findings to clinical treatment for $HK1^-HK2^+$ cancers, several steps will be required: (1) $shHK2^{DOX}$ HK2 inhibition needs to be replaced by a selective HK2 inhibitor. GlaxoSmithKline recently reported their development of HK2-preferental inhibitors [10]. (2) DPI stood out among all screened compounds as the best synergistic partner with HK2 knockdown in $HK1^-HK2^+$ liver cancer cells. Although DPI has been extensively tested in pre-clinical animal models [28, 41–44], its safety in human subjects is not known. Clinical drugs with ETC-targeting effects, such as metformin [45] and papaverine [46], will need to be examined for their abilities to replace DPI in the combination therapy. (3) Doses, schedules, and routes of administration of the therapeutic agents involved in the triple combination will need optimization; the dosages in this study for xenograft tumor analyses were based on the previously reported single-agent dosages in mouse studies [28, 47]. Because of the synergistic effects, the required dosage of each agent for optimal combination therapy may well be lower than those used in these initial studies.

Conclusions

We identified the $HK1^-HK2^+$ cancer subsets existing among a wide variety of cancer types. HK2 is the only active HK isoform driving glycolysis in the $HK1^-HK2^+$ subsets of cancers. The combination therapy we have developed specifically reduced the cellular ATP level in these $HK1^-HK2^+$ cancer cells to a level incompatible with cell survival. In conclusion, we suggest that reduction of ATP levels to a level that will no longer support the survival of $HK1^-HK2^+$ cancer cells can be clinically exploited as a targeted, precision medicine for $HK1^-HK2^+$ tumors, regardless of their tissue of origin.

Additional files

Additional file 1: Figure S1. $HK1^-HK2^+$ cancer cells are highly sensitive to HK2 knockdown-induced growth inhibition. **Figure S2.** DPI synergizes with HK2 knockdown or inhibition in $HK1^-HK2^+$ liver cancer cells. **Figure S3.** DPI synergizes with HK2 silencing/inhibition by targeting mitochondrial complex I in $HK1^-HK2^+$ liver cancer cells. **Figure S4.** HK isoform expression in Hep3B/$shHK2^{DOX}$ xenograft tumors with DOX and/or DPI treatments. **Figure S5.** Inhibition of fatty acid oxidation sensitizes $HK1^-HK2^+$ liver cancer cells to the HK2 inhibition/DPI combination. **Figure S6.** Modulation of $HK1^-HK2^+$ liver cancer cellular metabolism by the HK2i/DPI/PER combination. **Figure S7.** PER as a single agent does not have a significantly detectable effect on growth of subcutaneous Hep3B/$shHK2^{DOX}$ tumors. (PPTX 782 kb)

Additional file 2: Table S1. The list of 119 FDA-approved oncology drugs provided by the National Cancer Institute (NCI) tested for synergy with DOX treatment in Hep3B/$shHK2^{DOX}$ cells. **Table S2.** Synergy between HK2 inhibition and DPI. (DOCX 44 kb)

Abbreviations

CT: Computed tomography; DOX: Doxycycline; DPI: Diphenyleneiodonium; ETC: Electron transport chain; FAO: Fatty acid oxidation; FDG: Fluorodeoxyglucose; HK: Hexokinase; PER: Perhexiline; PET: Positron emission tomography

Acknowledgements

We thank Drs. Caius Radu and Sotirios Tetradis for the insightful comments and advice on the research. We thank Drs. Diane M. Simeone (NYU Langone Health), Andrew E. Aplin (Thomas Jefferson University), and Ethan V. Abel (University of Michigan) for the gift of the DOX-inducible shRNA system.

Funding

Shili Xu is a FY15 Horizon Awardee (W81XWH-16-1-0162) supported by the DoD Peer Reviewed Cancer Research Program. TGG is supported by an American Cancer Society Research Scholar Award (RSG-12-257-01-TBE). HRH is supported by the Phelps Family Foundation and the Crump Family Foundation.

Authors' contributions

SX and HH conceived the study, designed the experiments, and wrote the paper. SX performed or participated in all experiments. AC and HD participated in experiments and helped in the design of in vitro and in vivo experiments. DB and LS performed mass spectrometry and data analysis on metabolite samples and Seahorse respirometry assay and data analysis on oxygen consumption rates in conjunction with TGG and OS. RD provided facilities, guidance, and assistance in designing and performing high-throughput screens. JL provided expertise, guidance, and participation in the PET analyses. All authors critically evaluated the manuscript. All authors read and approved the final manuscript.

Competing interests

The authors declare that they have no competing interests.

Author details

[1]Department of Molecular and Medical Pharmacology, David Geffen School of Medicine, University of California, Los Angeles, Los Angeles, CA 90095, USA. [2]Department of Biological Chemistry, David Geffen School of Medicine, University of California, Los Angeles, Los Angeles, CA 90095, USA. [3]UCLA Metabolomics Center, David Geffen School of Medicine, University of California, Los Angeles, Los Angeles, CA 90095, USA. [4]Crump Institute for Molecular Imaging, David Geffen School of Medicine, University of California, Los Angeles, Los Angeles, CA 90095, USA. [5]Jonsson Comprehensive Cancer Center, David Geffen School of Medicine, University of California, Los Angeles, Los Angeles, CA 90095, USA. [6]Division of Endocrinology, Department of Medicine, David Geffen School of Medicine, University of California, Los Angeles, Los Angeles, CA 90095, USA. [7]California NanoSystems Institute, David Geffen School of Medicine, University of California, Los Angeles, Los Angeles, CA 90095, USA. [8]Molecular Biology Institute, David Geffen School of Medicine, University of California, Los Angeles, Los Angeles, CA 90095, USA.

References

1. Yu Y. Molecular classification and precision therapy of cancer: immune checkpoint inhibitors. Front Med. 2018;12:229–35.
2. Drilon A, et al. A next-generation TRK kinase inhibitor overcomes acquired resistance to prior TRK kinase inhibition in patients with TRK fusion-positive solid tumors. Cancer Discov. 2017;7:963–72.
3. Drilon A, et al. Efficacy of larotrectinib in TRK fusion-positive cancers in adults and children. N Engl J Med. 2018;378:731–39.
4. Schulze A, Harris AL. How cancer metabolism is tuned for proliferation and vulnerable to disruption. Nature. 2012;491:364–73.
5. Wilson JE. Isozymes of mammalian hexokinase: structure, subcellular localization and metabolic function. J Exp Biol. 2003;206:2049–57.
6. Patra KC, et al. Hexokinase 2 is required for tumor initiation and maintenance and its systemic deletion is therapeutic in mouse models of cancer. Cancer Cell. 2013;24:213–28.
7. Wang L, et al. Hexokinase 2-mediated Warburg effect is required for PTEN- and p53-deficiency-driven prostate cancer growth. Cell Rep. 2014;8:1461–74.
8. Anderson M, Marayati R, Moffitt R, Yeh JJ. Hexokinase 2 promotes tumor growth and metastasis by regulating lactate production in pancreatic cancer. Oncotarget. 2016;8:56081–94.
9. Wolf A, et al. Hexokinase 2 is a key mediator of aerobic glycolysis and promotes tumor growth in human glioblastoma multiforme. J Exp Med. 2011;208:313–26.
10. Lin H, et al. Discovery of a novel 2,6-disubstituted glucosamine series of potent and selective hexokinase 2 inhibitors. ACS Med Chem Lett. 2016;7:217–22.
11. DeWaal D, et al. Hexokinase-2 depletion inhibits glycolysis and induces oxidative phosphorylation in hepatocellular carcinoma and sensitizes to metformin. Nat Commun. 2018;9:446.
12. Weinberg SE, Chandel NS. Targeting mitochondria metabolism for cancer therapy. Nat Chem Biol. 2015;11:9–15.
13. Carracedo A, Cantley LC, Pandolfi PP. Cancer metabolism: fatty acid oxidation in the limelight. Nat Rev Cancer. 2013;13:227–32.
14. Roessler S, et al. A unique metastasis gene signature enables prediction of tumor relapse in early-stage hepatocellular carcinoma patients. Cancer Res. 2010;70:10202 12.
15. Schulze K, et al. Exome sequencing of hepatocellular carcinomas identifies new mutational signatures and potential therapeutic targets. Nat Genet. 2015;47:505–11.
16. Barretina J, et al. The Cancer Cell Line Encyclopedia enables predictive modelling of anticancer drug sensitivity. Nature. 2012;483:603–7.
17. Rahib L, et al. Projecting cancer incidence and deaths to 2030: the unexpected burden of thyroid, liver, and pancreas cancers in the United States. Cancer Res. 2014;74:2913–21.
18. Som P, et al. A fluorinated glucose analog, 2-fluoro-2-deoxy-D-glucose (F-18): nontoxic tracer for rapid tumor detection. J Nucl Med. 1980;21:670–5.
19. Czernin J, Phelps ME. Positron emission tomography scanning: current and future applications. Annu Rev Med. 2002;53:89–112.
20. Chou TC, Talalay P. Quantitative analysis of dose-effect relationships: the combined effects of multiple drugs or enzyme inhibitors. Adv Enzym Regul. 1984;22:27–55.
21. Kurtoglu M, et al. Under normoxia, 2-deoxy-D-glucose elicits cell death in select tumor types not by inhibition of glycolysis but by interfering with N-linked glycosylation. Mol Cancer Ther. 2007;6:3049–58.
22. Cross AR, Jones OT. The effect of the inhibitor diphenylene iodonium on the superoxide-generating system of neutrophils. Specific labelling of a component polypeptide of the oxidase. Biochem J. 1986;237:111–6.
23. Stuehr DJ, et al. Inhibition of macrophage and endothelial cell nitric oxide synthase by diphenyleneiodonium and its analogs. FASEB J. 1991;5:98–103.
24. Lambert AJ, Buckingham JA, Boysen HM, Brand MD. Diphenyleneiodonium acutely inhibits reactive oxygen species production by mitochondrial complex I during reverse, but not forward electron transport. Biochim Biophys Acta. 2008;1777:397–403.
25. Laplante M, Sabatini DM. mTOR signaling in growth control and disease. Cell. 2012;149:274–93.
26. Wakil SJ, Abu-Elheiga LA. Fatty acid metabolism: target for metabolic syndrome. J Lipid Res. 2009;50(Suppl):S138–43.
27. Brand MD, Nicholls DG. Assessing mitochondrial dysfunction in cells. Biochem J. 2011;435:297–312.
28. Doroshow JH, et al. Effects of iodonium-class flavin dehydrogenase inhibitors on growth, reactive oxygen production, cell cycle progression, NADPH oxidase 1 levels, and gene expression in human colon cancer cells and xenografts. Free Radic Biol Med. 2013;57:162–75.
29. Vander Heiden MG, DeBerardinis RJ. Understanding the intersections between metabolism and cancer biology. Cell. 2017;168:657–69.
30. Li X, et al. A splicing switch from ketohexokinase-C to ketohexokinase-A drives hepatocellular carcinoma formation. Nat Cell Biol. 2016;18:561–71.
31. Ma R, et al. Switch of glycolysis to gluconeogenesis by dexamethasone for treatment of hepatocarcinoma. Nat Commun. 2013;4:2508.
32. Ricciardi MR, et al. Targeting the leukemia cell metabolism by the CPT1a inhibition: functional preclinical effects in leukemias. Blood. 2015;126:1925–9.
33. Park JH, et al. Fatty acid oxidation-driven Src links mitochondrial energy reprogramming and oncogenic properties in triple-negative breast cancer. Cell Rep. 2016;14:2154–65.
34. Metallo CM, Vander Heiden MG. Understanding metabolic regulation and its influence on cell physiology. Mol Cell. 2013;49:388–98.
35. Yuan HX, Xiong Y, Guan KL. Nutrient sensing, metabolism, and cell growth control. Mol Cell. 2013;49:379–87.
36. van Horssen R, et al. Modulation of cell motility by spatial repositioning of enzymatic ATP/ADP exchange capacity. J Biol Chem. 2009;284:1620–7.
37. Klingenberg M. The ADP and ATP transport in mitochondria and its carrier. Biochim Biophys Acta. 2008;1778:1978–2021.
38. Wright RH, et al. ADP-ribose-derived nuclear ATP synthesis by NUDIX5 is required for chromatin remodeling. Science. 2016;352:1221–5.
39. Glancy B, et al. Mitochondrial reticulum for cellular energy distribution in muscle. Nature. 2015;523:617–20.
40. Maruta H, et al. The involvement of ATP produced via (ADP-ribose)n in the maintenance of DNA replication apparatus during DNA repair. Biol Pharm Bull. 2007;30:447–50.
41. Holland PC, Clark MG, Bloxham DP, Lardy HA. Mechanism of action of the hypoglycemic agent diphenyleneiodonium. J Biol Chem. 1973;248:6050–6.
42. Bloxham DP. The relationship of diphenyleneiodonium-induced hypoglycaemia to the specific covalent modification of NADH-ubiquinone oxidoreductase. Biochem Soc Trans. 1979;7:103–6.

43. Kono H, et al. Diphenyleneiodonium sulfate, an NADPH oxidase inhibitor, prevents early alcohol-induced liver injury in the rat. Am J Physiol Gastrointest Liver Physiol. 2001;280:G1005–12.
44. Gustot T, et al. Differential liver sensitization to toll-like receptor pathways in mice with alcoholic fatty liver. Hepatology. 2006;43:989–1000.
45. Wheaton WW, et al. Metformin inhibits mitochondrial complex I of cancer cells to reduce tumorigenesis. Elife. 2014;3:e02242.
46. Morikawa N, Nakagawa-Hattori Y, Mizuno Y. Effect of dopamine, dimethoxyphenylethylamine, papaverine, and related compounds on mitochondrial respiration and complex I activity. J Neurochem. 1996;66:1174–81.
47. Schnell SA, et al. Therapeutic targeting of HES1 transcriptional programs in T-ALL. Blood. 2015;125:2806–14.

9

CD38 is methylated in prostate cancer and regulates extracellular NAD$^+$

Jack Mottahedeh[1], Michael C. Haffner[2,3], Tristan R. Grogan[4], Takao Hashimoto[1], Preston D. Crowell[5], Himisha Beltran[6,7], Andrea Sboner[7,8,9], Rohan Bareja[7,9,10], David Esopi[2], William B. Isaacs[2,3,11], Srinivasan Yegnasubramanian[2,12], Matthew B. Rettig[13,14,15,16], David A. Elashoff[4,15], Elizabeth A. Platz[2,17,18,19], Angelo M. De Marzo[2,3,11,18], Michael A. Teitell[15,20,21,22] and Andrew S. Goldstein[1,14,15,21,22*]

Abstract

Background: Cancer cell metabolism requires sustained pools of intracellular nicotinamide adenine dinucleotide (NAD$^+$) which is maintained by a balance of NAD$^+$ hydrolase activity and NAD$^+$ salvage activity. We recently reported that human prostate cancer can be initiated following oncogene expression in progenitor-like luminal cells marked by low expression of the NAD$^+$-consuming enzyme CD38. CD38 expression is reduced in prostate cancer compared to benign prostate, suggesting that tumor cells may reduce CD38 expression in order to enhance pools of NAD$^+$. However, little is known about how CD38 expression is repressed in advanced prostate cancer and whether CD38 plays a role in regulating NAD$^+$ levels in prostate epithelial cells.

Methods: CD38 expression, its association with recurrence after prostatectomy for clinically localized prostate cancer, and DNA methylation of the CD38 promoter were evaluated in human prostate tissues representing various stages of disease progression. CD38 was inducibly over-expressed in benign and malignant human prostate cell lines in order to determine the effects on cell proliferation and levels of NAD$^+$ and NADH. NAD$^+$ and NADH were also measured in urogenital tissues from wild-type and CD38 knockout mice.

Results: CD38 mRNA expression was reduced in metastatic castration-resistant prostate cancer compared to localized prostate cancer. In a large cohort of men undergoing radical prostatectomy, CD38 protein expression was inversely correlated with recurrence. We identified methylation of the CD38 promoter in primary and metastatic prostate cancer. Over-expression of wild-type CD38, but not an NAD$^+$ hydrolase-deficient mutant, depleted extracellular NAD$^+$ levels in benign and malignant prostate cell lines. However, expression of CD38 did not significantly alter intracellular NAD$^+$ levels in human prostate cell lines grown in vitro and in urogenital tissues isolated from wild-type and CD38 knockout mice.

Conclusions: CD38 protein expression in prostate cancer is associated with risk of recurrence. Methylation results suggest that CD38 is epigenetically regulated in localized and metastatic prostate cancer tissues. Our study provides support for CD38 as a regulator of extracellular, but not intracellular, NAD$^+$ in epithelial cells. These findings suggest that repression of CD38 by methylation may serve to increase the availability of extracellular NAD$^+$ in prostate cancer tissues.

Keywords: Prostate, CD38, NAD$^+$, Methylation

* Correspondence: AGoldstein@mednet.ucla.edu
[1]Department of Molecular, Cell & Developmental Biology, University of California Los Angeles, Los Angeles, CA, USA
[14]Department of Urology, David Geffen School of Medicine, University of California Los Angeles, Los Angeles, CA, USA

Background

More than 164,000 men in the USA are estimated to be newly diagnosed with prostate cancer in 2018 and greater than 29,000 men in the USA will die of prostate cancer this year [1]. While the 5-year survival rate of patients with low-grade localized prostate cancer is high, men with metastatic prostate cancer suffer from a 30% 5-year survival rate, as tumors become increasingly difficult to treat [1]. Most patients with advanced metastatic prostate cancer are treated with therapies targeting the androgen signaling axis, which can be initially effective but tumors eventually recur in a lethal castration-resistant state [2]. A key reason why advanced prostate cancer is so difficult to treat is that disease progression and treatment resistance is associated with epithelial plasticity [3, 4], loss of differentiated luminal epithelial features [5], and gain of a stem/progenitor-like transcriptional program [6–8]. Changes in gene expression are also associated with a gain of functional progenitor capacity in treatment-resistant disease [9, 10].

We have isolated basal [11, 12] and luminal progenitor [7] cells from human prostate epithelium and demonstrated that tumors initiate in progenitor cells following oncogene expression, using an in vivo tissue regeneration and human prostate transformation assay [13]. We found that CD38 could separate progenitor-enriched ($CD38^{lo}$) from differentiated ($CD38^{hi}$) luminal cells in the human prostate [7] based on differences in colony-forming [14], sphere-forming [12], and organoid-forming [15] capacity. The $CD38^{hi}$ cells expressed high levels of luminal differentiation markers including androgen receptor (AR) and AR target genes, while the $CD38^{lo}$ cells showed evidence of NFkB signaling and expression of the anti-apoptotic factor BCL2 [7]. Following oncogene expression and transplantation, the $CD38^{lo}$ luminal progenitors could give rise to highly proliferative tumors [7]. Given that basal cells are also $CD38^{lo}$, we identified an inverse correlation between CD38 expression and progenitor activity.

CD38 is a glycoprotein that regulates cellular nicotinamide adenine dinucleotide (NAD^+) metabolism through the hydrolysis of NAD^+ into nicotinamide and cyclic ADP Ribose (cADPR) [16, 17]. CD38 is linked to calcium signaling through the production of cADPR [18]. CD38 localization has been reported both on the cell surface and in intracellular compartments [18, 19]. Increased expression of CD38 is found in diverse hematological malignancies where it serves as a therapeutic target on the cell surface [20–23]. However, little is known about CD38 function in epithelial tissues. Deletion of CD38 in kidney epithelial cells initiates an epithelial-mesenchymal transition with loss of epithelial markers P-cadherin and ZO-1 and gain of mesenchymal markers desmin and α-smooth muscle actin [24]. In a limited cohort, a few studies have reported loss of CD38 expression in prostate cancer [25–27]. We have confirmed and extended these findings on a larger cohort of tissue samples, demonstrating that CD38 expression is inversely correlated with disease pathology, from benign prostate tissue to prostatic intraepithelial neoplasia (PIN) to low-grade cancer to high-grade cancer [7]. Using a global CD38 knockout mouse, Aksoy et al. reported significantly elevated NAD^+ levels in multiple tissues including brain, heart, lung, and liver extracts compared to WT animals [28]. As mice age, NAD^+ levels decline in several tissues which is associated with a decline in mitochondrial and adult stem cell function [29]. Interestingly, CD38 knockout mice are protected from an age-related decline in NAD^+ levels [20]. These data suggest that loss of CD38 in prostate cancer may contribute to elevated NAD^+ levels in tumor tissues.

NAD^+ is a metabolic co-factor and electron carrier that is critically important for both glycolysis and oxidative phosphorylation, as well as for the NAD^+-dependent deacetylases in the sirtuin family [30]. In order to supply sufficient pools of this metabolic co-factor, NAD^+ is generated from precursors including tryptophan, nicotinic acid, nicotinamide, and nicotinamide riboside (NR) through multiple pathways [31]. In the salvage pathway, nicotinamide phosphoribosyl-transferase (NAMPT) converts nicotinamide into nicotinamide mononucleotide (NMN) which can be further processed by nicotinamide mononucleotide adenylyltransferase (NMNAT) into NAD^+. Expression of NAMPT is elevated in prostate cancer tissues, and inhibition of NAMPT, through shRNA-mediated knockdown or small molecules, impairs proliferation of prostate cancer cell lines [32]. While intracellular NAD^+ levels maintain vital functions for epithelial cells, extracellular NAD^+ may function in immune suppression. Addition of NAD^+, but not nicotinamide or cADPR, has been shown to inhibit T cell proliferation, cytotoxic activity, and survival through the P2X7 receptor [33, 34]. This process has been termed NAD^+-induced cell death [35] and has been observed in multiple T cell subsets [33, 36]. Modulation of the immune microenvironment can have a significant impact on tumor progression and metastasis [37]. Several key questions remain unanswered, including (1) What is the level of CD38 expression in metastatic castration-resistant prostate cancer? (2) What mechanisms are responsible for low expression of CD38 in primary and metastatic prostate cancer? and (3) What are the functional consequences of CD38 expression in benign and malignant prostate epithelial cells? In this study, we address these questions using a range of approaches to evaluate prostate cancer tissues and cell lines.

Methods

Methylation analysis

Locus-specific DNA methylation analyses were performed as described by Yegnasubramanian et al. with minor modifications [38]. Patient samples used in this study were described previously [39, 40]. In brief, DNA sample concentrations were determined by a spectrophotometer and validated by quantitative real-time PCR. DNA samples were digested with AluI and HhaI (New England Biolabs). Enrichment reactions containing 20 μl of magnetic Tylon beads (Clontech), 10 μg of recombinant MBD2-MBD (Clontech), and 200 ng of unmethylated self-ligated pCR2.1 vector (Invitrogen) were assembled in enrichment buffer (4% glycerol, 1 mM $MgCl_2$, 0.5 mM EDTA, 0.5 mM DTT, 120 mM NaCl, 10 mM Tris–HCl (pH 7.4), 0.2% Tween-20, and protease inhibitors) and incubated for 1 h at room temperature. After immobilization of magnetic beads, the supernatants containing unbound MBD2-MBD polypeptides were discarded and digested DNA samples were diluted in 100 μl of enrichment buffer and incubated with MBD2-MBD-coated beads for 12 h at room temperature under gentle shaking. Beads and associated DNA complexes were then immobilized by magnetization and washed three times with enrichment buffer. Precipitated DNA containing methylated DNA fragments were eluted in water by heating to 95 °C for 15 min. Eluted DNA was then subjected to quantitative real-time PCR using the IQ SYBR Green Supermix (Biorad) using CD38-F: ATCCTCGTCGTGGTGCTC and CD38-R: CTTAGTCGCCAACCCACCT primers. Male white blood cell (WBC) genomic DNA was in vitro treated with M.SssI (NEB) to obtain a fully methylated control. Untreated male WBC DNA served as a negative control. For quantitative assessment of locus-specific methylation levels, C_t values of the samples of interest were normalized to C_t values of the positive control (SssI) and calculated methylation indices (ranging from 0.0 to 1.0) were used to derive methylation heatmaps. For in silico analysis of TCGA data correlating mRNA expression (RNA-seq, RSEM z-scores) and methylation (Infinium Human Methylation 450k BeadChip analysis) in primary prostate cancer samples, data were obtained from Cancer Genome Atlas Research Network [41] and were analyzed using cBioPortal [42]. Prostate cancer cell lines CWR22rv1, DU145, LNCaP, and LAPC4 were treated with 100 nM, 500 nM decitabine, or solvent (DMSO) for 4 days. Expression of *CD38* was determined by quantitative real-time PCR using primers:

CD38-F GCTCAATGGATCCCGCAGTA
CD38-R GGATCCTGGCATAAGTCTCTGG
GAPDH-F CCATCAAGTCCACAACACGGTTGC TGTA
GAPDH-R GTCTTATGACCACTGTCCATGCCA TCAC

Expression from RNA sequencing

RNA-seq data from the Weill Cornell Cohort included 164 samples: 31 benign prostate, 74 localized prostate cancer (PCa), and 41 CRPC-Adeno, and 18 CRPC-NE cases [43–45]. Tissue extraction from frozen material and RNA-seq processing and sequencing was performed according to the protocols previously described [43–45]. All reads were independently aligned with STAR_2.4.0f1 [46] for sequence alignment against the human genome build hg19, downloaded via the UCSC genome browser [http://hgdownload.soe.ucsc.edu/goldenPath/hg19/bigZips/], and SAMTOOLS v0.1.19 [47] for sorting and indexing reads. Cufflinks (2.0.2) [48] was used to quantify expression levels for all annotated genes in Gencode v19 [49] GTF annotation file. Expression levels are described by FPKM (fragment per kilobase of exonic regions per million mapped reads). Since the sequenced samples from the published cohorts were processed using different library preps, batch normalization was done using Combat from sva bioconductor package [50].

Tissue microarrays

The PSA progression tissue microarray was obtained through the Prostate Cancer Biorepository Network (PCBN) and has been previously described [51, 52]. For the majority of patients included, four cancer cores and two benign cores are included, and we plotted the mean score for each man's cancer or benign tissue cores. Immunohistochemical staining was performed as described [7] using antibodies against CD38 (LifeSpan BioSciences, LS-A9696). Staining scores were calculated by multiplying the percentage of CD38+ cells (from 0 to 100%) by the intensity of staining (from 0 to 3), as determined by a pathologist (M.A.T.). such that composite scores ranged from 0 to 300.

Statistical methods

Patient characteristics were summarized using means/SD and frequencies/percentages and then formally compared between recurrence/non-recurrence patients using paired *t* tests or McNemar's tests as appropriate (Table 1). The distribution of the average CD38 scores between cancer/benign biopsy cores were compared using a Wilcoxon test. The association between CD38 and recurrence was assessed using conditional logistic regression, taking into account the matching factors [53] (age, race, Gleason, pathologic stage) and adjusting for pre-operative PSA and surgical margin status. Three models were run, each with the covariates mentioned above and CD38 as above the median (1.25) in cancer cores, above the median (195) in benign cores, and above the median in both benign and cancer cores. For our validation data (UCLA-TMA [54]), we computed the same groups (above/below median using cancer median of 36.7 and benign median of 160) and constructed Kaplan Meier curves to assess recurrence-free survival between groups using the Breslow test. Statistical analyses were run using SAS 9.2 (SAS institute, Cary, NC,

Table 1 Patient characteristics in PSA progression tissue microarray

Characteristic	No recurrence ($n = 499$)	Recurrence ($n = 499$)	p value
Age at surgery	59.0 (6.0)	58.8 (6.3)	Matched
Race			Matched
AA	39 (7.8%)	47 (9.4%)	
White	440 (88.2%)	426 (85.4%)	
Other	11 (2.2%)	19 (3.8%)	
Gleason sum			Matched
5	3 (0.6%)	3 (0.6%)	
6	69 (13.8%)	68 (13.6%)	
7	314 (62.9%)	305 (61.1%)	
8	113 (22.6%)	123 (24.6%)	
S stage			Matched
1	67 (13.4%)	66 (13.2%)	
2	260 (52.1%)	260 (52.1%)	
3	172 (34.5%)	173 (34.7%)	
Pre-op PSA	11.0 (8.3)	12.3 (10.2)	0.026
Surgical margins +	110 (22.0%)	176 (35.3%)	< 0.001

The PSA progression tissue microarray contains tissue cores from 499 men who developed biochemical recurrence and 499 controls who did not develop recurrence, matched based on age, race, Gleason sum, and pathologic stage. Patient characteristics were summarized using means/ standard deviation and frequencies/percentages

USA). Relative NAD^+/protein or NAD^+/DNA levels were compared between groups using the two-sample t test. All statistical tests were two-tailed. $^*p < 0.05$, $^{**}p < 0.005$, $^{***}p < 0.0005$, and $^{****}p < 0.0001$ were computed using GraphPad Prism software.

Engineering expression of CD38

Using MGC Human CD38 sequence-verified cDNA (Clone ID: 4309086, Dharmacon) as a template, we amplified full-length CD38 with forward primer (GTAC AGCGCTGAGTTCGAACCATGGCCAACTGCGA) and reverse primer (GTACAGCGCTCTCGAGCTAGATCT CAGATGTGCA) and cloned into the inducible pSTV lentiviral vector using the AFE1 restriction site and Afe1 (New England Biolabs). The E226Q point mutant was generated by using QuickChange Lightning Site-Directed Mutagenesis Kit (Agilent) according to manufacturer's protocol with forward primer (GTTGCAAATTATGG ACTTGCACACTCCCAAAAGTGCT) and reverse primer (AGCACTTTTGGGAGTGTGCAAGTCCATAATT TGCAAC). CD38 expression is under the control of the Tet Response Element, which allows gene induction following addition of doxycycline (Dox, Sigma). In the same vector, GFP is constitutively expressed under the human ubiquitin promoter, allowing for isolation of highly transduced cells by fluorescence-activated cell sorting.

Cell lines, lentiviral transduction, and proliferation assays

Cell lines used in this study (RWPE1, LNCaP, DU145, PC3) were purchased from the ATCC and cultured in the recommended media. Cells were grown on plates coated with 0.01% poly-l-Lysine (Sigma) to enhance attachment. Cell lines were transduced at high MOI, expanded for 4–7 days of growth, and sorted for GFP expression using a BD FACS ARIA II prior to initial experiments. Cultures were expanded and maintain in the absence of Dox unless otherwise indicated. To measure cellular growth, cells were plated onto black wall clear bottom tissue culture plates. One hundred microliters of cells diluted at final concentration of 20,000–60,000/ml under different experimental conditions was plated. At different time points, 11 μl of 0.5 mg/ml of Resazurin-Na salt (alamarBlue) diluted in media was added to wells of interest and plates were continued to be incubated at 37 °C. Exactly 1 h later, total fluorescence was measured using a Tecan plate reader (Infinite M1000) with 555 ± 7 nm excitation and 590 ± 10 nm emission. Four different spots/well were measured, and third highest value was used for analysis. To measure cellular growth by increase in total DNA content, the media containing Resazurin was removed and cells were lysed by addition of 50 μl of buffer (0.1% SDS, 20 mM NaOH, and 1 mM EDTA) and returned to 37 °C incubator for additional data points. A day after the last data point was collected, 100 μl of buffer (30 mM Tris-HCl pH 7.4 and 6 μg/ml of Hoechst-33342) is added to wells, gently mixed by tapping the plate and incubated at 37 °C overnight. The next day, plates were given time to come to room temperature and analyzed using plate reader with 355 ± 10 nm excitation and 465 ± 10 nm emission.

Western blot

Cells grown in the absence of doxycycline were plated with 0 or 20 ng/ml of Dox added at the time of seeding for a total of 4 days. To collect protein, media was removed and cells were washed with HBSS and lysed in 300 μl of RIPA buffer and protease inhibitor (Roche). Cells were scraped from the plate, moved to Eppendorf tubes, and spun at 17,000×g for 10 min prior to storing the samples at − 20 °C. Total protein was determined using the BCA assay and ~ 5 μg of protein was separated on a 4–12% Bis-Tris PAGE. Proteins were transferred onto PVDF membranes and probed with primary antibodies followed by HRP conjugated secondary antibodies and detected with HRP chemiluminescence. Primary antibodies used were CD38 (Santa Cruz sc-374650), Alpha-tubulin (Developmental Studies Hybridoma Bank #12G10), NAMPT (Cell Signaling D7V5J), and NAPRT (Proteintech 13549-1-AP).

NAD^+/ NADH measurement from cell cultures

Cells were cultured in 24-well plates. Prior to NAD^+/ NADH measurement, media was removed and cells were washed with 500 µl of HBSS. Shortly after HBSS removal, 200 µl of 1:1 mixture of 0.4% SDS + 80 mM NaOH:PBS is added. After 10–15 min incubation at room temperature, the pH is adjusted by adding 400 µl of 18 mM HCl. DNA from cells was sheered by passing through a 25-G needle. 60 µl of the homogenate was transferred into mini-PCR tubes; we added 15 µl of 0.5 M HCl (for NAD^+) or NaOH (for NADH) and tubes were incubated at 60 °C for 15 min. Tubes were cooled and 50 µl of buffer (300 mM Tris-base +160mMNaOH or 300 mM Tris-base +160 mM HCl) was added for NAD^+ or NADH respectively. NAD^+/NADH was measured independently using NAD^+/NADH-Glo Assay (Promega) and normalized based on total protein and/or DNA. Protein concentrations were determined using 20 µl of homogenate with BCA assay. DNA concentrations were determined by mixing 60 µl of homogenate with 60 µl of 20 mM Tris-HCl, pH 7.4 and 10 µg/ml of Hoechst-33342, in Clear Bottom Black Polystyrene Microplates, against a DNA standard diluted in the same buffer. DNA to protein ratio was used to evaluate sample quality, purity, and well to well variation. Cellular permeabilization was achieved by addition of 100 µl of HBSS + 0.5% Triton X-100 after removal of HBSS wash solution. Plates are incubated for 15 min at room temperature prior to adding 200 µl of 1:1 mixture described above (0.4% SDS + 80 mM NaOH:PBS). Control wells received 200 µl of 1:1 mixture first, and after 15 min, 100 µl of HBSS +Triton X-100 was added. All wells were neutralized by addition of 300 µl of 25 mM HCl.

NAMPT inhibition with FK866

To see the effect of NAMPT inhibition on growth rate or NAD^+/NADH levels, cells were seeded in the presence of FK866 (Sigma) diluted in 100% EtOH and added to media to reach the concentration indicated. Media was changed with fresh drug every 48 h. Changes in total DNA measurements were used for growth rate analysis. NAD^+/NADH was measured on day 3.

Measurement of extracellular NAD^+ hydrolase activity

To test for extracellular NAD^+ hydrolase activity, transduced cells were seeded onto 24-well plates ± 20 ng/ml of Dox for a total of 4 days. Media was replaced with fresh media ± Dox 24 h prior to evaluation of NAD^+ hydrolase activity. Wells were washed with HBSS, and 200 µl of HBSS + 800 nM NAD^+ (Sigma, diluted in PBS) was added to each well and incubated at room temperature for 30 min. Media was removed from wells, centrifuged at 800×*g* for 10 min, and 60 µl was moved into a new tube and treated to measure NAD^+ by addition of 15 µl of 0.5 M HCl, heating, and neutralization. A serial dilution of starting material was also generated and treated under similar conditions as a standard. To measure the effect of extracellular NAD^+ on the internal pool: supernatant was removed, cells were washed with 1 ml of HBSS, and stopped by addition of 200 µl of 1:1 mixture (0.4% SDS + 80 mM NaOH:PBS) followed by HCl neutralization.

NAD^+/NADH measurements in mouse tissues

C57BL/6J (WT) and B6.129P2-Cd38tm1Lnd/J (CD38KO) mice were obtained from Jackson Labs and housed and bred under the care of the Division of Laboratory and Animal Medicine (DLAM) at UCLA according to approved protocols. To measure total NAD^+/NADH from prostate, seminal vesicles, and liver, tissues were obtained from adult mice (aged 8–16 weeks), rinsed with PBS, and stored in 0.8 ml PBS on ice. 0.8 ml of 0.4% SDS + 80 mM NaOH was added to each sample, and it was immediately sonicated on ice for 20–25 bursts (20-s pulses separated by 10 s) allowing complete dissociation of the tissue. Samples were maintained at room temperature to minimize additional precipitation. To study the contribution of seminal vesicle tissue without the fluid, seminal vesicles were cut on the coronal plane and fluid was pushed out. Remaining seminal vesicle tissues were rinsed with HBSS, placed into PBS on ice, and homogenized as described for total tissue. For DNA normalization, 200 µl of the sonicated homogenate was mixed with equal volume of 100 mM NaCl, 40 mM HCl, 20 mM Tris-HCl (pH 7.4), and 10 mM EDTA. 2.5 µl of Proteinase K (20 mg/ml, Thermo Scientific) was added to each tube, and the mixture was incubated at 55 °C for 2–3 h with shaking. Samples were allowed to come to room temperature and DNA was extracted with 500 µl of chloroform. Fifty microliters of the extracted samples is mixed with equal volume of 10 µg/ml of Hoechst (Invitrogen) for DNA measurement against a known DNA standard.

Isolation of total mouse prostate and seminal vesicle cells for flow cytometry and NAD^+ hydrolase activity

Total cells from prostate were obtained by modification of our published work [14]. The urogenital system was collected and placed in base media of RPMI (Gibco) + 10% FBS (Corning). Isolated prostates were moved onto a clean surface and minced using a razor blade. Tissue pieces were enzymatically digested in 1 mg/ml of Dispase (Gibco) and 1 mg/ml of collagenase type I (Gibco) diluted in base media and incubated at 37 °C on an orbital rocker for 60–90 min. Digested tissues are centrifuged at 800×*g* for 5 min and washed with PBS (Gibco). After 800×*g* centrifugation, PBS is removed, 500 µl of warm TryplE (Gibco) is added, and tubes are mixed and incubated at 37 °C water bath for 15 min. TryplE is inactivated by addition of 1.3 ml of base media. DNase I (Sigma) is added at a final concentration of 100 µg/ml, and tubes are incubated for an additional 10 min. The tissue is further dissociated mechanically using P-1000 pipet tips and passed through a 70-μm cell strainer. For flow cytometry, cells were stained with antibodies against mouse EpCAM-APC (clone G8.8, eBiosciences) and CD38-PE (clone 90, BioLegend) and evaluated using FACSDIVA software on a FACSCanto cytometer (BD Biosciences). To further purify viable seminal vesicle cells, 1× Percoll solution was made by adding 1 ml of 11× buffer (1100 mM Glycerol, 880 mM NaCl, 220 mM HEPES, and 4.4 mg/ml BSA) to 10 ml of Percoll (GE Life Sciences). After preparing a 1:1 mixture of cells suspended in 0.5 ml base media with 1× Percoll solution, samples are centrifuged at 800×*g* for 5 min. The supernatant containing cells floating at the top is moved to a new tube and is mixed at a 2:1 ratio with 4× buffer (4 ml of 11× buffer and 7 ml of RPMI + 10% FBS). The mixture is centrifuged at 3000×*g* for 5 min, and the supernatant is discarded. The pellet containing nearly 90–100% live cells is gradually increased in volume with base media. Cells suspend in base media are incubated at 37 °C for 30–40 min prior to analysis. To measure NAD^+ hydrolase activity of total cells, Percoll-purified seminal vesicle cells were centrifuged at 800×*g* for 5 min and washed once with HBSS. Using a 0.2-ml PCR tube, each sample (~ 500,000) was suspended in 50 μl of HBSS to which 50 μl of 2 nM of NAD^+-HBSS or HBSS was added. Samples were incubated in a 37 °C water bath for 50–60 min, with gentle mixing every 15 min. Cells were centrifuged at 800×*g* for 10 min, and 60 μl of the supernatant was used for NAD^+ measurement. To measure intracellular NAD^+, additional 20 μl of supernatant was removed from each tube and cells were washed with 180 μl of HBSS. After pelleting cells at 800×*g* for 10 min, most of the solution is removed and cells are suspended in 50 μl of HBSS followed by addition of 50 μl of 0.4% SDS and 200 mM HCl.

Collection of blood and purified liver cells from mice

Mice were euthanized by CO_2 inhalation and checked for the absence of response to pressure stimulus. Next, the chest cavity was exposed and 0.3–0.5 ml of blood was collected from the aorta using a 22-G needle and syringe pre-coated with (20 mg/ml) heparin. The blood was immediately moved to 0.5-ml tubes and centrifuged at 3000×*g* for 5 min in 4 °C. The supernatant was moved to a new tube and was further centrifuged at 17,000×*g* for 5 min. Finally, 40 μl of serum in duplicate was added to 10 μl of 0.5 M HCl, mixed, and stored on ice prior to starting the next animal. All animals used were 10–12 weeks of age. NAD^+ was measured as described above, comparing wild-type and CD38 knockout mice. After collecting blood for NAD^+ measurement, mice were perfused with 10 ml of HBSS. Liver tissue was moved to base media prior to dissociation. After mincing the liver, it was further digested in 5 ml of base media containing 0.5 mg/ml of Dispase and 0.5 mg/ml collagenase for 30–40 min at 37 °C on an orbital rocker. Partially dissociated tissues were pelleted, washed with PBS, digested with TryplE, neutralized, treated with DNase, diluted, and passed through 70-μM cell strainers. After centrifuging cells at 1000×*g*, the pellet was suspended in 1 ml of base media and was used for further Percoll purification, similar to seminal vesicle tissue described above. The final purified cell preparations contained less than 10% red blood cells. Percoll-purified seminal vesicle and liver cells were subjected to lysis and western blotting to analyze CD38 expression.

Results

CD38 mRNA is reduced in metastatic castration-resistant prostate cancer

We previously demonstrated that *CD38* mRNA and protein expression is reduced in primary prostate cancer [7], but the expression of *CD38* in metastatic prostate cancer is poorly defined. When comparing gene expression of metastatic prostate tumor samples recovered from autopsies to normal prostate, we identified *CD38* as significantly downregulated in metastases [55]. To further evaluate *CD38* expression in advanced disease, we interrogated transcriptional profiles of patient tissues representing benign prostate, primary prostate cancer, and castration-resistant prostate cancer (CRPC). The CRPC samples were subdivided into adenocarcinoma and neuroendocrine prostate cancer (NEPC) based on histological and molecular features [45]. RNA sequencing data indicates a clear trend with *CD38* mRNA expression lower in primary prostate cancer than in benign prostate, and further reduced in CRPC tissues (Fig. 1). Within CRPC subsets, *CD38* mRNA expression is lowest in NEPC tissues.

High expression of CD38 in prostate cancer is associated with reduced risk for recurrence

Based on low expression of *CD38* in CRPC samples, we hypothesized that CD38 protein expression in primary prostate cancer may be predictive of disease progression. We previously reported that low *CD38* mRNA expression in radical prostatectomy tissues is prognostic for biochemical recurrence and metastasis [7]. A recent study determined that combined expression of CD38 and ARG2 was prognostic for recurrence-free survival in a Stanford tissue cohort, while low expression of CD38 was associated with recurrence-free survival in the Canary tissue cohort [56]. We evaluated CD38 expression in the PSA progression tissue microarray (TMA) [51, 52] which contains prostatectomy tissues from 499 patients who developed biochemical recurrence as well as 499 control patients who did not develop recurrence, matched on age, race, pathological stage (T2, T3a, T3b, etc.), and Gleason sum (Table 1).

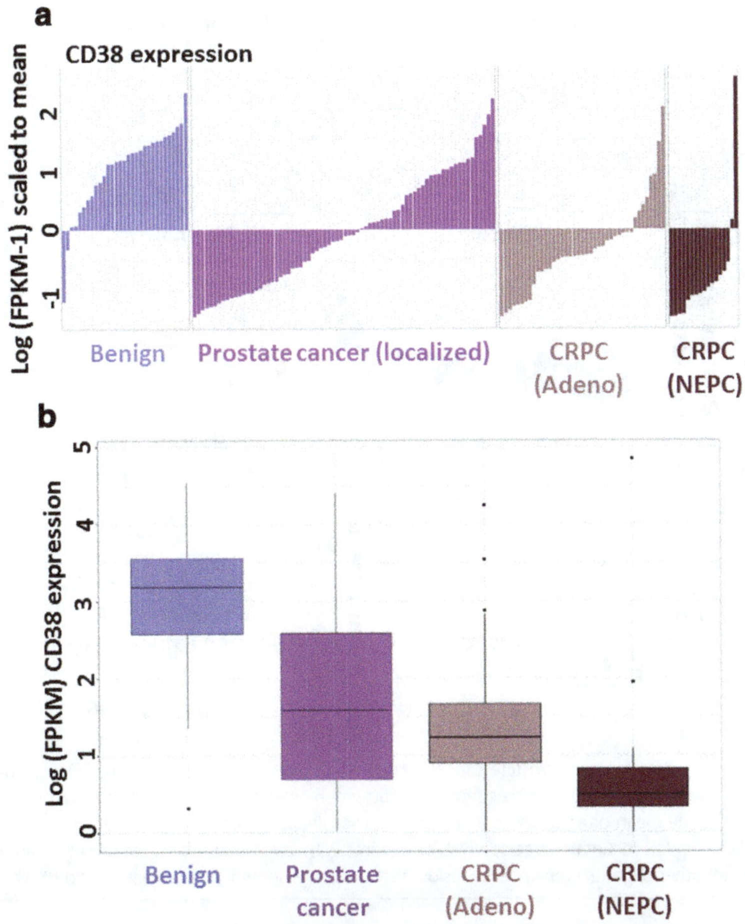

Fig. 1 Reduced expression of *CD38* in metastatic prostate cancer. **a** Waterfall plot indicating relative *CD38* mRNA expression from RNA sequencing of benign prostate, localized prostate cancer, metastatic castration-resistant prostate cancer (CRPC) with an adenocarcinoma (adeno) phenotype and metastatic CRPC with a neuroendocrine prostate cancer (NEPC) phenotype. Expression levels are presented as Log of FPKM-1 (Fragments Per Kilobase Million) values and scaled to the mean of all values shown. **b** Box plot corresponding to samples from **a** presented as Log of FPKM values

Overall, cancer tissues contained significantly lower CD38 staining scores than normal prostate (Fig. 2a–c). When cancer samples were split into two groups defined as above or below the median CD38 staining score, we found that higher CD38 (above the median) in cancer specimens was statistically significantly inversely associated with risk of recurrence (OR = 0.76, 95% CI 0.59–0.98, $p = 0.031$) (Table 2). These data are consistent with mRNA expression [7] and the Stanford/Canary tissue cohorts [56], indicating that low CD38 is associated with risk of recurrence. Gleason sum was not found to be a significant predictor of recurrence (Table 2) in this TMA, likely because the recurrence and no recurrence groups were well matched based on Gleason sum (Table 1).

When we analyzed the study looking only at normal (cancer-adjacent) glands, we did not find a statistically significant association between CD38 staining scores and recurrence (Table 2). However, when combining CD38 scores in normal and cancer, we found that high expression of CD38 (above the median) in both normal and cancer tissues is significantly associated with a reduced risk of recurrence ($p = 0.018$) when compared to all other combinations (above median cancer and below median normal, below median cancer and above median normal, below median cancer and below median normal). We found that high expression of CD38 in normal and cancer tissues is associated with a 21% lower risk of recurrence (OR = 0.79, 95% CI 0.63–0.98, $p = 0.037$) compared to patients who do not have high CD38 in both. We analyzed a separate TMA [54] for CD38 expression and observed a similar pattern, with high (above the median) expression for CD38 in both benign and cancer tissues associated with reduced risk of recurrence (Fig. 2d).

Evidence for epigenetic regulation of CD38 in prostate cancer

To test if *CD38* is regulated epigenetically by CpG methylation, we first performed in silico analysis and

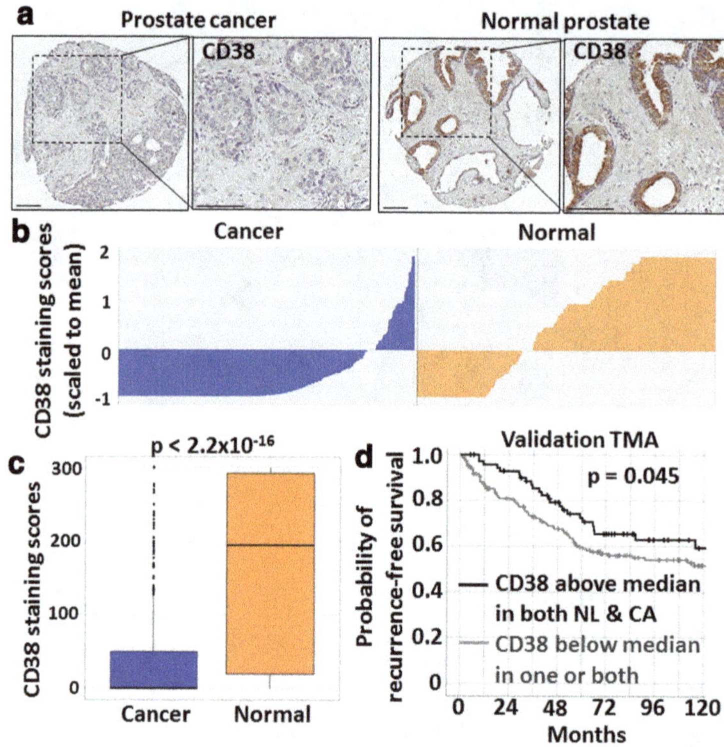

Fig. 2 Association of CD38 protein expression with prostate cancer recurrence. **a** Representative images of CD38 staining in normal and cancer cores from the PSA progression tissue microarray. Scale bars represent 100 μm. **b** Waterfall plot representing composite CD38 staining scores in normal and cancer cores scaled to the mean of all values. **c** Box plot of composite CD38 staining scores. Statistics represent Welch Two Sample *t* test. **d** Kaplan-Meier plot of biochemical recurrence-free survival for patients with CD38 staining scores greater than the median in both normal and cancer cores compared to all other patients (remainder). Breslow test *p* value is shown, with a hazard ratio of 0.71

identified a CpG island in close proximity to the transcriptional start site of *CD38*. Furthermore, re-analysis of publicly available reduced representation bisulfite sequencing (RRBS) data [57] for the prostate cancer cell line LNCaP demonstrated that dense CpG methylation was present around the transcriptional start site and in the first exon of *CD38* (Fig. 3a). To further investigate the methylation status of *CD38* in prostate cancer cell lines and clinical specimens, we used a previously described and extensively validated combined methylation-sensitive restriction enzyme digestion and methylated-DNA precipitation assay (COMPARE-MS) [38, 58, 59]. Whereas benign primary

Table 2 Higher CD38 is associated with a lower risk of recurrence after prostatectomy for clinically localized disease

Characteristic	Model 1 Odds ratio (95% CI)	*p* value	Model 2 Odds ratio (95% CI)	*p* value	Model 3 Odds ratio (95% CI)	*p* value
Age at surgery (years)	0.81 (0.70–0.93)	0.003	0.81 (0.71–0.93)	0.003	0.81 (0.71–0.93)	0.003
Caucasian (yes/no)	0.09 (0.02–0.41)	0.002	0.10 (0.02–0.45)	0.003	0.11 (0.02–0.49)	0.004
High Gleason sum (yes/no)	1.44 (0.08–27.4)	0.819	1.80 (0.10–34.1)	0.715	1.41 (0.07–26.7)	0.831
S stage (yes/no)	2.09 (0.26–16.59)	0.487	2.06 (0.25–17.00)	0.502	2.31 (0.25–21.07)	0.457
Pre-op PSA (1 unit)	1.01 (0.99–1.03)	0.227	1.01 (0.99–1.03)	0.282	1.01 (0.99–1.03)	0.274
Surgical margins (+/–)	2.33 (1.65–3.30)	< 0.001	2.25 (1.60–3.17)	< 0.001	2.37 (1.68–3.36)	< 0.001
CD38 above med. cancer	0.69 (0.52–0.91)	0.007	XX	XX	XX	XX
CD38 above med. benign	XX	XX	0.91 (0.69–1.20)	0.505	XX	XX
CD38 above med. for both	XX	XX	XX	XX	0.65 (0.48–0.88)	0.006

Three conditional logistic regression models were run, each with the covariates mentioned above and CD38 as above the median in cancer cores (model 1), above the median in benign cores (model 2), and above the median in both (model 3). Odds ratios and 95% confidence intervals were extracted from each model

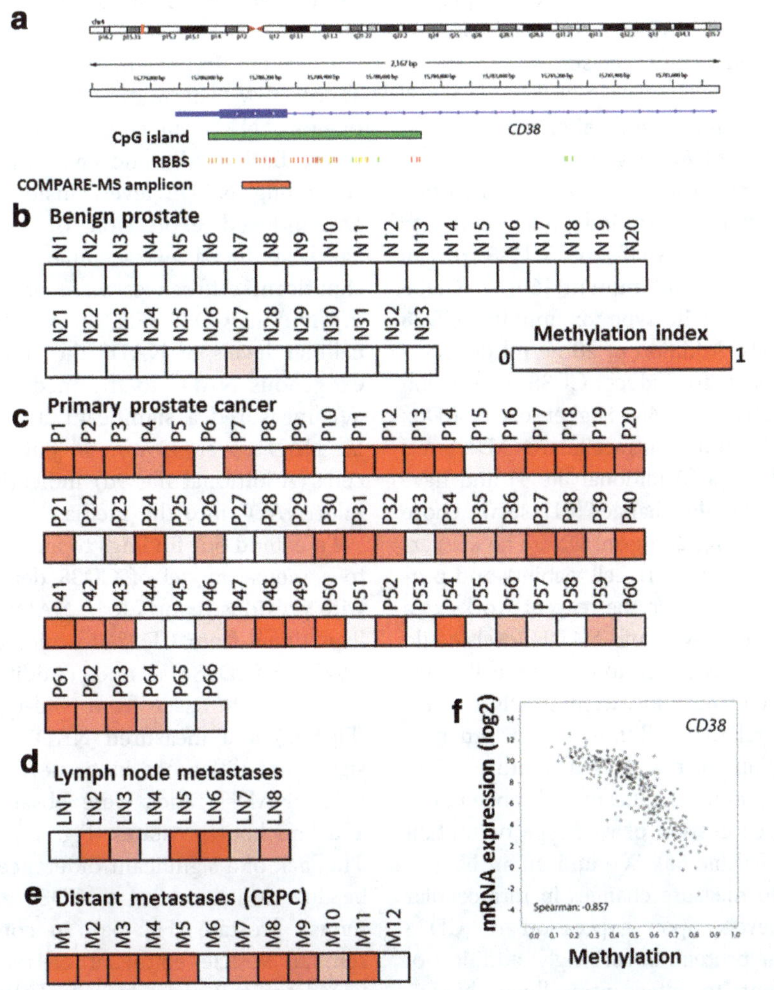

Fig. 3 The *CD38* locus undergoes CpG hypermethylation in prostate cancer. **a** Schematic representation of the *CD38* locus. Note that the CpG island (green box) extends downstream of the transcriptional start site into the first intron. In silico analysis of publicly available reduced representation bisulfite sequencing (RRBS) is shown below (heat map: red—dense methylation, green—no methylation). The location of the PCR amplicon used in subsequent COMPARE-MS experiments is indicated by the red box. **b**–**e** Methylation heat maps derived from COMPARE-MS analysis of benign prostate tissue (**b**), primary prostate cancers (**c**), and prostate cancer metastases (**d**, **e**) show hypermethylation of the CD38 in primary prostate cancer and prostate cancer metastases (heat map: red—dense methylation; white—no methylation). **f** In silico analysis of TCGA data reveals frequent hypermethylation of the *CD38* locus. Correlation plots of log2 mRNA expression (based on RNA-seq, RSEM z-scores) and methylation levels (based on Infinium Human Methylation 450k BeadChip analysis) in 333 primary prostate cancer samples

prostate epithelial cells (PrEC) and immortalized prostate epithelial cells (RWPE-1) showed no methylation, all prostate cancer cell lines (including LNCaP, LNCaP-abl, C4-2B, LAPC4, VCaP, DU145, PC3, and CWR22rv1) showed evidence of dense CpG methylation around the first exon of *CD38* (Additional file 1). Furthermore, analyses of clinical specimens showed low-level methylation in 2 of 33 benign prostate tissue samples; in contrast, 52 out of 66 primary carcinoma samples exhibited CpG methylation (Fig. 3b, c). Similarly, 6 out of 8 lymph node metastases and 10 out of 12 distant metastases showed methylation of *CD38* (Fig. 3d, e). These observations were further corroborated by in silico analyses of TCGA data [41] obtained using cBioPortal [42], which demonstrated high-level CpG methylation of the *CD38* locus, comparable to other known frequently methylated genes in prostate cancer such as *GSTP1* and *PTGS2* (Additional file 2). Importantly, these in silico analyses demonstrate a tight correlation between *CD38* methylation and mRNA expression (Fig. 3f). In addition, pharmacologic unmasking experiments using the DNA methyltransferase inhibitor 2′-deoxy-5-azacytidine (DAC) resulted in re-expression of *CD38* in a subset of cell lines with dense *CD38* CpG island methylation (Additional file 3), further supporting the notion that *CD38* expression is at least partially regulated by CpG methylation in prostate cancer. Taken together, these results suggest that the *CD38* locus undergoes hypermethylation changes that are present in primary tumors and maintained in regional and distant metastases.

CD38 expression does not significantly alter cell proliferation or intracellular NAD$^+$ levels

To assess the functional role of CD38 in prostate epithelial cells, we generated an inducible vector to engineer over-expression of wild-type CD38 or an NAD$^+$ hydrolase-deficient point mutant [60] of CD38 (E226Q). We introduced wild-type or mutant CD38 into benign RWPE1 cells. Addition of 20 ng/ml doxycycline (Dox) was sufficient to induce CD38 expression within 48 h by western blot (Fig. 4a). Higher levels of Dox caused a significant reduction in intracellular NAD$^+$ levels in non-transduced cell lines (Additional file 4) and have been associated with metabolic changes [61], so we chose to carry out our studies using 20 ng/ml Dox. The alamarBlue assay is often used to measure cell viability and proliferation in culture [62]. However, the reagent works as a redox indicator and altered NAD$^+$ and NADH levels could influence colorimetric changes used to quantify cell number. As an alternative to alamarBlue, we used DNA quantification to measure relative cell number in order to evaluate cell proliferation over 4 days in culture. With both approaches, we found no significant difference in cell proliferation following expression of wild-type or mutant CD38 (Fig. 4b, Additional file 5a). We utilized an NAD$^+$/NADH cycling assay to measure changes in intracellular NAD$^+$ and NADH levels upon expression of CD38 relative to total cellular protein. Surprisingly, addition of Dox was not sufficient to alter intracellular NAD$^+$, NADH, or NAD$^+$:NADH ratio (Fig. 4c–e). Results were replicated using LNCaP and DU145 prostate cancer cells expressing wild-type or mutant CD38 (Additional file 5b–e, Additional file 6a, b). CD38-expressing cells did not show an upregulation of NAMPT or NAPRT, two enzymes that can regenerate NAD$^+$ from precursors (Additional file 7a, b). Cells were treated with Triton-X100 to permeabilize cell membranes for 15 min prior to NAD$^+$/NADH measurements. Following permeabilization, cells expressing wild-type CD38, but not mutant CD38, demonstrated a dramatic reduction in NAD$^+$ levels (Fig. 4f, Additional file 6: Figure S6c,d). These findings suggest that wild-type CD38 exhibits NAD$^+$ hydrolase activity in permeabilized but not intact cells. Taken together, we find a lack of evidence to support CD38 as a significant regulator of intracellular NAD$^+$ levels or cell proliferation during short-term culture. Considerable depletion of intracellular NAD$^+$ and NADH levels by FK866, a small molecule inhibitor of NAMPT, was sufficient to impair cell proliferation of RWPE1, LNCaP, DU145, and PC-3 cells (Fig. 4g–i, Additional file 8a–i), similar to what has been reported for LNCaP and PC-3 cells [32].

CD38 expression promotes depletion of extracellular NAD$^+$

To evaluate extracellular NAD$^+$ hydrolase activity, we exposed WT or mutant CD38-expressing cells to exogenous NAD$^+$ in culture. Following 30 min, we collected both media and cell extracts and measured the remaining NAD$^+$ levels inside and outside of cells. Dox-induced expression of wild-type CD38 significantly reduced extracellular NAD$^+$ levels, while no significant differences were observed in cells expressing mutant CD38 (Fig. 4j, Additional file 6e, f). Intracellular levels of NAD$^+$ did not increase after adding exogenous NAD$^+$ to the media (Additional file 9a–c). We measured a significant net increase in extracellular NAD$^+$ over 30 min in culture from naïve LNCaP cells (Additional file 9d) indicating release of intracellular NAD$^+$ into the media.

To extend our findings to an in vivo system, we turned to a mouse model of CD38 deficiency [63]. Consistent with previous reports [64], NAD$^+$ levels were elevated in liver tissue from CD38−/− mice compared to wild-type C57BL/6 (CD38+/+) mice (Additional file 10a). We isolated prostate tissue from wild-type and CD38−/− mice (Fig. 5a) and measured NAD$^+$ and NADH levels. No significant difference in tissue NAD$^+$, NADH levels, or NAD$^+$:NADH ratios were observed between wild-type and knockout prostates (Fig. 5b, c, Additional file 10b). The lack of a significant difference in NAD$^+$ levels could be due to a low level of CD38 expression in wild-type mouse prostate (Fig. 5a). In contrast to the prostate, seminal vesicle epithelial cells express high levels of CD38 and this expression is abolished in knockout mice (Fig. 5a). Therefore, we reasoned that seminal vesicles may be a better model to assess the role of endogenous CD38 as a regulator of NAD$^+$ levels in urogenital tissues. Knockout seminal vesicles exhibited increased levels of NAD$^+$ and slightly elevated NAD$^+$:NADH ratios compared to CD38-expressing wild-type seminal vesicle tissues (Fig. 5d, Additional file 10c, d). Given that the seminal vesicles contain a large amount of fluid, we removed seminal fluid and measured NAD$^+$ levels in the remaining tissue. No significant difference in NAD$^+$ levels were observed in wild-type or knockout seminal vesicle tissues after removing the fluid (Fig. 5e), suggesting that external NAD$^+$ in fluid is likely to account for the increase in total tissue NAD$^+$ levels in knockout seminal vesicles. We measured NAD$^+$ levels in the blood of wild-type and knockout mice and found significantly elevated NAD$^+$ levels in the plasma of CD38-deficient mice (Additional file 9e). To assess the extracellular NAD$^+$ hydrolase activity, we treated purified seminal vesicle cells with exogenous NAD$^+$ and evaluated the remaining NAD$^+$ in the media after 1 h in culture. Knockout cells exhibited a significant deficiency in

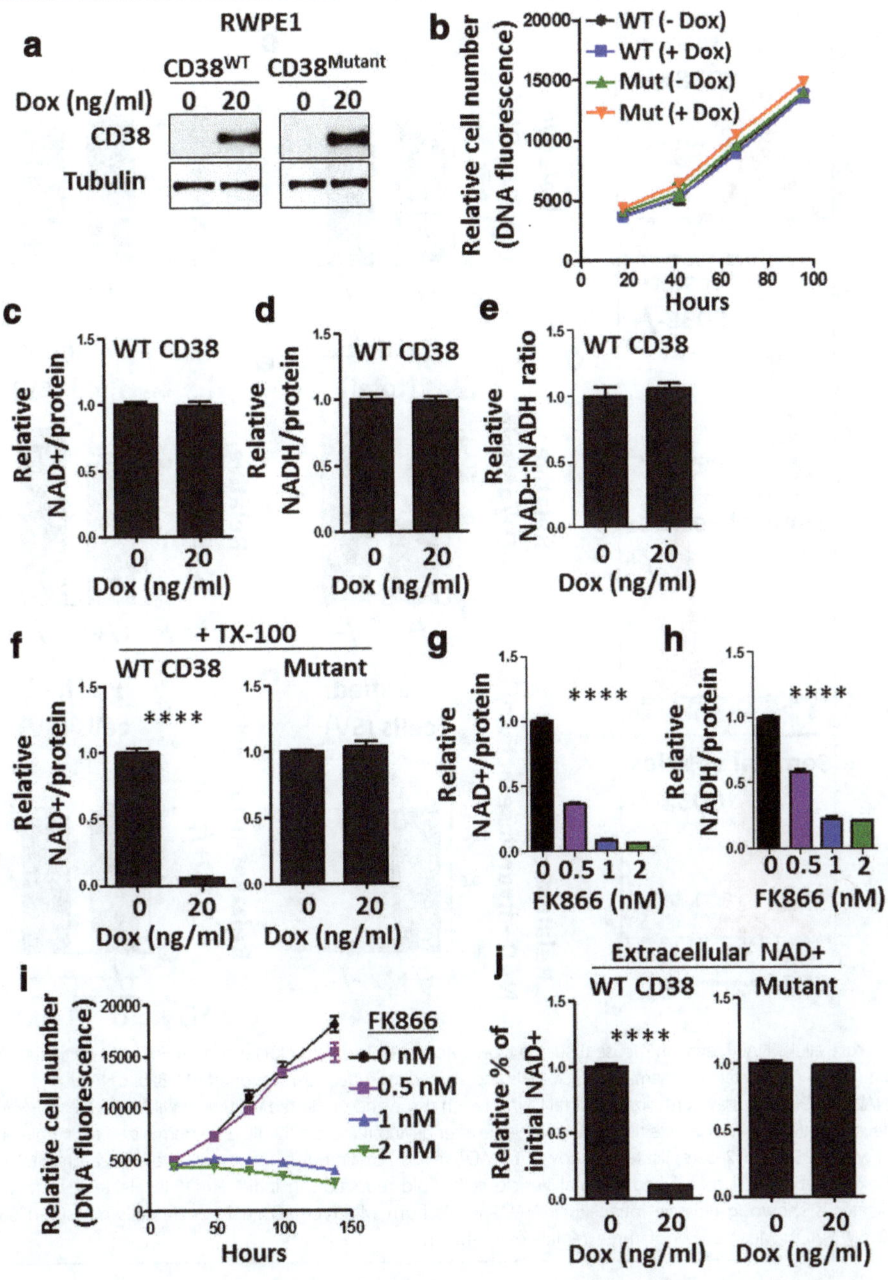

Fig. 4 CD38 regulates extracellular but not intracellular NAD$^+$ levels in RPWE1 cells. **a** Western blots demonstrate doxycyline (Dox) induced expression of wild-type (WT) or mutant (E226Q) CD38 in RWPE1 cells. Tubulin serves as a loading control. **b** Cell proliferation assay over 4 days in culture in the presence or absence of 20 ng/mL Dox. Relative cell number was assessed by measuring DNA fluorescence at 465 nm. 3–6 replicate wells per group per time point were measured. Plot shows mean ± standard error of the mean (SEM). **c**, **d** NAD$^+$ and NADH levels were measured relative to total protein in each sample and presented relative to no Dox (non-induced) sample. Mean ± SEM of four replicates is shown. **e** NAD$^+$:NADH ratio is calculated based on results shown in **c** and **d**. Mean ± SEM of four replicates is shown. **f** Cells were treated with Triton X-100 (TX-100) to permeabilize cells followed by NAD$^+$ measurements. NAD$^+$/protein is shown relative to no Dox. Mean ± SEM of four replicates is shown. **g–i** RWPE1 cells were treated with increasing concentrations of FK866 followed by NAD$^+$ (**g**) and NADH (**h**) measurements. Mean ± SEM of four replicates is shown. Newman-Keuls Multiple Comparison Test. **i** Cell proliferation assay over 4 days in culture in the presence of the indicated concentrations of FK866. DNA fluorescence represents relative cell number. 3–6 replicate wells per group per time point were measured. Plot shows mean ± standard error of the mean (SEM). **j** Relative NAD$^+$/protein levels in the media 30 min after the addition of 800 nM exogenous NAD$^+$. Mean ± SEM of four replicates is shown

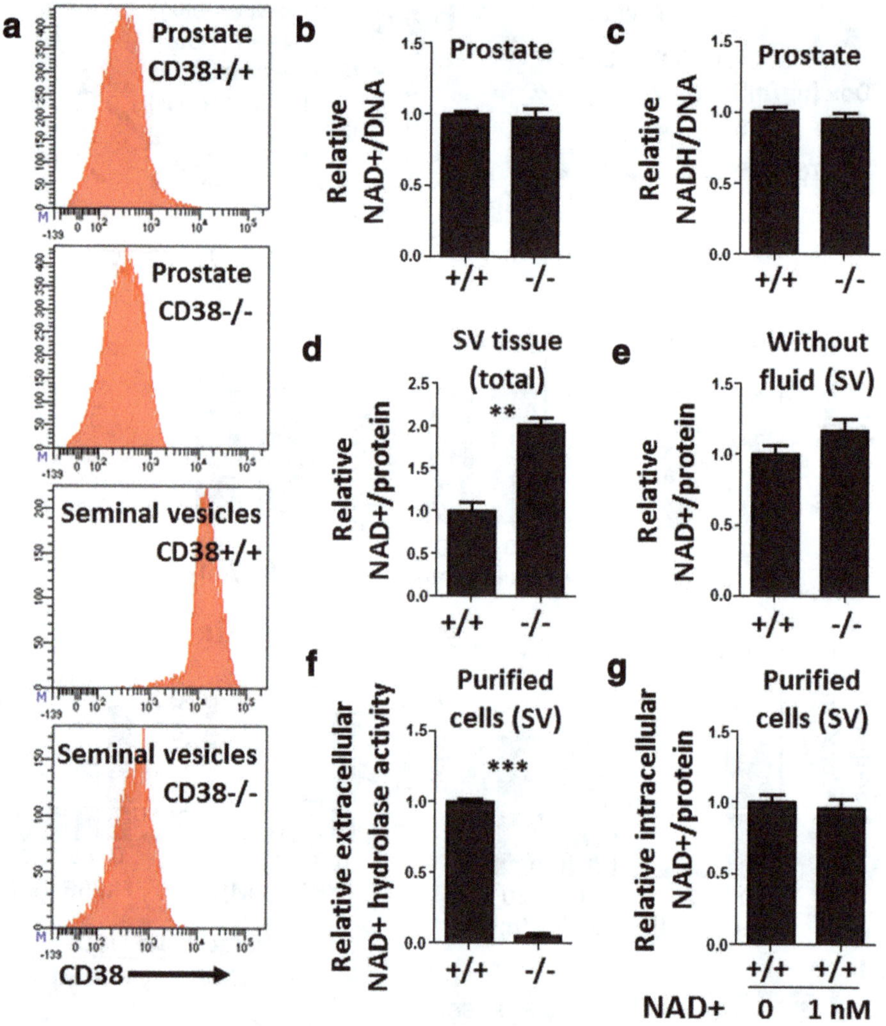

Fig. 5 CD38 regulates extracellular NAD$^+$ levels in mouse tissues. **a** Flow cytometry histogram plots gated on EpCAM+ epithelial cells from wild-type (CD38+/+) or knockout (CD38−/−) prostate and seminal vesicle cells and stained for surface expression of CD38. **b**, **c** NAD$^+$ and NADH levels were measured using the NAD$^+$/NADH-Glo assay normalized to total DNA in each tissue and presented relative to wild-type. Mean ± SEM of four replicates is shown. **d**, **e** NAD$^+$ levels in intact seminal vesicle tissue (**d**) or in tissue after having removed the fluid (**e**) normalized to protein and presented relative to wild-type. Mean ± SEM of 2–5 replicates is shown. **f** NAD$^+$ levels remaining in the media were measured 60 min after the addition of 800 nM exogenous NAD$^+$ to purified seminal vesicle cells. Fold reduction in initial NAD$^+$ levels, relative to wild-type, is shown. Mean ± SEM of duplicates is shown. **g** Relative intracellular NAD$^+$ levels from wild-type seminal vesicle cells measured 60 min after the addition of 0 or 800 nM NAD$^+$. Mean ± SEM of three replicates is shown

depleting extracellular NAD$^+$ compared to wild-type seminal vesicle cells (Fig. 5f). The addition of extracellular NAD$^+$ to seminal vesicle cells did not cause an increase in intracellular NAD$^+$ (Fig. 5g). These findings indicate that CD38 regulates extracellular NAD$^+$ levels, with little evidence for regulation of intracellular NAD$^+$, in mouse urogenital tissues and human prostate epithelial cell lines.

Discussion

NAD$^+$ is considered an important molecule associated with metabolism, health, and aging, in part through its role as a co-factor for sirtuins and poly-ADP-ribose polymerases (PARPs) [65, 66]. Repletion of NAD$^+$ in aging mice upon treatment with precursor molecules like nicotinamide riboside (NR) or nicotinamide mononucleotide (NMN) can reverse age-related tissue failure [29] and reduce the effects of diabetes [67]. NAD$^+$ likely plays a critical role in tumorigenesis, as depletion of intracellular NAD$^+$ levels by inhibition of NAMPT can impair prostate cancer cell proliferation [32], a result that we reproduced in our study.

CD38 is considered a regulator of intracellular NAD$^+$ levels [68]. Pharmacological inhibition of CD38 has been reported to increase intracellular NAD^+ levels [69]. A previous report in 293T cells showed that CD38 over-expression reduced intracellular NAD^+ levels by approximately 35% and this was associated with a reduced growth rate in vitro [70]. However, our results using NAMPT inhibitor FK866 indicate that even a 50% reduction in NAD^+ levels is not sufficient to impair cell proliferation of multiple human prostate cell lines (Fig. 4g–i, Additional file 8). Using mouse models, researchers have demonstrated increased NAD^+ levels in certain tissues lacking CD38 when compared to wild-type mice [28], which we validated in liver tissue (Additional file 10a). Interestingly, when NAD^+ levels were measured in various tissues from wild-type or knockout mice, including liver, adipose tissue, spleen, and skeletal muscle, only the liver showed a significant difference in adult mice younger than 32 months of age [64]. We found no difference in NAD^+ levels when comparing wild-type or CD38 knockout prostates from adult mice, 2–4 months of age. CD38 expression was considerably higher in cells isolated from seminal vesicles than from prostate (Fig. 5a) or liver (Additional file 10f), and we did find elevated NAD^+ levels in knockout seminal vesicle tissues. However, the trend was not observed after removing fluid, suggesting that elevated NAD^+ in knockout mice was likely due to differences in the extracellular fluid which make up a considerable portion of seminal vesicle tissues. By combining results from wild-type and CD38 knockout mice, as well as inducible over-expression in cell lines, we find a lack of evidence to support CD38 as a significant regulator of intracellular NAD^+ in prostate or seminal vesicles.

Several potential explanations may account for differences between published reports and our findings here. For tissues containing a large amount of fluid or blood, measurements of NAD^+ in whole tissues may be inconsistent with NAD^+ levels in purified cells from wild-type or CD38 knockout mice. Given that CD38 can rapidly deplete NAD^+ levels upon permeabilization, any attempts to extract NAD^+ from cells or tissues without immediately inactivating the CD38 enzymatic activity could lead to reductions in NAD^+ that are not reflective of NAD^+ levels in intact cells. Additionally, concentrations of doxycycline used to induce expression of CD38 can influence NAD^+ levels, as we found statistically significant reductions in intracellular NAD^+ levels simply by adding 40 or 80 ng/ml doxycycline to naïve RWPE1 and LNCaP cells (Additional file 4). Finally, CD38 may play a fundamentally different role in prostate and seminal vesicles than in the liver. It is not clear if increased NAD^+ levels in CD38 knockout liver tissues are due to the loss of intracellular or extracellular NAD^+ hydrolase activity. Given the amount of blood flowing through the liver, and the elevated NAD^+ levels in the blood of CD38 knockout mice, excess available NAD^+ may be taken up by knockout liver cells.

We find evidence to support CD38 as a regulator of extracellular NAD^+, suggesting that repression of CD38 expression in prostate cancer may serve to increase the pool of extracellular NAD^+. NAD^+ released from neurons can act as an inhibitory neurotransmitter in gastrointestinal muscles through P2Y receptors in multiple species [71, 72]. Prostate cancer cells release NAD^+ into the media (Additional file 9d), suggesting that NAD^+ may serve as an autocrine or paracrine signaling molecule for nearby epithelial or non-epithelial cell types in tumors. CD38 expression and extracellular NAD^+ hydrolase activity, or the absence of CD38 expression, might influence immune cell proliferation, activation, and survival. NAD^+ has been shown to inhibit both cytotoxic T cells [33] and regulatory T cells [36], indicating that the make-up of the immune environment may dictate potential immune-suppressing or immune-promoting effects of increased extracellular NAD^+. The relationship between prostate epithelial expression of CD38 and NAD^+-induced cell death has not been established. Additionally, a potential role of extracellular NAD^+ as a signaling molecule in vivo has yet to be investigated in prostate cancer. Further studies will be necessary to determine the effect of extracellular NAD^+ in the benign and tumor microenvironment. Outside of a functional role in prostate tumorigenesis, we and others have established CD38 as a marker of differentiated prostate luminal cells [7, 56], suggesting that loss of CD38 in prostate cancer may primarily serve as a marker of a de-differentiated or progenitor-like state.

Conclusions

Reduced expression of CD38 is common in prostate cancer and associated with recurrence after prostatectomy for clinically localized disease, but the mechanisms repressing CD38 expression are poorly understood. In this study, we identify CpG methylation in the *CD38* locus in primary and metastatic prostate cancer. Using inducible expression models in human prostate epithelial cell lines, we found that CD38 over-expression was not sufficient to impair cell proliferation in vitro or alter intracellular NAD^+ or NADH levels. Using a mouse model of CD38 deficiency, we did not find significant differences in intracellular NAD^+ levels between wild-type and CD38 knockout prostate or seminal vesicle tissues. However, we found that CD38 expression was sufficient to alter the levels of extracellular NAD^+, both in human cell lines and primary mouse cells. We therefore propose a model whereby repression of CD38 due to methylation enhances the extracellular pool of NAD^+ in prostate cancer.

Additional files

Additional file 1: CpG hypermethylation of *CD38* in prostate cancer cell lines. Related to Fig. 3, methylation heat maps derived from COMPARE-MS analysis of prostate cancer cell lines, referring to the PCR amplicon shown in Fig. 3a (heat map: red—dense methylation; white—no methylation). Note that male white blood cell DNA (WBC) and white blood cell DNA which was in vitro methylated by CpG Methyltransferase M.SssI (WBC SSSI) were used as negative and positive controls, respectively. (TIF 72 kb)

Additional file 2: In silico analysis of TCGA data correlating DNA methylation and mRNA expression of commonly methylated genes in prostate cancer. Correlation plots of log2 mRNA expression (based on RNA-seq, RSEM z-scores) and methylation levels (based on Infinium Human Methylation 450k BeadChip analysis) in 333 primary prostate cancer samples for *GSTP1* and *PTGS2. (TIF 122 kb)*

Additional file 3: Re-expression of *CD38* in prostate cancer cell lines after treatment with DNA methyltransferase inhibitor. Prostate cancer cell lines CWR22rv1, DU145, LNCaP, and LAPC4 were treated with 100 nM, 500 nM 5-aza-2'-deoxycytidine (decitabine, DAC), or solvent (DMSO) for 4 days. Expression of *CD38* was determined by quantitative real-time PCR. Note that a modest re-expression of *CD38* was observed in two (CWR22rv1, LAPC4) out of four cell lines. (TIF 124 kb)

Additional file 4: Effect of Dox on intracellular NAD^+ levels in RWPE1 and LNCaP cells. (a, b) Intracellular NAD^+ levels were measured relative to DNA measurements (a) or total cellular protein (b) in naïve RWPE1 (a) and LNCaP (b) cells exposed to varying concentrations of Dox. Results are presented relative to no Dox control. Plot shows mean of 4 replicates per time point ±SEM. Newman-Keuls Multiple Comparison Test. (TIF 67 kb)

Additional file 5: Effect of CD38 expression on RWPE1, LNCaP and DU145 cell proliferation. (a) RWPE1 cell proliferation evaluated using the alamarBlue reagent and measured based on relative absorbance. 0 or 20 ng/mL Dox was used over 4 days. Plots show mean of 3–6 replicates per time point ±SEM. (b, c) Western blot of LNCaP (b) and DU145 (c) cells expressing inducible wild-type or mutant (E226Q) CD38 with or without 20 ng/mL Dox. Tubulin is used as a loading control. (d, e) Cell proliferation evaluated using DNA measurements in LNCaP (d) and DU145 (e) cells. Plots show mean of 5 replicates per time point ± SEM. (TIF 107 kb)

Additional file 6: Effect of CD38 on intracellular/extracellular NAD^+ levels in LNCaP, DU145 cells. (a, b) NAD^+ levels were measured relative to total protein in LNCaP (a) and DU145 (b) cells expressing wild-type or mutant CD38 in the presence of 0 or 20 ng/mL Dox presented relative to no Dox (non-induced) sample. Mean ± SEM of 4 replicates is shown. (c, d) LNCaP (c) and DU145 (d) Cells were treated with Triton X-100 (TX-100) to permeabilize cells followed by NAD^+ measurements. NAD^+/protein is shown relative to no Dox. Mean ± SEM of 4 replicates is shown. (e, f) Relative NAD^+/protein levels in the media 30 min after the addition of 800 nM exogenous NAD^+ to LNCaP (e) and DU145 (f) cells. Mean ± SEM of 4 replicates is shown. (TIF 124 kb)

Additional file 7: Effect of CD38 on expression of enzymes involved in NAD^+ metabolism. (a, b) Western blots show expression of NAMPT, NAPRT and Tubulin (loading control) in Dox-induced wild-type CD38-expressing RWPE1 (a) and LNCaP (b) cells. (TIF 102 kb)

Additional file 8: NAMPT inhibitor FK866 depletes NAD^+ levels and impairs proliferation. (a, b, d, e, g, h) Intracellular NAD^+ and NADH levels were measured in the presence of the indicated concentrations of FK866 in LNCaP (a, b), DU145 (d, e) and PC3 (g, h) cells. Mean ± SEM of 4 replicates is shown. Newman-Keuls Multiple Comparison Test. (c, f, i) Cell proliferation assay over 4 days in culture in the presence of the indicated concentrations of FK866 in LNCaP (c), DU145 (f) and PC3 (i) cells. DNA fluorescence represents relative cell number. 3–6 replicate wells per group per time point were measured. Mean ± SEM is shown. (TIF 131 kb)

Additional file 9: Effect of extracellular NAD^+ on intracellular NAD^+ and NADH levels. (a, b) After the addition of exogenous NAD^+ to the media for 30 min, intracellular NAD^+ (a) and NADH (b) levels were measured in RWPE1 cells expressing wild-type or mutant CD38. Results are presented as NAD^+ or NADH relative to protein levels. 20 ng/mL Dox is presented in relation to no Dox (non-induced) samples. Mean ± SEM of 3 replicates is shown. (c) NAD^+:NADH ratio is calculated based on results shown in A and B. (d) Extracellular NAD^+ levels (normalized to total protein in the media) were measured using the NAD^+/NADH-Glo assay 30 min after the addition of fresh media containing 800 nM exogenous NAD^+ to naïve LNCaP cells. Mean ± SEM of 3 replicates is shown in the presence or absence of Dox. (TIF 94 kb)

Additional file 10: NAD^+ and NADH levels in wild-type and CD38 knockout mouse tissues. NAD^+ and NADH levels were measured using the NAD^+/NADH-Glo assay normalized to total DNA or protein in each tissue and presented relative to wild-type. (a) NAD^+/protein in livers of knockout compared to wild-type mice. (b) NAD^+:NADH ratio for prostate tissue is calculated based on results shown in Fig. 5b, c. (c) NADH levels for seminal vesicle tissue. (d) NAD^+:NADH ratio for seminal vesicle tissue is calculated based on results shown in Fig. 5d and Additional file 10c. Mean ± SEM of 2–4 replicates is shown. (e) NAD^+ levels were measured in equivalent volumes of plasma isolated from blood of 5 wild-type and 4 knockout mice. (f) Protein was isolated from purified liver or seminal vesicle cells obtained from wild-type adult male mice and probed with antibodies against CD38 or alpha-tubulin by western blot. (TIF 83 kb)

Acknowledgements
We thank Donghui Cheng for cell sorting. The monoclonal antibody 12G10 developed by The University of Iowa was obtained from the Developmental Studies Hybridoma Bank, created by the NICHD of the NIH and maintained at The University of Iowa, Department of Biology, Iowa City, IA 52242.

Funding
ASG is funded by the American Cancer Society (RSG-17-068-01-TBG), Department of Defense (W81XWH-13-1-0470), Margaret E. Early Medical Research Trust, NIH/NCI (P50CA092131/UCLA SPORE in Prostate Cancer), and support from UCLA's Jonsson Comprehensive Cancer Center, Broad Stem Cell Research Center, Clinical and Translational Science Institute, and Institute of Urologic Oncology. MCH is funded by a Prostate Cancer Foundation Young Investigator Award. YS is funded by a Prostate Cancer Foundation Challenge Award. HB is funded by Department of Defense (PC121341). MAT is funded by NIH/NCI R01CA185189. The research described was supported by NIH/National Center for Advancing Translational Science (NCATS) UCLA CTSI Grant Number UL1TR001881. Lentivirus was made at UCLA IMT core/Vector Core which is supported by CURE/P30 DK041301.

Authors' contributions
JM performed most of the experiments in cell lines, mouse tissues, and NAD^+/NADH measurements, analyzed results, and contributed to the writing of the manuscript. MCH conducted methylation experiments, analyzed results, and contributed to the writing and editing of the manuscript. TRG and DAE performed statistical analyses of the tissue microarrays and contributed to the writing and editing of the manuscript. TH and PDC performed immunohistochemistry and western blot experiments. HB, AS, and RB conducted analysis of CD38 expression in metastatic CRPC and contributed to the writing and editing of the manuscript. DE, WBI, and SY contributed to the methylation datasets, analysis, and editing of the manuscript. EAP and AMD provided the PSA progression tissue microarray, assisted with statistical considerations and analysis, and contributed to the writing and editing of the manuscript. MBR provided the validation set of tissue microarray slides. MAT scored CD38 expression in the tissue microarray and contributed to the editing of the manuscript. ASG is the corresponding author and oversaw all experiments, interpretation of results, and writing and editing of the manuscript. The manuscript was read and approved by all authors.

Competing interests
The authors declare that they have no competing interests.

Author details

[1]Department of Molecular, Cell & Developmental Biology, University of California Los Angeles, Los Angeles, CA, USA. [2]Sidney Kimmel Comprehensive Cancer Center at Johns Hopkins, Baltimore, MD, USA. [3]Department of Pathology, Johns Hopkins University School of Medicine, Baltimore, MD, USA. [4]Department of Medicine Statistics Core, University of California Los Angeles, Los Angeles, CA, USA. [5]Molecular Biology Interdepartmental Program, University of California Los Angeles, Los Angeles, CA, USA. [6]Department of Medicine, Division of Medical Oncology, Weill Cornell Medicine, New York, NY, USA. [7]Englander Institute for Precision Medicine, Weill Cornell Medicine, New York, NY, USA. [8]Department of Pathology and Laboratory Medicine, Weill Cornell Medicine, New York, NY, USA. [9]Institute for Computational Biomedicine, Weill Cornell Medicine, New York, NY, USA. [10]Department of Physiology and Biophysics, Weill Cornell Medicine, New York, NY, USA. [11]James Buchanan Brady Urological Institute, School of Medicine, Johns Hopkins University, Baltimore, MD, USA. [12]Departments of Oncology, Pathology, and Radiation Oncology and Molecular Radiation Sciences, Johns Hopkins University School of Medicine, Baltimore, MD, USA. [13]Division of Hematology-Oncology, Department of Medicine, David Geffen School of Medicine, University of California Los Angeles, Los Angeles, CA, USA. [14]Department of Urology, David Geffen School of Medicine, University of California Los Angeles, Los Angeles, CA, USA. [15]Jonsson Comprehensive Cancer Center, University of California Los Angeles, Los Angeles, CA, USA. [16]Veterans Administration Greater Los Angeles Healthcare System, Los Angeles, CA, USA. [17]Department of Epidemiology, Johns Hopkins Bloomberg School of Public Health, Baltimore, MD, USA. [18]Department of Oncology, Johns Hopkins University School of Medicine, Baltimore, MD, USA. [19]Department of Urology and the James Buchanan Brady Urological Institute, School of Medicine, Johns Hopkins University, Baltimore, MD, USA. [20]Department of Pathology & Laboratory Medicine, David Geffen School of Medicine, University of California Los Angeles, Los Angeles, CA, USA. [21]Broad Stem Cell Research Center, University of California Los Angeles, Los Angeles, CA, USA. [22]Molecular Biology Institute, University of California Los Angeles, Los Angeles, CA, USA.

References

1. Siegel RL, Miller KD, Jemal A. Cancer statistics, 2018. CA Cancer J Clin. 2018; 68(1):7–30.
2. Scher HI, Sawyers CL. Biology of progressive, castration-resistant prostate cancer: directed therapies targeting the androgen-receptor signaling axis. JClinOncol. 2005;23(32):8253–61.
3. Miao L, Yang L, Li R, Rodrigues DN, Crespo M, Hsieh JT, Tilley WD, de Bono J, Selth LA, Raj GV. Disrupting androgen receptor signaling induces snail-mediated epithelial-mesenchymal plasticity in prostate cancer. Cancer Res. 2017;77(11):3101–12.
4. Ware KE, Somarelli JA, Schaeffer D, Li J, Zhang T, Park S, Patierno SR, Freedman J, Foo WC, Garcia-Blanco MA, Armstrong AJ. Snail promotes resistance to enzalutamide through regulation of androgen receptor activity in prostate cancer. Oncotarget. 2016;7(31):50507–21.
5. Smith BA, Sokolov A, Uzunangelov V, Baertsch R, Newton Y, Graim K, Mathis C, Cheng D, Stuart JM, Witte ON. A basal stem cell signature identifies aggressive prostate cancer phenotypes. Proc Natl Acad Sci U S A. 2015; 112(47):E6544–52.
6. Markert EK, Mizuno H, Vazquez A, Levine AJ. Molecular classification of prostate cancer using curated expression signatures. Proc Natl Acad Sci U S A. 2011;108(52):21276–81.
7. Liu X, Grogan TR, Hieronymus H, Hashimoto T, Mottahedeh J, Cheng D, Zhang L, Huang K, Stoyanova T, Park JW, Shkhyan RO, Nowroozizadeh B, Rettig MB, Sawyers CL, Elashoff D, Horvath S, Huang J, Witte ON, Goldstein AS. Low CD38 identifies progenitor-like inflammation-associated luminal cells that can initiate human prostate cancer and predict poor outcome. Cell Rep. 2016;17(10):2596–606.
8. Zhang D, Jeter C, Gong S, Tracz A, Lu Y, Shen J, Tang DG. Histone 2B-GFP label-retaining prostate luminal cells possess progenitor cell properties and are intrinsically resistant to castration. Stem Cell Rep. 2018;10(1):228–42.
9. Qin J, Liu X, Laffin B, Chen X, Choy G, Jeter CR, Calhoun-Davis T, Li H, Palapattu GS, Pang S, Lin K, Huang J, Ivanov I, Li W, Suraneni MV, Tang DG. The PSA(−/lo) prostate cancer cell population harbors self-renewing long-term tumor-propagating cells that resist castration. Cell Stem Cell. 2012; 10(5):556–69.
10. Domingo-Domenech J, Vidal SJ, Rodriguez-Bravo V, Castillo-Martin M, Quinn SA, Rodriguez-Barrueco R, Bonal DM, Charytonowicz E, Gladoun N, de la Iglesia-Vicente J, Petrylak DP, Benson MC, Silva JM, Cordon-Cardo C. Suppression of acquired docetaxel resistance in prostate cancer through depletion of notch- and hedgehog-dependent tumor-initiating cells. Cancer Cell 2012;22(3):373–388.
11. Goldstein AS, Huang J, Guo C, Garraway IP, Witte ON. Identification of a cell of origin for human prostate cancer. Science. 2010;329(5991):568–71.
12. Goldstein AS, Lawson DA, Cheng D, Sun W, Garraway IP, Witte ON. Trop2 identifies a subpopulation of murine and human prostate basal cells with stem cell characteristics. Proc Natl Acad Sci U S A. 2008;105(52):20882–7.
13. Goldstein AS, Drake JM, Burnes DL, Finley DS, Zhang H, Reiter RE, Huang J, Witte ON. Purification and direct transformation of epithelial progenitor cells from primary human prostate. Nat Protoc. 2011;6(5):656–67.
14. Lukacs RU, Goldstein AS, Lawson DA, Cheng D, Witte ON. Isolation, cultivation and characterization of adult murine prostate stem cells. Nat Protoc. 2010;5(4):702–13.
15. Karthaus WR, Iaquinta PJ, Drost J, Gracanin A, van Boxtel R, Wongvipat J, Dowling CM, Gao D, Begthel H, Sachs N, Vries RGJ, Cuppen E, Chen Y, Sawyers CL, Clevers HC. Identification of multipotent luminal progenitor cells in human prostate organoid cultures. Cell. 2014;159(1):163–75.
16. Howard M, Grimaldi JC, Bazan JF, Lund FE, Santos-Argumedo L, Parkhouse RM, Walseth TF, Lee HC. Formation and hydrolysis of cyclic ADP-ribose catalyzed by lymphocyte antigen CD38. Science. 1993;262(5136):1056–9.
17. Zocchi E, Franco L, Guida L, Benatti U, Bargellesi A, Malavasi F, Lee HC, De Flora A. A single protein immunologically identified as CD38 displays NAD+ glycohydrolase, ADP-ribosyl cyclase and cyclic ADP-ribose hydrolase activities at the outer surface of human erythrocytes. Biochem Biophys Res Commun. 1993;196(3):1459–65.
18. Adebanjo OA, Anandatheerthavarada HK, Koval AP, Moonga BS, Biswas G, Sun L, Sodam BR, Bevis PJ, Huang CL, Epstein S, Lai FA, Avadhani NG, Zaidi M. A new function for CD38/ADP-ribosyl cyclase in nuclear Ca2+ homeostasis. Nat Cell Biol. 1999;1(7):409–14.
19. Shrimp JH, Hu J, Dong M, Wang BS, MacDonald R, Jiang H, Hao Q, Yen A, Lin H. Revealing CD38 cellular localization using a cell permeable, mechanism-based fluorescent small-molecule probe. J Am Chem Soc. 2014;136(15):5656–63.
20. Deckert J, Wetzel MC, Bartle LM, Skaletskaya A, Goldmacher VS, Vallee F, Zhou-Liu Q, Ferrari P, Pouzieux S, Lahoute C, Dumontet C, Plesa A, Chiron M, Lejeune P, Chittenden T, Park PU, Blanc V. SAR650984, a novel humanized CD38-targeting antibody, demonstrates potent antitumor activity in models of multiple myeloma and other CD38+ hematologic malignancies. Clin Cancer Res. 2014;20(17):4574–83.
21. Hurtado AM, Chen-Liang TH, Przychodzen B, Hamedi C, Munoz-Ballester J, Dienes B, Garcia-Malo MD, Anton AI, de Arriba F, Teruel-Montoya R, Ortuno FJ, Vicente V, Maciejewski JP, Jerez A. Prognostic signature and clonality pattern of recurrently mutated genes in inactive chronic lymphocytic leukemia. Blood Cancer J. 2015;5:e342.
22. Lokhorst HM, Plesner T, Laubach JP, Nahi H, Gimsing P, Hansson M, Minnema MC, Lassen U, Krejcik J, Palumbo A, van de Donk NW, Ahmadi T, Khan I, Uhlar CM, Wang J, Sasser AK, Losic N, Lisby S, Basse L, Brun N, Richardson PG. Targeting CD38 with Daratumumab monotherapy in multiple myeloma. N Engl J Med. 2015;373(13):1207–19.
23. Poret N, Fu Q, Guihard S, Cheok M, Miller K, Zeng G, Quesnel B, Troussard X, Galiegue-Zouitina S, Shelley CS. CD38 in hairy cell leukemia is a marker of poor prognosis and a new target for therapy. Cancer Res. 2015;75(18):3902–11.
24. Boini KM, Xia M, Xiong J, Li C, Payne LP, Li PL. Implication of CD38 gene in podocyte epithelial-to-mesenchymal transition and glomerular sclerosis. J Cell Mol Med. 2012;16(8):1674–85.
25. Kramer G, Steiner G, Fodinger D, Fiebiger E, Rappersberger C, Binder S, Hofbauer J, Marberger M. High expression of a CD38-like molecule in

normal prostatic epithelium and its differential loss in benign and malignant disease. J Urol. 1995;154(5):1636–41.
26. Liu AY, Roudier MP, True LD. Heterogeneity in primary and metastatic prostate cancer as defined by cell surface CD profile. Am J Pathol. 2004;165(5):1543–56.
27. Kramer G, Steiner GE, Sokol P, Mallone R, Amann G, Marberger M. Loss of CD38 correlates with simultaneous up-regulation of human leukocyte antigen-DR in benign prostatic glands, but not in fetal or androgen-ablated glands, and is strongly related to gland atrophy. BJU Int. 2003; 91(4):409–16.
28. Aksoy P, White TA, Thompson M, Chini EN. Regulation of intracellular levels of NAD: a novel role for CD38. Biochem Biophys Res Commun. 2006;345(4): 1386–92.
29. Zhang H, Ryu D, Wu Y, Gariani K, Wang X, Luan P, D'Amico D, Ropelle ER, Lutolf MP, Aebersold R, Schoonjans K, Menzies KJ, Auwerx J. NAD(+) repletion improves mitochondrial and stem cell function and enhances life span in mice. Science. 2016;352(6292):1436–43.
30. Aksoy P, Escande C, White TA, Thompson M, Soares S, Benech JC, Chini EN. Regulation of SIRT 1 mediated NAD dependent deacetylation: a novel role for the multifunctional enzyme CD38. Biochem Biophys Res Commun. 2006; 349(1):353–9.
31. Canto C, Menzies KJ, Auwerx J. NAD(+) metabolism and the control of energy homeostasis: a balancing act between mitochondria and the nucleus. Cell Metab. 2015;22(1):31–53.
32. Wang B, Hasan MK, Alvarado E, Yuan H, Wu H, Chen WY. NAMPT overexpression in prostate cancer and its contribution to tumor cell survival and stress response. Oncogene. 2011;30(8):907–21.
33. Wang J, Nemoto E, Kots AY, Kaslow HR, Dennert G. Regulation of cytotoxic T cells by ecto-nicotinamide adenine dinucleotide (NAD) correlates with cell surface GPI-anchored/arginine ADP-ribosyltransferase. J Immunol. 1994; 153(9):4048–58.
34. Bortell R, Moss J, McKenna RC, Rigby MR, Niedzwiecki D, Stevens LA, Patton WA, Mordes JP, Greiner DL, Rossini AA. Nicotinamide adenine dinucleotide (NAD) and its metabolites inhibit T lymphocyte proliferation: role of cell surface NAD glycohydrolase and pyrophosphatase activities. J Immunol. 2001;167(4):2049–59.
35. Seman M, Adriouch S, Scheuplein F, Krebs C, Freese D, Glowacki G, Deterre P, Haag F, Koch-Nolte F. NAD-induced T cell death: ADP-ribosylation of cell surface proteins by ART2 activates the cytolytic P2X7 purinoceptor. Immunity. 2003;19(4):571–82.
36. Hubert S, Rissiek B, Klages K, Huehn J, Sparwasser T, Haag F, Koch-Nolte F, Boyer O, Seman M, Adriouch S. Extracellular NAD+ shapes the Foxp3+ regulatory T cell compartment through the ART2-P2X7 pathway. J Exp Med. 2010;207(12):2561–8.
37. Hamid O, Robert C, Daud A, Hodi FS, Hwu WJ, Kefford R, Wolchok JD, Hersey P, Joseph RW, Weber JS, Dronca R, Gangadhar TC, Patnaik A, Zarour H, Joshua AM, Gergich K, Elassaiss-Schaap J, Algazi A, Mateus C, Boasberg P, Tumeh PC, Chmielowski B, Ebbinghaus SW, Li XN, Kang SP, Ribas A. Safety and tumor responses with lambrolizumab (anti-PD-1) in melanoma. N Engl J Med. 2013;369(2):134–44.
38. Yegnasubramanian S, Lin X, Haffner MC, DeMarzo AM, Nelson WG. Combination of methylated-DNA precipitation and methylation-sensitive restriction enzymes (COMPARE-MS) for the rapid, sensitive and quantitative detection of DNA methylation. Nucleic Acids Res. 2006;34(3):e19.
39. Yegnasubramanian S, Kowalski J, Gonzalgo ML, Zahurak M, Piantadosi S, Walsh PC, Bova GS, De Marzo AM, Isaacs WB, Nelson WG. Hypermethylation of CpG islands in primary and metastatic human prostate cancer. Cancer Res. 2004;64(6):1975–86.
40. Yegnasubramanian S, Wu Z, Haffner MC, Esopi D, Aryee MJ, Badrinath R, He TL, Morgan JD, Carvalho B, Zheng Q, De Marzo AM, Irizarry RA, Nelson WG. Chromosome-wide mapping of DNA methylation patterns in normal and malignant prostate cells reveals pervasive methylation of gene-associated and conserved intergenic sequences. BMC Genomics. 2011;12:313.
41. Cancer Genome Atlas Research N. The molecular taxonomy of primary prostate cancer. Cell. 2015;163(4):1011–25.
42. Gao J, Aksoy BA, Dogrusoz U, Dresdner G, Gross B, Sumer SO, Sun Y, Jacobsen A, Sinha R, Larsson E, Cerami E, Sander C, Schultz N. Integrative analysis of complex cancer genomics and clinical profiles using the cBioPortal. Sci Signal. 2013;6(269):pl1.
43. Beltran H, Rickman DS, Park K, Chae SS, Sboner A, MacDonald TY, Wang Y, Sheikh KL, Terry S, Tagawa ST, Dhir R, Nelson JB, de la Taille A, Allory Y, Gerstein MB, Perner S, Pienta KJ, Chinnaiyan AM, Wang Y, Collins CC, Gleave ME, Demichelis F, Nanus DM, Rubin MA. Molecular characterization of neuroendocrine prostate cancer and identification of new drug targets. Cancer Discov. 2011;1(6):487–95.
44. Chakravarty D, Sboner A, Nair SS, Giannopoulou E, Li R, Hennig S, Mosquera JM, Pauwels J, Park K, Kossai M, MacDonald TY, Fontugne J, Erho N, Vergara IA, Ghadessi M, Davicioni E, Jenkins RB, Palanisamy N, Chen Z, Nakagawa S, Hirose T, Bander NH, Beltran H, Fox AH, Elemento O, Rubin MA. The oestrogen receptor alpha-regulated lncRNA NEAT1 is a critical modulator of prostate cancer. Nat Commun. 2014;5:5383.
45. Beltran H, Prandi D, Mosquera JM, Benelli M, Puca L, Cyrta J, Marotz C, Giannopoulou E, Chakravarthi BV, Varambally S, Tomlins SA, Nanus DM, Tagawa ST, Van Allen EM, Elemento O, Sboner A, Garraway LA, Rubin MA, Demichelis F. Divergent clonal evolution of castration-resistant neuroendocrine prostate cancer. Nat Med. 2016;22(3):298–305.
46. Dobin A, Davis CA, Schlesinger F, Drenkow J, Zaleski C, Jha S, Batut P, Chaisson M, Gingeras TR. STAR: ultrafast universal RNA-seq aligner. Bioinformatics. 2013;29(1):15–21.
47. Li H, Handsaker B, Wysoker A, Fennell T, Ruan J, Homer N, Marth G, Abecasis G, Durbin R, Genome Project Data Processing S. The sequence alignment/ map format and SAMtools. Bioinformatics. 2009;25(16):2078–9.
48. Trapnell C, Roberts A, Goff L, Pertea G, Kim D, Kelley DR, Pimentel H, Salzberg SL, Rinn JL, Pachter L. Differential gene and transcript expression analysis of RNA-seq experiments with TopHat and cufflinks. Nat Protoc. 2012;7(3):562–78.
49. Derrien T, Johnson R, Bussotti G, Tanzer A, Djebali S, Tilgner H, Guernec G, Martin D, Merkel A, Knowles DG, Lagarde J, Veeravalli L, Ruan X, Ruan Y, Lassmann T, Carninci P, Brown JB, Lipovich L, Gonzalez JM, Thomas M, Davis CA, Shiekhattar R, Gingeras TR, Hubbard TJ, Notredame C, Harrow J, Guigo R. The GENCODE v7 catalog of human long noncoding RNAs: analysis of their gene structure, evolution, and expression. Genome Res. 2012;22(9):1775–89.
50. Leek JT, Johnson WE, Parker HS, Jaffe AE, Storey JD. The sva package for removing batch effects and other unwanted variation in high-throughput experiments. Bioinformatics. 2012;28(6):882–3.
51. Hempel HA, Cuka NS, Kulac I, Barber JR, Cornish TC, Platz EA, De Marzo AM, Sfanos KS. Low intratumoral mast cells are associated with a higher risk of prostate cancer recurrence. Prostate. 2017;77(4):412–24.
52. Toubaji A, Albadine R, Meeker AK, Isaacs WB, Lotan T, Haffner MC, Chaux A, Epstein JI, Han M, Walsh PC, Partin AW, De Marzo AM, Platz EA, Netto GJ. Increased gene copy number of ERG on chromosome 21 but not TMPRSS2-ERG fusion predicts outcome in prostatic adenocarcinomas. Mod Pathol. 2011;24(11):1511–20.
53. Breslow NE, Day NE. Statistical methods in cancer research. Volume I - The analysis of case-control studies. IARC Sci Publ. 1980;32:5–338.
54. Gollapudi K, Galet C, Grogan T, Zhang H, Said JW, Huang J, Elashoff D, Freedland SJ, Rettig M, Aronson WJ. Association between tumor-associated macrophage infiltration, high grade prostate cancer, and biochemical recurrence after radical prostatectomy. Am J Cancer Res. 2013;3(5):523–9.
55. Aryee MJ, Liu W, Engelmann JC, Nuhn P, Gurel M, Haffner MC, Esopi D, Irizarry RA, Getzenberg RH, Nelson WG, Luo J, Xu J, Isaacs WB, Bova GS, Yegnasubramanian S. DNA methylation alterations exhibit intraindividual stability and interindividual heterogeneity in prostate cancer metastases. Sci Transl Med. 2013;5(169):169ra110.
56. Sahoo D, Wei W, Auman H, Hurtado-Coll A, Carroll PR, Fazli L, Gleave ME, Lin DW, Nelson PS, Simko J, Thompson IM, Leach RJ, Troyer DA, True LD, McKenney JK, Feng Z, Brooks JD. Boolean analysis identifies CD38 as a biomarker of aggressive localized prostate cancer. Oncotarget. 2018;9(5): 6550–61.
57. Meissner A, Mikkelsen TS, Gu H, Wernig M, Hanna J, Sivachenko A, Zhang X, Bernstein BE, Nusbaum C, Jaffe DB, Gnirke A, Jaenisch R, Lander ES. Genome-scale DNA methylation maps of pluripotent and differentiated cells. Nature. 2008;454(7205):766–70.
58. Yegnasubramanian S, Haffner MC, Zhang Y, Gurel B, Cornish TC, Wu Z, Irizarry RA, Morgan J, Hicks J, DeWeese TL, Isaacs WB, Bova GS, De Marzo AM, Nelson WG. DNA hypomethylation arises later in prostate cancer progression than CpG island hypermethylation and contributes to metastatic tumor heterogeneity. Cancer Res. 2008;68(21):8954–67.
59. Sharad S, Ravindranath L, Haffner MC, Li H, Yan W, Sesterhenn IA, Chen Y, Ali A, Srinivasan A, McLeod DG, Yegnasubramanian S, Srivastava S, Dobi A, Petrovics G. Methylation of the PMEPA1 gene, a negative regulator of the androgen receptor in prostate cancer. Epigenetics. 2014;9(6):918–27.

60. Congleton J, Jiang H, Malavasi F, Lin H, Yen A. ATRA-induced HL-60 myeloid leukemia cell differentiation depends on the CD38 cytosolic tail needed for membrane localization, but CD38 enzymatic activity is unnecessary. Exp Cell Res. 2011;317(7):910–9.
61. Ahler E, Sullivan WJ, Cass A, Braas D, York AG, Bensinger SJ, Graeber TG, Christofk HR. Doxycycline alters metabolism and proliferation of human cell lines. PLoS One. 2013;8(5):e64561.
62. Page B, Page M, Noel C. A new fluorometric assay for cytotoxicity measurements in-vitro. Int J Oncol. 1993;3(3):473–6.
63. Cockayne DA, Muchamuel T, Grimaldi JC, Muller-Steffner H, Randall TD, Lund FE, Murray R, Schuber F, Howard MC. Mice deficient for the ecto-nicotinamide adenine dinucleotide glycohydrolase CD38 exhibit altered humoral immune responses. Blood. 1998;92(4):1324–33.
64. Camacho-Pereira J, Tarrago MG, Chini CCS, Nin V, Escande C, Warner GM, Puranik AS, Schoon RA, Reid JM, Galina A, Chini EN. CD38 dictates age-related NAD decline and mitochondrial dysfunction through an SIRT3-dependent mechanism. Cell Metab. 2016;23(6):1127–39.
65. Yoshino J, Baur JA, Imai SI. NAD(+) intermediates: the biology and therapeutic potential of NMN and NR. Cell Metab. 2018;27(3):513–28.
66. Rajman L, Chwalek K, Sinclair DA. Therapeutic potential of NAD-boosting molecules: the in vivo evidence. Cell Metab. 2018;27(3):529–47.
67. Yoshino J, Mills KF, Yoon MJ, Imai S. Nicotinamide mononucleotide, a key NAD(+) intermediate, treats the pathophysiology of diet- and age-induced diabetes in mice. Cell Metab. 2011;14(4):528–36.
68. Chini EN. CD38 as a regulator of cellular NAD: a novel potential pharmacological target for metabolic conditions. Curr Pharm Des. 2009; 15(1):57–63.
69. Escande C, Nin V, Price NL, Capellini V, Gomes AP, Barbosa MT, O'Neil L, White TA, Sinclair DA, Chini EN. Flavonoid apigenin is an inhibitor of the NAD+ ase CD38: implications for cellular NAD+ metabolism, protein acetylation, and treatment of metabolic syndrome. Diabetes. 2013;62(4): 1084–93.
70. Hu Y, Wang H, Wang Q, Deng H. Overexpression of CD38 decreases cellular NAD levels and alters the expression of proteins involved in energy metabolism and antioxidant defense. J Proteome Res. 2014;13(2):786–95.
71. Mutafova-Yambolieva VN, Hwang SJ, Hao X, Chen H, Zhu MX, Wood JD, Ward SM, Sanders KM. Beta-nicotinamide adenine dinucleotide is an inhibitory neurotransmitter in visceral smooth muscle. Proc Natl Acad Sci U S A. 2007;104(41):16359–64.
72. Hwang SJ, Durnin L, Dwyer L, Rhee PL, Ward SM, Koh SD, Sanders KM, Mutafova-Yambolieva VN. Beta-nicotinamide adenine dinucleotide is an enteric inhibitory neurotransmitter in human and nonhuman primate colons. Gastroenterology. 2011;140(2):608–617 e606.

Metabolic characterization of isocitrate dehydrogenase (IDH) mutant and IDH wildtype gliomaspheres uncovers cell type-specific vulnerabilities

Matthew Garrett[1†], Jantzen Sperry[2†], Daniel Braas[2,3], Weihong Yan[4], Thuc M. Le[2,5], Jack Mottahedeh[6], Kirsten Ludwig[6], Ascia Eskin[7], Yue Qin[6], Rachelle Levy[8], Joshua J. Breunig[8,9,10], Frank Pajonk[11,12], Thomas G. Graeber[2,3,12], Caius G. Radu[2,5,12], Heather Christofk[2,3,12,14], Robert M. Prins[1,2,12], Albert Lai[12,13], Linda M. Liau[1,12], Giovanni Coppola[6,13] and Harley I. Kornblum[2,6,12,14*]

Abstract

Background: There is considerable interest in defining the metabolic abnormalities of IDH mutant tumors to exploit for therapy. While most studies have attempted to discern function by using cell lines transduced with exogenous IDH mutant enzyme, in this study, we perform unbiased metabolomics to discover metabolic differences between a cohort of patient-derived IDH1 mutant and IDH wildtype gliomaspheres.

Methods: Using both our own microarray and the TCGA datasets, we performed KEGG analysis to define pathways differentially enriched in IDH1 mutant and IDH wildtype cells and tumors. Liquid chromatography coupled to mass spectrometry analysis with labeled glucose and deoxycytidine tracers was used to determine differences in overall cellular metabolism and nucleotide synthesis. Radiation-induced DNA damage and repair capacity was assessed using a comet assay. Differences between endogenous IDH1 mutant metabolism and that of IDH wildtype cells transduced with the IDH1 (R132H) mutation were also investigated.

Results: Our KEGG analysis revealed that IDH wildtype cells were enriched for pathways involved in de novo nucleotide synthesis, while IDH1 mutant cells were enriched for pathways involved in DNA repair. LC-MS analysis with fully labeled ^{13}C-glucose revealed distinct labeling patterns between IDH1 mutant and wildtype cells. Additional LC-MS tracing experiments confirmed increased de novo nucleotide synthesis in IDH wildtype cells relative to IDH1 mutant cells. Endogenous IDH1 mutant cultures incurred less DNA damage than IDH wildtype cultures and sustained better overall growth following X-ray radiation. Overexpression of mutant IDH1 in a wildtype line did not reproduce the range of metabolic differences observed in lines expressing endogenous mutations, but resulted in depletion of glutamine and TCA cycle intermediates, an increase in DNA damage following radiation, and a rise in intracellular ROS.

(Continued on next page)

* Correspondence: HKornblum@mednet.ucla.edu
†Equal contributors
[2]Department of Molecular and Medical Pharmacology, David Geffen School of Medicine, UCLA, Room 379 Neuroscience Research Building, 635 Charles E. Young Dr. South, Los Angeles, CA 90095, USA
[6]Department of Psychiatry and Biobehavioral Sciences and Semel Institute for Neuroscience & Human Behavior, UCLA, Room 379 Neuroscience Research Building, 635 Charles E. Young Dr. South, Los Angeles, CA 90095, USA

(Continued from previous page)

Conclusions: These results demonstrate that IDH1 mutant and IDH wildtype cells are easily distinguishable metabolically by analyzing expression profiles and glucose consumption. Our results also highlight important differences in nucleotide synthesis utilization and DNA repair capacity that could be exploited for therapy. Altogether, this study demonstrates that IDH1 mutant gliomas are a distinct subclass of glioma with a less malignant, but also therapy-resistant, metabolic profile that will likely require distinct modes of therapy.

Keywords: 2-hydroxyglutarate, Metabolism, Nucleotide, Radiation, Glioma

Background

Alteration in cellular metabolism is a key pathway to the development of cancer. Most oncogenes and tumor suppressors influence cellular metabolism, and there are examples of mutations in metabolic genes that become tumorigenic [1]. Homologous mutations in the metabolic enzymes isocitrate dehydrogenase 1 and 2 (*IDH1* and *IDH2*) are found in acute myelogenous leukemia, colon cancer and glioma [2]. In glioma, these mutations generally co-occur with either 1p/19q co-deletion or with mutations in *TP53*, the former with more oligodendrocytic characteristics and the latter with more astrocytic characteristics [3]. In contrast to metabolic mutations that involve a loss of function, IDH mutations were found to bestow a new enzymatic function of reducing alpha-ketoglutarate (a-KG) to 2-hydroxyglutarate (2-HG) [4]. In the presence of IDH mutations, the 2-HG molecule, normally found at low levels, can increase to millimolar amounts. Understandably, there has been considerable interest in what role this potential "oncometabolite" might have on cells. Given the structural similarity of the 2-HG molecule to a-KG, it was suspected that 2-HG may be a competitive inhibitor that blocked access to a-KG-dependent enzymes that regulate cell epigenetics [5, 6].

There has been considerable interest in defining what effects IDH mutations have on glioma cell biology, and what the discovery of an IDH mutation can tell us about a specific glioma. These questions are important for two reasons. The first reason comes from the rationale that if the IDH mutant enzyme changes the metabolic state of the cell, this may render the cell more or less vulnerable to certain types of therapy. For example, it has been reported that the IDH1mutation makes cells more vulnerable to radiation [7] or NAD+ depletion [8]. This issue has become even more clinically relevant with the discovery that the presence of IDH mutations can be diagnosed via imaging even prior to surgery [9]. The second reason comes from the observation that glioblastoma patients with IDH mutant tumors have prolonged survival compared to patients with IDH wildtype tumors and that there are now pharmacological inhibitors of the IDH mutant enzymes available that block 2-HG formation [10]. If it is the case that the IDH mutation is actually a metabolic burden to the cell, then use of these inhibitors may actually aid the tumor cell and accelerate growth. Studies using mutant IDH inhibitors in in vivo xenograft models have led to mixed results with one showing slowed growth [11] and another showing accelerated growth [8].

Attempts to focus on isolating metabolic differences between IDH mutant and IDH wildtype glioblastomas have historically suffered from an unproven assumption that the metabolic differences between IDH mutant and IDH wildtype tumors can be largely attributed to the presence or absence of the IDH mutation itself [12, 13]. However, more recent evidence suggests that IDH mutation may be one of the initial mutations to occur in those gliomas [14, 15]. Large-scale bioinformatics analyses of mutational, expression and epigenetic datasets reveal that IDH mutant and IDH wildtype tumors are different on a very fundamental level [16] and may have different cells of origin, and different paths of tumorigenesis. Unfortunately, attempts to study cells derived from endogenous IDH mutant tumors have been hampered by the difficulty involved in establishing and maintaining IDH mutant glioma cells in culture.

To address these issues, we have performed a metabolic analysis on a cohort of patient-derived IDH1 mutant and IDH wildtype tumor cells to determine differences between these groups that may potentially be exploitable for therapy. We demonstrate that when compared to IDH wildtype glioma cells and tumors, IDH1 mutant cells and tumors are enriched for gene sets associated with DNA repair, while wildtype cells have greater expression of gene sets associated with nucleotide biosynthesis. IDH1 mutant cells have metabolic profiles that are distinct from those of IDH wildtype cells and our findings indicate that at least some of these differences are not corrected by overexpression of mutant IDH1 in IDH wildtype cells. Functional studies surprisingly demonstrate that IDH1 mutant cells are better able to recover from radiation treatment and less prone to the effects of inhibition of de novo nucleotide biosynthesis. These findings indicate that IDH mutant and wildtype tumors may be responsive to different metabolically directed therapies and that the previously held views that IDH mutant tumors are highly radiosensitive may not be correct for all subsets of IDH mutant tumors and needs further exploration.

Methods

Collection of in vitro cultures

Samples were collected under institutional review board-approved protocols and graded by neuropathologists. We previously reported on gene expression analysis in these samples in all except one of the IDH mutants [17]. IDH wildtype samples were all from GBM. Of the seven IDH1 mutant cultures, five were from GBM, one from a grade III oligoastrocytoma and one from a grade II oligodendroglioma. Cultures were prepared as described previously [17]. Briefly, on the day of resection, samples were digested with papain. Acellular debris was removed and remaining cells were incubated in gliomasphere media (DMEM/F12 supplemented with B27, penicillin/ampicillin, heparin, EGF and bFGF) for several days until spheres began to form. Frozen stocks were made at passage 5 to maintain cells at low passage. One IDH1 mutant line, BT142, was obtained through ATCC [18, 19]. Relevant information pertaining to the cultures used for in vitro experiments is summarized in Additional file 1, which provides the characteristics of the patients and the tumor as reported by neuropathologists as well as data from comparative genomic hybridization and whole exome sequencing in the samples for which it was available. The majority of experiments were performed using the same 3 IDH WT lines (HK157, HK301, and HK308) and 3 IDH1 mutant lines (HK213, HK252, and HK322). Prior to the completion of data collection, the HK322 culture was lost. Therefore, two additional IDH1 mutant lines (BT142 and HK211) were included for the radiation experiments.

Whole exome sequencing and mutation analysis

Genomic DNA was extracted and fragmented by sonication using the Covaris acoustic disruptor (model E210, Covaris Inc.) to achieve an average fragment size of 200 base pairs. Two hundred nanograms of DNA from each sample were used for the construction of DNA libraries using Kapa Hyper DNA library prep kits and matched dual index adapters (Integrated DNA Technologies). Exome capture was performed using the Nimblegen SeqCap EZ Exome enrichment kit. Sequencing was performed on an Illumina HiSeq 4000 following the manufacturer's instructions. 65–70 million 120-base, paired-end reads were obtained per sample on average, with a 50× average depth of coverage within the targeted exome. Raw image files were processed with the Illumina CASAVA 1.8 software (Illumina, San Diego, CA).

Whole exome sequencing was analyzed using the Genome Analysis Toolkit (GATK) [20] pipeline. Briefly, short reads were aligned using the Burrows-Wheeler Aligner (BWA) [21]. SAMtools was used to convert between SAM and BAM file format, and Picard tools to sort alignments and mark duplicates. Variants were called using the GATK HaplotypeCaller function with the following parameters: variant index parameter 128,000; variant index type LINEAR; nda; maxAltAlleles 4; ERC GVCF; contamination 0.02. ANNOVAR [22] was used to annotate variants.

Copy number variation (CNV) analysis

DNA libraries were hybridized onto Affymetrix CytoScanHD arrays. We first processed the raw intensity CEL files using the R package affy2sv [23] to generate B-allele frequency (BAF) and log R ratio (LRR) values. Secondly, we used the PennCNV software (parameters: exome HMM model with gcmodel adjustment, filtered by 10 SNPs minimum 10 and with region length longer than 50 k) [24], the R package GenoCN (parameters: cnv-only snpInfo$PFB > 1; outputSNP 1; outputSeg TRUE) [25], and the R package Rawcopy (default parameters) [26] for CNV inference. CNV calls were obtained by integrating the output from all callers.

Gene set enrichment analysis

RNA was purified from 59 patient-derived gliomasphere cultures and hybridized to Affymetrix U133 Plus 2.0 arrays. For KEGG-based analysis, we collapsed gene expression probes based on enzyme activity (Enzyme Commission numbers [EC]) rather than on gene identity to avoid unequal representation of equivalent enzymatic function within pathways, thus emphasizing potential flux through the network. The metric used for gene ranking was the signal to noise ratio (SNR) between the IDH1 mutant and IDH1WT samples. The metric was calculated for all candidate probesets of each gene or enzymatic activity and the probeset with maximum absolute metric value was retained. Probeset annotation was based on UniGene build #201, and UniGene identifiers were mapped to each EC using the gene names provided by KEGG. Pathways with fewer than three or greater than 500 nodes represented by the data were excluded from the analysis. This resulted in 167 KEGG modules in the TCGA dataset and 186 modules in the gliomasphere data set.

Glucose/glutamine uptake

200,000 cells were plated in 3 ml of gliomasphere media and allowed to grow for 24 h. The cells were spun down and counted, and glucose and glutamine levels in the used media were measured using a NOVA Bioanalyzer and compared to blank control [27–29]. To evaluate the effects of IDH1 mutant inhibition on glucose/glutamine uptake, 5 μM of c227 was added to the culture 24 h before being harvested.

Cell proliferation studies (CFSE)

Cell proliferation of endogenous IDH1 mutant and IDH wildtype cultures was assessed using CFDA SE (CFSE;

carboxyfluoresceindiacetate, succinimidyl ester) cell tracer kit (Invitrogen) as described previously [30]. Briefly, spheres were dissociated with Accumax (Innovative Cell Technologies), stained with CFSE according to manufacturer suggestions, and grown for 5 days under normal gliomasphere conditions at a density of 100,000 cells/mL. Preparation for FACS analysis was performed according to manufacturer guidelines using 4% paraformaldehyde as a fixative. Following FACS acquisition, Proliferation Wizard Basic Model was used to assess proliferative populations within each sample and to generate average division times.

Liquid chromatography–mass spectrometry (LC-MS)

Cells were cultured for 24 h and rinsed with PBS, and either unlabeled media, 50% ^{13}C-glucose labeled media, or 50% ^{13}C-glutamine labeled media was added. After 24 h, cells were rinsed with ice-cold 150 mM NH_4AcO (pH 7.3), followed by addition of 400 μl cold methanol and 400 μl cold water. Cells were transferred to an Eppendorf tube, and 10 nmol norvaline (Sigma-Aldrich, N7502) as well as 400 μl chloroform was added to each sample. For the metabolite extraction, samples were vortexed for 5 min on ice and spun down, and the aqueous layer was transferred into a glass vial and dried. Metabolites were resuspended in 70% ACN and 5 μl loaded onto a Phenomenex Luna 3u NH_2 100A (150 × 2.0 mm) column. The chromatographic separation was performed on an UltiMate 3000 RSLC (Thermo Scientific) with mobile phases A (5 mM NH_4AcO pH 9.9) and B (ACN) and a flow rate of 300 μl/min. The gradient ran from 15% A to 95% A over 18 min, 9 min isocratic at 95% A, and re-equilibration for 7 min. Metabolite detection was achieved with a Thermo Scientific Q Exactive mass spectrometer run in polarity switching mode (+3.0 kV/−2.25 kV). TraceFinder 3.3 (Thermo Scientific) was used to quantify metabolites as the area under the curve using retention time and accurate mass measurements (< 3 ppm). Relative amounts of metabolites were calculated by summing up all isotopologues of a given metabolite and normalized to the internal standard and cell number. Clustering analysis was done in R.

Metabolic tracing using combined liquid chromatography and tandem mass spectrometry (LC-MS/MS)

Cell lines were grown in gliomasphere media supplemented with fully labeled ^{13}C-glucose and ^{13}C9,^{15}N3-dC. The cells were allowed to grow for 48 h at which point they were harvested and lysed. Genomic DNA was extracted using the Quick-gDNA MiniPrep kit (Zymo Research, D3021) and hydrolyzed to nucleosides using the DNA Degradase Plus kit (Zymo Research, E2021), following manufacturer-supplied instructions. In the final step of DNA extraction, 50 μL of water was used to elute the DNA into 1.5 mL Eppendorf tubes. A nuclease solution (5 μL; 10× buffer/DNA Degradase Plus™/water, 2.5/1/1.5, *v*/*v*/*v*) was added to 20 μL of the eluted genomic DNA in an HPLC injector vial. The samples were then incubated overnight at 37 °C. Samples (20 μL) were injected onto a porous graphitic carbon column (Thermo Fisher Scientific Hypercarb, 100 × 2.1 mm, 5 μm particle size) equilibrated in solvent A (water/acetonitrile/formic acid, 95/5/0.2, *v*/*v*/*v*) and eluted (200 μL/min) with an increasing concentration of solvent B (acetonitrile/water/formic acid, 90/10/0.2, *v*/*v*/*v*) using min/%B/flow rates (μL/min) as follows: 0/0/200, 5/0/200, 10/15/200, 20/15/200, 21/40/200, 25/50/200, 26/100/700, 30/100/700, 31/0/700, 34/0/700, 35/0/200. The effluent from the column was directed to the Agilent Jet Stream ion source connected to the triple quadrupole mass spectrometer (Agilent 6460) operating in the multiple reaction monitoring mode using previously optimized settings. The peak areas for each nucleosides and nucleotides (precursor→fragment ion transitions) at predetermined retention times were recorded using the software supplied by the instrument manufacturer (Agilent MassHunter). To evaluate the effects of IDH1 mutant inhibition on glucose glutamine labeling, 5 μM of c227 was initially added to the culture and then re-added following PBS wash.

Deoxythymidine (dT) treatment

To evaluate the effects of nucleotide synthesis inhibition, a group of cells were grown in gliomasphere media and subjected to 1 mM dT treatment and allowed to grow for 4 days. At this point the cells were harvested, stained with DAPI, and subjected to flow cytometry analysis to determine cell cycle distribution.

Radiation

To determine the extent of DNA damage following radiation, gliomaspheres were dissociated, plated at 1×10^5 cells/mL, and subjected to a 10 Gy dose of radiation using an X-ray irradiator (Gulmay Medical, Atlanta, GA) (5.519 Gy/min; 250 kV; a 4-mm Be, a 3-mm Al, and a 1.5-mm Cu filter). Neutral-buffered Oxiselect Comet Assay Kit (Cell Biolabs) was used to assess DNA damage according to manufacturer's instructions. For the c227 comet experiments presented in Additional file 2, IDH1 mutant cells were treated with 5 μM c227 or control for 48 h prior to irradiation (10 Gy) and comet analysis as described above. Radiation-induced apoptosis was measured at 4 days after treatment using TUNEL staining. To determine effects of growth following radiation, cell lines were plated at 2×10^5 cells in 3 ml of gliomasphere media. They were then subjected to the indicated doses of radiation (0, 2, 6, and 10 Gy) and allowed to recover for a minimum of 4 days. When the control group of each cell line was ready to be passaged, all samples from that line were dissociated with Accumax (Innovated Cell Tech.), counted on a Countess Automated Cell Counter (Invitrogen, C10227) using 0.4% trypan blue, and compared to the non-irradiated control group. Each bar on the graph (dose of radiation) is the average percent of control based on a minimum of three independent replicates (Error bars = ± SEM). The growth curve experiments following radiation presented in Additional file 3 were carried out in a similar manner with the following exceptions. All cell lines were plated at an initial density of 2×10^5 cells per 3 ml and given a single 10 Gy dose of radiation or control (0 Gy). When the fastest growing sample was ready to be passaged, all cultures from each group were dissociated, counted, and then replated at 2×10^5 cells. This was repeated three times in order to generate the growth curve presented in Additional file 3. Three IDH WT and three IDH1 mutant cultures were used for each group. Data is based on three independent replicates.

IDH1 mutant overexpression/ROS measurement

cDNA for the IDH1 mutant gene (R132H) was cloned into a lentiviral vector and transfected into HK308 cell line. This vector encodes a murine orthologue and was found to maintain better and more consistent expression of the mutant protein and 2-HG than a human vector (data not shown). Five hundred thousand IDH1WT cells were dissociated and plated in 3 ml of neurosphere mediated, infected with the lentivirus, and allowed to grow for 2 weeks. The cells were sorted for GFP and again allowed to grow and form spheres. All experiments were done within 6 weeks of infection. Overexpression of the IDH1 mutant protein was confirmed by western blot and 2-HG measurement. IDH1 mutant and IDH wild-type cells were allowed to grow in gliomasphere media. They were then collected, stained with CellROX reagents (Thermo Fisher), and analyzed by flow cytometry. The total ROS level was the integration of the area under the curve as previously described [31].

Statistical analysis

Statistical analyses were performed using the GraphPad Prism software. Sample comparisons and level of significance were determined using the ANOVA model and two-tailed Student's t tests where appropriate. All quantitative data presented are the mean ± standard error of the mean (SEM) unless otherwise noted. Experiments were performed in triplicate, with calculation of 95% confidence interval and p values in relevant comparisons.

Results

KEGG GSEA analysis

Expression data from 59 gliomasphere lines (52 IDH WT GBM and 7 IDH1 mutant) was subjected to Gene Set Enrichment Analysis (GSEA) using KEGG gene modules [32, 33]. Microarray data (GSE98995) is from data described in Laks et al. [17]. A similar comparative analysis was performed on IDH1 mutant and IDH WT tumor samples in the TCGA dataset (183 IDH1WT, 19 IDH1mut). Each KEGG module was assigned a normalized enrichment score (NES) for each dataset and then plotted (Fig. 1, Additional file 4). We noted a positive correlation between the gliomasphere and TCGA datasets giving confidence that our in vitro cells are a good model for in vivo tumors.

There were fewer modules enriched in the IDH1 mutant group in both the TCGA (37/167 gene set modules) as well as our gliomasphere data set (50/186 gene set modules). To identify some potential target metabolic pathways, we used a cut-off enrichment value of 1.2. Even with this liberal cut-off, we only identified four modules that were enriched in IDH1 mutant cells in both data sets. Of these four, the "Homologous Recombination" and "Nucleotide Base Excision Repair" modules were selected for further study due to the clinical relevance in terms of response to radiation. In contrast, there were 35 modules that were enriched in IDH WT cells (Fig. 1, Additional file 4). The "Pentose Phosphate Pathway" and "Amino Sugar and Nucleotide Sugar Metabolism" were selected for further study to determine if IDH1WT cells are in fact more dependent on the de novo pathway of nucleotide synthesis.

Metabolic profile

To assess the differences found in the expression analysis, and to investigate any further metabolic differences between groups, a cohort of IDH WT and IDH1 mutant lines were selected for further study. Key mutations and CNVs of the five IDH1 mutant cultures and three IDH WT cultures that were most intensively studied are listed in Additional file 1. Of note, 4 of 5 of our IDH mutant cultures had pathogenic TP53 mutations and only one (BT142, obtained from ATCC) was 1p/19q co-deleted (Additional file 1). Sample 322 was lost prior to detailed analysis, but clinical cytogenetics of the primary tumor demonstrated that it was not 1p/19q co-deleted, despite it being an oligodendroglioma.

A cohort of 18 IDH WT and 5 IDH1 mutant cultures were subjected to a panel of metabolic measurements including glucose uptake, glutamine uptake, and lactate production rates. Glucose uptake rate was significantly higher in IDH WT cells although there was no significant difference in the lactate production to glucose uptake ratio, suggesting that both cohorts are highly glycolytic. The net glutamine uptake rate for all cells tested was near zero (Fig. 2a–c). Consistent with these differences in glucose uptake, IDH wildtype cells grew faster than IDH1 mutant cells (Additional file 5).

To further define the different utilization of these metabolites, we performed LC-MS on three IDH WT (HK157, HK301, and HK308) and three IDH1 mutant

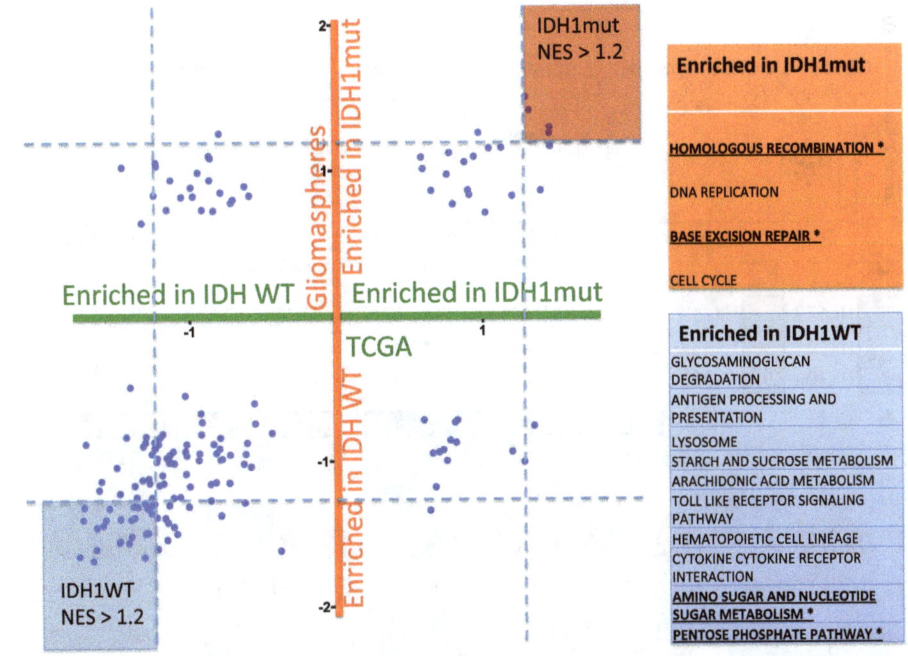

Fig. 1 KEGG Gene Set Enrichment Analysis. Plot of expression data from TCGA (167 KEGG modules) and our gliomasphere dataset (186 KEGG modules). Each KEGG module was assigned a normalized enrichment score (NES) in either the IDH1 mutant or IDH1WT group. Each blue dot represents a different module. The enrichment score for a particular module in the TCGA data is plotted along the X-axis and that associated with the gliomasphere dataset for the same module is plotted on the Y-axis. Thus, a module that is highly enriched in IDH1 mutants compared to wildtype in both datasets would be in the upper right corner and modules highly enriched in IDH wildtype in both datasets would be in the lower left hand corner. Differentially enriched modules (NES > 1.2), listed on the right, were identified as potential candidates for further investigation

(HK213, HK252, and HK322) lines with both fully labeled ^{13}C glucose and fully labeled ^{13}C glutamine. We then defined a single percent label for each metabolite and performed hierarchical clustering to identify if these six cell lines naturally partitioned into groups. Consistent with the observed differences in glucose uptake, IDH1 mutant and IDH WT samples partitioned into separate groups when assessed for glucose labeling (Fig. 2d). Applying hierarchical clustering to the samples according to glutamine labeling or total metabolite amount did not distinguish the samples into distinct groups.

Since glucose labeling could distinguish between IDH1 mutant and IDH WT samples, we performed t tests and compiled a list of all metabolites that had an uncorrected p value < 0.05. Thirty-two metabolites fulfilled this criterion of differential glucose labeling. Of these 32 metabolites, there was a significant over-representation of nucleotide precursors (9/32 chi-square $p < 0.007$). Interestingly, all of the nucleotide precursors showed increased glucose labeling in the IDH WT group (Fig. 2e, Additional file 6).

De novo versus salvage nucleotide synthesis

Because our gene expression and metabolomics results are consistent with elevated nucleotide metabolism in IDH WT cells, we decided to investigate further whether IDH WT cells are more dependent on de novo nucleotide synthesis than IDH1 mutant cells. We profiled the de novo and salvage contribution to deoxycytidine triphosphate incorporation into newly replicated DNA using labeled ^{13}C glucose (to denote de novo) and labeled [^{13}C9,^{15}N3]dC (to denote salvage). Using the same set of three IDH WT lines and three IDH1 mutant lines, we found that while all samples utilized both pathways, the IDH WT samples used primarily de novo synthesis while the IDH1 mutant samples used both pathways relatively equally (Fig. 3a, b). To identify if this difference had functional relevance, we utilized high levels of deoxythymidine (dT), an inhibitor of the de novo pathway [34] to determine if there is any differential response between the two groups. Predicting that this inhibitor would have an effect on the ability of cells to pass through S phase, we treated cells for 4 days (~ 1 doubling time) with dT and then performed cell cycle analysis using DAPI. All cell lines showed an increase in the number of cells in S phase; however, in the IDH1 mutant samples, cells were better able to pass through S phase and proceed with cell division. In contrast, at the end of the 4-day treatment period, almost all IDH wildtype cells were found in the S phase (Fig. 3c).

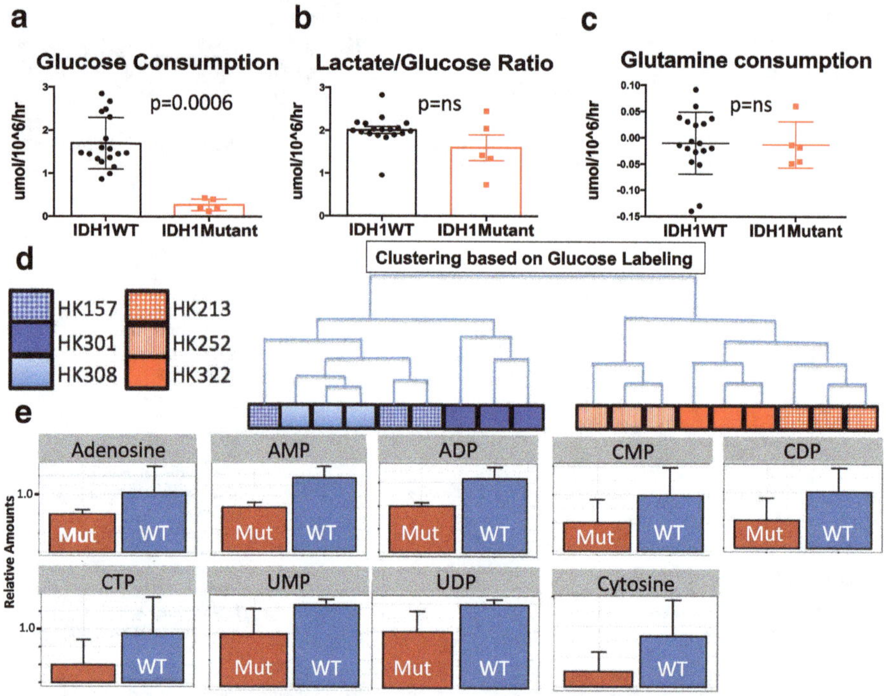

Fig. 2 Metabolic profile of IDH1 mutant and wildtype cells. **a–c** Quantification of glucose and glutamine consumption as well as the ratio of glucose consumed to lactate produced. Measurements were acquired using NOVA ($N = 18$ IDH WT and 5 IDH1 mutant). Statistical significance was determined by Student's *t* test. **d** Clustering of three IDH1 mutant and three IDH wildtype lines according to LC-MS glucose labeling (IDHWTs: blue, IDH1 mutants: red). A glucose labeling index for each of the 159 metabolites analyzed was calculated for all 6 cell lines followed by non-hierarchical clustering analysis. Each line was run in triplicate and all samples are shown. **e** Quantification of glucose labeling among nucleotide precursors by group. Relative amounts of metabolites were calculated by summing up all isotopologues of a given metabolite and normalized to the internal standard and cell number

DNA repair in response to radiation

Having discovered that GSEA expression analysis accurately predicted that IDH1 mutant cells are less dependent on de novo nucleotide synthesis than are the IDH wildtype cells that we studied, we next turned to the modules that we found to be enriched in IDH1 mutant cells, namely modules involved with DNA repair and cellular response to radiation. Using a comet assay, we first tested whether there was a difference in the amount of DNA damage incurred from a given dose of radiation and how quickly that DNA was repaired. For these experiments, we studied two of our IDH1/TP53 mutant lines as well as BT142, a highly studied IDH1 mutant that is 1p/19q-co-deleted but that also bears a TP53 mutation [18, 19]. At a dose of 10 Gy, significantly more IDH WT cells showed signs of DNA damage as compared to IDH1 mutant cells at all time points tested (Fig. 4a, b). In IDH1 mutant cells, DNA damage peaked immediately after exposure to radiation, but that damage was largely repaired within 4 h. Damage in IDH wildtype cells peaked after the first hour post-radiation and followed a similar trend with regard to repair. To examine repair dynamics, we next restricted our focus only to those cells with sustained measurable damage (comet tails) and then calculated tail moment length at different time points (0, 60, 120, and 240 min) to assess which group more efficiently repairs DNA. Again, the IDH1 mutant cultures showed significantly less initial damage following radiation and were able to resolve DNA breaks more quickly (Fig. 4c). However, there was no significant difference in DNA damage between IDH1 mutant and wildtype cells by the final time point of the assay.

We assessed the extent of apoptotic cell death using the TUNEL assay but saw relatively low levels of TUNEL staining and no significant difference between the two groups (Additional file 7). However, when we examined the ability of cells to grow after radiation, we again found that IDH1 mutant cells were better able to re-enter the cell cycle and divide as compared to IDH WT cells (Fig. 4d). To ensure that these effects were not due to differences in growth rate between IDH1 mutant and wildtype cells, we repeated the experiment from Fig. 4d but performed a growth curve assay over several passages to compare effects of high dose radiation (10 Gy) on growth (Additional file 3). This analysis confirmed that IDH1 mutants once again grow better following radiation and are able to continue to proliferate after several passages. Meanwhile, IDH wildtype cultures are unable to sustain growth past the first week following this high dose of radiation. In all, these data suggest that the

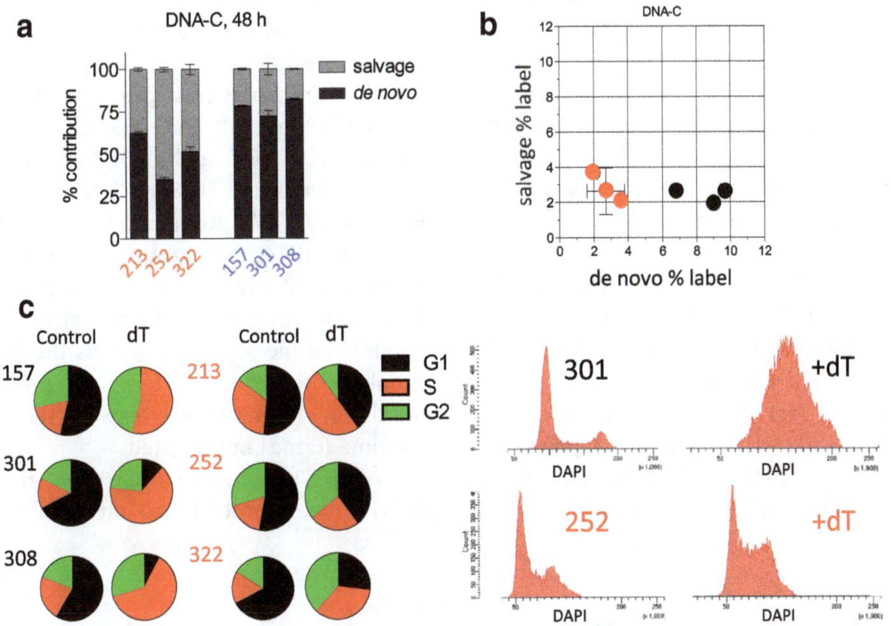

Fig. 3 IDH1 mutant cells utilize de novo and salvage pathways for nucleotide biosynthesis. **a**, **b** Quantification of de novo nucleotide synthesis and salvage pathway utilization by LC-MS with labeled glucose and nucleotides. **a** The relative contribution of each pathway plotted in bar graph format. **b** The same data plotted two-dimensionally. Error bars represent ± STDEV. **c** Cell cycle analysis by flow cytometry (DAPI) following 4-day treatment with 1 mM deoxythymidine (dT) or control (left: distribution of cells in G1, S phase, and G2; right: representative histograms of cell cycle distribution for IDH1 mutant and WT cultures following dT treatment)

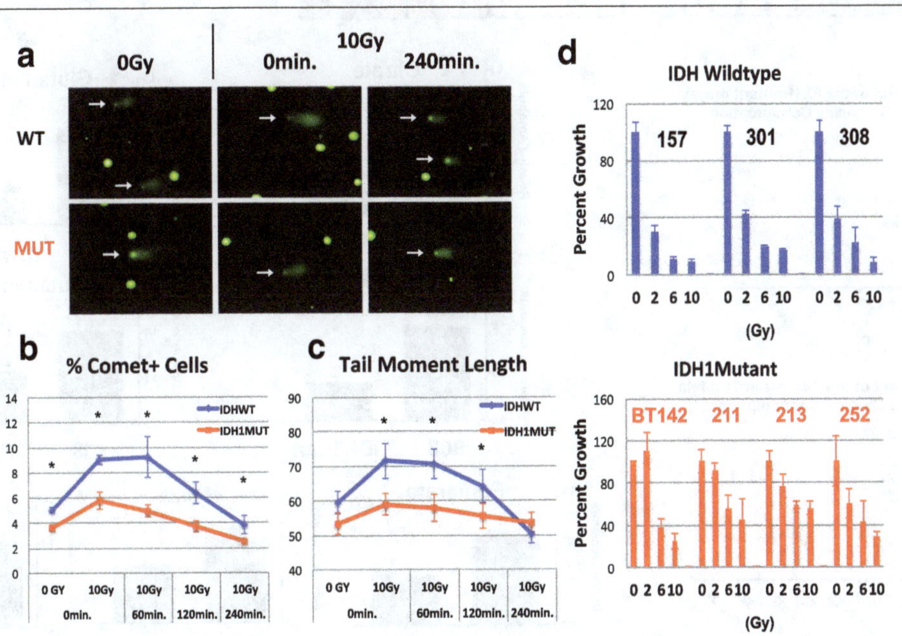

Fig. 4 IDH1 mutant cells show diminished vulnerability to radiation. **a**–**c** Assessment of DNA damage and repair by comet analysis following irradiation (10 Gy). **a** Representative images of cells following comet assay. White arrows indicate cells with comets. **b** Graph showing the percent of cells with comets. Comet number was calculated for each line individually and then averaged by group. **c** Tail moment length for each comet was calculated as the length from the center of the comet head to the center of the tail. Tail moment length was calculated for each line individually and then averaged by group. Significance levels were calculated by ANOVA followed by post hoc t tests. Asterisks denote $p < 0.05$, error bars: ± SEM. **d** Quantification of the effects of increasing doses of radiation (0, 2, 6, and 10 Gy) on culture growth as described in the "Methods" section. Graphs represent cell counts normalized to non-irradiated controls

effects of radiation on growth are not simply due to differences in growth rates between IDH wildtypes and mutants.

IDH1 mutant overexpression as a model for IDH1 mutant glioma

IDH1 mutant overexpression in an IDH1WT background makes those cells more vulnerable to radiation [7]. With our new result that endogenous IDH1 mutant cells are less vulnerable to radiation than the IDH WT cells tested, it appeared that the IDH1 mutation itself was not the sole determinant driving the difference between these two groups. To further test this hypothesis, we overexpressed the IDH1 mutant protein in an IDH WT background (HK308 + IDH1mut) and pharmacologically inhibited the IDH1 mutant protein in an endogenous IDH1 mutant cell line (HK213 + c227). We used LC-MS to confirm 2-HG production and inhibition respectively (Additional file 8). Once we confirmed the appropriate effects on 2-HG production, we repeated the glucose-uptake clustering analysis to see if this artificial IDH1 mutant line (HK308 + IDH1mut) clustered with the IDH WT or the IDH1 mutant groups (Fig. 5a). We found that the HK308 + IDH1mut samples clustered with the IDH WT group and the HK213 + c227 clustered with the IDH1mut group. More specifically, neither IDH1 mutant overexpression nor the c227 inhibitor led to a change in glucose labeling of nucleotide precursors (Additional file 9). This supports the hypothesis that the simple presence of IDH1 mutant protein or 2-HG was not driving the difference between these two groups over the time frames investigated.

We next investigated what effect the presence of the IDH1 mutant protein had on cellular metabolism. We

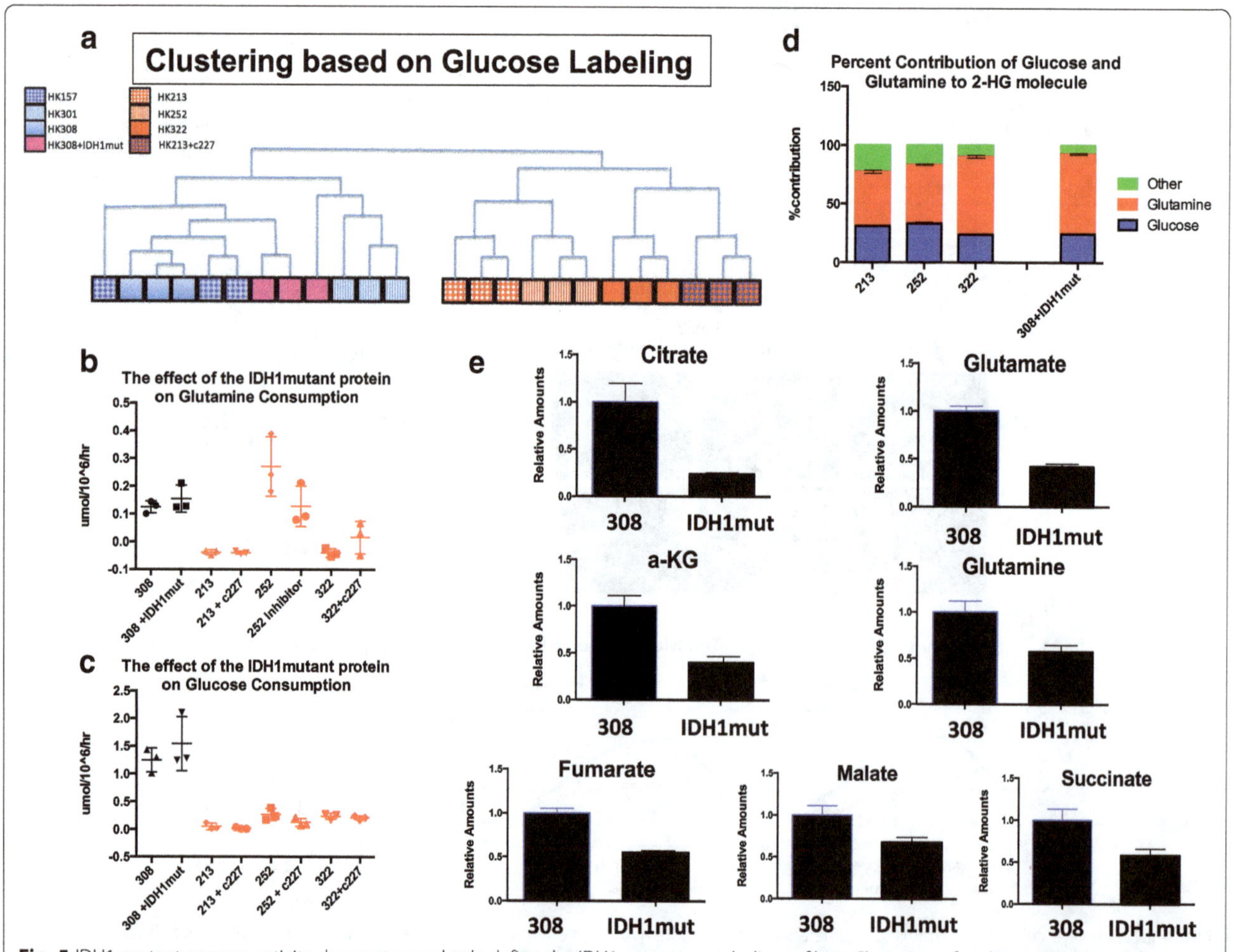

Fig. 5 IDH1 mutant enzyme activity does not completely define the IDH1 mutant metabolic profile. **a** Clustering of eight samples based on LC-MS glucose labeling as described in Fig. 2. Analysis includes the same cohorts of IDH1 mutant and wildtype cultures with the addition of IDH1 mutant overexpression in an IDH WT line and inhibition of the endogenous mutant enzyme (308 + IDH1mut and 213 + c227 respectively). **b, c** Quantification of glutamine and glucose consumption with IDH1 mutant overexpression and inhibition. **d** Contribution of glucose and glutamine to 2-HG production in endogenous and transduced IDH1 mutants. **e** Effects of IDH1 mutant overexpression on glutamine and TCA cycle intermediates quantified using LC-MS. $p < 0.05$ for all seven metabolites shown. Error bars denote ± SEM

examined the effects on glutamine and glucose consumption and found that neither the addition nor inhibition of the endogenous IDH1 mutant enzyme influenced the consumption of either metabolite (Fig. 5b, c). This was a surprising result given that the expression of the IDH1 mutant enzyme leads to production of high levels of 2-hydroxyglutarate and presumed consumption of alpha-ketoglutarate. To investigate this further, we used LC-MS tracing with labeled glucose and glutamine to determine how the cell makes 2-HG. Both endogenous IDH1 mutants and our overexpression model primarily used glutamine to make 2-HG (Fig. 5d). However, given that we did not observe an increase in the amount of glutamine consumption with the addition of the IDH1 mutant gene, we hypothesized that the cells may be depleted of glutamine. Consistent with this prediction, we saw significantly lower levels of glutamine as well as all TCA cycle intermediates when the IDH1 mutant gene was overexpressed (Fig. 5e). In a recent study, Li et al. found that elevating 2-HG levels leads to a significant accumulation of succinate with corresponding decreases in fumarate and malate [35]. Interestingly, we observed decreased levels of succinate and increases in fumarate and malate with 2-HG inhibition (c227) in an endogenous IDH1 mutant line (HK213). However, this did not accurately reflect the differences between endogenous IDH1 mutant and IDH wildtype cells which had roughly comparable levels of glutamine and TCA cycle intermediates (Additional file 10), suggesting that the IDH1 mutation is well-compensated for in the cells that carry it.

In order to further identify potential differences between the endogenous IDH1 mutant and overexpression models, as well as to help clarify differences between our observations of radiation sensitivity from previous reports [7], we repeated our radiation experiments on HK308 with and without overexpression of the IDH1 mutant enzyme. Overexpression of the mutation in this IDH wildtype line resulted in greater DNA damage and decreased repair immediately following radiation (Fig. 6a–c). These results are contrary to what was observed when comparing endogenous IDH1 mutants to IDH wildtype cell lines (Fig. 4). IDH1 mutant overexpression did, however, result in better growth following radiation. One possible explanation for this finding is that exogenous expression of the IDH1 mutant enzyme in HK308 leads to significantly slower growth and this may give the cell more time to repair any DNA

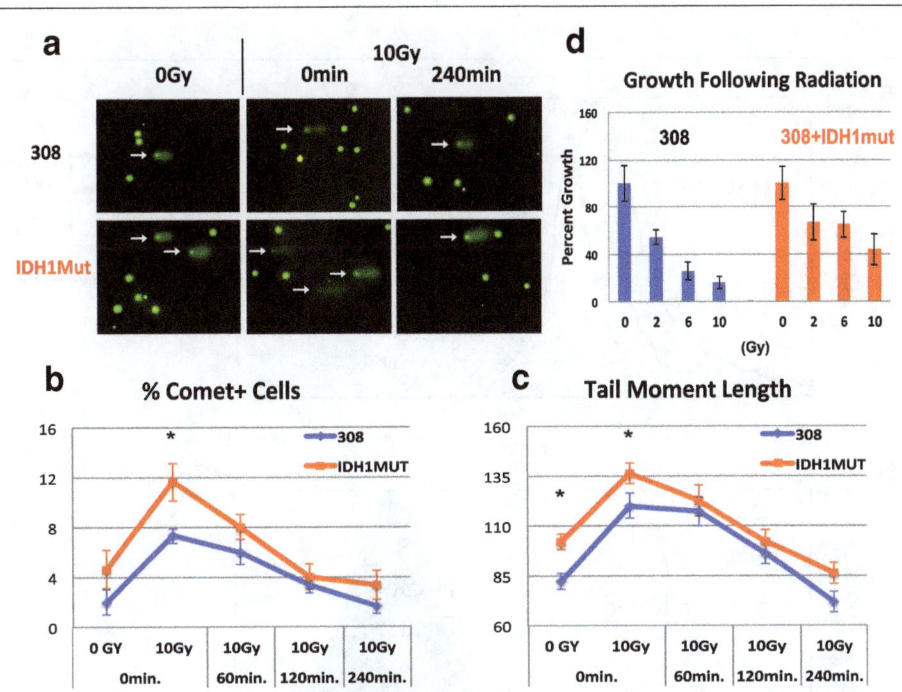

Fig. 6 IDH1 mutant overexpression does not accurately mimic the DNA repair capacity of endogenous mutants. **a**–**c** Assessment of DNA damage and repair by comet analysis following radiation (10 Gy). **a** Representative images of cells following comet assay. White arrows point to cells with comets. **b** Graph shows the percent of cells with comets. Comet number was calculated for each line individually and then averaged by group. **c** Tail moment length for each comet is calculated as the length from the center of the comet head to the center of the tail. Tail moment length was calculated for each line individually and then averaged by group. **d** Quantification of the effects of increasing doses of radiation (0, 2, 6, and 10 Gy) on culture growth as described in the "Methods" section. Graphs represent cell counts normalized to non-irradiated controls. Significance levels were calculated by ANOVA followed by post hoc *t* tests. Asterisks denote $p < 0.05$, Error bars: ± SEM

damage before re-entering the cell cycle. We also investigated the effects of IDH1 mutant inhibition (c227) on radiation-induced DNA damage and repair (Additional file 2). This analysis did not reveal any increase in DNA damage on a per cell basis, as measured by tail moment length. Interestingly though, we did see a more global increase in DNA damage in the c227-treated cells as shown by the increased number of comet+ cells. This treatment did not fully reverse the phenotype to that of IDH wildtype, however. One interpretation of these results is that endogenous IDH1 mutants are adapted to high levels of 2-HG which actually serve a protective role against DNA damage. On the other hand, IDH wildtype cells transduced with the mutant enzyme are not adapted to the dramatically increased levels of 2-HG, resulting in the opposite effect.

Finally, we examined the effect of the IDH1 mutant enzyme on reactive oxygen species (ROS) levels. Interestingly, studies have reported mixed results regarding the effect of the IDH1 mutation on ROS with different results in different cell types [36, 37]. We found that the endogenous IDH1 mutant lines had significantly higher ROS levels than the IDH WT lines (Fig. 7a). This appears to be due to the IDH1 mutation itself, because when we overexpressed the IDH1 mutant enzyme in HK308, the ROS levels increased significantly (Fig. 7b).

Discussion

Many groups have attempted to determine the effect of the IDH1 mutation on host cells as a way to discover metabolic vulnerabilities that may be exploited for therapy. Endogenous IDH1 mutant glioma cells are difficult to grow and maintain in culture—indeed, we lost one line during the process of these experiments—and thus, the first experiments to determine the effect of the IDH1 mutation on cells involved exogenous overexpression of the IDH1 mutant gene in an IDH WT background and performing mass spectroscopy to find differences in the levels of the various metabolites [13, 19, 38–40]. While many of these studies had overlapping findings (e.g., a decrease in glutamine and glutamate levels), other findings were more variable and seemed to depend on the cell model being used. Additionally, many of these in vitro differences did not translate to ex vivo patient tumor tissue [41].

Consistent with the aforementioned studies, we also saw a decrease in glutamine and glutamate with exogenous IDH1 mutant overexpression. However, there was no difference in glutamine, glutamate, or any TCA cycle intermediates between IDH wildtype cells and endogenous IDH1 mutant cells. This suggests that endogenous IDH1 mutant cells may be able to compensate for many of the effects of the IDH1 mutant enzyme itself. One possible explanation for this is that IDH1 mutant glioma

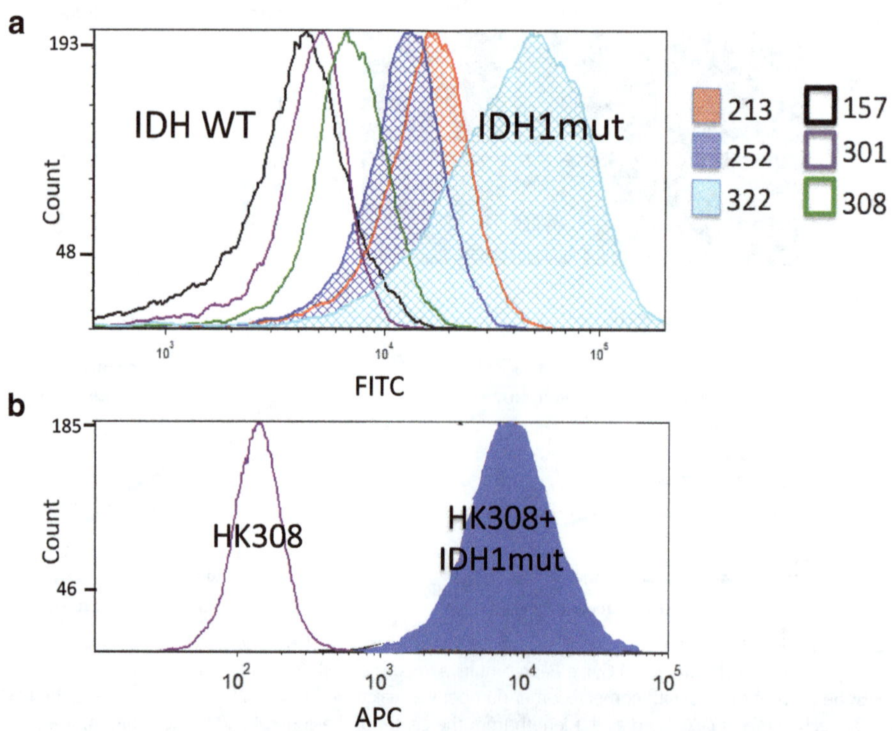

Fig. 7 IDH1 mutant enzyme leads to higher ROS levels. **a** Histogram displaying ROS levels of three IDH1 mutant and three IDH1 wildtype gliomaspheres measured using flow cytometry (CellROX Green). **b** Similar ROS analysis of an IDH WT line (HK308) with and without IDH1 mutant overexpression (CellROX Deep Red). Results shown are from individual experiments. Three replicates yielded identical findings

cells and IDH wildtype glioma cells are derived from different cell types with different properties. However, it is also possible that given enough time, the exogenous IDH1 mutant model would also be able to compensate for the IDH1 mutant enzyme and increase its glutamine and glutamate levels.

Another approach to determine the metabolic effect of the IDH1 mutation on glioma cells is to inhibit the IDH1 mutation in an endogenous IDH1 mutant line. Both the current study and the prior study of Tateishi et al. [8] found a mixed effect of the IDH1 mutant inhibitor on TCA cycle intermediates, with citrate being significantly increased in both studies. In our study, we used a relatively short incubation period (24 h) with the c227 inhibitor in order to isolate the differences in metabolic flux from the changes in gene expression that are associated with 2-HG and aberrant methylation. Although the Tateishi study did not find any significant changes in global methylation with prolonged c227 inhibitor treatment, they did find an increase in NADH levels likely due to increased Naprt1 expression and NAD synthesis. We did not see this change over our shorter time course, and in fact, we saw decreased NADH levels with c227 treatment.

A current challenge in IDH mutant research stems from the variability in methodological approaches used which can significantly alter findings. Identifying potential shortcomings of each will greatly improve the reliability of results. For example, by restricting comparisons to purely isogenic cell lines with or without IDH1 mutant enzyme overexpression or inhibition, the conclusions are limited to the effect of the IDH1 mutant enzyme itself and ignore differences between IDH1 mutant and IDH wildtype tumors that may be independent of the IDH1 mutation. Furthermore, metabolites do not act independently but function as parts of larger pathways. Using only the total cellular levels of various metabolites, it is difficult to draw any conclusions about particular pathways. In this study, we utilized multiple methods to identify cell-type specific vulnerabilities. By using expression data and metabolic tracing studies, we were readily able to distinguish several pathways as well as labeling patterns that clearly distinguished IDH1 mutant from IDH wildtype cells. This distinctive metabolic signature was intrinsic to the cell itself, was retained even with pharmacological inhibition of the IDH1 mutant enzyme, and was not seen in the exogenous overexpression model.

Further evidence of cell culture model variability between IDH mutant studies can be seen from two additional reports published during the preparation of this manuscript, Sulkowski et al. and Lu et al. [42, 43], which demonstrated a diminished capacity for DNA damage repair in IDH1 mutant cells citing deficiencies in homologous recombination and compromised PARP-mediated DNA repair. We observed greater DNA damage and a similar decreased capacity for DNA repair only when using an IDH1 mutant overexpression model. In contrast, our results indicate greater DNA repair capacity in IDH1 mutant cells following radiation. One potential explanation could be that our cultures represent only a subset of IDH1 mutant tumors. Most, if not all, contain endogenous IDH1 R132H mutations and mutant TP53, an important protein that itself may play a large role in mediating many of the observed effects independent of the IDH1 mutant enzyme. Furthermore, the IDH wildtype GBM cultures that were selected as controls could influence the differences observed. While both of these prior studies utilize exogenously transduced IDH mutations, which may have different characteristics, one report did also utilize glioma cells with endogenous mutations for some of their key experiments [42]. However, it is not clear whether these mutant lines are similar to ours with respect to their other mutations. Furthermore, the endogenous mutant cultures from the prior report were propagated in serum, while ours are continuously maintained in serum-free conditions. The differences among these studies have important ramifications for therapy. If, as we propose, IDH1 mutants have a greater capacity for DNA repair following radiation, then radiation therapy may have diminished efficacy. Further study will be required to resolve these differences.

Many of the clinical trials that guide current treatment protocols for glioblastoma were conducted before the discovery of the IDH mutation and thus included a majority of IDH wildtype and a minority of IDH mutant patients. With evidence mounting that IDH mutant gliomas have very different cellular characteristics, it is unclear whether the results of these trials can be generalized to IDH mutant tumors. In particular, the results of this study show that IDH1 mutant gliomas are less vulnerable to radiation-induced DNA damage which draws into question the efficacy of radiation therapy for this subset of tumors. This result was surprising when combined with the fact that exogenous IDH1 mutant overexpression makes cells more vulnerable to radiation [7] and that the IDH1 mutant enzyme significantly increases the amount of reactive oxygen species in the cell. While the cytotoxic and cytostatic mechanisms of radiation are multi-factorial, one of the main mechanisms is DNA damage through the indirect production of free radicals [44]. One possible explanation for the decreased DNA damage seen in IDH mutant cells following radiation is that in order to survive this mutation, IDH mutant cells must develop buffering mechanisms against high levels of reactive oxygen species. This adaptation in turn could make them more resistant to radiation induced DNA damage.

The clinical evidence for the efficacy of radiation in IDH1 mutant gliomas is mixed. In one study, IDH1 mutant tumors seemed to show a better radiographic response following radiation [45]. However, another trial found that for supratentorial low-grade gliomas (of which the majority are likely IDH mutant) high-dose radiation had worse survival than low-dose radiation [46]. It is possible that both findings are correct and that radiographic response may not correlate with clinical survival. Conversely, it is possible that IDH mutant tumors are maximally sensitive to low-dose radiation and higher doses do not provide any further benefit.

Our studies of nucleotide metabolism have potential implications for therapeutics. The availability of nucleotides for DNA synthesis can be a rate-limiting step in cellular proliferation [47]. Nucleotides are synthesized through either de novo or *salvage pathways*. Pharmacologically, the de novo pathway can be inhibited by high concentrations of dT and the salvage pathway can be inhibited by a novel class of compounds [34]. Our data suggest that IDH1 mutant tumors, in contrast to the majority of GBM, utilize this salvage pathway and would hence require both pathways to be inhibited in therapeutic strategies employing inhibition of nucleotide biosynthesis.

A limitation to the current study is that, while gene expression studies are performed using both cultured cells and data derived directly from IDH mutant tumors in vivo, our functional results are obtained from in vitro studies. Very few studies have investigated a spectrum of IDH mutant gliomas in vivo. This is undoubtedly due to the difficulty in propagating these cells in xenograft models. Although not shown, the cells we have utilized did not form xenografts in immunodeficient mice, either in the brain or subcutaneously. The reasons for this are unknown, but suggest that the establishment of tumors from endogenous IDH1 mutants requires host-derived factors that are not present in our model systems. While our findings present novel hypotheses and avenues for future studies, some caution must be taken prior to applying our results directly to clinical trials.

Conclusions

With evidence mounting that IDH mutant gliomas constitute a distinct subclass that follows an independent path of tumorigenesis [48], we endeavored to characterize metabolic differences between IDH1 mutant and IDH wildtype gliomas. Our data are consistent with this concept and provide evidence that some of the distinctions may not be directly related to the IDH1 mutation itself. Furthermore, our data suggest that while IDH1 mutant gliomas may have a less malignant phenotype, they may also be relatively resistant to certain therapies, including radiation.

Additional files

Additional file 1: Patient-derived gliomasphere culture characteristics. Relevant patient information and clinical characteristics for the primary, patient-derived gliomasphere cultures used in this study. Summary of selected copy-number alterations and mutations are also shown. (PDF 42 kb)

Additional file 2: 2-HG inhibition with c227 moderately increases DNA damage following radiation but does not reverse the IDH1 mutant phenotype to an IDH wildtype phenotype. A-B. Assessment of DNA damage and repair by comet analysis following irradiation (10 Gy). HK252 was treated for 48 h with 5 μM c227 or control prior to comet analysis and compared to the IDH WT line HK157. A. Similar analysis of tail moment length as conducted in Fig. 4. B. Graph showing the percent of cells with comets as explained in Fig. 4. All error bars represent ± SEM. (PDF 46 kb)

Additional file 3: IDH1 mutant cells are better able to proliferate following radiation than IDH wildtype cells. A. Growth curve following radiation (0 and 10 Gy) shows average fold increases in cell number between IDH wildtype and IDH1 mutant groups over three passages. Each group consists of three IDH1 mutant and three IDH wildtype cultures respectively. Growth curves were generated from individual cell counts at each time point. B. Identical growth curve as shown in (A), however, the non-irradiated groups have been removed for better visual comparison between irradiated IDH mutant and wildtype groups. Error bars represent ± STDEV. (PDF 51 kb)

Additional file 4: KEGG gene set enrichment analysis of IDH1 mutant and wildtype gliomaspheres. Thirty-five modules were enriched in IDH wildtypes compared to four modules in IDH1 mutants. (PDF 79 kb)

Additional file 5: IDH wildtype cells show faster growth rate compared to IDH1 mutant cells. Six IDH wildtype and five IDH1 mutant gliomasphere cultures were assessed for proliferation rate by flow cytometry using carboxyfluorescein succinimidyl ester (CFSE). ($p < 0.05$). (PDF 19 kb)

Additional file 6: Glucose labeling of metabolites. Glucose fractional contribution was computed for all 159 metabolites. Metabolites that were significantly different between groups (uncorrected *t* test $p < 0.05$) are shown here. (PDF 137 kb)

Additional file 7: Radiation leads to low levels of TUNEL staining in gliomaspheres. Representative images and quantification of cells stained for TUNEL positivity 4 days after exposure to increasing doses of radiation. There is no significant difference between groups. Error bars represent ± SEM. (PDF 2212 kb)

Additional file 8: IDH1 mutant overexpression leads to high levels of 2-HG and the c227 inhibitor is an effective inhibitor of 2-HG formation. IDH wildtype gliomaspheres transduced with the IDH1 mutant enzyme (308 + IDH1mut) and endogenous IDH1 mutant cells treated with 5 μM c227 inhibitor (213 + c227) for 24 h are compared to their respective controls (308 and 213) for 2-HG levels as determined by LC-MS. Data represent the means ± SEM of three replicates per condition. (PDF 22 kb)

Additional file 9: IDH1 mutant enzyme does not affect glucose labeling of nucleotide precursors. Cells were treated and analyzed as described for Supporting Figure S4 in order to determine the percent labeling of nucleotide precursors. There is no significant difference when comparing IDH1 mutant overexpression or endogenous mutant inhibition to their respective controls. (PDF 64 kb)

Additional file 10: Effects of pharmacologic inhibition of the IDH1 mutant enzyme on TCA cycle intermediates. Cells were analyzed as described in Supporting Figure S5. Left: Metabolites with significantly different percent glucose labeling of metabolites in the endogenous IDH1 mutant line 213 treated with c227 inhibitor or control ($p < 0.05$). Right: Percent labeling from endogenous IDH1 mutant and IDH wildtype groups for metabolites that were not significantly different. (PDF 206 kb)

Abbreviations

2-HG: 2-hydroxyglutarate; a-KG: Alpha-ketoglutarate; dT: Deoxythymidine; GSEA: Gene set enrichment analysis; IDH: Isocitrate dehydrogenase; LC-MS: Liquid chromatography–mass spectrometry; PARP: Poly ADP ribose polymerase; ROS: Reactive oxygen species; TCA cycle: Tricarboxylic acid cycle; TP53: Tumor protein 53

Acknowledgements
Not applicable.

Funding
This work was supported in whole or part by National Institute of Health (NIH) Grants: NS052563 (H.I.K.), the UCLA SPORE in Brain Cancer (P50 CA211015); the Dr. Miriam and Sheldon G. Adelson Medical Research Foundation; J.J.B was supported by a Research Scholar Grant, RSG-16-217-01-TBG from the American Cancer Society and by NIH Grant R33 CA202900. We acknowledge the support of the NINDS Informatics Center for Neurogenetics and Neurogenomics P30 NS062691 (G.C).

Authors' contributions
MG and JS are equal contributors to this manuscript and conducted most of the experiments, analyzed results, and wrote most of the paper. DB helped conduct and analyze the results for the labeled glucose LC-MS experiments. WY and TGG helped perform GSEA analysis. TML and CGR provided the experimental outline and assisted with the LC-MS/MS nucleotide synthesis experiments. JM and AE assisted with culture propagation and maintenance. KL assisted with radiation experiments. YQ and GC performed exome and CNV analysis. RL and JJB generated and provided the IDH1 mutant overexpression vector. FP provided valuable insight and assistance with radiation experiments. HC assisted with overall experimental design and provided materials and insight into NOVA experiments. RMP, AL, and LML assisted with experimental design, interpretation of data, and manuscript preparation. HIK is the corresponding author and oversaw all experimental design, interpretation of results, and preparation of this manuscript. All authors read and approved the final manuscript for publication.

Competing interests
The authors declare that they have no competing interests.

Author details
[1]Department of Neurosurgery, and the Interdepartmental Program in the Neurosciences, University of California, Los Angeles, CA 90095, USA. [2]Department of Molecular and Medical Pharmacology, David Geffen School of Medicine, UCLA, Room 379 Neuroscience Research Building, 635 Charles E. Young Dr. South, Los Angeles, CA 90095, USA. [3]UCLA Metabolomics Center, UCLA, Los Angeles, USA. [4]Department of Chemistry and Biochemistry, UCLA, Los Angeles, USA. [5]Ahmanson Translational Imaging Division, UCLA, Los Angeles, USA. [6]Department of Psychiatry and Biobehavioral Sciences and Semel Institute for Neuroscience & Human Behavior, UCLA, Room 379 Neuroscience Research Building, 635 Charles E. Young Dr. South, Los Angeles, CA 90095, USA. [7]Department of Human Genetics, UCLA, Los Angeles, USA. [8]Board of Governors Regenerative Medicine Institute, Cedars-Sinai Medical Center, Los Angeles, CA, USA. [9]Samuel Oschin Comprehensive Cancer Center, Cedars-Sinai Medical Center, Los Angeles, CA, USA. [10]Department of Biomedical Sciences, Cedars-Sinai Medical Center, Los Angeles, CA, USA. [11]Department of Radiation Oncology, David Geffen School of Medicine at UCLA, Los Angeles, USA. [12]Jonsson Comprehensive Cancer Center, UCLA, Room 379 Neuroscience Research Building, 635 Charles E. Young Dr. South, Los Angeles, CA 90095, USA. [13]Department of Neurology, UCLA, Los Angeles, USA. [14]Eli and Edythe Broad Center of Regenerative Medicine and Stem Cell Research, UCLA, Room 379 Neuroscience Research Building, 635 Charles E. Young Dr. South, Los Angeles, CA 90095, USA.

References
1. King A, Selak MA, Gottlieb E. Succinate dehydrogenase and fumarate hydratase: linking mitochondrial dysfunction and cancer. Oncogene. 2006;25(34):4675–82.
2. Parsons DW, Jones S, Zhang X, Lin JC, Leary RJ, Angenendt P, Mankoo P, Carter H, Siu IM, Gallia GL, et al. An integrated genomic analysis of human glioblastoma multiforme. Science. 2008;321(5897):1807–12.
3. Lai A, Kharbanda S, Pope WB, Tran A, Solis OE, Peale F, Forrest WF, Pujara K, Carrillo JA, Pandita A, et al. Evidence for sequenced molecular evolution of IDH1 mutant glioblastoma from a distinct cell of origin. J Clin Oncol. 2011;29(34):4482–90.
4. Dang L, White DW, Gross S, Bennett BD, Bittinger MA, Driggers EM, Fantin VR, Jang HG, Jin S, Keenan MC, et al. Cancer-associated IDH1 mutations produce 2-hydroxyglutarate. Nature. 2009;462(7274):739–44.
5. Turcan S, Rohle D, Goenka A, Walsh LA, Fang F, Yilmaz E, Campos C, Fabius AW, Lu C, Ward PS, et al. IDH1 mutation is sufficient to establish the glioma hypermethylator phenotype. Nature. 2012;483(7390):479–83.
6. Saha SK, Parachoniak CA, Ghanta KS, Fitamant J, Ross KN, Najem MS, Gurumurthy S, Akbay EA, Sia D, Cornella H, et al. Mutant IDH inhibits HNF-4alpha to block hepatocyte differentiation and promote biliary cancer. Nature. 2014;513(7516):110–4.
7. Li S, Chou AP, Chen W, Chen R, Deng Y, Phillips HS, Selfridge J, Zurayk M, Lou JJ, Everson RG, et al. Overexpression of isocitrate dehydrogenase mutant proteins renders glioma cells more sensitive to radiation. Neuro-Oncology. 2013;15(1):57–68.
8. Tateishi K, Wakimoto H, Iafrate AJ, Tanaka S, Loebel F, Lelic N, Wiederschain D, Bedel O, Deng G, Zhang B, et al. Extreme vulnerability of IDH1 mutant cancers to NAD+ depletion. Cancer Cell. 2015;28(6):773–84.
9. Pope WB, Prins RM, Albert Thomas M, Nagarajan R, Yen KE, Bittinger MA, Salamon N, Chou AP, Yong WH, Soto H, et al. Non-invasive detection of 2-hydroxyglutarate and other metabolites in IDH1 mutant glioma patients using magnetic resonance spectroscopy. J Neuro-Oncol. 2012;107(1):197–205.
10. Deng G, Shen J, Yin M, McManus J, Mathieu M, Gee P, He T, Shi C, Bedel O, McLean LR, et al. Selective inhibition of mutant isocitrate dehydrogenase 1 (IDH1) via disruption of a metal binding network by an allosteric small molecule. J Biol Chem. 2015;290(2):762–74.
11. Rohle D, Popovici-Muller J, Palaskas N, Turcan S, Grommes C, Campos C, Tsoi J, Clark O, Oldrini B, Komisopoulou E, et al. An inhibitor of mutant IDH1 delays growth and promotes differentiation of glioma cells. Science. 2013;340(6132):626–30.
12. Izquierdo-Garcia JL, Cai LM, Chaumeil MM, Eriksson P, Robinson AE, Pieper RO, Phillips JJ, Ronen SM. Glioma cells with the IDH1 mutation modulate metabolic fractional flux through pyruvate carboxylase. PLoS One. 2014;9(9):e108289.
13. Grassian AR, Parker SJ, Davidson SM, Divakaruni AS, Green CR, Zhang X, Slocum KL, Pu M, Lin F, Vickers C, et al. IDH1 mutations alter citric acid cycle metabolism and increase dependence on oxidative mitochondrial metabolism. Cancer Res. 2014;74(12):3317–31.
14. Johnson BE, Mazor T, Hong C, Barnes M, Aihara K, McLean CY, Fouse SD, Yamamoto S, Ueda H, Tatsuno K, et al. Mutational analysis reveals the origin and therapy-driven evolution of recurrent glioma. Science. 2014;343(6167):189–93.
15. Watanabe T, Nobusawa S, Kleihues P, Ohgaki H. IDH1 mutations are early events in the development of astrocytomas and oligodendrogliomas. Am J Pathol. 2009;174(4):1149–53.
16. Eckel-Passow JE, Lachance DH, Molinaro AM, Walsh KM, Decker PA, Sicotte H, Pekmezci M, Rice T, Kosel ML, Smirnov IV, et al. Glioma groups based on 1p/19q, IDH, and TERT promoter mutations in tumors. N Engl J Med. 2015;372(26):2499–508.
17. Laks DR, Crisman TJ, Shih MY, Mottahedeh J, Gao F, Sperry J, Garrett MC, Yong WH, Cloughesy TF, Liau LM, et al. Large-scale assessment of the gliomasphere model system. Neuro-Oncology. 2016;18(10):1367–78.
18. Luchman HA, Stechishin OD, Dang NH, Blough MD, Chesnelong C, Kelly JJ, Nguyen SA, Chan JA, Weljie AM, Cairncross JG, et al. An in vivo patient-derived model of endogenous IDH1-mutant glioma. Neuro-Oncology. 2012;14(2):184–91.
19. Izquierdo-Garcia JL, Viswanath P, Eriksson P, Cai L, Radoul M, Chaumeil MM, Blough M, Luchman HA, Weiss S, Cairncross JG, et al. IDH1 mutation induces reprogramming of pyruvate metabolism. Cancer Res. 2015;75(15):2999–3009.
20. McKenna A, Hanna M, Banks E, Sivachenko A, Cibulskis K, Kernytsky A, Garimella K, Altshuler D, Gabriel S, Daly M, et al. The genome analysis toolkit: a MapReduce framework for analyzing next-generation DNA sequencing data. Genome Res. 2010;20(9):1297–303.
21. Li H, Durbin R. Fast and accurate long-read alignment with burrows-wheeler transform. Bioinformatics. 2010;26(5):589–95.
22. Wang K, Li M, Hakonarson H. ANNOVAR: functional annotation of genetic variants from high-throughput sequencing data. Nucleic Acids Res. 2010;38(16):e164.
23. Hernandez-Ferrer C, Quintela Garcia I, Danielski K, Carracedo A, Perez-Jurado LA. Gonzalez JR. affy2sv: an R package to pre-process Affymetrix CytoScan HD and 750K arrays for SNP, CNV, inversion and mosaicism calling. BMC Bioinformatics. 2015;16:167.
24. Wang K, Li M, Hadley D, Liu R, Glessner J, Grant SF, Hakonarson H, Bucan M. PennCNV: an integrated hidden Markov model designed for high-resolution

copy number variation detection in whole-genome SNP genotyping data. Genome Res. 2007;17(11):1665–74.
25. Sun WTZ. genoCN: genotyping and copy number study tools. In: R package version 1.28.0; 2010.
26. Mayrhofer M, Viklund B, Isaksson A. Rawcopy: improved copy number analysis with Affymetrix arrays. Sci Rep. 2016;6:36158.
27. Derfus GE, Abramzon D, Tung M, Chang D, Kiss R, Amanullah A. Cell culture monitoring via an auto-sampler and an integrated multi-functional off-line analyzer. Biotechnol Prog. 2010;26(1):284–92.
28. Thai M, Graham NA, Braas D, Nehil M, Komisopoulou E, Kurdistani SK, McCormick F, Graeber TG, Christofk HR. Adenovirus E4ORF1-induced MYC activation promotes host cell anabolic glucose metabolism and virus replication. Cell Metab. 2014;19(4):694–701.
29. Thai M, Thaker SK, Feng J, Du Y, Hu H, Ting Wu T, Graeber TG, Braas D, Christofk HR. MYC-induced reprogramming of glutamine catabolism supports optimal virus replication. Nat Commun. 2015;6:8873.
30. Visnyei K, Onodera H, Damoiseaux R, Saigusa K, Petrosyan S, De Vries D, Ferrari D, Saxe J, Panosyan EH, Masterman-Smith M, et al. A molecular screening approach to identify and characterize inhibitors of glioblastoma stem cells. Mol Cancer Ther. 2011;10(10):1818–28.
31. Wan XS, Zhou Z, Kennedy AR. Adaptation of the dichlorofluorescein assay for detection of radiation-induced oxidative stress in cultured cells. Radiat Res. 2003;160(6):622–30.
32. Kanehisa M, Goto S. KEGG: Kyoto Encyclopedia of Genes and Genomes. Nucleic Acids Res. 2000;28(1):27–30.
33. Subramanian A, Tamayo P, Mootha VK, Mukherjee S, Ebert BL, Gillette MA, Paulovich A, Pomeroy SL, Golub TR, Lander ES, et al. Gene set enrichment analysis: a knowledge-based approach for interpreting genome-wide expression profiles. Proc Natl Acad Sci U S A. 2005;102(43):15545–50.
34. Laks DR, Ta L, Crisman TJ, Gao F, Coppola G, Radu CG, Nathanson DA, Kornblum HI. Inhibition of nucleotide synthesis targets brain tumor stem cells in a subset of glioblastoma. Mol Cancer Ther. 2016;15(6):1271–8.
35. Li F, He X, Ye D, Lin Y, Yu H, Yao C, Huang L, Zhang J, Wang F, Xu S, et al. NADP(+)-IDH mutations promote hypersuccinylation that impairs mitochondria respiration and induces apoptosis resistance. Mol Cell. 2015;60(4):661–75.
36. Sasaki M, Knobbe CB, Itsumi M, Elia AJ, Harris IS, Chio II, Cairns RA, McCracken S, Wakeham A, Haight J, et al. D-2-hydroxyglutarate produced by mutant IDH1 perturbs collagen maturation and basement membrane function. Genes Dev. 2012;26(18):2038–49.
37. Barker CA, Bishop AJ, Chang M, Beal K, Chan TA. Valproic acid use during radiation therapy for glioblastoma associated with improved survival. Int J Radiat Oncol Biol Phys. 2013;86(3):504–9.
38. Reitman ZJ, Duncan CG, Poteet E, Winters A, Yan LJ, Gooden DM, Spasojevic I, Boros LG, Yang SH, Yan H. Cancer-associated isocitrate dehydrogenase 1 (IDH1) R132H mutation and d-2-hydroxyglutarate stimulate glutamine metabolism under hypoxia. J Biol Chem. 2014;289(34):23318–28.
39. Reitman ZJ, Jin G, Karoly ED, Spasojevic I, Yang J, Kinzler KW, He Y, Bigner DD, Vogelstein B, Yan H. Profiling the effects of isocitrate dehydrogenase 1 and 2 mutations on the cellular metabolome. Proc Natl Acad Sci U S A. 2011;108(8):3270–5.
40. Chaumeil MM, Larson PE, Woods SM, Cai L, Eriksson P, Robinson AE, Lupo JM, Vigneron DB, Nelson SJ, Pieper RO, et al. Hyperpolarized [1-13C] glutamate: a metabolic imaging biomarker of IDH1 mutational status in glioma. Cancer Res. 2014;74(16):4247–57.
41. Ohka F, Ito M, Ranjit M, Senga T, Motomura A, Motomura K, Saito K, Kato K, Kato Y, Wakabayashi T, et al. Quantitative metabolome analysis profiles activation of glutaminolysis in glioma with IDH1 mutation. Tumour Biol. 2014;35(6):5911–20.
42. Sulkowski PL, Corso CD, Robinson ND, Scanlon SE, Purshouse KR, Bai H, Liu Y, Sundaram RK, Hegan DC, Fons NR, et al. 2-Hydroxyglutarate produced by neomorphic IDH mutations suppresses homologous recombination and induces PARP inhibitor sensitivity. Sci Transl Med. 2017:9(375).
43. Lu Y, Kwintkiewicz J, Liu Y, Tech K, Frady LN, Su YT, Bautista W, Moon SI, MacDonald J, Edwend MG, et al. Chemosensitivity of IDH1 mutant gliomas due to an impairment in PARP1-mediated DNA repair. Cancer Res. 2017; 77(7):1709–18.
44. Sevilla MD, Becker D, Kumar A, Adhikary AG, Ion-Beam Irradiation of DNA. Free radical mechanisms, electron effects, and radiation chemical track structure. Radiat Phys Chem Oxf Engl. 2016;1993(128):60–74.
45. Tran AN, Lai A, Li S, Pope WB, Teixeira S, Harris RJ, Woodworth DC, Nghiemphu PL, Cloughesy TF, Ellingson BM. Increased sensitivity to radiochemotherapy in IDH1 mutant glioblastoma as demonstrated by serial quantitative MR volumetry. Neuro-Oncology. 2014;16(3):414–20.
46. Shaw E, Arusell R, Scheithauer B, O'Fallon J, O'Neill B, Dinapoli R, Nelson D, Earle J, Jones C, Cascino T, et al. Prospective randomized trial of low- versus high-dose radiation therapy in adults with supratentorial low-grade glioma: initial report of a north central cancer treatment group/radiation therapy oncology group/eastern cooperative oncology group study. J Clin Oncol. 2002;20(9):2267–76.
47. Mannava S, Grachtchouk V, Wheeler LJ, Im M, Zhuang D, Slavina EG, Mathews CK, Shewach DS, Nikiforov MA. Direct role of nucleotide metabolism in C-MYC-dependent proliferation of melanoma cells. Cell Cycle. 2008;7(15):2392–400.
48. Cancer Genome Atlas Research N, Brat DJ, Verhaak RG, Aldape KD, Yung WK, Salama SR, Cooper LA, Rheinbay E, Miller CR, Vitucci M, et al. Comprehensive, integrative genomic analysis of diffuse lower-grade gliomas. N Engl J Med. 2015;372(26):2481–98.

11

Bortezomib resistance in multiple myeloma is associated with increased serine synthesis

Esther A. Zaal[1], Wei Wu[1], Gerrit Jansen[2], Sonja Zweegman[3], Jacqueline Cloos[3,4] and Celia R. Berkers[1*]

Abstract

Background: The proteasome inhibitor bortezomib (BTZ) is successfully applied in the treatment of multiple myeloma, but its efficacy is restricted by the wide-spread occurrence of resistance. Metabolic alterations play an important role in cancer development and aid in the cellular adaptation to pharmacologically changed environments. Metabolic changes could therefore play an essential role in the development of drug resistance. However, specific metabolic pathways that can be targeted to improve bortezomib therapy remain unidentified.

Methods: We elucidated the metabolic mechanisms underlying bortezomib resistance by using mass spectrometry-based metabolomics and proteomics on BTZ-sensitive and BTZ–resistant multiple myeloma cell lines as well as in a set of CD138+ cells obtained from multiple myeloma patients.

Results: Our findings demonstrate that a rewired glucose metabolism sustains bortezomib resistance. Mechanistically, this results in higher activity of both the pentose phosphate pathway and serine synthesis pathway, ultimately leading to an increased anti-oxidant capacity of BTZ-resistant cells. Moreover, our results link both serine synthesis pathway activity and expression of 3-phosphoglycerate dehydrogenase (PHGDH), which catalyzes the rate-limiting step of serine synthesis, to bortezomib resistance across different BTZ-resistant multiple myeloma cell lines. Consistently, serine starvation enhanced the cytotoxicity of bortezomib, underscoring the importance of serine metabolism in the response to BTZ. Importantly, in CD138+ cells of clinically bortezomib refractory multiple myeloma patients, PHGDH expression was also markedly increased.

Conclusions: Our findings indicate that interfering with serine metabolism may be a novel strategy to improve bortezomib therapy and identify PHGDH as a potential biomarker for BTZ resistance.

Keywords: Metabolism, Drug resistance, Bortezomib, Multiple myeloma, PHGDH

Background

The proteasome inhibitor bortezomib (BTZ) is widely used in the treatment of multiple myeloma (MM) [1, 2]. The proteasome is a large intracellular protease complex, composed of a 20S core particle and two 19S regulatory particles. The 20S core particle consists of two outer rings of α-subunits and two inner rings of β-subunits. Three of these β-subunits, termed β1, β2, and β5 are catalytically active [3]. They can be replaced by the three interferon inducible subunits β1i, β2i, and β5i to form immunoproteasomes. BTZ acts by inhibiting primarily the β5/β5i subunits and to a lesser extent the β1/β1i subunits [4]. The resulting imbalance between production and degradation of proteins leads to the accumulation of (regulatory) proteins, causing endoplasmic reticulum stress and activation of the unfolded protein response. Proteasome inhibition eventually causes apoptosis in malignant cells via multiple pathways, including overproduction of reactive oxygen species [5–7].

Despite good clinical results of initial treatment, many patients eventually relapse from BTZ therapy [7–9]. Resistance is associated with mutations in the binding pocket of the β5 subunit (*PSMB5*), resulting in impaired binding of the drug [10–12], upregulation of the proteasomal

* Correspondence: c.r.berkers@uu.nl
[1]Biomolecular Mass Spectrometry and Proteomics, Bijvoet Center for Biomolecular Research and Utrecht Institute of Pharmaceutical Sciences, Utrecht University, Padualaan 8, 3584 CH Utrecht, The Netherlands

machinery, and a change in the ratio of (immuno) proteasomal subunits [13–15]. However, how relevant PSMB5 mutations are in relapsed patients remains unclear [16] and more recent studies suggest that other mechanisms are involved in BTZ resistance, such as the unfolded protein response and vesicular exocytosis of ubiquitinated proteins [5, 17–20].

Targeting metabolism is emerging as a promising strategy for cancer therapy [21–23]. Metabolic alterations have been linked to resistance to chemotherapeutic agents [24–27] and may also play a role in the (lack of) response to BTZ. In particular, higher glycolytic activity has been found to lower BTZ sensitivity under hypoxic conditions [28] and BTZ resistant cells were found to have proteomic changes in redox and energy metabolism [29]. However, specific metabolic targets that can serve to augment responses to BTZ therapy remain unidentified.

In this study, we aimed to identify altered metabolic pathways in BTZ-resistant MM cells that drive resistance. By using mass spectrometry and tracer-based metabolomics combined with proteomics, we show that BTZ-resistant cells adapt their glucose metabolism. Mechanistically, this metabolic rewiring results in higher activity of both the pentose phosphate pathway (PPP) and serine synthesis pathway (SSP) and ultimately leads to an increased anti-oxidant capacity of BTZ-resistant cells. We also demonstrate that serine starvation enhances the effect of BTZ and that 3-phosphoglycerate dehydrogenase (PHGDH), which catalyzes the rate limiting step in the SSP, is upregulated across different BTZ-resistant MM cells. Our results indicate that serine metabolism is associated with BTZ resistance and that interfering with this pathway may be a novel strategy to improve BTZ therapy.

Methods

Reagents

The proteasome activity probe Me_4BodipyFL-Ahx_3L_3VS was a gift from Huib Ovaa (Leiden University Medical Center, The Netherlands). Bortezomib (BTZ) and carfilzomib (CFZ) were purchased from Selleck Chemicals. All solvents were obtained from Biosolve. All other chemicals were obtained from Sigma-Aldrich, unless stated otherwise.

Cell culture

Human multiple myeloma RPMI-8226 wild type (WT) cells were purchased from ATCC. BTZ-resistant cells were obtained as described previously [11]. AMO-1 and ARH-77 WT, BTZ- and CFZ-resistant cells were kindly provided by C. Driessen (Kantonsspital St. Gallen, Switzerland). Cells were maintained in suspension culture in RPMI-1640 (Lonza) medium supplemented with 2 mM L-glutamine (Lonza), 10% fetal bovine serum (FBS) (Gibco) and 100 μg/ml penicillin/streptomycin (Lonza) and were kept at 37 °C in humidified 5% CO_2 atmosphere. BTZ- and CFZ-resistant cells were continuously cultured in the presence of BTZ or CFZ as previous described [11, 13]. Cells were cultured without drugs 4–6 days prior to experiments. Media were supplemented with 10% FBS and 100 μg/ml penicillin/streptomycin unless stated otherwise.

Proteasome activity profiling

Proteasome activity was measured using Me_4BodipyFL-Ahx_3L_3VS as described previously [30]. Cells were suspended in triplicate at a density of 1×10^6 cells/ml in RPMI-1640 medium and incubated with the indicated concentrations of BTZ at 37 °C for 1 h, followed by a 1-h incubation with 500 nM Me_4BodipyFL-Ahx_3L_3VS. Cells were collected by centrifugation, washed with PBS and lysed for 30 min in NP40 lysis buffer (50 mM Tris, pH 7.4, 150 mM NaCl, 1% NP40) at 4 °C, followed by centrifugation at 14,000*g* to remove membrane fractions, nuclei and cell debris. Protein concentrations were determined using the Bradford assay (Bio-rad) and equal amounts of protein were denatured by boiling in XT Sample buffer (Bio-rad) with 9% β-mercaptoethanol. Proteins were separated on a 4–12% SDS-PAGE gel (Bio-rad) and fluorescence was measured with a Typhoon scanner (GE Healthcare) ($\lambda_{ex}/\lambda_{em}$ = 488/526 nm). Protein loading was confirmed with a coomassie blue stain.

Cell viability and cell growth assays

Cells were suspended in triplicate at a density of $2–5 \times 10^5$ cells/ml in RPMI-1640 medium in 96-well plates and incubated with drugs at the indicated concentrations for 24–48 h. Cell growth was monitored continuously with the IncuCyte live-cell imager system. Images were automatically acquired every 2 h for 1–2 days. Pictures were analyzed using the IncyCyte Zoom software. Cell growth was defined as the amount of cell doublings per 24/48 h and calculated based on increase of confluency. Cell death was assessed after 24–48 h by incubating each well with 30 μM propidium iodide and measuring fluorescence after 15 min using the IncuCyte live-cell imager system. Cell death was calculated based on the area of the fluorescent signal, normalized to confluency of the wells. Cell viability was measured in parallel after 24–48 h by incubation of cells with 50 μM resazurin for an additional 2 h, after which absorption was measured at 570 nm and 600 nm using a Multiskan GO microplate reader (Thermo Scientific). Results were calculated by subtraction of background absorbance at 600 nm from absorbance at 570 nm.

Liquid chromatrography—mass spectrometry (LC-MS)-based metabolomics

For all experiments, cells were diluted in fresh medium 16–24 h prior to the start of experiments. ^{13}C–tracer experiments were performed as described [31, 32], with minor changes. At the start of all experiments, cells were counted and centrifuged for 5 min at 1400 rpm to remove the old medium. Cells were then resuspended in DMEM containing 8 mM [U-^{13}C]D-glucose (Cambridge Isotopes) at a density of 1 × 10^6 cells/ml, unless indicated otherwise. After 4 or 8 h, samples were washed with PBS and harvested by centrifugation for 5 min at 1000*g* at 4 °C. At these timepoints, cells had recovered from centrifugation and reached pseudo-steady state, without nutrients being depleted from the culture media. For all analyzed metabolites, (near) isotopic steady state was reached at these time points. In addition, samples were harvested after 24 h to analyze serine levels in the cells. Because at this point some nutrients were depleted, no other metabolites were analyzed in these samples. Metabolites were extracted by adding 100–200 μl ice-cold MS lysis buffer (methanol/acetonitrile/uLCMS H_2O (2:2:1)) to the cell pellets. To measure extracellular metabolites, medium samples were obtained prior to harvesting cells at 8 or 24 h. Metabolites were extracted by diluting 10 μl medium in 1 mL MS lysis buffer. To measure differences in extracellular metabolites in different BTZ-resistant cell lines, cells were resuspended at a density of 1 × 10^6 cells/ml in in Minimal Essential Medium (MEM), supplemented with 1 mM L-glutamine, 0.2 mM L-serine and 0.2 mM L-glycine. Medium samples were obtained after 8 h and metabolites were extracted as described above. For serine starvation experiments, medium was formulated to match the composition of DMEM [31]. Medium consisted of MEM, supplemented with additional 1× MEM vitamins, 1× MEM amino acids, 10% dialyzed FBS and glucose up to 25 mM, in the presence or absence of 0.4 mM L-serine. Cells were resuspended at a density of 0.7 × 10^6 in triplicate wells and were pre-incubated for 24 h in the presence or absence of serine. After 24 h, cells were centrifuged at 1400 rpm for 5 min and media was replaced with matched media containing [U-^{13}C]D-glucose. After an additional 4 h, cells were harvested as described above.

Metabolites were analyzed by LC-MS (see Additional file 1: methods for details). Metabolites were identified based on exact mass within 5 ppm and further validated by concordance with retention times of standards. Peak areas of identified metabolites were in their respective linear range of detection. Metabolites were quantified using LCquan software (Thermo Scientific). Because cells were resuspended at equal cell densities, no substantial cell growth occurred between 0 and 8 h, and growth rates between resistant and sensitive cell lines were comparable up to 24 h, samples were assumed to contain equal cell numbers. Peak intensities were additionally normalized based on median peak intensity to correct for technical variations during mass spectrometry analysis. Isotopomer distributions were corrected for natural abundance and data are plotted as relative peak area compared to WT cells under control conditions.

DHA uptake assay

Cells were suspended at a density of 0.5 × 10^6 cells in 200 μl in MEM supplemented with 1 mM L-glutamine and 0.2 mM L-serine. Cells were incubated with 5 mM dehydroascorbic acid (DHA) for 5 min at 37 °C. DHA uptake was terminated by addition of 1.5 ml cold PBS. Cells were centrifuged at 1000*g* for 5 min at 4 °C and lysed in 75 μl MS lysis buffer. Samples were centrifuged at 16.000*g* for 15 min at 4 °C to remove precipitated proteins and cell debris and the supernatants were collected for LC-MS analysis.

GSH/GSSG ratio

Cells were suspended at a density of 2.5 × 10^6 cells/ml in triplicate wells of 12-well plates and incubated in the indicated conditions. Cells were washed with cold PBS and lysed in 10 mM HCl by two freeze/thaw cycles. Proteins were precipitated by addition of 1% 5-sulfosalicylic acid and pelleted by centrifugation at 4 °C for 10 min at 8000*g*. The ratio of reduced to oxidized glutathione (GSH/GSSG) in the supernatant was measured using the quantification kit for oxidized and reduced glutathione (Sigma-Aldrich) according to the manufacturer's instructions.

Proteomics

Cells were suspended in RPMI medium at a density of 1 × 10^6 cells/ml and incubated for 2 h. Three replicates of 5 × 10^6 cells were washed with PBS and centrifuged for 5 min at 4 °C. Cell pellets were lysed at room temperature by gentle vortexing in 8 M urea, 50 mM ammonium bicarbonate, 2% Triton X-100 and 0.1% SDS, supplemented with phosphatase inhibitor (PhosSTOP, Roche) and protease inhibitor (cOmplete mini EDTA-free, Roche). Total lysates were reduced in 4 mM dithiothreitol (DTT), alkylated in 8 mM iodoacetamide, and digested sequentially at 37 °C with 1:75 LysC (Wako) and 1:50 Trypsin (Sigma-Aldrich) for 4 and 12 h, respectively. Digested peptides were acidified with 0.1% formic acid (FA) and purified by strong cation exchange STAGE tips, using loading buffer 80% ACN, 0.1% FA and elution buffer 0.5 M ammonium acetate, 20% ACN, 0.1% FA. Eluted peptides were dried by vacuum concentrator and 2 μg equivalent of peptides was analyzed in 3 h reverse phase separation on the UHPLC 1290 system (Agilent) coupled to an Orbitrap Q Exactive Plus mass spectrometer (Thermo Scientific). See Additional file 1: methods for details.

Immunoblotting

For drug treatment, cells were resuspended in RPMI medium at a density of 1 × 10^6 cells/ml and incubated for 8 h with the indicated concentrations of BTZ. Cells were lysed in a buffer containing 8 M urea and 50 mM ammonium bicarbonate, supplemented with phosphatase- and protease inhibitor. Protein content was determined using the Bradford assay (Bio-rad) and equal amounts of protein were denatured by boiling in XT Sample buffer (Bio-rad) with 15 mM DTT. Proteins were separated on a 12% % SDS-PAGE gel (Bio-rad) and electroblotted onto PVDF membranes. The antibodies used were 3-phosphoglycerate dehydrogenase (PHGDH, Sigma-Aldrich), phosphoserine-aminotransferase antibody (PSAT1, Abcam), phosphoserine phosphatase antibody (PSPH, Abcam), and Tubulin antibody (Santa Cruz). For patient samples, protein loading was confirmed with a coomassie blue stain of the membrane.

Multiple myeloma patient samples

CD138-positive cells, isolated from bone marrow of 6 MM patients at diagnosis and during (BTZ) therapy, were available from the Hematology biobank. Patient characteristics are presented in Additional file 1: Table S1. Research was approved by the Medical Ethics Committee of the VU University Medical Center and all patients gave written informed consent.

Results

Bortezomib resistance in MM cells is not solely driven by adaptation of the proteasome itself

To study BTZ resistance, we compared human BTZ-sensitive RPMI-8226 wild-type (WT) MM cells with two BTZ-resistant cell lines (BTZ/7 and BTZ/100), which grow in the presence of 7 and 100 nM BTZ, respectively [11]. Cell viability assays showed the 48-h IC_{50} values towards BTZ to be 7.3 ± 2.4 nM, 25.3 ± 6.6 nM and 231.9 ± 73 nM in the WT, BTZ/7, and BTZ/100 cell lines, respectively (Fig. 1a), in line with previous reports [11, 33]. Comparable IC_{50} values were found by analyzing the cell growth of these cell lines, and also cell death assays using propidium iodide showed similar trends (Additional file 1: Figure S1a). BTZ-resistant cells displayed cross-resistance towards the proteasome inhibitor carfilzomib (CFZ), but not to the chemotherapeutic drugs methotrexate (folate antagonist) and melphalan (alkylating agent) (Additional file 1: Figure S1b). This suggests that the observed adaptations are related to proteasome inhibitor resistance rather than multidrug resistance, as also previously described for THP-1 cells [10].

Next, we evaluated the proteasome activity in these cells with and without BTZ treatment using the cell-permeable fluorescent proteasome activity probe $Me_4BodipyFL-Ahx_3L_3VS$. In this assay, the fluorescence intensity directly correlates to the proteasome (subunit) activity, which can be visualized using SDS-PAGE [30]. Without BTZ treatment, both BTZ/7 and BTZ/100 cells showed reduced activity of the β2i subunit, a relative upregulation of the β2 activity and a lower total proteasome activity compared to WT cells (Fig. 1b), consistent with published reports [11, 33, 34]. BTZ treatment decreased total proteasome activity in a dose dependent manner with 50% proteasome inhibition at 107.5 ± 56 nm for the BTZ/100 cells and 10.3 ± 4.1 nM and 15.1 ± 0.9 nM in the WT and BTZ/7 cells, respectively (Fig. 1c, Additional file 1: Figure S1c). Whereas the onset of β2 inhibition was shifted towards higher BTZ concentrations in the BTZ/100 cells, only small differences were observed in the onset of β1/5 inhibition between sensitive and resistant cell lines

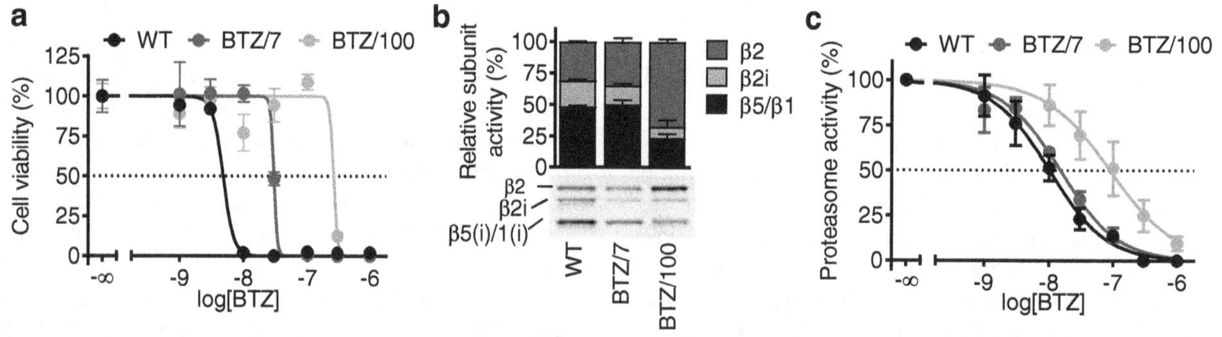

Fig. 1 Bortezomib resistance is not solely driven by adaptations of the proteasome. **a** Cell viability of RPMI-8226 wild type (WT) and bortezomib-resistant (BTZ/7 and BTZ/100) cells after a 48-h treatment with increasing concentrations of bortezomib. Results represent % cell viability ± SD compared to non-treated controls of a representative experiment (*n* = 3). **b** In gel fluorescence measurements of a representative experiment showing proteasome activity profiles of RPMI-8226 WT, BTZ/7, and BTZ/100 cells after a 1-h incubation with proteasome activity probe $Me_4BodipyFL-Ahx_3L_3VS$ (lower panel). Quantification of gel images, with subunit activity plotted as of total proteasome activity. Results represent averages of 3 independent experiments (upper panel). **c** Total proteasome activity of RPMI-8226 WT, BTZ/7 and BTZ/100 cells after a 2-h incubation with increasing concentrations of bortezomib, compared to non-treated controls. Results represent quantification of gel images obtained by a 1-h incubation with $Me_4BodipyFL-Ahx_3L_3VS$. Results represent averages of 3 independent experiments. BTZ = bortezomib

(Additional file 1: Figure S1c). These results suggest that upregulation of β2 activity is one of the main proteasomal driving forces of BTZ resistance in RPMI-8226 cells. However, in contrast to WT cells, both resistant cell lines still show survival at 50% proteasome inhibition, in line with earlier results [29]. This indicates that in order to survive BTZ treatment, BTZ/7, and BTZ/100 cells not only change the proteasome itself, but also adapt to survive under conditions of continuous proteasome inhibition.

Bortezomib-resistant cells have an enhanced activity of the pentose phosphate pathway

Because metabolic alterations are increasingly recognized as a driving force in drug resistance, we next investigated whether such metabolic changes drive adaptation to continuous proteasome inhibition in BTZ-resistant MM cells. BTZ sensitivity has been linked to higher glycolytic activity under hypoxic conditions [28]. However, many metabolic pathways branch off from glycolysis, including the tricarboxylic acid (TCA) cycle, pentose phosphate pathway (PPP) and nucleotide synthesis pathway. Hence, to get a more comprehensive insight into the altered glucose metabolism in BTZ resistant cells, we first mapped the glucose metabolism in both resistant and sensitive cells by performing ^{13}C–glucose tracer experiments. To this end, WT and BTZ/100 cells were grown in the presence of 8 mM [U-^{13}C]-glucose and the incorporation of ^{13}C–carbon from glucose in downstream metabolites was followed over time using mass spectrometry. In addition, changes in extracellular metabolites levels were analyzed. A centrifugation step—which disturbs the cells—is unavoidable to resuspend cells in [U-^{13}C]-glucose medium and cells will only reach pseudo-steady state hours after being resuspended. Therefore, early time points (less than 4 h) were excluded from the analysis. As expected, BTZ/100 cells displayed both an increased uptake of glucose from and increased secretion of lactate into the culture medium, indicative of a higher glycolytic activity (Fig. 2a, b). In addition, BTZ/100 cells displayed higher intracellular levels of ^{13}C–glucose, as well as higher levels of ^{13}C–pyruvate and ^{13}C–lactate (Fig. 2c), supporting higher glycolytic activity. No differences in the amount of ^{13}C–citrate were observed between cell lines, suggesting no change in glucose flux to the TCA cycle (Fig. 2c). In contrast, sedoheptulose-7-phosphate (S7P), an intermediate of the PPP, was one of the most upregulated metabolites in BTZ/100 cells compared to WT cells. Substantially increased levels of de novo synthesized $^{13}C_7$ –labeled S7P (M+7) were present in BTZ/100 cells, indicating a higher PPP activity in resistant cells (Fig. 2c). Moreover, higher amounts of M+4 and M+6 isotopomers of S7P were present in BTZ/100 cells, which are indicative of increased PPP cycling and further support the higher PPP activity in these cells. After 8 h, the S7P levels dropped in both cell lines, suggesting that the cells temporarily raised their PPP activity in response to some type of stress, most likely the centrifugation of the cells. We therefore hypothesize that bortezomib-resistant cells have a higher basal PPP activity as well as a higher capability to increase PPP activity in response to stress [35].

To investigate whether these findings are general features of BTZ-resistant cells, we repeated the MS analysis on BTZ-sensitive AMO-1 multiple myeloma cells and its BTZ- and CFZ-resistant counterparts and included RPMI-8226 cells as a reference. We also included BTZ-resistant ARH-77 cells, which have a different origin (plasmocytoid lymphoma) in these analyses (Additional file 1: Figure S2a-c) [13, 29]. Whereas BTZ-resistant AMO-1 and RPMI-8226 cells all showed higher glucose uptake, lactate secretion and PPP activity compared to sensitive cells, AMO-1 CFZ/90 cells did not show these metabolic changes. Notably, overexpression of the drug efflux transporter ABCB1/P-glycoprotein, for which carfilzomib is a bona fide substrate, is an important underlying mechanism of carfilzomib resistance in CFZ/90 AMO-1 [29, 36]. It is thus likely that these cells do not require metabolic adaptations to oppose proteasome inhibitor induced apoptosis. ARH-77 BTZ-resistant cells on the other hand showed an opposite effect on glucose uptake, lactate secretion and PPP metabolism. Together, these findings show that BTZ-resistant MM cells have higher PPP activity compared to sensitive cells, and suggest that this effect is specific for bortezomib as well as for multiple myeloma.

Enhanced pentose phosphate pathway activity increases the anti-oxidant capacity of bortezomib-resistant cells

The PPP provides both ribose for purine nucleotide synthesis and NADPH, which cells use for maintaining intracellular redox balance [35]. Since oxidative stress plays a role in the mechanism of action of BTZ, and BTZ/100 cells showed only moderately increased levels of the purines AMP and GMP (Fig. 2c), we hypothesized that BTZ-resistant cells increase their PPP activity predominantly to increase their anti-oxidant defenses and counteract the effect of the drug. Indeed, BTZ-resistant RPMI-8226 cells showed significantly higher concentrations of total glutathione, an important cellular antioxidant (Fig. 3a). Significantly higher levels of intracellular reduced glutathione (GSH) were also found in BTZ-resistant AMO-1 cells as compared to BTZ-sensitive AMO-1 cells (Additional file 1: Figure S2d). RPMI-8226 BTZ/100 cells were also less sensitive to hydrogen peroxide (H_2O_2) compared to WT cells (IC_{50} 256 μM vs. 67 μM) (Fig. 3b). When BTZ/100 cells were exposed to H_2O_2 after a 24-h preincubation with the PPP inhibitor trans-androsterone (TA), the IC_{50} of H_2O_2 shifted from 579 μM to 358 μM (Fig. 3c), confirming that resistance to

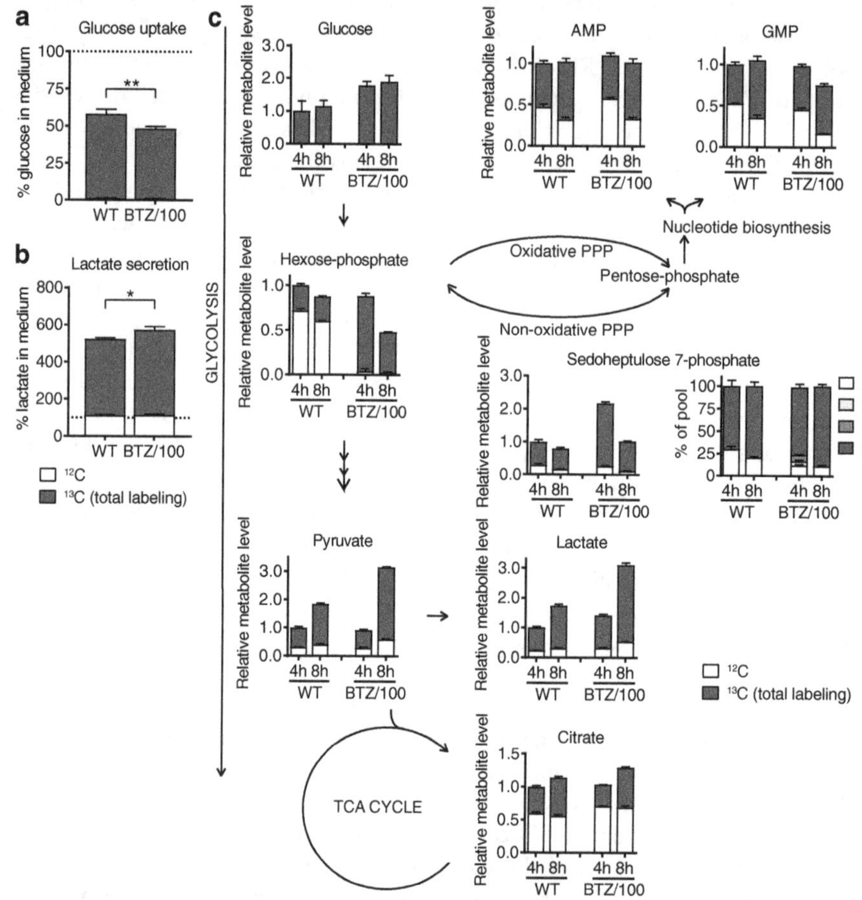

Fig. 2 Bortezomib-resistant cells have an enhanced activity of the pentose phosphate pathway. Intra- and extracellular metabolite analysis of RPMI-8226 wild type (WT) and bortezomib resistant (BTZ/100) cells. Cells were suspended in DMEM containing 8 mM [U-^{13}C] D-glucose. **a, b** Media samples were collected after 8 h, followed by LC-MS analysis of extracellular glucose (**a**) and lactate (**b**). Results represent % peak area ± SD compared to cell-free media ($n = 3$). Unpaired t-tests were performed (* = $p < 0.05$, ** = $p < 0.01$,). **c** Intracellular metabolites were extracted after 4 and 8 h and analyzed by LC-MS. Data are means ± SD ($n = 3$) of unlabeled (white) and ^{13}C- labeled metabolites (gray). AMP = adenosine monophosphate, GMP = guanosine monophosphate, PPP = pentose phosphate pathway, TCA = tricarboxylic acid

oxidizing agents in these cells is at least partly mediated through their increased PPP activity. Furthermore, we found that the GSH/GSSG ratio was increased in BTZ/100 cells compared to WT cells (Fig. 3d), indicative of an increased anti-oxidant capacity. Finally, the ability of cells to reduce dehydroascorbate (DHA, oxidized vitamin C) to ascorbic acid (AA) can be used as a tool to analyze cellular redox status [37]. DHA is rapidly taken up by the glucose transporters GLUT1 and GLUT3 and subsequently reduced either spontaneously or by GSH- and NADPH-dependent enzymes. As a consequence, DHA reduction is coupled to the ability of cells to regenerate NADPH and GSH [37]. We therefore developed an MS assay to measure the intracellular reduction of DHA to AA (Fig. 3e). Exposure to DHA resulted in similar intracellular levels of DHA in both WT and BTZ/100 cells. In contrast, significantly higher levels of AA were found in BTZ-resistant cells, indicating an increased conversion of DHA to AA. Because reduction of DHA will help maintain a DHA gradient over the cell membrane that favors transport [38], total DHA plus AA levels are also higher in the BTZ-resistant cells. Moreover, whereas DHA exposure decreased GSH/GSSG ratio in WT cells compared to control conditions, this ratio remained stable in BTZ/100 cells (Fig. 3d). These data indicate that the WT cells lack the capacity to regenerate GSH and NADPH, which renders them more sensitive to oxidative stress compared to the resistant cells.

Bortezomib-resistant cells have a higher activity of the serine synthesis pathway

The serine synthesis pathway (SSP), in which serine is synthesized from 3-phosphoglycerate, is another pathway that branches off from glycolysis and that is involved in both

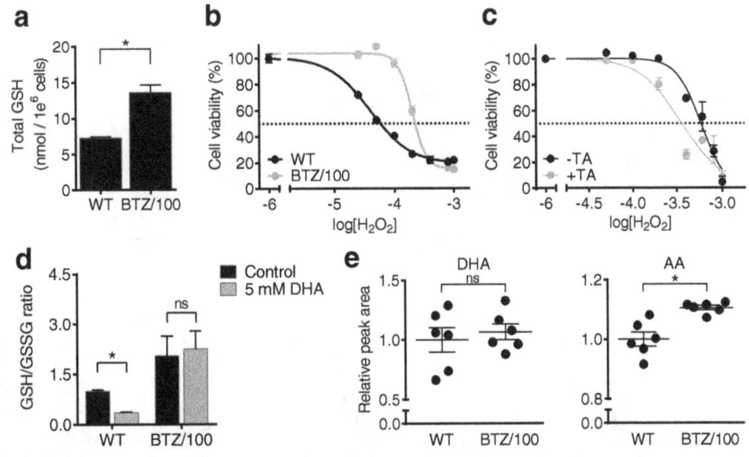

Fig. 3 Enhanced pentose phosphate pathway activity increases the anti-oxidant capacity of bortezomib-resistant cells. **a** Total GSH levels of RPMI-8226 wild type (WT) and bortezomib resistant (BTZ/100) cells. Data are means ± SD (n = 3) **b** Cell viability of RPMI-8226 WT and BTZ/100 cells after a 16-h treatment with increasing concentrations of H_2O_2. Results represent mean cell viability ± SD compared to non-treated controls (n = 3). **c** Cell viability of RPMI-8226 BTZ/100 cells after treatment for 24 h with 50 μM trans-androsterone (TA), followed by 24 h with increasing concentrations of H_2O_2. Results represent mean cell viability ± SD compared to non-treated control (n = 3). **d** GSH/GSSG ratio of RPMI-8226 WT and BTZ/100 cells after 5 min treatment with 5 mM DHA. Data are means ± SD (n = 3). **e** Analysis of intracellular levels of DHA (left panel) and AA (right panel) in RPMI-8226 WT and BTZ/100 cells. Cells were treated with 5 mM DHA or vehicle for 5 min and subjected to LC-MS analyses. Data are means ± SD (n = 3). Two-way ANOVA tests were performed (ns = not significant, * = $p < 0.05$). AA = ascorbic acid, DHA = dehydroascorbic acid, GSH = glutathione, TA = trans-androsterone

NADPH regeneration and GSH production. We therefore questioned whether BTZ-resistant cells also showed increased activity of the SSP. To investigate the basal activity of the SSP in BTZ sensitive and resistant cells, we performed tracer experiments in DMEM containing 8 mM ^{13}C–glucose and normal levels of (unlabeled) ^{12}C–serine. As the activity of the SSP is controlled primarily by the demand for serine and is only activated when serine is depleted from the extracellular environment [31, 39–43], we expected only low levels of de novo serine synthesis under these conditions. Indeed, both RPMI-8226 WT and BTZ/100 cells contained predominantly ^{12}C serine, obtained from the culture medium, and only small amounts of ^{13}C–serine (M+1, M+2, and M+3) (Fig. 4a). However, the levels of M+3 serine, which is synthesized de novo from glucose through the SSP [44], were higher in resistant cells compared to wild-type cells, indicative of a higher basal activity of the SSP in these cells. Moreover, BTZ/100 cells displayed a higher uptake of serine from the cell culture medium compared to the WT cells (Fig. 4b). Serine was almost depleted from the culture media of BTZ/100 cells after 24 h, resulting in substantially lower serine levels 24 h after fresh medium was added to the cells (Fig. 4a, b). Although the intracellular data should be interpreted with care, as other nutrients are also depleted at 24 h, these data do indicate that BTZ/100 cells have an increased demand for serine compared to WT cells, which is met by increasing both serine synthesis and serine uptake.

Next, we investigated how BTZ-sensitive and -resistant cells behaved under conditions of serine starvation, when upregulation of the SSP would be a requirement to survive. To this end, cells were grown in the presence or absence of serine and glycine (SG), first for 24 h in the presence of [U-^{12}C]-glucose, and subsequently for 4 h using [U-^{13}C]-glucose, as described elsewhere [31]. To reduce extra stress on the cells and ensure ample glucose supply throughout the experiment, we supplemented the cell culture medium with 25 mM glucose instead of 8 mM. These higher glucose levels did however not affect serine synthesis, at least under serine-fed conditions (compare Fig. 4a, 4-h time point, to Fig. 4c and Additional file 1: Figure S3a). In both WT and BTZ/100 cells, serine starvation resulted in a decrease in both total serine levels and ^{13}C–serine levels (Fig. 4c, Additional file 1: Figure S3a), probably reflecting the rapid conversion of serine to further downstream metabolites [39]. Although total glycine and GSH levels also decreased in both cell lines during serine starvation (Additional file 1: Figure S3a), higher levels of ^{13}C–glycine and ^{13}C–GSH were found in BTZ/100 cells (Fig. 4c), indicating that the SSP can be activated to a higher extent in resistant cells compared to WT cells. Additionally, BTZ-resistant cells were able to maintain higher levels of GSH during serine starvation (Additional file 1: Figure S3a), supporting our findings that they have higher anti-oxidant capacity.

Given that cells with high SSP activity are able to proliferate in the absence of extracellular serine [44], we next hypothesized that especially WT cells, that have low SSP activity, would be sensitive to serine starvation both in the absence and presence of BTZ. Indeed, serine starvation lowered the viability of WT cells to less than 50%, while

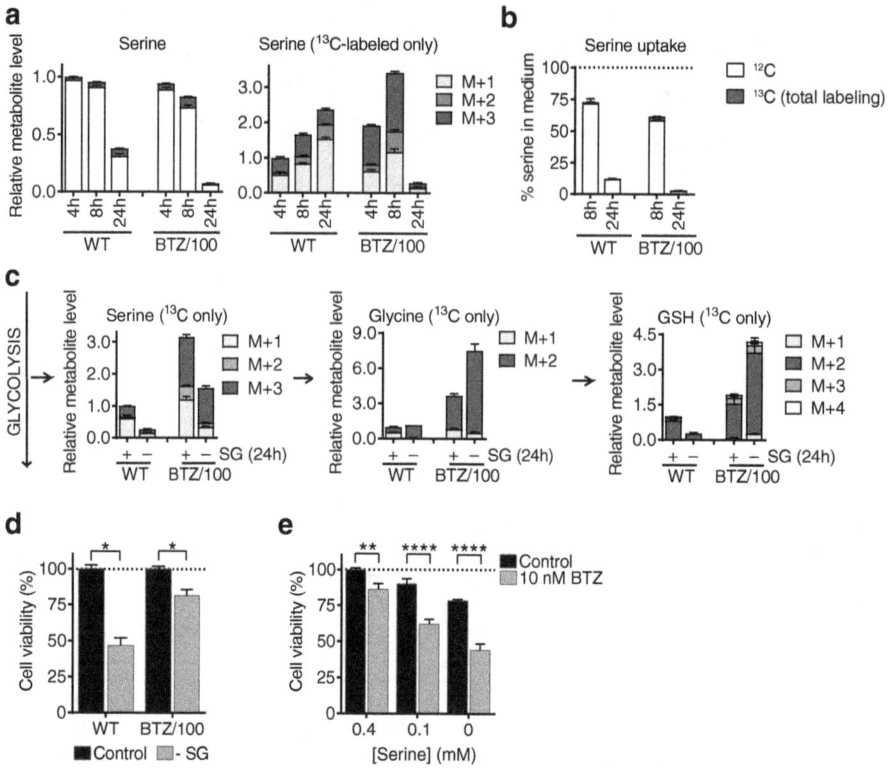

Fig. 4 Bortezomib resistant cells have a higher activity of the serine synthesis pathway. **a, b** Intra- and extracellular analysis of serine levels of RPMI-8226 wild type (WT) and bortezomib resistant (BTZ/100) cells. Cells were suspended in DMEM containing 8 mM [U-^{13}C] D-glucose. Intracellular metabolites were extracted after 4, 8 and 24 h and analyzed by LC-MS (**a**). Data are means ± SD (n = 3) of unlabeled (white) and ^{13}C- labeled serine (left panel). Labeled serine was plotted as M+1, M+2 and M+3 isotopomers (right panel). Media samples were collected after 8 and 24 h, followed by LC-MS analysis of extracellular serine (**b**). Results represent % peak area ± SD compared to non-treated media (n = 3). **c** Intracellular metabolite analysis of RPMI-8226 WT and BTZ/100 cells in the presence or absence of extracellular serine and glycine (–SG). Cells were grown complete medium in the presence or absence of 0.4 mM serine. After 24 h, media were replaced with matched media containing 20 mM [U-^{13}C] D-glucose and intracellular metabolites were extracted after 4 h, followed by LC-MS analysis. Data are means ± SD (n = 3) of labeled metabolites. **d** Cell viability of RPMI-8226 WT and BTZ/100 cells after 48 h of serine starvation (–SG). Results represent mean cell viability ± SD compared to non-treated control (n = 3). **e** Cell viability of RPMI-8226 WT cells after 48 h in 0.4 mM, 0.1 mM or no serine, including 24 h of 10 nM bortezomib. Results represent mean cell viability ± SD compared to non-treated control (n = 3). One-way ANOVA tests were performed (ns = not significant, * = $p < 0.05$, ** = $p < 0.01$, **** = $p < 0.0001$). BTZ = bortezomib, GSH = glutathione

BTZ/100 cells remained over 75% viable after 48 h of serine starvation (Fig. 4d), likely because they compensate for the lack of serine through serine synthesis. At the same time, serine starvation significantly increased the amount of cell death in WT cells, but not in BTZ/100 cells (Additional file 1: Figure S3b). Importantly, a 24-h serine starvation prior to BTZ treatment increased the cytotoxic effect of BTZ on WT cells (Fig. 4e). These data not only confirm that the presence of serine is important in the defense mechanism of cells against BTZ, but also suggests that serine starvation could be combined with BTZ to increase the efficacy of treatment in BTZ-sensitive patients.

Bortezomib resistance correlates to the expression of PHGDH

Having established the importance of both the PPP and SSP in the response of cells to BTZ, we next asked whether these differences were also found on the protein level. Hence, we performed proteomics on WT, BTZ/7 and BTZ/100 cells and quantified >3500 proteins, 395 of which were classified as metabolic enzymes (Fig. 5a, Additional file 1: Figure S4a, Tables S2 and S3). The highest upregulated metabolic enzyme in both BTZ/7 and BTZ/100 cells was 3-phosphoglycerate dehydrogenase (PHGDH; fold change (FC) = 11.27 and 7.86, respectively), the first and rate-limiting enzyme in the SSP, underscoring the importance of the SSP in the response to BTZ. In agreement with our findings, overexpression of PHGDH has previously been associated with an increased glucose flux through the SSP and the ability to proliferate in the absence of extracellular serine [44, 45]. Of the other SSP enzymes, phosphoserine aminotransferase 1 (PSAT1) was downregulated in BTZ/100 cells, while the proteomics data showed no change in the expression of

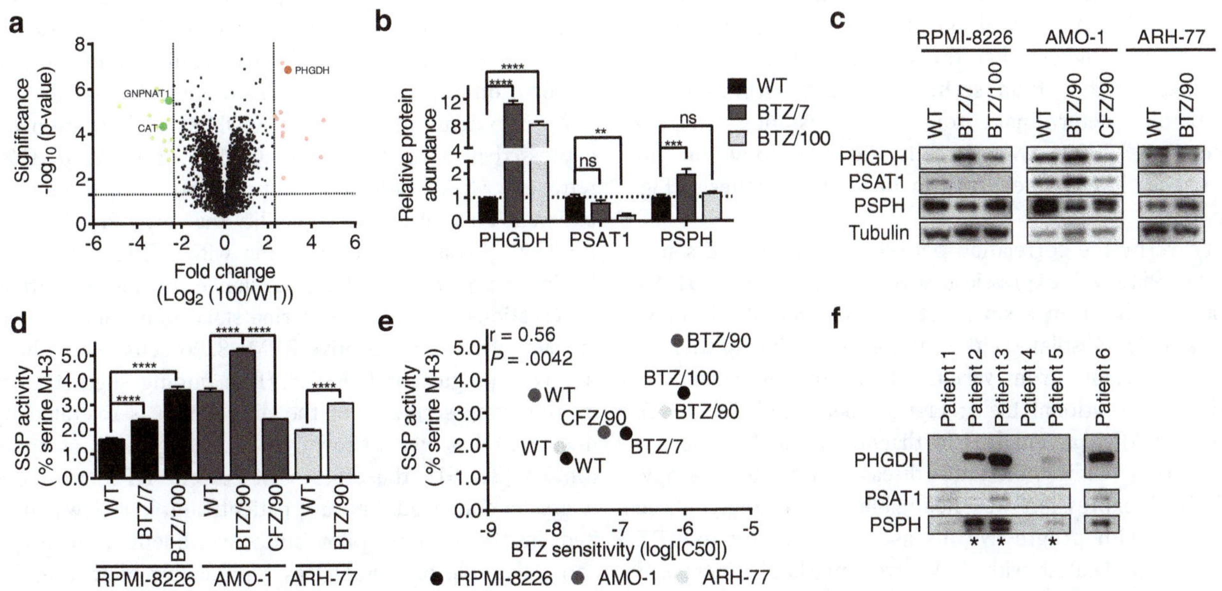

Fig. 5 Bortezomib resistance correlates to the expression of PHGDH. **a** Graphical representation of quantitative proteomics data. Proteins are ranked in volcano plot according to their statistically *p*-value (y-axis) and relative abundance ratio between RPMI-8226 wild type (WT) and bortezomib resistant (BTZ/100 cells) (x-axis). Colored spots represent significantly upregulated (red) or downregulated (green) proteins in BTZ/100 cells with at least a 5-fold change. Significantly regulated metabolic enzymes are marked. **b** Quantitative proteomics data of enzymes involved in the serine synthesis pathway. Data represents means ± SD ($n = 3$). **c** Immunoblot of 3-phosphoglycerate dehydrogenase (PHGDH), phosphoserine aminotransferase 1 (PSAT1), phosphoserine phosphatase (PSPH) and Tubulin expression in RPMI-8226, AMO-1 and ARH-77 bortezomib-sensitive and -resistant cells. **d** Fractions of serine M+3 in RPMI-8226, AMO-1 and ARH-77 bortezomib-sensitive and -resistant cells. Data represent % serine M+3 of total serine ± SD ($n = 3$). One-way ANOVA tests were performed (**** = $p < 0.0001$). **e** Correlation between serine M+3 fractions and bortezomib sensitivity in RPMI-8226, AMO-1 and ARH-77 bortezomib-sensitive and -resistant cells. IC_{50}s were determined in cell viability assay after 48 h of increasing concentrations of bortezomib. Pearson correlation $r = 0.56$ ($p = .0042$). **f** Immunoblot of PHGDH, PSAT1 and PSPH in isolated CD138+ plasma cells from diagnosed multiple myeloma patients ($n = 6$). Patients with progressive disease/refractory to BTZ-containing therapy are indicated with *. PHGDH is blotted on a separate membrane. BTZ = bortezomib, CFZ = carfilzomib, PHGDH = 3-phosphoglycerate dehydrogenase, PSAT1 = phosphoserine aminotransferase 1, PSPH = phosphoserine phosphatase, SSP = serine synthesis pathway

phosphoserine phosphatase (PSPH) in BTZ/100 cells compared to WT cells (Fig. 5b). However, since PHGDH is the rate-limiting enzyme in the SSP, the much higher PHGDH levels in BTZ/100 cells should allow for higher rates of serine synthesis in these cells. An 8-h treatment with BTZ had no effect on SSP enzyme levels in either cell line (Additional file 1: Figure S4b), suggesting that the higher levels of PHGDH in BTZ/100 cells are not resulting from decreased proteasomal degradation of PHGDH but rather from an increase in PHGDH protein synthesis. Amongst the moderately upregulated metabolic enzymes (FC 1.5–5) in BTZ/100 cells were 6-phosphogluconolactonase (PGLS; FC = 1.61) and transketolase (TKT1; FC = 1.53), enzymes involved in NADPH production through PPP. In addition, glutamate-cysteine ligase (GCLC; FC = 1.51) and cystathione γ-lyase (CTH; FC = 2.27), both important enzymes in GSH synthesis, were upregulated. These results are in line with the increased anti-oxidant capacity of resistant cells and further validate the metabolomics results described above.

To validate that higher expression of PHGDH as well as higher SSP activity are general features of BTZ-resistant cells, we performed a western blot for all SSP enzymes on our panel of BTZ- and CFZ-resistant cells (Fig. 5c). In all resistant cell lines, one or more SSP enzymes were upregulated. Both BTZ-resistant RPMI-8226 and AMO-1 cells showed higher expression of PHGDH compared to their sensitive counterparts, AMO-1 BTZ/90 cells showed increased expression of PSAT1, while ARH-77 BTZ/90 cells showed higher expression of PSPH (Fig. 5c). In addition, we profiled the activity of the SSP in these 8 cell lines by measuring the abundance of $^{13}C_3$-serine (M+3) after incubation with [U-^{13}C]-glucose (Fig. 5d). All BTZ-resistant cells showed a higher M+3 serine fraction compared to their WT counterparts, in line with higher expression of SSP enzymes in BTZ-resistant cells. Moreover, we observed a significant correlation between the serine M+3 fraction and the 48-h IC_{50} towards BTZ in these cell lines (Fig. 5e). In the RPMI-8226 and AMO-1 BTZ-resistant cells, the increase in SSP activity was accompanied by an increased uptake of extracellular serine (Additional file 1: Figure S4c). However, no difference in serine uptake was seen in ARH-77 cells, and no significant correlation was found between serine uptake and the 48-h IC_{50} towards BTZ (Additional file 1: Figure S4d). Together, these data suggest that the ability to perform serine synthesis rather than serine uptake is an important metabolic determinant for BTZ resistance. As expected, CFZ/90 AMO-1 cells did not show an increase in PHGDH expression or serine synthesis (Fig. 5c, d).

To verify the correlation between SSP and BTZ sensitivity, PHGDH expression was examined in CD138+ plasma cells from a small set (n = 6) of multiple myeloma patients isolated either at diagnosis, during therapy or after relapse from various therapeutic interventions (Fig. 5f, Additional file 1: Figure S3e, f and Table S1). For one MM patient (#1) at diagnosis, and for one patient (#4) with metastatic disease prior to therapy, PHGDH expression was negligible. Interestingly, three patients with progressive disease or refractory to BTZ therapy (indicated with *) showed markedly increased PHGDH expression, which was accompanied by higher PSPH expression but not PSAT1 expression. Notably, patient #6, that never received BTZ, but relapsed on melphalan, prednisone, lenalidomide therapy also displayed high PHGDH and PSPH expression. These results suggest that (BTZ)-therapy resistance in MM is associated with increased PHDGH expression in CD138 + cells.

Discussion

Metabolic alterations may play an essential role in the development of cellular resistance against anticancer drugs [24–27]. In the present study, we therefore aimed to identify metabolic mechanisms underlying BTZ resistance in MM. Here, we demonstrate for the first time that BTZ resistance in MM cells is sustained by metabolic rewiring, particularly of serine metabolism. Using tracer-based metabolomics, we show that the SSP has significantly increased activity in BTZ-resistant MM and plasmocytoid lymphoma cell lines. Importantly, we also observed a strong correlation between SSP activity and the ability of cells to withstand increasing BTZ concentrations in all BTZ-resistant cell lines tested.

The SSP is involved in NADPH regeneration and in the production of precursors for nucleotide and glutathione synthesis, and has been shown to be an important pathway to sustain cancer growth and proliferation [42, 43]. PHGDH, the first and rate-limiting enzyme of the SSP, is often overexpressed in cancer and has been linked to tumorigenesis as well as poor diagnosis in different cancers [45–48], identifying PHGDH as an interesting pharmaceutical target [47, 49, 50]. Using proteomics, we show that PHGDH is the highest upregulated metabolic enzyme in BTZ-resistant RPMI-8226 MM cells, and Western blots confirm that also in other BTZ-resistant cell lines one or more SSP enzymes are upregulated. The status of known regulators of the SSP in bortezomib resistance remains to be investigated.

We also demonstrate that PHGDH and PSPH are overexpressed in a small panel of CD138+ cells from BTZ-refractory MM patients compared to BTZ-responsive patients. This raises the possibility that high PHGDH expression, possibly in combination with PSPH expression, could be predictive of BTZ resistance. In line with these observations, we find that serine starvation enhances the efficacy of BTZ in sensitive RPMI-8226 cells, which have not yet upregulated PHGDH. This finding suggests that by removing serine from the diet, which is tolerated by mice and has been shown to reduce growth of some tumors [31, 51], the efficacy of current BTZ treatment might be enhanced. Because patient sample size was limited in the current pilot study, confident conclusions about the role of PHGDH as a predictive biomarker for bortezomib response cannot be drawn at this point. However, the results in patient-derived CD138+ cells underscore our findings in cell lines and warrant further research with a larger, controlled patient cohort to validate the use of PHGDH as a diagnostic tool to determine BTZ sensitivity in MM and other hematologic diseases. Notably, one patient that never received BTZ but was relapsing on melphalan, prednisone and lenalidomide, also displayed high PHGDH expression, raising the possibility that the observed changes in metabolism are also associated with other ROS-inducing agents. BTZ-resistant RPMI-8226 cells indeed show cross-resistance to CFZ, as has also been reported for AMO-1 cells [29], suggesting that the observed metabolic changes confer cross-resistance to other proteasome inhibitors to a certain extent, as expected. However, our data also show that BTZ-resistant RPMI-8226 cells do not display cross-resistance to either methotrexate or melphalan, both of which increase intracellular ROS levels, suggesting that the observed metabolic changes are specific for proteasome inhibitor resistance.

In addition to changes in the SSP, we find that the influx of glucose into the PPP is increased in BTZ-resistant MM cell lines. Proteomics experiments confirm that several proteins involved in both the PPP and in GSH metabolism are upregulated in BTZ resistant cells, in line with previous reports [29]. These metabolic alterations ultimately result in an increased anti-oxidant capacity of BTZ-resistant cells, as evidenced by a lower susceptibility to H_2O_2-induced oxidative stress, a higher GSH/GSSG ratio, and an increased ability to convert DHA to AA. Likely, this increased anti-oxidant capacity functions to protect resistant cells from BTZ-induced oxidative stress [6, 52]. Remarkably, increased PPP metabolism was not observed in ARH-77 plasmocytoid lymphoma cells. A recent report shows that BTZ resistance in leukemia was mediated through exocytosis of polyubiquitinated proteins [20], which may eliminate the need for extensive metabolic rewiring to induce resistance. The same holds true for CFZ-resistant cells, in which overexpression of ABCB1/P-glycoprotein has been described as an important mechanism of resistance [29]. It thus seems likely that the ability of cells to employ other mechanisms of resistance regulates the extent of metabolic resistance. Altered serine metabolism, however, occurred in all resistant cell lines tested. Our data therefore strongly support the hypothesis that altered serine metabolism is one of the core mechanisms of resistance, together with changes in proteasome abundance and composition. The clear correlation that we observe between PHGDH expression, SSP activity and BTZ sensitivity encourage further studies to determine whether increased SSP activity is causally related to BTZ resistance and whether PHGDH can be targeted to overcome BTZ resistance.

Conclusions

Here, we have identified specific metabolic mechanisms underlying bortezomib resistance. In particular, our results imply that bortezomib resistance is associated with high activity of the serine synthesis pathway and overexpression of PHGDH. Interfering with serine metabolism, either by removal of serine from the diet or by PHGDH inhibition, could potentially increase the efficacy of bortezomib treatment in both sensitive and resistant patients. In addition, we propose PHGDH expression as a novel biomarker of bortezomib response.

Additional file

Additional file 1: Supplemental information. Supplemental Methods; **Figure S1.** Response of RPMI-8226 WT, BTZ/7 and BTZ/100 cells to bortezomib and other chemotherapeutic agent; **Figure S2.** Intra- and extracellular metabolite analysis of BTZ- and CFZ-resistant cell lines; **Figure S3.** Response to serine starvation of RPMI-8226 WT and BTZ/100 cells; **Figure S4.** Bortezomib resistance correlates to the expression of PHGDH; **Table S1.** Characteristics of multiple myeloma patients; **Table S2.** Upregulated metabolic enzymes in RPMI-8226 BTZ/100 and BTZ/7 cells compared to WT; **Table S3.** Downregulated metabolic enzymes in RPMI-8226 BTZ/100 and BTZ/7 cells compared to WT. (PDF 6298 kb)

Abbreviations

AA: Ascorbic acid; BTZ: Bortezomib; CFZ: Carfilzomib; DHA: Dehydroascorbic acid; FBS: Fetal bovine serum; FC: Fold change; GSH: Glutathione; GSSG: Glutathione disulfide; H2O2: Hydrogen peroxide; MEM: Minimal essential medium; MM: Multiple myeloma; PHGDH: 3-phosphoglycerate dehydrogenase; PPP: Pentose phosphate pathway; PSAT1: Phosphoserine aminotransferase 1; PSPH: Phosphoserine phosphatase; S7P: Sedoheptulose-7-phosphate; SSP: Serine synthesis pathway; TA: Trans-androsterone; TCA: Tricarboxylic acid; WT: Wild type

Acknowledgements

The authors would like to thank Pieter Langerhorst, Klaas Vermaas, and Haley Baptist for technical assistance, Huib Ovaa for providing Me_4BodipyFL-Ahx_3L_3VS, Christoph Driessen for providing BTZ- and CFZ-resistant cell lines, and Albert Heck for constructive discussions.

Funding

CRB was supported by VENI grant (project 722.013.009) from the Netherlands Organization for Scientific Research (NWO).

Authors' contributions

CRB and EAZ developed this study, designed the experiments and wrote the manuscript. EAZ and WW performed the experiments. EAZ, CRB, WW, GJ, SZ, and JC performed data analysis and interpretation. All authors reviewed the results and approved the final version of the manuscript.

Competing interests

All authors declare that they have no competing interests.

Author details

[1]Biomolecular Mass Spectrometry and Proteomics, Bijvoet Center for Biomolecular Research and Utrecht Institute of Pharmaceutical Sciences, Utrecht University, Padualaan 8, 3584 CH Utrecht, The Netherlands. [2]Amsterdam Rheumatology and Immunology Center—Location VUMC, VU University Medical Center, Amsterdam, The Netherlands. [3]Department of Hematology, VU University Medical Center, Amsterdam, The Netherlands. [4]Pediatric Oncology/Hematology, VU University Medical Center, Amsterdam, The Netherlands.

References

1. Moreau P, Richardson PG, Cavo M, Orlowski RZ, San Miguel JF, Palumbo A, et al. Proteasome inhibitors in multiple myeloma: 10 years later. Blood. 2012; 120:947–59.
2. Anderson KC. The 39th David A. Karnofsky Lecture: bench-to-bedside translation of targeted therapies in multiple myeloma. J Clin Oncol. 2012;30: 445–52.
3. Raynes R, Pomatto LCD, Davies KJA. Degradation of oxidized proteins by the proteasome: Distinguishing between the 20S, 26S, and immunoproteasome proteolytic pathways. Mol Aspects Med. 2016;50:41–55.
4. Berkers CR, Ovaa H. Drug discovery and assay development in the ubiquitin-proteasome system. Biochem Soc Trans. 2010;38(Pt 1):14–20.
5. Obeng EA, Carlson LM, Gutman DM, Harrington WJ, Lee KP, Boise LH. Proteasome inhibitors induce a terminal unfolded protein response in multiple myeloma cells. Blood. 2006;107:4907–16.
6. Lipchick BC, Fink EE, Nikiforov MA. Oxidative stress and proteasome inhibitors in multiple myeloma. Pharmacol Res. 2016;105:210–5.
7. Niewerth D, Jansen G, Assaraf YG, Zweegman S, Kaspers GJL, Cloos J. Molecular basis of resistance to proteasome inhibitors in hematological malignancies. Drug Resist Updat. 2015;18:18–35.
8. McConkey DJ, Zhu K. Mechanisms of proteasome inhibitor action and resistance in cancer. Drug Resist Updat. 2008;11:164–79.
9. Orlowski RZ, Kuhn DJ. Proteasome inhibitors in cancer therapy: Lessons from the first decade. Clin Cancer Res. 2008;14:1649–57.
10. Oerlemans R, Franke NE, Assaraf YG, Cloos J, van Zantwijk I, Berkers CR, et al. Molecular basis of bortezomib resistance: proteasome subunit beta5 (PSMB5) gene mutation and overexpression of PSMB5 protein. Blood. 2008; 112:2489–99.
11. Franke NE, Niewerth D, Assaraf YG, van Meerloo J, Vojtekova K, van Zantwijk CH, et al. Impaired bortezomib binding to mutant β5 subunit of the proteasome is the underlying basis for bortezomib resistance in leukemia cells. Leukemia. 2012;26:757–68.
12. de Wilt LHAM, Jansen G, Assaraf YG, van Meerloo J, Cloos J, Schimmer AD, et al. Proteasome-based mechanisms of intrinsic and acquired bortezomib resistance in non-small cell lung cancer. Biochem Pharmacol. 2012;83:207–17.
13. Rückrich T, Kraus M, Gogel J, Beck A, Ovaa H, Verdoes M, et al. Characterization of the ubiquitin-proteasome system in bortezomib-adapted cells. Leukemia. 2009;23:1098–105.
14. Balsas P, Galán-Malo P, Marzo I, Naval J. Bortezomib resistance in a myeloma cell line is associated to PSMβ5 overexpression and polyploidy. Leuk Res. 2012;36:212–8.

15. Niewerth D, Kaspers GJL, Jansen G, van Meerloo J, Zweegman S, Jenkins G, et al. Proteasome subunit expression analysis and chemosensitivity in relapsed paediatric acute leukaemia patients receiving bortezomib-containing chemotherapy. J Hematol Oncol. 2016;9:82.
16. Lichter DI, Danaee H, Pickard MD, Tayber O, Sintchak M, Shi H, et al. Sequence analysis of β-subunit genes of the 20S proteasome in patients with relapsed multiple myeloma treated with bortezomib or dexamethasone. Blood. 2012;120:4513–6.
17. Ling SCW, Lau EKK, Al-Shabeeb A, Nikolic A, Catalano A, Iland H, et al. Response of myeloma to the proteasome inhibitor bortezomib is correlated with the unfolded protein response regulator XBP-1. Haematologica. 2012;97:64–72.
18. Leung-Hagesteijn C, Erdmann N, Cheung G, Keats JJ, Stewart AK, Reece DE, et al. Xbp1s-negative tumor B cells and pre-plasmablasts mediate therapeutic proteasome inhibitor resistance in multiple myeloma. Cancer Cell. 2013;24:289–304.
19. Driessen C, Kraus M, Joerger M, Rosing H, Bader J, Hitz F, et al. Treatment with the HIV protease inhibitor nelfinavir triggers the unfolded protein response and may overcome proteasome inhibitor resistance of multiple myeloma in combination with bortezomib: a phase I trial (SAKK 65/08). Haematologica. 2016;101:346–55.
20. Franke NE, Kaspers GL, Assaraf YG, van Meerloo J, Niewerth D, Kessler FL, et al. Exocytosis of polyubiquitinated proteins in bortezomib-resistant leukemia cells: a role for MARCKS in acquired resistance to proteasome inhibitors. Oncotarget. 2016;7:74779–96.
21. Ward PS, Thompson CB. Metabolic reprogramming: a cancer hallmark even warburg did not anticipate. Cancer Cell. 2012;21:297–308.
22. Vander Heiden MG, Cantley LC, Thompson CB. Understanding the Warburg effect: the metabolic requirements of cell proliferation. Science. 2009;324: 1029–33.
23. Galluzzi L, Kepp O, Vander Heiden MG, Kroemer G. Metabolic targets for cancer therapy. Nat Rev Drug Discov. 2013;12:829–46.
24. Liu H, Liu Y, Zhang J-T. A new mechanism of drug resistance in breast cancer cells: fatty acid synthase overexpression-mediated palmitate overproduction. Mol Cancer Ther. 2008;7:263–70.
25. Zhao Y, Liu H, Liu Z, Ding Y, Ledoux SP, Wilson GL, et al. Overcoming trastuzumab resistance in breast cancer by targeting dysregulated glucose metabolism. Cancer Res. 2011;71:4585–97.
26. Stäubert C, Bhuiyan H, Lindahl A, Broom OJ, Zhu Y, Islam S, et al. Rewired metabolism in drug-resistant leukemia cells: a metabolic switch hallmarked by reduced dependence on exogenous glutamine. J Biol Chem. 2015;290: 8348–59.
27. Baenke F, Chaneton B, Smith M, Van Den Broek N, Hogan K, Tang H, et al. Resistance to BRAF inhibitors induces glutamine dependency in melanoma cells. Mol Oncol. 2016;10:73–84.
28. Maiso P, Huynh D, Moschetta M, Sacco A, Aljawai Y, Mishima Y, et al. Metabolic signature identifies novel targets for drug resistance in multiple myeloma. Cancer Res. 2015;75:2071–82.
29. Soriano GP, Besse L, Li N, Kraus M, Besse A, Meeuwenoord N, et al. Proteasome inhibitor-adapted myeloma cells are largely independent from proteasome activity and show complex proteomic changes, in particular in redox and energy metabolism. Leukemia. 2016;30:2198–207.
30. Berkers CR. van Leeuwen FWB, Groothuis T a, Peperzak V, van Tilburg EW, Borst J, et al. Profiling proteasome activity in tissue with fluorescent probes. Mol Pharm. 2007;4:739–48.
31. Maddocks ODK, Berkers CR, Mason SM, Zheng L, Blyth K, Gottlieb E, et al. Serine starvation induces stress and p53-dependent metabolic remodelling in cancer cells. Nature. 2013;493:542–6.
32. Buescher JM, Antoniewicz MR, Boros LG, Burgess SC, Brunengraber H, Clish CB, et al. A roadmap for interpreting (13)C metabolite labeling patterns from cells. Curr Opin Biotechnol. 2015;34:189–201.
33. Niewerth D, van Meerloo J, Jansen G, Assaraf YG, Hendrickx TC, Kirk CJ, et al. Anti-leukemic activity and mechanisms underlying resistance to the novel immunoproteasome inhibitor PR-924. Biochem Pharmacol. 2014;89:43–51.
34. Kraus M, Rückrich T, Reich M, Gogel J, Beck A, Kammer W, et al. Activity patterns of proteasome subunits reflect bortezomib sensitivity of hematologic malignancies and are variable in primary human leukemia cells. Leukemia. 2007;21:84–92.
35. Kuehne A, Emmert H, Soehle J, Winnefeld M, Fischer F, Wenck H, et al. Acute Activation of Oxidative Pentose Phosphate Pathway as First-Line Response to Oxidative Stress in Human Skin Cells. Mol Cell. 2015;59:359–71.
36. Verbrugge SE, Assaraf YG, Dijkmans Ba C, Scheffer GL, Al M, den Uyl D, et al. Inactivating PSMB5 mutations and P-glycoprotein (multidrug resistance-associated protein/ATP-binding cassette B1) mediate resistance to proteasome inhibitors: ex vivo efficacy of (immuno)proteasome inhibitors in mononuclear blood cells from patients with. J Pharmacol Exp Ther. 2012;341:174–82.
37. Bohndiek SE, Kettunen MI, Hu D, Kennedy BWC, Boren J, Gallagher FA, et al. Hyperpolarized [1-13C]-ascorbic and dehydroascorbic acid: vitamin C as a probe for imaging redox status in vivo. J Am Chem Soc. 2011;133:11795–801.
38. Corti A, Casini AF, Pompella A. Cellular pathways for transport and efflux of ascorbate and dehydroascorbate. Arch Biochem Biophys. 2010;500:107–15.
39. Labuschagne CF, van den Broek NJF, Mackay GM, Vousden KH, Maddocks ODK. Serine, but not glycine, supports one-carbon metabolism and proliferation of cancer cells. Cell Rep. 2014;7:1248–58.
40. Maddocks ODK, Labuschagne CF, Adams PD, Vousden KH. Serine Metabolism Supports the Methionine Cycle and DNA/RNA Methylation through De Novo ATP Synthesis in Cancer Cells. Mol Cell. 2016;61:210–21.
41. Tedeschi PM, Markert EK, Gounder M, Lin H, Dvorzhinski D, Dolfi SC, et al. Contribution of serine, folate and glycine metabolism to the ATP. NADPH and purine requirements of cancer cells Cell Death Dis. 2013;4:e877.
42. Locasale JW. Serine, glycine and one-carbon units: cancer metabolism in full circle. Nat Rev Cancer. 2013;13:572–83.
43. Amelio I, Cutruzzolá F, Antonov A, Agostini M, Melino G. Serine and glycine metabolism in cancer. Trends Biochem Sci. 2014;39:191–8.
44. Mullarky E, Lucki NC, Beheshti Zavareh R, Anglin JL, Gomes AP, Nicolay BN, et al. Identification of a small molecule inhibitor of 3-phosphoglycerate dehydrogenase to target serine biosynthesis in cancers. Proc Natl Acad Sci U S A. 2016;113:1778–83.
45. DeNicola GM, Chen P-H, Mullarky E, Sudderth JA, Hu Z, Wu D, et al. NRF2 regulates serine biosynthesis in non-small cell lung cancer. Nat Genet. 2015; 47:1475–81.
46. Pollari S, Käkönen S-M, Edgren H, Wolf M, Kohonen P, Sara H, et al. Enhanced serine production by bone metastatic breast cancer cells stimulates osteoclastogenesis. Breast Cancer Res Treat. 2011;125:421–30.
47. Mullarky E, Mattaini KR, Vander Heiden MG, Cantley LC, Locasale JW. PHGDH amplification and altered glucose metabolism in human melanoma. Pigment Cell Melanoma Res. 2011;24:1112–5.
48. Locasale JW, Grassian AR, Melman T, Lyssiotis CA, Mattaini KR, Bass AJ, et al. Phosphoglycerate dehydrogenase diverts glycolytic flux and contributes to oncogenesis. Nat Genet. 2011;43:869–74.
49. Possemato R, Marks KM, Shaul YD, Pacold ME, Kim D, Birsoy K, et al. Functional genomics reveal that the serine synthesis pathway is essential in breast cancer. Nature. 2011;476:346–50.
50. Pacold ME, Brimacombe KR, Chan SH, Rohde JM, Lewis CA, Swier LJYM, et al. A PHGDH inhibitor reveals coordination of serine synthesis and one-carbon unit fate. Nat Chem Biol. 2016;12:452–8.
51. Maddocks ODK, Athineos D, Cheung EC, Lee P, Zhang T, van den Broek NJF, et al. Modulating the therapeutic response of tumours to dietary serine and glycine starvation. Nature. 2017;544:372–6.
52. Du Z-X, Zhang H-Y, Meng X, Guan Y, Wang H-Q. Role of oxidative stress and intracellular glutathione in the sensitivity to apoptosis induced by proteasome inhibitor in thyroid cancer cells. BMC Cancer. 2009;9:56.

12

Hepatocellular carcinoma-associated hypercholesterolemia: involvement of proprotein-convertase-subtilisin-kexin type- 9 (PCSK9)

Dipti Athavale[1], Surbhi Chouhan[1], Vimal Pandey[1,2], Shyamananda Singh Mayengbam[1], Snahlata Singh[1] and Manoj Kumar Bhat[1*]

Abstract

Background: PCSK9 regulates low-density lipoprotein cholesterol (LDLc) level and has been implicated in hypercholesterolemia. Aberrant plasma lipid profile is often associated with various cancers. Clinically, the relationship between altered serum lipid level and hepatocellular carcinoma (HCC) has been documented; however, the underlying cause and implications of such dyslipidemia remain unclear.

Methods: The present study includes the use of HepG2 tumor xenograft model to study the potential role of glucose (by providing 15% glucose via drinking water) in regulating PCSK9 expression and associated hypercholesterolemia. To support in vivo findings, in vitro approaches were used by incubating HCC cells in culture medium with different glucose concentrations or treating the cells with glucose uptake inhibitors. Impact of hypercholesterolemia on chemotherapy was demonstrated by exogenously providing LDLc followed by appropriate in vitro assays.

Results: We observed that serum and hepatic PCSK9 level is decreased in mice which were provided with glucose containing water. Interestingly, serum and tumor PCSK9 level was upregulated in HepG2-tumor-bearing mice having access to water containing glucose. Additionally, elevated LDLc is detected in sera of these mice. In vitro studies indicated that PCSK9 expression was increased by high glucose availability with potential involvement of reactive oxygen species (ROS) and sterol regulatory element binding protein-1 (SREBP-1). Furthermore, it is also demonstrated that pre-treatment of cells with LDLc diminishes cytotoxicity of sorafenib in HCC cells.

Conclusion: Taken together, these results suggest a regulation of PCSK9 by high glucose which could contribute, at least partly, towards understanding the cause of hypercholesterolemia in HCC and its accompanied upshots in terms of altered response of HCC cells towards cancer therapy.

Keywords: Hepatocellular carcinoma, Hypercholesterolemia, Glucose, PCSK9, Sorafenib

* Correspondence: manojkbhat@nccs.res.in; manojkbhat62@gmail.com
[1]Laboratory No. 6, National Centre for Cell Science, Savitribai Phule Pune University Campus, Ganeshkhind, Pune 411 007, India
Full list of author information is available at the end of the article

Background

Proprotein-convertase-subtilisin-kexin type-9 (PCSK9) is a serine protease, primarily synthesized by the liver. Following the autocatalysis in endoplasmic reticulum, it is secreted as a catalytically inert heterodimer consisting of c-terminal domain and a non-covalently bound pro-domain [1–3]. Extracellular PCSK9 binds and targets low-density lipoprotein receptor (LDLR) towards lysosomal degradation thus, restricting its recycling to the cell surface [1]. There is a tight correlation between serum PCSK9 and low-density lipoprotein cholesterol (LDLc) level in humans as PCSK9 is a post-transcriptional inhibitor of LDLR [4]. Apart from the mutations in LDLR and apolipoprotein B (ApoB), the gain of function mutation in PCSK9 gene is implicated in autosomal dominant familial hypercholesterolemia [3]. Several studies highlight the involvement of PCSK9 in imparting advantages to certain cancer types. PCSK9, also known as neural apoptosis-regulated convertase 1 (NARC1), exhibits an anti-apoptotic function in lung cancer and neuroglioma cells [5, 6]. It is demonstrated to be involved in metastasis such that its deficiency reduces melanoma metastasis due to lower circulatory cholesterol level [7]. Moreover, it induces hyperlipidemia which promotes tumor growth [8].

Hepatocellular carcinoma (HCC), the most common form of primary liver cancer, is the sixth largest cancer type based on the number of incidences worldwide [9]. It is more prevalent in Asia and accounts for 75% of all liver cancer cases [10]. Chronic viral hepatitis, history of alcohol consumption, fatty liver disorders, and metabolic syndrome led cirrhosis are the major risk factors for HCC [11]. With poor prognosis and limited treatment options, liver cancer is ranked fourth for cancer-related deaths [9, 12]. Currently, sorafenib, a multi-kinase inhibitor, is the primary chemotherapeutic agent for HCC treatment [13]. However, resistance to sorafenib is emerging and multiple mechanisms have been proposed [14].

Although hepatitis B (HBV) and C (HCV) virus infections are causative factors for HCC pathogenesis, other non-viral factors like obesity or type 2 diabetes mellitus (T2DM) are emerging as independent risk factors. Obesity or T2DM-promoted influx of nutrients (sugars, free fatty acids), pro-inflammatory cytokines, adipokines, and insulin resistance cause chronic low-grade inflammation in the liver. This can accelerate development cascade of liver diseases like non-alcoholic fatty liver disease (NAFLD), non-alcoholic steatohepatits (NASH), and cirrhosis, ultimately leading to HCC [15, 16]. Cancer cells rewire their cellular metabolism to enhance glucose uptake to support rapid reproduction [17]. Hyperglycemia, a common manifestation of diabetes or obesity, renders an advantageous access of glucose to cancer cells, thus directly or indirectly contributing to the risk and progression of tumors [18–20].

The effect of different nutrients on tissue gene expression and serum PCSK9 has been studied extensively. Various dietary lipids either did not change or lowered serum PCSK9 in healthy human subjects [21]. However, the role of glucose in the regulation of PCSK9 expression remains elusive. Considering the co-existence of HCC and metabolic syndromes which are often associated with the persistent nutritional overload, altered PCSK9 regulation is indeed a possibility. On these lines, we hypothesized that glucose could have effect on PCSK9 expression in HCC tumor which may have implications in altering LDLc level in the host. By modulating glucose availability, serum and tissue expression of PCSK9 was analyzed in the presence and absence of HCC-xenograft. In vitro studies were also focused on validating the in vivo observation and evaluating its possible consequence on the response towards chemotherapy.

Methods

Cell lines and cell culture

Human hepatocellular carcinoma cell lines HepG2 and Hep3B were procured from ATCC (Manassas, VA, USA) and were maintained at our in-house cell repository at National Centre for Cell Science (NCCS), Pune, India. HuH-7 cell line was obtained from Dr. Ralf Bartenschlager (University of Heidelberg, Germany). Cells were cultured in Dulbecco's modified Eagle medium (DMEM) supplemented with 10% heat-inactivated fetal bovine serum (life technologies, CA, USA), penicillin (100 U/ml), and streptomycin (100 μg/ml) (Invitrogen Life Technologies, CA, USA) and maintained in a humidified atmosphere of 5% CO_2 at 37 °C. Cells were intermittently checked for their typical morphology.

Chemicals and antibodies

D-glucose, D-mannitol, glutamine, sodium pyruvate, sodium lactate, 2-deoxyglucose, crystal violet, fasentin, fatostatin, catalase, lipoprotein-deficient serum (LPDS), vinculin antibody (V9131) and thiazolyl blue tetrazolium bromide (MTT) were purchased from Sigma-Aldrich (MO, USA). Cytochalasin B was purchased from MP Biomedicals (OH, USA). Recombinant PCSK9 protein was purchased from BioLegend (CA, USA). LDLc was purchased from Lee Biosolutions (Missouri, USA) and reconstituted as per manufacturer's instruction. PCSK9 (sc-66996), Transferrin Receptor (TfR; sc-7087), PCNA (sc-56), β-actin (sc-1615), procaspase 3 (sc-7272), SREBP-1 (sc-8984), SREBP-2 (sc-5603), GAPDH (sc-20357), Histone H1 (sc-10806), pERK (sc-7383), ERK (sc-154), Insulin (sc-8033), HRP-conjugated secondary antibodies, and sorafenib (sc-357801A) were purchased from Santa Cruz Biotechnology (CA, USA). LDLR (ab-30532) antibody was purchased from Abcam (MA, USA). Antibody for PARP (9542) was purchased from Cell Signaling Technology

(MA, USA). Mouse PCSK9 antibody (AF-3985) was purchased from R&D Systems (MN, USA). Low-density lipoprotein from human plasma, DiI complex (DiI-LDL), was purchased from Life Technologies (OR, USA). BD Matrigel™ was purchased from BD Biosciences (MA, USA).

Animal experiment

All animal experiments were performed as per the requirement and guidelines of the Committee for the Purpose of Control and Supervision of Experiments on Animals (CPCSEA), Government of India, and after obtaining permission of the Institutional Animal Ethics Committee (IAEC). Six- to 8-week-old male NOD/SCID mice were divided into four groups ($n = 6$ per group). Mice from group I and group III had access to drinking water without glucose while mice from group II and group IV were supplied with 15% glucose via drinking water throughout the experiment [19]. After 15 days, mice from group III and group IV were subcutaneously (s.c.) injected with HepG2 cells (5×10^6/mouse) along with matrigel. Once the tumors were palpable, bi-dimensional measurements were taken with Vernier Caliper every third day. Tumor volume (mm^3) was calculated with the formula (width^2 × length) × 0.52. For glucose tolerance test (GTT), mice from group I and group II were fasted for 6 h, and blood glucose was measured with ACCU-CHEK Active glucometer (Roche diagnostics, Germany) and considered as basal glucose at 0 min. Mice were injected with glucose (3 g/ kg) intraperitoneally, and blood glucose level was measured at 30 min, 60 min, 90 min, and 120 min. At the end of the experiment, mice were fasted for 4 h and sacrificed by CO_2 euthanasia. Subcutaneous tumor and liver were excised and stored at − 80 °C for further assays.

Serum biochemistry

Before euthanizing the experimental mice from all the groups, blood was collected by orbital sinus puncture. Serum lipid parameters such as LDLc, total cholesterol (TC), and triglycerides (TG) were estimated as described previously [22].

In vitro treatments

HCC cells seeded in 6-well plates were cultured in DMEM with low glucose (LG; 5 mM) or high glucose (HG; 25 mM) along with concentrations of inhibitors and substrates as indicated, and cells were processed for relevant functional assays. Plasmid expressing hPCSK9 was a kind gift from Dr. Jay Horton (UT South-western, TX, USA). HepG2 cells were transfected with empty vector or hPCSK9 plasmid using Lipofectamine 2000 (Life technologies, OR, USA) for 8 h. Post-transfection, HepG2 cells were cultured in HG for 48 h and overexpression of PCSK9 was checked by Western blotting.

Indirect ELISA

Sera from mice or lyophilized culture media from HepG2 cells treated with LG or HG were used to coat ELISA plates at 4 °C overnight. The plates were then processed as described previously [23]. Standard curves with different concentrations of recombinant hPCSK9 and mPCSK9 were prepared to quantify concentration of secretory PCSK9.

Quantitative reverse transcription PCR (RT-qPCR)

Total RNA from HepG2 cells and tissues was isolated with TRIzol™ (Invitrogen, CA, USA). Complementary DNA was prepared from 2 μg of total RNA as described previously [23]. Subsequently, RT-qPCR was performed using MESA GREEN SYBR MIX (Eurogentech, Belgium) with specific primer sets (Additional file 1: Table S1). The following thermal conditions were used: step 1: 95 °C for 2 min, step 2: 95 °C for 15 s, step 3: 55 °C for 20 s, and step 4: 72 °C for 20 s, and $2^{-\Delta\Delta ct}$ method was used to calculate fold change in gene expression.

Immunoblotting

Whole cell or tissue samples were lysed in ice-cold RIPA buffer as described earlier [24]. Membrane, cytosolic, and nuclear fractions were prepared as described earlier [25, 26]. After protein quantitation using Coomassie Plus Protein Assay Reagent (Thermo Scientific, IL, USA), 50–100 μg of protein samples were resolved on 8–10% of SDS-PAGE and transferred to nitrocellulose membranes. Membranes were blocked and further probed with indicated primary and HRP-conjugated secondary antibodies. Immunoreactive bands were visualized using luminescence detection reagent (Santa Cruz Biotechnology, CA, USA) and quantified with ImageJ software.

Glucose estimation

After culturing HepG2 cells for mentioned time period in DMEM with indicated glucose concentration, supernatant was collected and the residual glucose in the spent medium was estimated with GOD-POD-based glucose assay kit (Spinreact, Spain) according to the manufacturer's instructions.

Immunofluorescence staining

HepG2 cells were seeded on multi-well chambered slides (MP Biomedicals, OH, USA). Cells were treated as mentioned in pertinent figure legends and processed for staining as described previously [27]. Cells were analyzed under Zeiss LSM 510 microscope, and images were processed by LSM image analysis software (Carl Zeiss, Germany).

Reactive oxygen species (ROS) measurement

Cellular ROS generation on treating cells with LG, HG, or HG + catalase was measured with 2, 7-dichlorofluorescein diacetate (DCFDA) dye. Cells were incubated with 5 μM of DCFDA at 37 °C for 30 min. The fluorescence of DCFDA was measured on FL1 channel on flow cytometer (FACS Calibur, Becton Dickinson, USA). Data were analyzed using Cell Quest Pro software (Becton Dickinson, California, USA) for 10,000 cells.

LDL uptake assay

HepG2 cells were grown on 12-well plates or multi-well chambered slides (MP Biomedicals, OH, USA). Following the treatment of LG or HG medium or transfection of hPCSK9 plasmid, cells were processed for LDL uptake assay by either FACS or confocal microscopy as described earlier [28]. Briefly, DiI-LDL (10 μg/ml) was added at the end of the treatment for 2 h. Cells were washed with PBS and processed for either the measurement of DiI-LDL fluorescence in FL2 channel on flow cytometer (FACS Calibur, Becton Dickinson, USA) or fixed with 3% paraformaldehyde, mounted with UltraCruz® mounting medium (Santa Cruz Biotechnology, USA), and images were acquired on Zeiss LSM 510 microscope.

MTT assay

Cells (2×10^3 cells/ well) were seeded in 96-well plates and allowed to adhere. After 24 h, cells were treated with vehicle, LDLc, or sorafenib as per experimental requirements. At the end of the treatments, medium was removed and MTT solution (1 mg/ml) was added to each well, and plates were incubated for 4 h at 37 °C. Isopropanol (100 μl) was added to solubilize formazan crystals, and absorbance was recorded at 570 nm.

Long-term survival assay

Cells (5×10^2 cells/well) were seeded in 24-well plates and treated with vehicle, LDLc, or sorafenib as mentioned in respective figure legend. After completion of treatment, medium was removed, fresh medium was added to each well and cells were cultured for another 10 days by changing medium every third day. Thereafter, cells were fixed and stained with crystal violet, and images were taken using Olympus digital camera (Tokyo, Japan).

Statistical analysis

All data are presented as mean ± standard deviation (SD) or mean ± standard error of the mean (SEM) as mentioned. Statistical comparison was performed by unpaired two-tailed Student's t test by using Sigma Plot (Systat Software Inc., CA, USA). Statistical significance was accepted at $P < 0.05$ level ($^{*}p < 0.05$, $^{**}p < 0.01$, $^{***}p < 0.001$).

Results

PCSK9 expression is increased upon supplementation of glucose in vivo

To evaluate the effect of glucose on PCSK9 expression and its consequences in HCC, NOD/SCID male mice were divided into four groups. Mice from group I and group III had access to drinking water without glucose. Mice from group II and group IV were exposed to 15% glucose via drinking water throughout the experiment. Group III and group IV mice were injected with HepG2 cells subcutaneously, and tumor progression was measured. Glucose tolerance test (GTT) performed in mice from group I and group II indicated increased blood glucose levels in group II as compared to group I, implying that glucose feeding impairs blood glucose clearance and increases its availability (Fig. 1a). Additionally, glucose feeding enhanced the tumor progression in group IV, as compared to group III (Fig. 1b). Therefore, it is likely that excess glucose available to animals may be a contributory factor towards rapid proliferation of HCC cells in group IV. By ELISA, higher serum PCSK9 level was detected in mice from group IV compared to group III (Fig. 1c). Since, the antibody used in ELISA has a cross-reactivity to mouse PCSK9, to distinguish between host and graft-secreted PCSK9, murine PCSK9 level in the serum was quantified with mouse-specific antibody by ELISA. Interestingly, murine PCSK9 level was reduced in serum of non-tumor-bearing mice from group II as compared to group I (Fig. 1d). Although, increased levels of murine PCSK9 were noted in group III and group IV as compared with group I and group II, it did not change between group III and group IV (Fig. 1d). No changes in the serum insulin level were observed upon glucose feeding. Also, insulin did not induce PCSK9 expression in LG and HG medium in HepG2 cells (Additional file 2: Figure S1A and B). To seek a clear understanding of the effect of glucose on xenograft-secreted PCSK9, mRNA and protein levels of PCSK9 in tumor tissue were analyzed by qPCR and Western blot, respectively. Figure 1e shows that, mRNA expression of PCSK9 was increased significantly in tumor tissues of mice from group IV as compared to group III. Also, tumor tissue from group IV had an increase in PCSK9 protein level as compared to group III (Fig. 1f). However, in tumor tissue lysates, LDLR level remained unaltered between group III and group IV (Fig. 1f). Overall, these observations imply that elevated serum PCSK9 level detected in group IV might be contributed by HepG2-xenograft.

Next, lipid parameters were measured in serum collected from group III and group IV. Elevated serum LDLc, total cholesterol, and triglycerides were detected in sera of mice from group IV as compared to group III (Fig. 2a). Serum LDLc level is sensitive towards hepatic

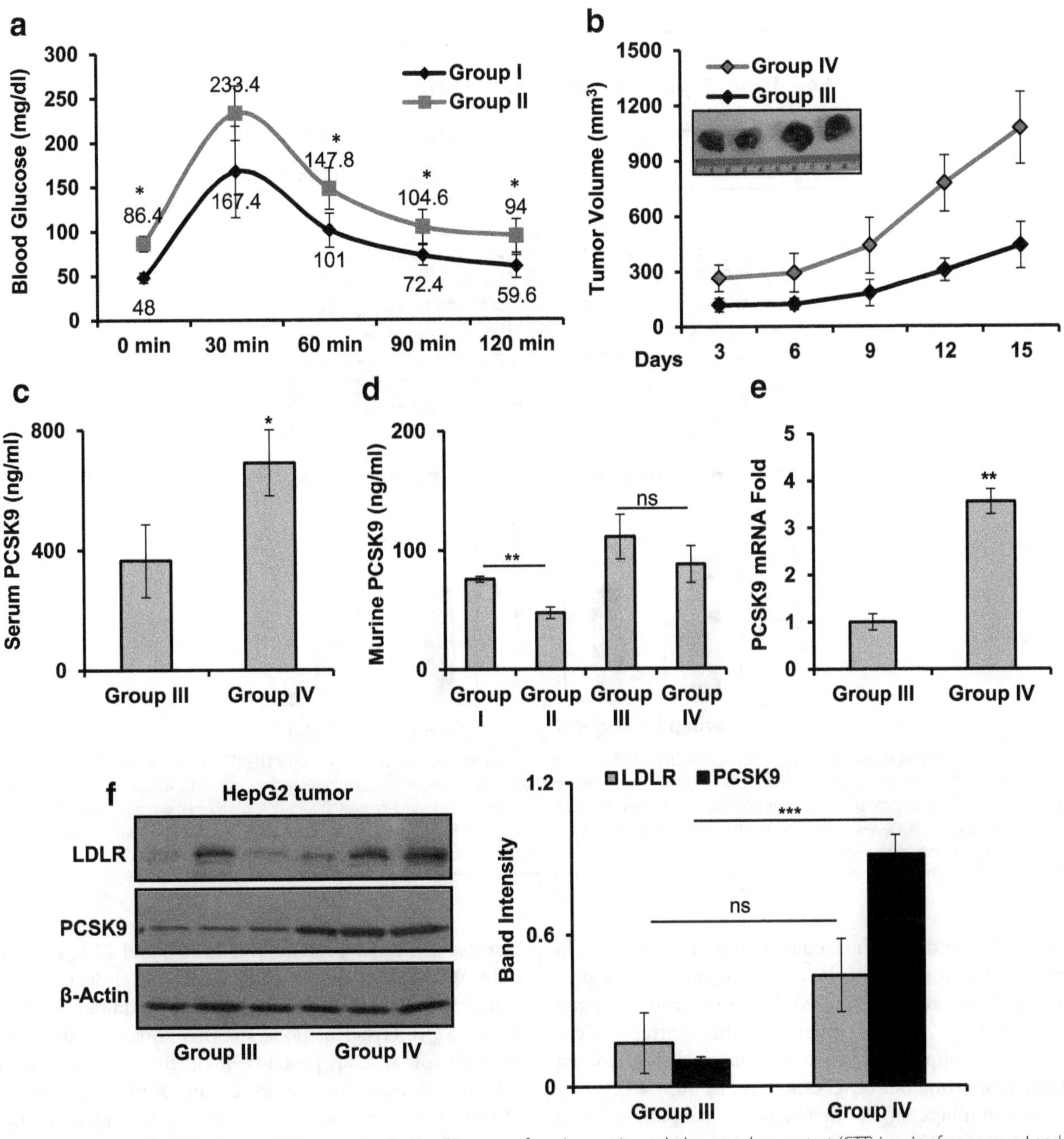

Fig. 1 Glucose availability induces PCSK9 expression in HepG2-xenografts. **a** Intraperitoneal glucose tolerance test (GTT) in mice from group I and group II. **b** Tumor progression in group III and group IV, after injecting HepG2 cells (5×10^6) subcutaneously. **c** Individual serum samples collected from group III and group IV were subjected to ELISA to quantify circulatory PCSK9 levels. **d** Individual serum samples collected from group I, group II, group III, and group IV were subjected to ELISA to quantify murine PCSK9 levels. **e** PCSK9 transcripts in three representative tumor tissue samples from group III and group IV were analyzed by qRT-PCR. **f** Tumor or liver tissue lysates from three representative samples were resolved by SDS-PAGE and LDLR, and PCSK9 protein levels were analyzed by immunoblot. Band intensities were measured by densitometry and normalized with β-actin. The results are given as means ± standard deviation; $^*p < 0.05$, $^{**}p < 0.01$, $^{***}p < 0.001$ denote significant differences in the groups; ns non-significant

LDLR availability, and slight alteration in its level could have consequences on serum lipid profile [29, 30]. Moreover, human PCSK9 infusion in murine system effectively reduces hepatic LDLR and elevates serum LDLc [31, 32]. Therefore, LDLR protein levels in the liver and tumor tissues were analyzed. An increase in the hepatic LDLR protein was noted in glucose-fed mice from group II as compared to group I (Fig. 2b, left panel). The level of hepatic LDLR decreased in group IV as compared to group III (Fig. 2b, right panel and Additional file 2:

a

Parameter	Group III	Group IV
Low density lipoprotein cholesterol	44.37 ± 2.31	68.71 ± 6.17*
Total Cholesterol	64.12 ± 4.38	82.94 ± 6.31*
Triglycerides	30.32 ± 2.3	62.66 ±19.87*

b

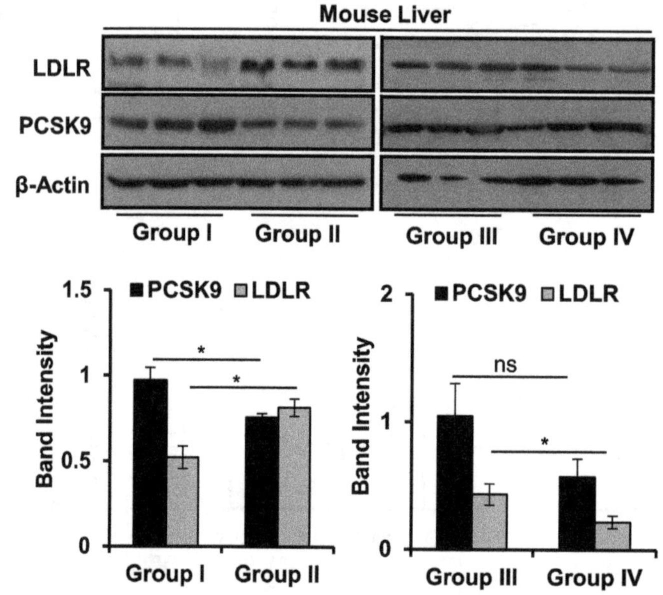

Fig. 2 Glucose feeding differentially alters hepatic PCSK9 and LDLR protein level in presence and absence of HepG2-tumors. **a** Low-density lipoprotein cholesterol (mg/dl), total cholesterol (mg/dl), and triglycerides (mg/dl) in serum samples were estimated using kits as per the manufacturer's instructions. **b** Mouse liver homogenates from groups I and II (left panel) and groups III and IV (right panel) were resolved by SDS-PAGE, LDLR and PCSK9 levels were analyzed by Western blot. Band intensities were measured by densitometry and normalized with β-actin. The results are given as means ± standard deviation; *$p < 0.05$ denote significant differences in the groups; ns non-significant

Figure S1C and D), thus contributing for the rise in serum LDLc in group IV. However, hepatic PCSK9 protein level remained unaltered between group III and group IV (Fig. 2b, right panel). On the contrary, it decreased in group II as compared to group I (Fig. 2b, left panel) supporting our observation in Fig. 1d.

These findings imply that glucose supplementation modulates PCSK9 and LDLR levels in mice with and without HepG2 xenograft. PCSK9 derived from tumor-graft increases on glucose feeding and likely to be associated with development of hypercholesterolemia in xenograft-bearing mice from group IV as compared to group III.

Glucose modulates PCSK9 expression in HCC cells

To corroborate above stated findings in vitro, human hepatoma cells, HepG2, HuH-7, and Hep3B, were cultured in increasing glucose concentrations (1 mM, 5 mM, and 25 mM) and the level of PCSK9 protein was analyzed. HepG2 and HuH-7 cells exhibited a glucose-dependent increase in PCSK9 protein level at 12 h and 24 h, respectively. Whereas in Hep3B cells, PCSK9 level decreased at higher glucose concentration at 24 h (Additional file 3: Figure S2A). Hyper osmotic stress is known to affect expression of several proteins [33]; therefore, mannitol (Mann; 20 mM) was used as an osmolarity control. PCSK9 level remained comparable to low glucose (LG; 5 mM) upon adjusting the osmolarity with mannitol suggesting that hyperosmolarity associated with high glucose (HG; 25 mM) had minimal effect on glucose-induced PCSK9 protein expression (Fig. 3a and Additional file 3: Figure S2B). Further, in HepG2 cells cultured in HG, PCSK9 mRNA level was significantly upregulated as compared to LG, at 12 h (Fig. 3b). PCSK9 being a secretory protein, its extracellular level in culture medium was measured by ELISA. A significant increase in secretory as well as intracellular PCSK9 was detected in HG as compared to LG culture condition at 12 h and 24 h (Fig. 3c). Also, the percentage of glucose availability decreased in LG and HG medium during 0 h to 24 h; however, it remained

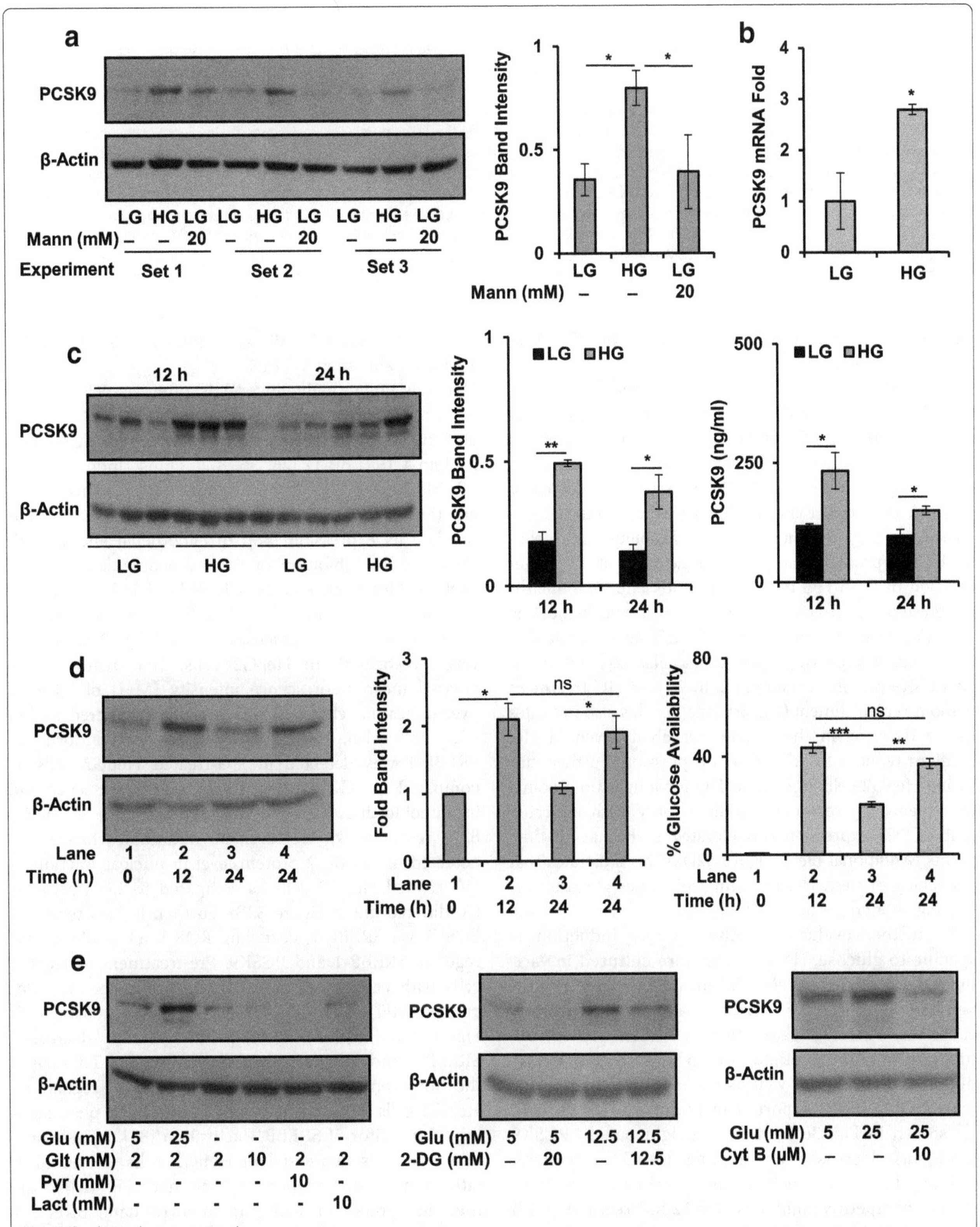

Fig. 3 (See legend on next page.)

(See figure on previous page.)

Fig. 3 Glucose-dependent regulation of PCSK9 in HCC cells. **a** HepG2 cells were cultured in LG, HG, and LG + Mannitol (Mann) for 12 h. Expression of PCSK9 protein was examined by immunoblot in three independent sets of experiments. Band intensities were measured by densitometry and normalized with β-actin. **b** HepG2 cells were cultured in LG and HG for 12 h. PCSK9 mRNA level was quantified by qRT-PCR. **c** HepG2 cells were cultured in LG and HG for 12 h and 24 h. Immunoblot analysis was performed with total protein lysates. PCSK9 protein band intensities were quantified by densitometry and normalized to β-actin. Extracellular PCSK9 in culture supernatant was quantified by ELISA. **d** HepG2 cells were seeded in 35-mm plates and allowed to adhere. LG medium was added in all the plates for 24 h. Then, LG medium was removed and cells were incubated in HG medium for 12 h and 24 h, respectively. HG medium was replaced with fresh HG medium after 12 h, and the plate was incubated for further 12 h (lane 4). Whole cell lysates were subjected for immunoblotting to analyze expression of PCSK9. Band intensities were quantified by densitometry and normalized to β-actin. Glucose remaining in the culture supernatant was estimated at each time point. **e** HepG2 cells were treated with indicated concentrations of glucose (Glu), glutamine (Glt), pyruvate (pyr), lactate (lact) 2-deoxyglucose (2-DG), and cytochalasin B (CytB) for 12 h and expression of PCSK9 was analyzed by Western blot. Bar graphs represent mean ± SEM; $n = 3$; $^*p < 0.05$, $^{**}p < 0.01$ denote significant differences in the groups; ns non-significant

significantly higher in HG as compared to LG (Additional file 3: Figure S2C).

Having demonstrated the glucose-stimulated expression of PCSK9, its specific dependency on glucose was further evaluated. HepG2 cells when cultured in LG medium for 24 h, not only glucose availability in the medium was reduced but also cellular PCSK9 expression was decreased (Fig. 3d, lane 1 of right and left panel, respectively). Increase in the percent glucose availability and cellular PCSK9 protein expression was detected at 12 h after addition of fresh HG medium (Fig. 3d, lane 2). Similarly, replenishing fresh HG medium after 12 h and incubating HepG2 cells for the next 12 h (Fig. 3d, lane 4), resulted in a significant increase in glucose availability and cellular PCSK9 protein, as compared to 24 h of HG treatment without replenishment (Fig. 3d, lane 3). This also indicates that a decrease in the glucose availability even in HG medium reduces PCSK9 protein expression. Further, culturing HepG2 cells in LG and HG for longer time points by replenishing respective medium every 12 h indicated that PCSK9 expression was elevated in HG at all time points (Additional file 3: Figure S2D). This illustrates that restocking of fresh HG medium replenishes glucose thus causing an increase in PCSK9 protein.

To further evaluate whether PCSK9 induction is specific to glucose, HepG2 cells were cultured in various other carbon sources. Culturing HepG2 cells individually in glutamine, pyruvate and lactate did not cause any detectable alteration in PCSK9 protein expression in absence of glucose up to 12 h (Fig. 3e). A number of specific as well as non-specific glucose uptake inhibitors are reported in literature [19, 34, 35]. As shown in Fig. 3e (middle and right panel), PCSK9 level was decreased on treating HepG2 cells with 2-deoxyglucose (competitive inhibitor) or cytochalasin B (non-competitive inhibitor) for 12 h. Treatment with fasentin (GLUT1 inhibitor) resulted in the reduction in PCSK9 level in a dose-dependent manner (Additional file 3: Figure S2E). Thus, the above stated findings suggest that induction of PCSK9 expression is specific to glucose availability and uptake.

Glucose stimulates PCSK9 expression via ROS and SREBP-1 without alteration in LDLR

Hyperglycemia (high glucose) is often associated with overproduction of reactive oxygen species (ROS). It is also known to induce sterol regulatory element binding protein-1 (SREBP-1) [25, 36, 37]. Transcription factors, SREBP-1 and SREBP-2, bind to the sterol response element (SRE) in the promoter region of PCSK9 gene and regulate its expression [38]. In endothelial and smooth muscle cells, inhibition of ROS, downregulates PCSK9 protein. Moreover, increased ROS level is implicated in upregulating SREBP-1 [39, 40]. Thus, involvement of ROS and SREBP-1 in glucose-induced PCSK9 expression was investigated. In HepG2 cells, HG treatment increased mean fluorescence intensity (MFI) of DCFDA dye, indicating elevated ROS level as compared to LG (Fig. 4a). Also, increased level of nuclear form of SREBP-1 was detected in HG-treated HepG2 cells as compared to LG treatment by immunofluorescence and immunoblotting (Fig. 4b and Additional file 4: Figure S3A, respectively). However, no noticeable change was detected in SREBP-2 protein level in nuclear fraction of HG-treated HepG2 cells as compared to LG treatment (Additional file 4: Figure S3B). Further, if ROS regulates PCSK9 via SREBP-1, curtailing ROS level would downregulate SREBP-1 and PCSK9. Pre-treatment of HepG2 cells with catalase (CATA), a ROS scavenger [41], decreased MFI of DCFDA dye in HG (Additional file 5: Figure S4A and B). Subsequently, it also decreased SREBP-1 and PCSK9 protein level (Fig. 4c). To analyze the involvement of SREBP-1 in PCSK9 regulation, HepG2 cells were treated with fatostatin, a pharmacological inhibitor of SREBP-1 activation [37]. PCSK9 protein level was decreased in HepG2 cells treated with fatostatin in dose-dependent manner (Fig. 4d). Further, in agreement with the in vitro data, SREBP-1 level was upregulated in tumor tissue lysates of mice from group IV in comparison with group III (Fig. 4e).

Subsequently, to study if glucose regulates LDLR via PCSK9, LDLR level and its activity under LG and HG

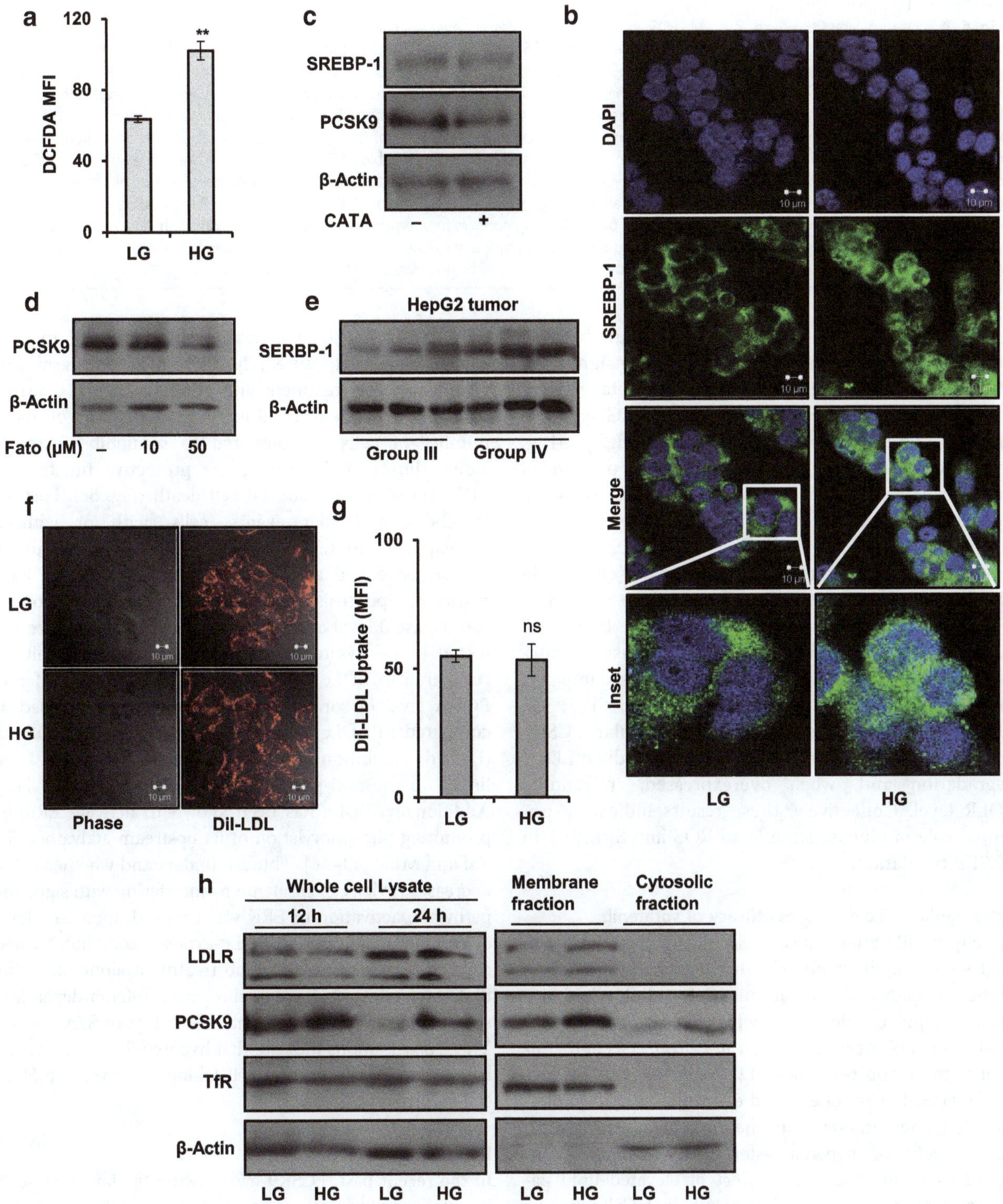

Fig. 4 (See legend on next page.)

(See figure on previous page.)

Fig. 4 Glucose stimulates PCSK9 expression via ROS and SREBP-1 but does not alter LDLR. **a** Measurement of ROS level in HepG2 cells treated with LG and HG medium for 12 h. **b** Immunofluorecence staining of SREBP-1 in HepG2 cells cultured in LG and HG for 12 h (Scale bar = 10 μm). **c** HepG2 cells were pre-treated with 1500 U/ml of catalase (CATA) for 3 h; subsequently, HG treatment was given for 6 h. Whole cell lysates were resolved by SDS-PAGE and SREPB-1; PCSK9 and β-actin protein levels were analyzed by immunoblot. **d** HepG2 cells were pre-treated with indicated concentrations of fatostatin (Fato) for 3 h, subsequently HG treatment was given for 6 h. Whole cell lysates were resolved by SDS-PAGE. PCSK9 and β-actin protein levels were analyzed by immunoblot. **e** Tumor tissue homogenates of three representative samples from group III and group IV were resolved on SDS-PAGE, and SREBP-1 protein level was analyzed by Western blot. **f** Whole cell lysates were prepared from HepG2 cells treated with LG and HG for 12 h and 24 h, respectively, or membrane and cytosolic fractions were prepared from HepG2 cells treated with LG and HG for 24 h by replenishing respective medium after 12 h. Expression of PCSK9 and LDLR were analyzed by immunoblot. Transferring receptor (TfR) and β-actin were included in the Western blot as loading controls for membrane and cytosolic fractions. **g, h** HepG2 cells were incubated in LG and HG medium for 12 h and processed for DiI-LDL uptake assay either by FACS or confocal staining. All bar graphs represent means ± SEM; $^{**}p < 0.01$ denotes significant differences between the groups; ns non-significant

culture conditions were checked by immunoblotting and DiI-LDL uptake assay, respectively. No significant changes in LDLR level or DiI-LDL uptake were detected in HepG2 cells cultured under LG and HG for 12 h (Additional file 6: Figure S5A and Fig. 4f, g, respectively). Further, expression of LDLR protein, in whole cell lysates and membrane-cytosolic fractions, were analyzed at different time points by Western blot. Despite changes in the level of PCSK9 in whole cell lysate or membrane-cytosolic fractions, changes in LDLR level were not detected at 12 h and 24 h (Fig. 4h). However, overexpressing human PCSK9 in HepG2 cells by transient transfection caused reduction in LDLR level and DiI-LDL uptake as compared to control (Additional file 6: Figure S5B and C) [1, 32]. This observation suggested that extracellular PCSK9 present in HG medium is insufficient to induce LDLR degradation and, when overexpressed, it reduces LDLR level. Collectively, these results indicate a potential role of glucose stimulated ROS and SREBP-1 in PCSK9 regulation.

Extracellular LDLc decreases efficacy of sorafenib

Rapidly proliferating cancer cells satisfy their lipid and cholesterol requirements by either increasing the uptake of dietary lipids or reprogramming intracellular lipid biogenesis. Lipid droplets (LD) which consist of excessive lipids and cholesterol are stored in cancer cells and contribute to chemo-resistance [42]. Very few studies have investigated impact of elevated extracellular lipid parameters on chemotherapy. In the present in vivo study, development of hypercholesterolemic phenotype impelled us to investigate the effect of elevated lipid parameters on the efficacy of sorafenib in HCC cells. To mimic hypercholesterolemic condition in vitro, cells were provided with LDL cholesterol exogenously and evaluated for the response to sorafenib [43]. Based on initial screening experiments and literature, sorafenib (5 μM) and LDLc (100 μg/ml) concentrations were selected for HepG2 and HuH-7 cells (Additional file 7: Figure S6). Upon sorafenib treatment, survival increased significantly in LDLc exposed cells compared to cells without LDLc exposure (Fig. 5a, b). In long-term survival assay, pre-treatment and presence of LDLc during sorafenib treatment resulted in the survival of more number of cells as compared to sorafenib treatment alone, thus complementing the protective function of LDLc on sorafenib-induced cell death (Fig. 5c). Further, to check molecular events, cells, with or without pre-exposure to LDLc, were treated with sorafenib in the presence and absence of LDLc for 48 h and hallmarks of apoptosis were analyzed. Downregulation of procaspase 3 level and increased PARP cleavage were detected in the lysates of cells treated with sorafenib as compared to LDLc exposed cells treated with sorafenib. PCNA level in sorafenib-treated cells was decreased as compared to LDLc exposed cells treated with sorafenib (Fig. 5d). Inhibition of RAF/MEK/ERK pathway has been linked to the anti-proliferative action of sorafenib [11]. Additionally, LDLc has been shown to activate ERK by promoting phosphorylation of its upstream activators like Raf and MEK [43–46]. Thus, to understand whether LDLc decreases toxicity of sorafenib by interfering with signaling pathways, activation of ERK was checked. Increased level of pERK was detected in LDLc-exposed sorafenib-treated cells as compared to sorafenib treatment alone, implying that extracellular LDLc can abrogate sorafenib-dependent signal transduction (Additional file 8: Figure S7A and B). These observations indicate that hypercholesterolemia can hamper sorafenib-induced cell killing and promote HCC cell survival.

Discussion

In the recent past, PCSK9 has drawn attention because of its role in dyslipidemia and proposition of it being a target in the management of hypercholesterolemia associated with cardiovascular disease [47]. Nutritional status, pertaining to either fasting and feeding or various dietary interventions, has been reported to alter circulatory PCSK9 level in humans [48, 49]. Also, a study by Cariou et al. indicated an obvious relation between sugar-rich diet and serum PCSK9 level [46]. In the present study, to mimic the elevated blood

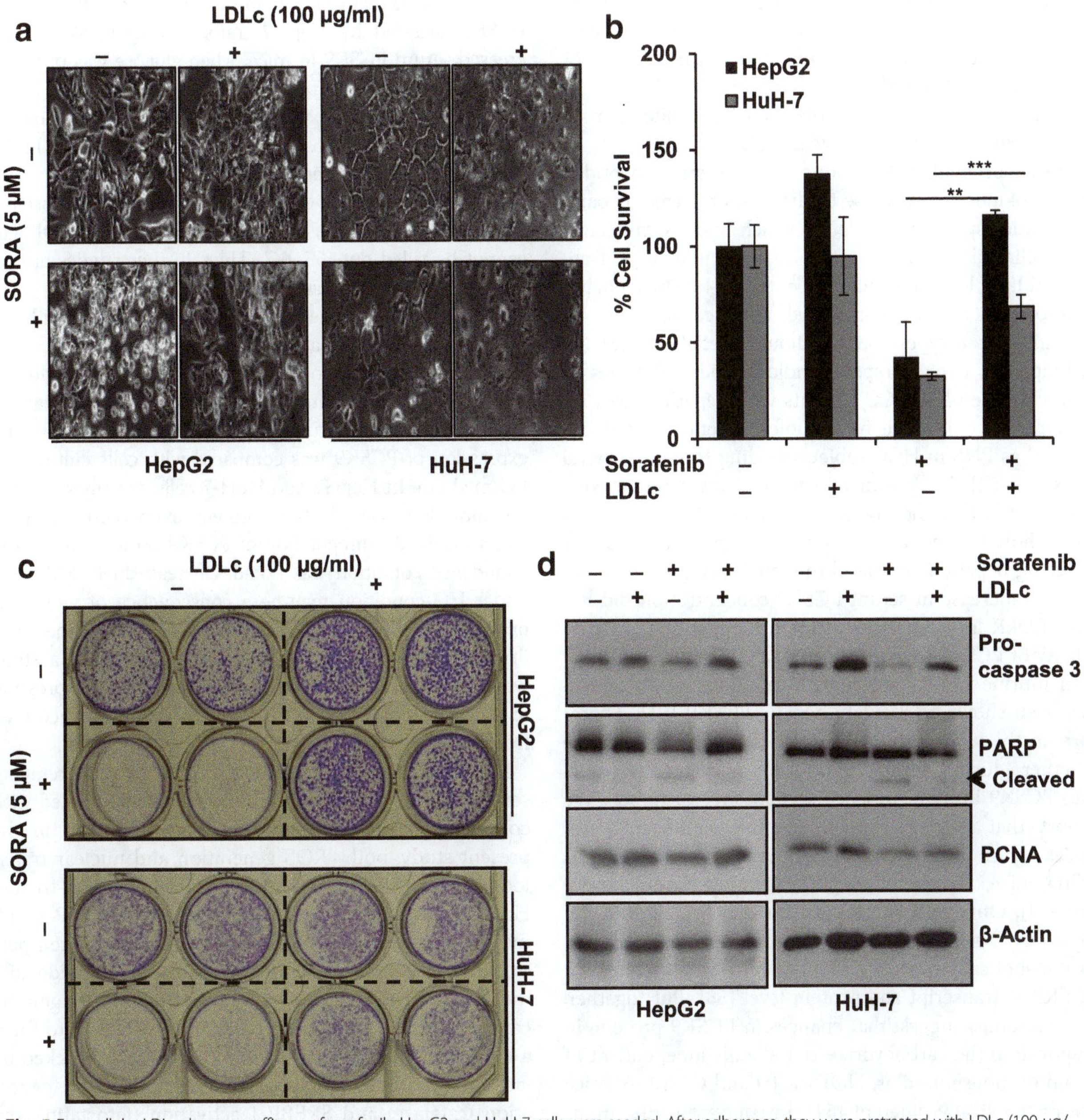

Fig. 5 Extracellular LDLc decreases efficacy of sorafenib. HepG2 and HuH-7 cells were seeded. After adherence, they were pretreated with LDLc (100 μg/ml) in 5% LPDS for 24 h, followed by 5 μM of sorafenib (SORA) treatment for the next 48 h in the presence or absence of LDLc as indicated and processed as follows: **a** Cell images were taken by Olympus (DP-71) camera (magnification × 20). **b** Percentage of cell survival was determined using MTT assay. Vehicle-treated cells served as control and OD values of control were considered as 100% viable. Error bars represent variations within the wells of an experiment. **c** Long-term cell survival assay. **d** Whole cell lysates were resolved on SDS-PAGE, subjected to immunoblot analysis and expression of procaspase-3, cleaved PARP; PCNA were analyzed. β-Actin was used as loading control. Bar graph represents means ± standard deviation; $^{**}p < 0.01$, $^{***}p < 0.001$ denotes significant differences between the groups

glucose condition; drinking water containing glucose was provided, and its impact on PCSK9 expression was studied in HepG2-xenografted mice. Analyzing serum PCSK9 in tumor-bearing mice revealed that glucose feeding significantly upregulated its level. Since the mRNA and protein levels of PCSK9 were elevated in tumor tissues of glucose provided, tumor-bearing mice than the tumor-bearing mice without glucose feeding, the transcriptional regulation of PCSK9 by glucose is likely to be responsible for the enhanced serum level of PCSK9. Hyperinsulinemia is often linked with sugar-rich diet feeding [50, 51]; however, in present study, serum insulin levels did not alter upon glucose feeding which concurs with earlier reports [52, 53]. It should also be noted that even though insulin induced

PCSK9 expression in rat/mouse hepatoma cells and primary hepatocytes [51, 54], it exhibited either neutral or inhibitory effect on serum PCSK9 in human subjects [55, 56]. Therefore, together with our observations, in this report, it is unlikely that insulin contributes to any alteration in PCSK9 expression in HepG2 xenograft.

Tumor-originated secretions of hormones, peptides, and cytokines can give rise to disorders referred as paraneoplastic syndromes (PNS) which can significantly affect clinical outcomes [57]. Various studies report abnormal lipid level in cancer patients and hyper/hypocholesterolemia can be considered as a consequence of certain cancer types [58]. Although detail studies are lacking, few clinical reports indicate reduced levels of total cholesterol in HCC patients with hepatitis virus infection [59, 60], while hypercholesterolemia was documented as PNS in HCC subjects leading to poor survival rates [61, 62]. In agreement with the latter, our in vivo data reveals that the presence of HepG2-tumor induces hypercholesterolemia upon glucose supplementation by reducing hepatic LDLR level in graft-bearing mice. However, an increase in serum PCSK9 concentration did not alter LDLR level in HepG2-tumor, highlighting the specificity of PCSK9 towards hepatic LDLR [63].

In murine physiology, nutritional status of an animal has been shown to regulate hepatic PCSK9 [51]. Therefore, in the work outlined here, it is essential to analyze whether glucose feeding modulates endogenous (murine) PCSK9 in both presence and absence of tumor. We report that glucose supplementation significantly reduces serum and hepatic PCSK9 protein level in NOD/SCID mice, devoid of HepG2-xenograft (group II vs. group I). Our observation correlates fairly well with the report by Dong et al., in which feeding fructose-rich diet to metabolically normal C57BL/6J mice reduced hepatic PCSK9 at transcript and protein level [53]. Put together, these findings suggest that changes in PCSK9 protein, in response to the carbohydrate-rich diet, is independent of strain of mouse used as, NOD/SCID and C57BL/6J mice are metabolically different [64]. In contrast to the minimum changes in hepatic LDLR as reported by Dong et al., in the present study, upregulation in hepatic LDLR protein was noted in mice without tumor-graft on glucose feeding. This difference can be due to either extended duration (2 months) of glucose feeding or differential response of liver towards glucose feeding as compared to 3 weeks of fructose feeding. Further, consistent with earlier study [8], in this work, we report increase in serum levels of murine PCSK9 in presence of tumor as compared to mice without tumor (Fig. 1d). Together with the previous literature and our observations regarding effect of sugar on PCSK9 expression, it can be concluded that, in mice physiology, high-sugar/carbohydrate feeding decreases PCSK9 protein. This strengthens our hypothesis that rather than the endogenous PCSK9, the PCSK9 secreted by HepG2-grafts is responsible for increased serum PCSK9 in mice, when glucose was provided and may be involved in reducing hepatic LDLR level in the host. The findings reported here do not exclude the involvement of other post-translational regulators of LDLR like IDOL (inducible degrader of LDL receptor). Liver X receptor (LXR) regulates expression of IDOL and glucose being an inducer of LXR; the role of glucose-LXR-IDOL axis cannot be ruled out [65, 66]. Thus, further studies are required to reveal such association if any.

In vitro studies in the present work also concur with the in vivo observation that PCSK9 expression is induced by glucose availability. Considering the exacerbated glucose uptake property of cancer cells, high glucose availability was maintained by culturing HCC cells in HG medium and expression of PCSK9 was compared with cells cultured in LG medium. In HepG2 and HuH-7 cells, treatment of HG medium, increased PCSK9 protein expression while, in Hep3B cells, downregulation of PCSK9 protein, in glucose abundance condition was noted. Decrease in PCSK9 level under HG-condition may be a consequence of viral genome integration in Hep3B cells [67] and needs further confirmation. This proposition gained strength from a study which reported a significantly decreased PCSK9 expression in HCC tissue samples, and majority of them were acquired from hepatitis virus B/C-infected HCC patients [68].

Hyperglycemia induced ROS generation, can regulate several signaling pathways, and has also been linked with complications in diabetes and obesity [69]. As, in the present study, both ROS generation and nuclear translocation of SREBP-1 were enhanced in HG-treated HepG2 cells, involvement of glucose-ROS-SREBP-1 link may be a possibility in PCSK9 regulation. Hydrogen peroxide formed by the action of cellular superoxide dismutase is further converted to water and oxygen by catalase enzyme [41]. The process of proteolysis to form a mature form of SREBP-1 from precursor is blocked by fatostatin [70]. By employing inhibitor of ROS generation (catalase) and SREBP-1 activation (fatostatin), the present study points towards a role of ROS and SREBP-1 in PCSK9 regulation under HG which warrants further evaluation.

Metabolic rewiring supports not only proliferation of tumor cells but also the enzymes involved in these networks confer therapeutic resistance to cancer cells [71]. In addition to these peculiar cellular modifications, host-derived factors which are induced by tumor can also amend chemotherapeutic response. For instance, our recent studies showed that resistin, which is primarily secreted by tumor-infiltrated host macrophages, arrests colon cancer cells in G1 phase and hampers 5-fluorouracil uptake [23]. Similarly, in the present study, tumor-induced hypercholesterolemia in the host can have an implication in chemotherapy. Mounting evidences support the idea that cholesterol-rich extracellular milieu imparts proliferative and aggressive phenotype to cancer cells [22, 45, 46]. Moreover, we have earlier reported that cholesterol can affect the functional outcome of anticancer drugs in various cancer cell types [72, 73]. Thus, considering the profound effect of cholesterol in cancer cell growth and response towards chemotherapy, it is clinically relevant to investigate the effect of extracellular LDLc on efficacy of sorafenib. Studies have tried to find a mechanistic association between lipid-enriched cellular pathways and low response rate to cancer therapy. Plasma LDLc is uptaken by LDLR through receptor-mediated endocytosis, and indeed silencing LDLR potentiates conventional chemotherapy [74]. A shift towards de novo lipogenesis was reported to be involved in tumor relapse after sorafenib withdrawal [75]. Adding to these findings, we report elevated extracellular LDLc impairs the efficacy of sorafenib towards HCC cells. Sorafenib as well as its metabolites have strong binding affinities to plasma proteins such as human serum albumin, α and β-gluobulins, and LDL. Binding of sorafenib to plasma proteins is implicated in limiting its uptake and pharmacological/ toxicological responses [76, 77]. Serum PCSK9 level is positively correlated with plasma LDL [4]. In the present report, increase in LDL fraction due to altered PCSK9 level or hypercholesterolemia (independent of PCSK9 signaling) would increase the probability of sorafenib binding to LDL, thus reducing the fraction of drug available for uptake by the tumor cells.

Collectively, these observations suggest that intracellular lipogenic networks as well as lipid-rich extracellular milieu can influence chemotherapeutic outcome in cancer cells. Further detailed mechanistic studies regarding LDLc promoted diminished sensitivity of HCC cells to sorafenib would help in strategizing newer combination therapies in the treatment of HCC.

Conclusions

Overall, this study illustrates tumor-secreted PCSK9 is induced by glucose availability, and its possible involvement in causing hypercholesterolemia in HCC. As shown in the schematic table (Fig. 6a), upon glucose feeding, PCSK9 level in serum as well as in tumor tissue was elevated in mice with tumor-graft (group IV) as compared to tumor-bearing mice without glucose feeding (group III). Also, group IV had a higher serum LDLc, partially owing to the decrease in hepatic LDLR level in these mice as compared to group III. Mice from group II had decreased levels of serum and hepatic PCSK9 while upregulated level of hepatic LDLR protein when compared with mice from group I. Overall, these

a

	High Glucose availability	
	Group II (Vs. Group I)	Group IV (Vs. Group III)
Serum	PCSK9↓	PCSK9↑ LDLc↑
Liver	PCSK9↓ LDLR↑	PCSK9# LDLR↓
Tumor tissue	NA	PCSK9↑ LDLR#

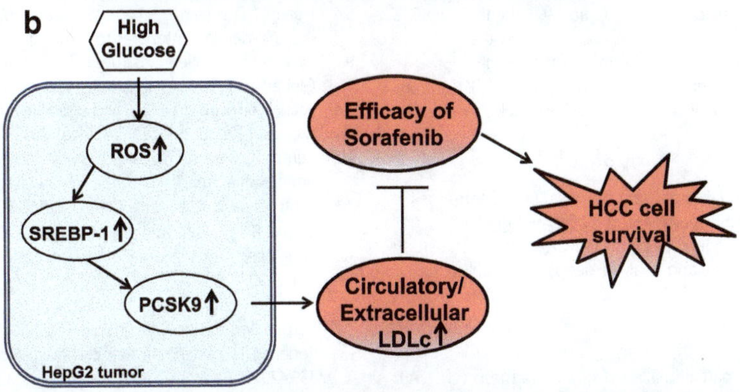

Fig. 6 Schematic illustration. **a** Table summarizes levels of LDLc and PCSK9 in serum, LDLR and PCSK9 protein in liver and tumor tissues of mice from group II and group IV when compared with group I and group III respectively. NA denotes not applicable, and the number sign denotes non-significant change. **b** The proposed model demonstrate HG-driven changes in HepG2 tumor leading to increased expression of PCSK9 and associated hypercholesrolemia which can further lead to HCC cell survival by decreasing the efficacy of sorafenib

observations would help in understanding the association between abnormal plasma lipid level and HCC in humans. Additionally, a specific interrelation among the etiology of HCC, blood glucose, and PCSK9 needs to be explored in future. Figure 6b demonstrates a proposed model, linking glucose-induced expression of PCSK9 to its upstream regulators; ROS and SREBP-1 and downstream consequence like hypercholesterolemia can decrease efficacy of sorafenib in HCC cells. Therefore, controlling systemic cholesterol level, prior to sorafenib treatment, may have clinical implications in HCC patients.

Additional files

Additional file 1: Table S1. Primer pair sets (DOCX 13 kb)

Additional file 2: Figure S1. Effect of glucose feeding on serum insulin and hepatic LDLR levels. (DOCX 120 kb)

Additional file 3: Figure S2. Glucose specificity of PCSK9 regulation (DOCX 114 kb)

Additional file 4: Figure S3. Effect of glucose on SREBP-1 and SREBP-2 (DOCX 50 kb)

Additional file 5: Figure S4. Effect of catalase on ROS generation in HG (DOCX 21 kb)

Additional file 6: Figure S5. Effect of glucose and PCSK9 overexpression on LDLR (DOCX 118 kb)

Additional file 7: Figure S6. Screening of sorafenib and LDLc concentration (DOCX 76 kb)

Additional file 8: Figure S7. Effect of LDLc on sorafenib mediated signaling (DOCX 112 kb)

Abbreviations

2-DG: 2-Deoxyglucose; CATA: Catalase; CytB: Cytochalasin B; Fato: Fatostatin; Glt: Glutamine; Glu: Glucose; HCC: Hepatocellular carcinoma; HG: High glucose; Lact: Lactate; LDLc: Low-density lipoprotein cholesterol; LDLR: Low-density lipoprotein receptor; LG: Low glucose; Mann: Mannitol; PCSK9: Proprotein-convertase-subtilisin-kexin type-9; Pyr: Pyruvate; ROS: Reactive oxygen species; SORA: Sorafenib; SREBP-1: Sterol regulatory element binding protein

Acknowledgements

The authors thank Dr. S.C. Mande, Director, NCCS, Pune, India, for being very supportive and giving all the encouragement to carry out this work. D.A. thanks the Department of Biotechnology (DBT); S.C. and V.P. thank Council for Scientific and Industrial Research (CSIR); S.S.M. and S.S. thank the University Grants Commission (UGC), New Delhi, India, for research fellowship. The support from the Experimental Animal Facility (EAF), Central Instrumental Facility, and technical staff of NCCS is also duly acknowledged.

Funding

This work was supported by an Intramural Grant from National Centre for Cell Science (NCCS) funded by the Department of Biotechnology (DBT), Government of India. The funding agencies had no involvement in the study design, data collection, interpretation, and analysis, decision to publish, or writing of the manuscript.

Note

This work was carried out for the partial fulfillment of a Ph.D. thesis (of D. A.) to be submitted to Savitribai Phule Pune University, Pune, India. Parts of this work were presented in the following meetings: "World Congress on Cancer", February 2018, Rajasthan, India; "EMBO workshop: Metabolic Disorders and Liver Cancer", April 2017, Palma de Mallorca, Spain; "International Conference on Cancer research", November 2015, NCCS, Pune, India, and "International Symposium on Molecular Pathways to Therapeutics: Paradigms and Challenges in Oncology", February, 2015, ACTREC-TMC, Navi Mumbai, India.

Authors' contributions

Experiments were conceived and designed by MKB and DA. Experiments were primarily performed by DA with contribution from SSM, SS, and SC. VP contributed towards initial data generation. DA and MKB wrote the manuscript. All authors read, reviewed, edited, and approved the final manuscript.

Competing interests

The authors declare that they have no competing interest.

Author details

[1]Laboratory No. 6, National Centre for Cell Science, Savitribai Phule Pune University Campus, Ganeshkhind, Pune 411 007, India. [2]Present address: Laboratory of Neuroscience, Department of Biotechnology & Bioinformatics, School of Life Sciences, University of Hyderabad, Hyderabad, Telangana 500046, India.

References

1. Benjannet S, Rhainds D, Essalmani R, Mayne J, Wickham L, Jin W, et al. NARC-1/PCSK9 and its natural mutants: zymogen cleavage and effects on the low density lipoprotein (LDL) receptor and LDL cholesterol. J Biol Chem. 2004;279:48865–75.
2. Seidah NG, Benjannet S, Wickham L, Marcinkiewicz J, Jasmin SB, Stifani S, et al. The secretory proprotein convertase neural apoptosis-regulated convertase 1 (NARC-1): liver regeneration and neuronal differentiation. Proc Natl Acad Sci. 2003;100:928–33.
3. Abifadel M, Varret M, Rabès JP, Allard D, Ouguerram K, Devillers M, et al. Mutations in PCSK9 cause autosomal dominant hypercholesterolemia. Nat Genet. 2003;34:154–6.
4. Horton JD, Cohen JC, Hobbs HH. PCSK9: a convertase that coordinates LDL catabolism. J Lipid Res. 2009;50:172–7.
5. Xu X, Cui Y, Cao L, Zhang Y, Yin Y, Hu X. PCSK9 regulates apoptosis in human lung adenocarcinoma A549 cells via endoplasmic reticulum stress and mitochondrial signaling pathways. Exp Ther Med. 2017;13:1993–9.
6. Piao MX, Bai JW, Zhang PF, Zhang YZ. PCSK9 regulates apoptosis in human neuroglioma u251 cells via mitochondrial signaling pathways. Int J Clin Exp Pathol. 2015;8:2787–94.
7. Sun X, Essalmani R, Day R, Khatib AM, Seidah NG, Prat A. Proprotein convertase subtilisin/kexin type 9 deficiency reduces melanoma metastasis in liver. Neoplasia. 2012;14:1122–31.
8. Huang J, Li L, Lian J, Schauer S, Vesely PW, Kratky D, et al. Tumor-induced hyperlipidemia contributes to tumor growth. Cell Rep. 2016;15:336–48.
9. Fitzmaurice C, Allen C, Barber RM, Barregard L, Bhutta ZA, Brenner H, et al. Global, regional, and national cancer incidence, mortality, years of life lost, years lived with disability, and disability-adjusted life-years for 32 cancer groups, 1990 to 2015. JAMA Oncol. 2017;3:524–48.
10. Petrick JL, Braunlin M, Laversanne M, Valery PC, Bray F, McGlynn KA. International trends in liver cancer incidence, overall and by histologic subtype, 1978–2007. Int J Cancer. 2016;139:1534–45.
11. Le GM, Biagini MR, Tarocchi M, Polvani S, Galli A. Chemotherapy for hepatocellular carcinoma: the present and the future. World J Hepatol. 2017;9:907–20.
12. Torre LA, Islami F, Siegel RL, Ward EM, Jemal A. Global cancer in women: burden and trends. Cancer Epidemiol Biomark Prev. 2017;26:444–57.
13. Roberts LR. Sorafenib in liver cancer–just the beginning. N Engl J Med. 2008; 359:420–2.
14. Zhai B, Sun XY. Mechanisms of resistance to sorafenib and the corresponding strategies in hepatocellular carcinoma. World J Hepatol. 2013;5:345–52.

15. Reeves HL, Zaki MYW, Day CP. Hepatocellular carcinoma in obesity, type 2 diabetes, and NAFLD. Dig Dis Sci. 2016;61:1234–45.
16. Yang JD, Mohamed HA, Cvinar JL, Gores GJ, Roberts LR, Kim WR. Diabetes mellitus heightens the risk of hepatocellular carcinoma except in patients with hepatitis c cirrhosis. Am J Gastroenterol. 2016;111:1573–80.
17. Hanahan D, Weinberg RA. Hallmarks of cancer: the next generation. Cell. 2011;144:646–74.
18. Ryu TY, Park J, Scherer PE. Hyperglycemia as a risk factor for cancer progression. Diabetes Metab J. 2014;38:330–6.
19. Chouhan S, Singh S, Athavale D, Ramteke P, Pandey V. Glucose induced activation of canonical Wnt signaling pathway in hepatocellular carcinoma is regulated by DKK4. Sci Rep. 2016;6:1–15.
20. Cohen DH, LeRoith D. Obesity, type 2 diabetes, and cancer: the insulin and IGF connection. Endocr Relat Cancer. 2012;19:27–45.
21. Krysa JA, Ooi TC, Proctor SD, Vine DF. Nutritional and lipid modulation of PCSK9: effects on cardiometabolic risk factors. J Nutr. 2017;147:473–81.
22. Malvi P, Chaube B, Pandey V, Vijayakumar V, Boreddy PR, Mohammad N, et al. Obesity induced rapid melanoma progression is reversed by orlistat treatment and dietary intervention: role of adipokines. Mol Oncol. 2015;9: 689–703.
23. Singh S, Chouhan S, Mohammad N, Bhat MK. Resistin causes G1 arrest in colon cancer cells through upregulation of SOCS3. FEBS Lett. 2017;591:1371–82.
24. Pandey V, Vijayakumar MV, Ajay AK, Malvi P, Bhat MK. Diet-induced obesity increases melanoma progression: involvement of Cav-1 and FASN. Int J Cancer. 2012;130:497–508.
25. Pandey V, Chaube B, Bhat MK. Hyperglycemia regulates MDR-1, drug accumulation and ROS levels causing increased toxicity of carboplatin and 5-fluorouracil in MCF-7 cells. J Cell Biochem. 2011;112:2942–52.
26. Nishiumi S, Ashida H. Rapid preparation of a plasma membrane fraction from adipocytes and muscle cells: application to detection of translocated glucose transporter 4 on the plasma membrane. Biosci Biotechnol Biochem. 2007;71:2343–6.
27. Singh S, Bhat MK. Carboplatin induces apoptotic cell death through downregulation of constitutively active nuclear factor-κB in human HPV-18 E6-positive HEp-2 cells. Biochem Biophys Res Commun. 2004;318:346–53.
28. Vijayakumar MV, Pandey V, Mishra GC, Bhat MK. Hypolipidemic effect of fenugreek seeds is mediated through inhibition of fat accumulation and upregulation of LDL receptor. Obesity. 2010;18:667–74.
29. Urban D, Pöss J, Böhm M, Laufs U. Targeting the proprotein convertase subtilisin/kexin type 9 for the treatment of dyslipidemia and atherosclerosis. J Am Coll Cardiol. 2013;62:1401–8.
30. Jeon H, Blacklow SC. Structure and physiologic function of the low-density lipoprotein receptor. Annu Rev Biochem. 2005;74:535–62.
31. Grefhorst A, McNutt MC, T a L, Horton JD. Plasma PCSK9 preferentially reduces liver LDL receptors in mice. J Lipid Res. 2008;49:1303–11.
32. Lagace TA, Curtis DE, Garuti R, Mcnutt MC, Park SW, Prather HB, et al. Secreted PCSK9 decreases the number of LDL receptors in hepatocytes and in livers of parabiotic mice. J Clin Invest. 2006;116:2995–3005.
33. Madonna R, Giovannelli G, Confalone P, Renna FV, Geng Y-J, De Caterina R. High glucose-induced hyperosmolarity contributes to COX-2 expression and angiogenesis: implications for diabetic retinopathy. Cardiovasc Diabetol. 2016;15:18–32.
34. Wood TE, Dalili S, Simpson CD, Hurren R, Mao X, Saiz FS, et al. A novel inhibitor of glucose uptake sensitizes cells to FAS-induced cell death. Mol Cancer Ther. 2008;7:3546–55.
35. Takemura A, Che XF, Tabuchi T, Moriya S, Miyazawa K, Tomoda A. Enhancement of cytotoxic and pro-apoptotic effects of 2-aminophenoxazine-3-one on the rat hepatocellular carcinoma cell line dRLh-84, the human hepatocellular carcinoma cell line HepG2, and the rat normal hepatocellular cell line RLN-10 in combination with with 2-deoxy-D-glucose. Oncol Rep. 2012;27:347–55.
36. Hasty AH, Shimano H, Yahagi N, Amemiya-Kudo M, Perrey S, Yoshikawa T, et al. Sterol regulatory element-binding protein-1 is regulated by glucose at the transcriptional level. J Biol Chem. 2000;275:31069–77.
37. Uttarwar L, Gao B, Ingram AJ, Krepinsky JC. SREBP-1 activation by glucose mediates TGF-β upregulation in mesangial cells. AJP Ren Physiol. 2012;302: 329–41.
38. Horton JD, Shah NA, Warrington JA, Anderson NN, Park SW, Brown MS, et al. Combined analysis of oligonucleotide microarray data from transgenic and knockout mice identifies direct SREBP target genes. Proc Natl Acad Sci. 2003;100:12027–32.
39. Sekiya M, Hiraishi A, Touyama M, Sakamoto K. Oxidative stress induced lipid accumulation via SREBP1c activation in HepG2 cells. Biochem Biophys Res Commun. 2008;375:602–7.
40. Ding Z, Liu S, Wang X, Deng X, Fan Y, Sun C, et al. Hemodynamic shear stress via ROS modulates pcsk9 expression in human vascular endothelial and smooth muscle cells and along the mouse aorta. Antioxid Redox Signal. 2015;22:760–71.
41. Bai J, Cederbaum AI. Catalase protects HepG2 cells from apoptosis induced by DNA-damaging agents by accelerating the degradation of p53. J Biol Chem. 2003;278:4660–7.
42. Beloribi-Djefaflia S, Vasseur S, Guillaumond F. Lipid metabolic reprogramming in cancer cells. Oncogene. 2016;5:189–201.
43. Naito S, Makhov P, Astsaturov I, Golovine K, Tulin A, Kutikov A, et al. LDL cholesterol counteracts the antitumour effect of tyrosine kinase inhibitors against renal cell carcinoma. Br J Cancer. 2017;116:1203–7.
44. Pintus G, Tadolini B, Posadino AM, Sanna B, Debidda M, Carru C, et al. PKC/Raf/MEK/ERK signaling pathway modulates native-LDL-induced E2F-1 gene expression and endothelial cell proliferation. Cardiovasc Res. 2003;59:934–44.
45. Rodrigues C, Domingues G, Matias I, Matos J, Fonseca I, de Almeida JM, et al. LDL-cholesterol signaling induces breast cancer proliferation and invasion. Lipids Health Dis. 2014;13:1–9.
46. Wang C, Li P, Xuan J, Zhu C, Liu J, Shan L, et al. Cholesterol enhances colorectal cancer progression via ROS elevation and MAPK signaling pathway activation. Cell Physiol Biochem. 2017;42:729–42.
47. Seidah NG. Proprotein convertase subtilisin kexin 9 (PCSK9) inhibitors in the treatment of hypercholesterolemia and other pathologies. Curr Pharm Des. 2013;19:3161–72.
48. Persson L, Cao G, Ståhle L, Sjöberg BG, Troutt JS, Konrad RJ, et al. Circulating proprotein convertase subtilisin kexin type 9 has a diurnal rhythm synchronous with cholesterol synthesis and is reduced by fasting in humans. Arterioscler Thromb Vasc Biol. 2010;30:2666–72.
49. Cariou B, Langhi C, Le Bras M, Bortolotti M, Lê K-A, Theytaz F, et al. Plasma PCSK9 concentrations during an oral fat load and after short term high-fat, high-fat high-protein and high-fructose diets. Nutr Metab (Lond). 2013;10:4–15.
50. Cao D, Lu H, Lewis TL, Li N. Intake of sucrose-sweetened water induces insulin resistance and exacerbates memory deficits and amyloidosis in a transgenic mouse model of Alzheimer disease. J Biol Chem. 2007;282: 36275–82.
51. Costet P, Cariou B, Lambert G, Lalanne F, Lardeux B, Jarnoux AL, et al. Hepatic PCSK9 expression is regulated by nutritional status via insulin and sterol regulatory element-binding protein 1c. J Biol Chem. 2006; 281:6211–8.
52. Nyman LR, Tian L, Hamm DA, Schoeb TR, Gower BA, Nagy TR, et al. Long-term effects of high-fat or high-carbohydrate diets on glucose tolerance in mice with heterozygous carnitine palmitoyltransferase-1a deficiency. Nutr Diabetes. 2011;1:e14 1–11.
53. Dong B, Bahadur A, Azhar S, Seidah NG, Liu J. High-fructose feeding promotes accelerated degradation of hepatic LDL receptor and hypercholesterolemia in hamsters via elevated circulating PCSK9 levels. Atherosclerosis. 2015;239:364–74.
54. Type SK, Miao J, Manthena PV, Haas ME, Ling AV, Shin D, et al. Role of insulin in the regulation of proprotein convertase. Arter Thromb Vasc Bio. 2015;35:1589–96.
55. Kappelle PJ, Lambert G, Dullaart RP. Plasma proprotein convertase subtilisin – kexin type 9 does not change during 24 h insulin infusion in healthy subjects and type 2 diabetic patients. Atherosclerosis. 2011;214:432–5.
56. Awan Z, Dubuc G, Faraj M, Dufour R, Seidah NG, Davignon J, et al. The effect of insulin on circulating PCSK9 in postmenopausal obese women. Clin Biochem. 2014;47:1033–9.
57. Pelosof LC, Gerber DE. Paraneoplastic syndromes: an approach to diagnosis and treatment. Mayo Clin Proc. 2010;85:838–54.
58. Munir R, Usman H, Hasnain S, Smans K, Kalbacher H, Zaidi N. Atypical plasma lipid profile in cancer patients: cause or consequence? Biochimie. 2014;102:9–18.
59. Khattab MA, Eslam M, Mousa YI, Ela-Adawy N, Fathy S, Shatat M, et al. Association between metabolic abnormalities and hepatitis C-related hepatocellular carcinoma. Ann Hepatol. 2012;11:487–94.
60. Chen Z, Keech A, Collins R, Slavin B, Chen J, Campbell TC, et al. Prolonged infection with hepatitis B virus and association between low blood cholesterol concentration and liver cancer. BMJ. 1993;306:890–4.

61. Qu Q, Wang S, Chen S, Zhou L, Rui JA. Prognostic role and significance of paraneoplastic syndromes in hepatocellular carcinoma. Am Surg. 2014;80:191–6.
62. Luo JC, Hwang SJ, Wu JC, Lai CR, Li CP, Chang FY, et al. Clinical characteristics and prognosis of hepatocellular carcinoma patients with paraneoplastic syndromes. Hepato-Gastroenterology. 2002;49:1315–9.
63. Luo Y, Warren L, Xia D, Jensen H, Sand T, Petras S, et al. Function and distribution of circulating human PCSK9 expressed extrahepatically in transgenic mice. J Lipid Res. 2009;50:1581–8.
64. Chaparro RJ, Konigshofer Y, Beilhack GF, Shizuru JA, McDevitt HO, Chien YH. Nonobese diabetic mice express aspects of both type 1 and type 2 diabetes. Proc Natl Acad Sci U S A. 2006;103:12475–80.
65. Mitro N, Mak PA, Vargas L, Godio C, Hampton E, Molteni V, et al. The nuclear receptor LXR is a glucose sensor. Nature. 2007;445:219–23.
66. Zelcer N, Hong C, Boyadjian R, Tontonoz P. LXR regulates cholesterol uptake through Idol-dependent ubiquitination of the LDL receptor. Science. 2009; 325:100–4.
67. Huang P, Zhuang B, Zhang H, Yan H, Xiao Z, Li W, et al. Hepatitis B virus X protein (HBx) is responsible for resistance to targeted therapies in hepatocellular carcinoma: ex vivo culture evidence. Clin Cancer Res. 2015;21:4420–30.
68. Bhat M, Skill N, Marcus V, Deschenes M, Tan X, Bouteaud J, et al. Decreased PCSK9 expression in human hepatocellular carcinoma. BMC Gastroenterol. 2015;15:176–86.
69. Marseglia L, Manti S, D'Angelo G, Nicotera A, Parisi E, Di Rosa G, et al. Oxidative stress in obesity: a critical component in human diseases. Int J Mol Sci. 2015;16:378–400.
70. Kamisuki S, Mao Q, Abu-Elheiga L, Gu Z, Kugimiya A, Kwon Y, et al. A small molecule that blocks fat synthesis by inhibiting the activation of SREBP. Chem Biol. 2009;16:882–92.
71. Zhao Y, Butler EB, Tan M. Targeting cellular metabolism to improve cancer therapeutics. Cell Death Dis. 2013;4(e532):1–10.
72. Mohammad N, Malvi P, Meena A, Singh S, Chaube B, Vannuruswamy G, et al. Cholesterol depletion by methyl-β-cyclodextrin augments tamoxifen induced cell death by enhancing its uptake in melanoma. Mol Cancer. 2014; 13:204–16.
73. Mohammad N, Vikram Singh S, Malvi P, Chaube B, Athavale D, Vanuopadath M, et al. Strategy to enhance efficacy of doxorubicin in solid tumor cells by methyl-β-cyclodextrin: involvement of p53 and Fas receptor ligand complex. Sci Rep. 2015;5:11853–66.
74. Guillaumond F, Bidaut G, Ouaissi M, Servais S, Gouirand V, Olivares O, et al. Cholesterol uptake disruption, in association with chemotherapy, is a promising combined metabolic therapy for pancreatic adenocarcinoma. Proc Natl Acad Sci. 2015;112:2473–8.
75. Sounni NE, Cimino J, Blacher S, Primac I, Truong A, Mazzucchelli G, et al. Blocking lipid synthesis overcomes tumor regrowth and metastasis after antiangiogenic therapy withdrawal. Cell Metab. 2014;20:280–94.
76. Schuhmacher J, Kohlsdorfer C, Bühner K, Brandenburger T, Kruk R. High-throughput determination of the free fraction of drugs strongly bound to plasma proteins. J Pharm Sci. 2004;93:816–30.
77. Villarroel MC, Pratz KW, Xu L, Wright JJ, Smith BD, Rudek MA. Plasma protein binding of sorafenib, a multi kinase inhibitor: in vitro and in cancer patients. Investig New Drugs. 2012;30:2096–102.

13

Mutant IDH1 gliomas downregulate phosphocholine and phosphoethanolamine synthesis in a 2-hydroxyglutarate-dependent manner

Pavithra Viswanath[1], Marina Radoul[1], Jose Luis Izquierdo-Garcia[2,3], Hema Artee Luchman[4], J. Gregory Cairncross[5], Russell O. Pieper[6], Joanna J. Phillips[6] and Sabrina M. Ronen[1*]

Abstract

Background: Magnetic resonance spectroscopy (MRS) studies have identified elevated levels of the phospholipid precursor phosphocholine (PC) and phosphoethanolamine (PE) as metabolic hallmarks of cancer. Unusually, however, PC and PE levels are reduced in mutant isocitrate dehydrogenase 1 (IDHmut) gliomas that produce the oncometabolite 2-hydroxyglutarate (2-HG) relative to wild-type IDH1 (IDHwt) gliomas. The goal of this study was to determine the molecular mechanism underlying this unusual metabolic reprogramming in IDHmut gliomas.

Methods: Steady-state PC and PE were quantified using ^{31}P-MRS. To quantify de novo PC and PE synthesis, we used ^{13}C-MRS and measured flux to ^{13}C-PC and ^{13}C-PE in cells incubated with [1,2-^{13}C]-choline and [1,2-^{13}C]-ethanolamine. The activities of choline kinase (CK) and ethanolamine kinase (EK), the enzymes responsible for PC and PE synthesis, were quantified using ^{31}P-MR-based assays. To interrogate the role of 2-HG, we examined IDHwt cells incubated with 2-HG and, conversely, IDHmut cells treated with the IDHmut inhibitor AGI-5198. To examine the role of hypoxia-inducible factor 1-α (HIF-1α), we silenced HIF-1α using RNA interference. To confirm our findings in vivo and in the clinic, we studied IDHwt and IDHmut orthotopic tumor xenografts and glioma patient biopsies.

Results: De novo synthesis of PC and PE was reduced in IDHmut cells relative to IDHwt. Concomitantly, CK activity and EK activity were reduced in IDHmut cells. Pharmacological manipulation of 2-HG levels established that 2-HG was responsible for reduced CK activity, EK activity, PC and PE. 2-HG has previously been reported to stabilize levels of HIF-1α, a known regulator of CK activity. Silencing HIF-1α in IDHmut cells restored CK activity, EK activity, PC and PE to IDHwt levels. Our findings were recapitulated in IDHmut orthotopic tumor xenografts and, most importantly, in IDHmut patient biopsies, validating our findings in vivo and in the clinic.

Conclusions: This study identifies, to our knowledge for the first time, a direct role for 2-HG in the downregulation of CK and EK activity, and thereby, PC and PE synthesis in IDHmut gliomas. These results highlight the unusual reprogramming of phospholipid metabolism in IDHmut gliomas and have implications for the identification of MRS-detectable metabolic biomarkers associated with 2-HG status.

Keywords: IDH1 mutation, 2-Hydroxyglutarate, Metabolic reprogramming, Magnetic resonance spectroscopy, Phosphocholine, Phosphoethanolamine, Choline kinase, Ethanolamine kinase, HIF-1α, Brain tumors

* Correspondence: sabrina.ronen@ucsf.edu
[1]Department of Radiology and Biomedical Imaging, University of California San Francisco, 1700 4th Street, Box 2532. Byers Hall 3rd Floor, Suite, San Francisco, CA 94143, USA

Background

Mutations in isocitrate dehydrogenase 1 (*IDH1*) are characteristic of low-grade gliomas and secondary upgraded glioblastomas [1]. The wild-type IDH1 (IDHwt) enzyme converts isocitrate to α-ketoglutarate (α-KG), while the mutant IDH1 (IDHmut) enzyme converts α-KG to the oncometabolite 2-hydroxyglutarate (2-HG). By competitively inhibiting the activity of α-KG-dependent dioxygenases such as prolyl hydroxylases, JmJc-domain histone demethylases, and the TET family of 5-methylcytosine hydroxylases, 2-HG induces alterations in epigenetics and cell signaling that ultimately drive tumorigenesis [1, 2].

The IDH1 mutation also induces metabolic reprogramming that often differs from that observed in IDHwt gliomas [3]. For instance, the Warburg effect, characterized by increased glucose uptake and lactate production, is a metabolic feature of cancer cells, including IDHwt gliomas [4]. However, IDHmut gliomas downregulate lactate production compared to IDHwt [5, 6]. Likewise, elevated phospholipid metabolism is a hallmark of cancer. Phosphocholine (PC) and phosphoethanolamine (PE) are intermediates in the synthesis of phosphatidylcholine (PtdCho) and phosphatidylethanolamine (PtdE), which are quantitatively the most important phospholipids in the cell [7]. Levels of PC, and oftentimes PE, are elevated in every cancer studied to date, including IDHwt gliomas [8, 9]. This effect is typically mediated by overexpression and increased activity of choline kinase (CK) and, less frequently, ethanolamine kinase (EK), the enzymes that phosphorylate choline and ethanolamine to PC and PE, respectively (Fig. 1a) [8–10]. Unusually, however, we and others have previously found that steady-state PC levels are reduced in IDHmut cells relative to IDHwt [11, 12], while Esmaeili et al. showed reduced levels of PE in IDHmut gliomas relative to IDHwt [13].

Magnetic resonance spectroscopy (MRS) is a non-invasive metabolic imaging modality that can be used to quantify metabolism in cells, animals, and patients [14]. ^{1}H- and ^{31}P-MRS quantify steady-state metabolite levels, whereas ^{13}C-MRS monitors metabolic fluxes [15]. ^{31}P-MRS can detect PC and PE as well as the phospholipid breakdown products glycerophosphocholine (GPC) and glycerophosphoethanolamine (GPE). ^{1}H-MRS detects total choline (tCho)-containing metabolites comprised of choline, PC, and GPC. Elevated levels of PC and tCho can be detected using MRS in most tumors compared to normal tissue, including high-grade IDHwt glioblastomas, and have emerged as non-invasive imaging biomarkers of cancer [16–18]. The reduction in PC and PE observed in IDHmut gliomas was therefore considered as unusual and with potential for serving as an indicator of IDH status [3, 11–13].

The goal of this study was to investigate the molecular mechanism driving the modulation of PC and PE levels in IDHmut gliomas in order to potentially validate these compounds as metabolic imaging biomarkers of the IDH mutation [11–13]. Using genetically engineered and patient-derived cell models as well as orthotopic tumor xenografts, we show that 2-HG production in IDHmut gliomas leads to reduced CK and EK activity and thereby reduced PC and PE synthesis and steady-state levels. Our data indicates that this effect is mediated by hypoxia inducible factor-1α (HIF-1α). Importantly, we confirmed our findings in glioma patient biopsies, highlighting their clinical relevance. Collectively, our study illuminates the mechanism underlying the unusual downregulation of choline and ethanolamine metabolism in IDHmut gliomas and also points to the potential and challenges associated with PC and PE as biomarkers of these tumors.

Methods

Cell culture

The generation and characterization of U87 and NHA cells expressing IDHwt (U87IDHwt and NHAIDHwt) or IDH1 R132H mutant enzyme (U87IDHmut and NHAIDHmut) have been previously described [11]. Briefly, all cell lines were maintained between passages 15 and 30 in Dulbecco's modified Eagle's medium (DMEM) supplemented with 10% fetal calf serum, 2 mM glutamine, and 100 U/ml penicillin and streptomycin under normoxic conditions. In addition, the medium was supplemented with 28 μM choline (the normal concentration of choline in DMEM is 28 μM and, therefore, the final concentration of choline was 56 μM) and 56 μM ethanolamine in order to mimic the conditions used in our ^{13}C-MRS studies (see below). We established that the addition of choline and ethanolamine as described above did not alter the growth as determined by cell counting or proliferation as measured in doubling time of our cells for at least 15 passages. Nor did the addition of choline and ethanolamine alter total PC and PE levels as determined by examination of ^{31}P-MRS data from cell extracts as well as bioreactors. The BT54 patient-derived model was provided by H.A.L and J.G.C and cultured as neurospheres in serum-free medium as previously described [19] and the Neurocult medium supplemented with a concentration of 56 μM choline and 56 μM ethanolamine. All cell lines were routinely tested for mycoplasma contamination and authenticated by short tandem repeat fingerprinting (Cell Line Genetics) and assayed within 6 months of authentication.

Cell treatments

IDHwt and IDHmut siHIF-1α cells were treated with 1 mM D-2-HG (Sigma-Aldrich) for 24 h. U87IDHwt and U87IDHmut siHIF-1α cells were permeabilized with 0.01% digitonin (Sigma-Aldrich) in phosphate-buffered saline (PBS) for 10 min prior to treatment. IDHmut cells were treated with 10 μM AGI-5198 for 72 h. DMSO was used as vehicle control in all cases.

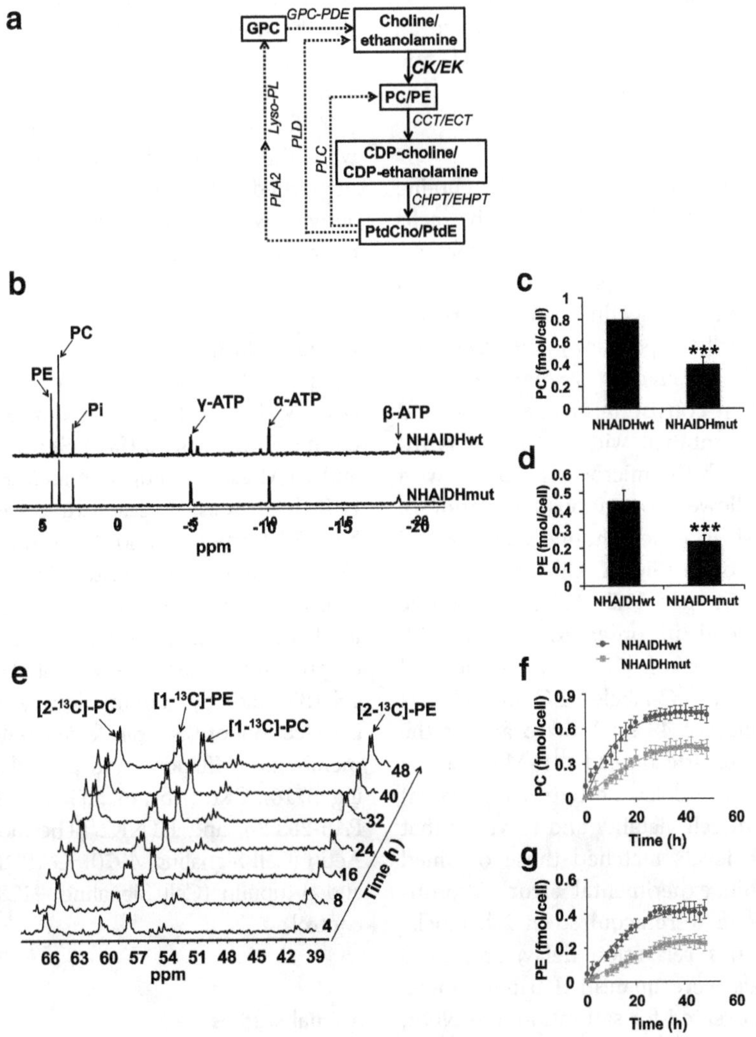

Fig. 1 PC and PE synthesis is downregulated in IDHmut glioma cells. **a** Metabolic pathways of choline and ethanolamine phospholipid metabolism in mammalian cells. CK, choline kinase; EK, ethanolamine kinase; CCT, CTP:PC cytidylyltransferase; ECT, CTP:PE cytidylyltransferase; CHPT, choline phosphotransferase; EHPT, ethanolamine phosphotransferase; PLA2, phospholipase A2; Lyso-PL, lyso-phospholipase. Straight lines represent the phospholipid synthetic pathways while dotted lines represent the degradation pathways. **b** Representative ^{31}P-MR spectra of the aqueous fraction of cell extracts in the NHA model. Pi, inorganic phosphate; ATP, adenosine triphosphate. PC (**c**) and PE (**d**) levels in the NHA model. **e** Representative ^{13}C-MR spectra showing the build-up of [1-^{13}C]-PC, [2-^{13}C]-PC, [1-^{13}C]-PE, and [2-^{13}C]-PE over 48 h in live NHAIDHmut cells in an MR-compatible bioreactor. Representative non-linear kinetic fits of de novo synthesis of [1-^{13}C]-PC (**f**) and [2-^{13}C]-PE (**g**) in the NHA model

RNA interference

SMARTpool siRNA (Dharmacon, GE) against human HIF-1α (M-004018-05) and non-targeting siRNA pool #2 (D-001206-14-05) were transfected according to manufacturer's instructions. Briefly, 2×10^6 U87 or NHA cells, or 2.5×10^6 BT54 cells as neurospheres, were seeded in a 150-mm dish. Twenty-four hours later, cells were transfected with 25 nM siRNA using DharmaFECT 4 transfection reagent (GE) and were incubated at 37 °C for an additional 72 h prior to harvesting for further studies.

MRS of cell extracts

Metabolite extraction was performed using the dual-phase methanol-chloroform extraction method [11], and spectra were recorded on a 500-MHz spectrometer (Bruker) equipped with a Triple Resonance CryoProbe. ^{1}H-MR spectra (1D water presaturation ZGPR sequence, 90° flip angle, 3 s relaxation delay, 256 acquisitions), proton-decoupled ^{13}C-MR spectra (30° flip angle, 3 s relaxation delay, 2048 acquisitions) and proton-decoupled ^{31}P-MR spectra (30° flip angle, 2.6 s relaxation delay, 1440 acquisitions) were acquired; peak integrals were quantified using Mnova (Mestrelab), corrected for saturation effects, and normalized to cell number and to an external reference (trimethylsilyl propionate for ^{1}H- and ^{13}C-MR and methylene diphosphonic acid for ^{31}P).

MRS of live cells

^{13}C-MRS studies to quantify flux from [1,2-^{13}C]-choline and [1,2-^{13}C]-ethanolamine to PC and PE in live cells were performed on a 600-MHz Bruker spectrometer using a 10-mm broadband probe as previously described [20]. Cells were grown on fibronectin-coated microcarrier beads (Pronectin-F, Pall Corporation) and assembled into an MR-compatible bioreactor system [20, 21]. Briefly, a perfusion system consisting of one inflow and two outflow lines was combined with a 10-mm NMR tube at the bottom of which the microcarrier beads with cells were placed. This allowed continuous circulation of culture medium (DMEM) in which choline was replaced with 56 μM [1,2-^{13}C]-choline (Sigma-Aldrich) to measure PC synthesis, and 56 μM [1,2-^{13}C]-ethanolamine (Sigma-Aldrich) was added in order to measure PE synthesis. The incorporation of [1,2-^{13}C]-choline and [1,2-^{13}C]-ethanolamine into ^{13}C-labeled PC and PE was monitored over the course of 48 h. Prior to and at the end of every study, proton-decoupled ^{31}P-MR spectra (30° flip angle, 3 s relaxation delay, and 1024 transients) were obtained to confirm cell viability and to verify that steady-state PC and PE levels matched those obtained from cell extracts (within experimental error). Proton-decoupled ^{13}C-MR spectra were acquired in 2 h blocks using a 30° flip angle, 6 s relaxation delay, and 2400 transients. Peak integrals were quantified using Mnova (Mestrelab Research), corrected for saturation and NOE, and normalized to cell number and to a metabolite of known concentration (1.59 mM inorganic phosphate for ^{31}P-MR spectra and 5 mM [1-^{13}C]-glucose added to the medium for this purpose for ^{13}C-MR spectra). The build-up of ^{13}C-labeled PC and PE over time was analyzed using a non-linear kinetic model (GraphPad Prism) that assumes that PC and PE are primarily generated by choline/ethanolamine phosphorylation [20]. Therefore, the kinetics of PC build-up are expected to follow the equation $^{13C}PC(t) = A\ (1-e^{-kt})$ where ^{13C}PC represents ^{13}C-labeled PC at time point t, A represents the asymptotic value of the ^{13}C-labeled pool of PC, i.e., the total steady state PC pool, and k is the pseudo-first-order rate constant for CK. A similar equation was used to quantify PE build-up and obtain a pseudo-first-order rate constant for EK.

CK and EK activity

CK activity was determined using ^{31}P-MR spectroscopy as described earlier [22]. A similar assay was developed for determining EK activity: cells or tumor tissue were lysed in buffer (10 mM glycylglycine, pH 8, 2 mM dithiothreitol) and lysate added to reaction mix (60 mM glycylglycine, pH 8, 3 mM ethanolamine, 4 mM ATP, and 4 mM $MgCl_2$). Proton-decoupled ^{31}P-MR spectra (30° flip angle, 2.6 s relaxation delay, 128 transients) were then acquired every 5 min and PE concentration quantified from peak integrals as described above. EK activity was measured by linear regression of the time course of PE production.

Western blotting

Cells (~ 10^7) were lysed by sonication in RIPA buffer (25 mM Tris-HCl pH 7.6, 150 mM NaCl, 1% NP-40, 1% sodium deoxycholate, 0.1% SDS) containing 150 nM aprotinin and 1 μM each of leupeptin and E64 protease inhibitor. For HIF-1α analysis, nuclear extracts were prepared using the NE-PER fractionation kit (Thermo-Fisher Scientific) according to manufacturer's instructions. Lysates were cleared by centrifugation at 14,000 rpm for 15 min at 4 °C and boiled in SDS-PAGE sample buffer (95 °C for 10 min). Total cellular protein (~ 20 μg) was separated on a 10% polyacrylamide gel (Bio-Rad) by sodium dodecyl sulphate polyacrylamide gel electrophoresis, transferred onto Immobilon-FL PVDF membrane (Millipore) and probed for HIF-1α (Cell Signaling, 3716), CKα (Abcam, ab38290), ETNK1 (Thermo-Fisher, PA5-28325), and ETNK2 (Thermo-Fisher, PA5-38807). β-Actin (Cell Signaling, 4970), GAPDH (Cell Signaling, 2118), and β-tubulin (Cell Signaling, 2128) were used as loading control.

Animal studies

Animal studies were conducted in accordance with the University of California Institutional Animal Care and Use Committee (IACUC) guidelines under protocol number AN101013. U87IDHwt and U87IDHmut cells (3×10^5cells/10 μl) were intracranially injected into athymic nu/nu mice (Simonsen Laboratories) by the free-hand technique. T2-weighted MR imaging used to monitor tumor volume was performed on a 14.1-T vertical MR system (Agilent Technologies) equipped with a single-channel ^{1}H coil. Images were acquired using a multislice spin-echo sequence with the following parameters: time-to-echo 20 ms; repetition time 1200 ms; field of view 25×25 mm^2; matrix 512×256; slice thickness 1.0 mm; and number of averages 2. Tumor contours in each axial slice were drawn manually, and tumor volume was determined as a sum of the areas multiplied by slice thickness using in-house MR software (SIVIC). When the tumors reached ~ 100 mm^3, the animals were sacrificed and tumor tissue snap frozen for metabolic and biochemical analysis ($n = 5$ for U87IDHwt, $n = 7$ for U87IDHmut).

DNA hypermethylation

Analysis of methylation of CHKA, ETNK1, and ETNK2 genes was performed as previously described [6]. Briefly, genomic DNA was isolated; bisulfite was converted using the EZ DNA MethylationKit (Zymo Research) and processed on Infinium Human Methylation 450 bead arrays (Illumina). Probes that were significantly different between IDHwt and IDHmut cells were identified using the Limma (moderated *t* test) approach as described previously [23, 24]. The ratio between methylated probe intensity and total probe intensity, which can be interpreted as the percentage of methylation, was designated as the beta (β) value and used to calculate the $\Delta\beta$ values (the difference between IDHmut and IDHwt cells) for each gene.

Patient samples

Flash-frozen human tumor tissue ($n = 4$ IDHwt, $n = 3$ IDHmut), with no patient-identifying information, was obtained in compliance with informed consent policy from the UCSF Brain Tumor Center Biorepository and Pathology Core. The Committee on Human Research at UCSF approved sample use, and the Institutional Review Board at UCSF approved research. Tumors were considered IDHmut if they were immunopositive with the anti-IDH1 R132H antibody (DIA-H09, Dianova) and IDHwt if negative for IDH1 mutation, EGFR amplification, and/or PTEN loss as determined clinically by FISH.

TCGA data analysis

Mean normalized *z*-scores for *CHKA*, *ETNK1*, and *ETNK2* mRNA expression (RNA Seq V2 RSEM dataset) and DNA methylation (HM450 dataset) were calculated from data for low-grade glioma (grades II and III) patient biopsies deposited in the larger TCGA database (http://cancergenome.nih.gov) and downloaded via the CBio Portal (http://www.cbioportal.org) [25, 26].

Statistical analysis

All experiments were performed on a minimum of five samples and results presented as mean ± standard deviation. Statistical significance was assessed using an unpaired two-tailed Student's *t* test assuming unequal variance with $p < 0.05$ considered significant. "*" represents $p < 0.05$, "**" represents $p < 0.01$, and "***" represents $p < 0.005$. NS indicates that there is no statistically significant difference.

Results

PC and PE synthesis is downregulated in IDHmut glioma cells

We examined PC and PE synthesis in two cell models, a U87 glioblastoma-based model and an immortalized normal human astrocyte (NHA) model. In each case, the cells were genetically engineered to express either IDHwt or IDH1 R132H mutant enzyme [11]. Using ^{1}H-MRS, we previously reported that steady-state PC levels were reduced in IDHmut cells relative to IDHwt [11]. Separately, Esmaeili et al. used ^{31}P-MRS to show that steady-state PE was reduced in IDHmut gliomas relative to IDHwt [13]. Here, we used ^{31}P-MR analysis of cell extracts (Fig. 1b) to confirm both of these findings in our models. Steady-state PC as well as PE were significantly reduced in IDHmut cells relative to IDHwt in both NHA (Fig. 1c, d) and U87 (Additional file 1: Figure S1A-B) models. We also confirmed that steady-state PC pool sizes as determined by ^{31}P-MRS matched the values previously determined by ^{1}H-MRS in both our NHA and U87 models (Additional file 1: Figure S1C-D).

We then used ^{13}C-MRS to monitor PC and PE synthesis in live cells perfused with [1,2-^{13}C]-choline and [1,2-^{13}C]-ethanolamine over 48 h (Fig. 1e). This time course was chosen because steady-state pools of PC and PE were filled by 48 h (as determined by comparing to our ^{31}P-MRS data, Additional file 1: Figure S1E-H) while breakdown products of PtdCho and PtdE such as ^{13}C-GPC and ^{13}C-GPE were below detection, indicating that ^{13}C-labeled PC and PE was generated primarily de novo from extracellular ^{13}C-choline and ^{13}C-ethanolamine. The kinetic fits for PC and PE build-up are shown in Fig. 1f, g for the NHA model and in Additional file 1: Figure S1I-J for the U87 model. The pseudo-first-order rate constant for CK dropped significantly by 40% from 0.08 ± 0.007 h^{-1} in NHAIDHwt to 0.05 ± 0.004 h^{-1} in NHAIDHmut and by 39% from 0.1 ± 0.008 h^{-1} in U87IDHwt to 0.06 ± 0.007 h^{-1} in U87IDHmut. Similarly, the pseudo-first-order rate constant for EK decreased significantly by 50% from 0.06 ± 0.005 h^{-1} to 0.03 ± 0.004 h^{-1} in the NHA model and by 40% from 0.08 ± 0.005 h^{-1} to 0.05 ± 0.003 h^{-1} in the U87 model.

CK activity and EK activity are reduced in IDHmut glioma cells

Next, we examined the expression and activity of CK and EK, the enzymes responsible for PC and PE synthesis (Fig. 1a) in our models. In mammalian cells, CK exists in three isoforms, CKα1 and CKα2 (encoded by the *CHKA* gene) and CKβ (*CHKB* gene), of which the α but not β isoforms have been associated with malignant transformation [9, 10]. In our IDHmut cells, CKα expression was significantly reduced relative to IDHwt (Fig. 2a, b). Using a ^{31}P-MR-based assay (Fig. 2c), we also measured CK activity in cell lysates and found a significant reduction in IDHmut cells relative to IDHwt in both NHA (61%, Fig. 2d) and U87 (60%, Fig. 2e) models.

EK is encoded by the *ETNK1* and *ETNK2* genes [27, 28]. We were unable to detect expression of ETNK1 or ETNK2 using commercially available antibodies in our models (data not shown). Nonetheless, measurement of EK, or EK-like

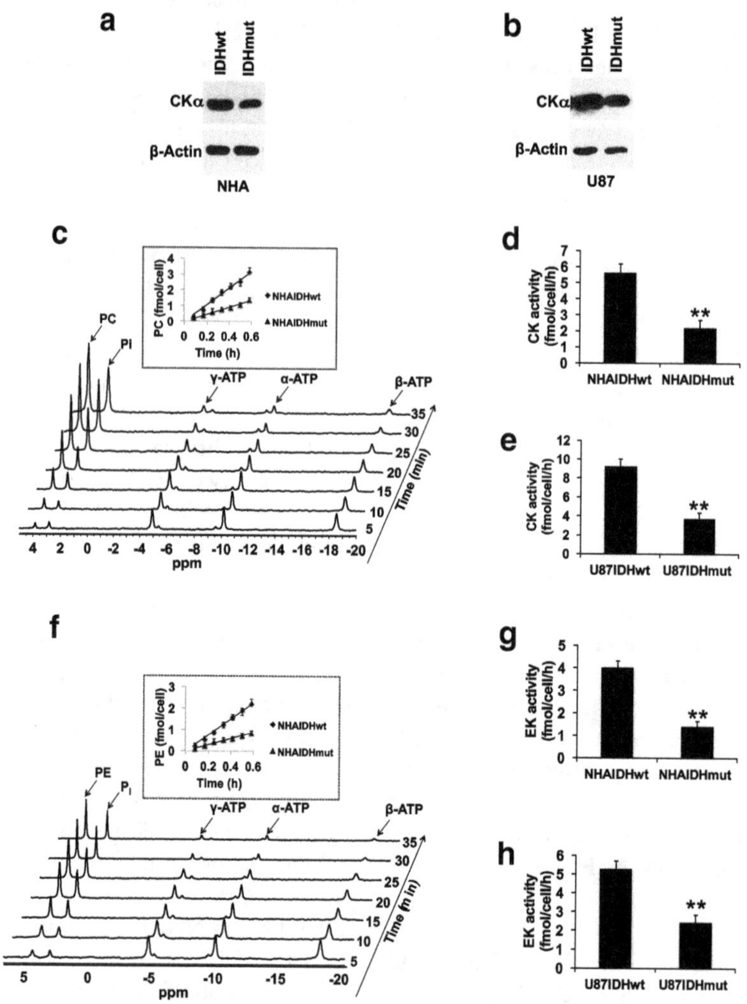

Fig. 2 CK activity and EK activity are downregulated in IDHmut glioma cells. CKα expression in the NHA (**a**) and U87 (**b**) models. **c** Representative ^{31}P-MR assay for CK activity showing PC build-up following addition of cell lysate to a reaction mix containing choline and ATP. The inset shows the rate of PC production in the NHA model. Quantification of CK activity in the NHA (**d**) and U87 (**e**) models. **f** Representative ^{31}P-MR assay for EK activity showing PE build-up following addition of cell lysate to a reaction mix containing ethanolamine and ATP. The inset shows the rate of PE production in the NHA model. Quantification of EK activity in the NHA (**g**) and U87 (**h**) models

activity in cell lysates (Fig. 2f), showed a significant reduction in IDHmut cells relative to IDHwt in both NHA (65%, Fig. 2g) and U87 (54%, Fig. 2h) models.

2-HG mediates the reduction in CK activity and EK activity as well as PC and PE levels

In an effort to link our results to the IDH1 mutation, we pharmacologically manipulated the presence of 2-HG and examined choline and ethanolamine metabolism in IDHwt cells incubated with 2-HG or in IDHmut cells treated with the IDHmut enzyme inhibitor AGI-5198 [29, 30]. PC and PE levels were reduced in IDHwt cells treated with 2-HG in both NHA (Fig. 3a, b) and U87 (Additional file 1: Figure S2A-B) models. Conversely, inhibiting 2-HG production by treating IDHmut cells with AGI-5198 restored PC and PE to levels similar to those observed in IDHwt cells. Concomitantly, CKα expression, CK activity, and EK activity were reduced in a manner linked to the presence of 2-HG in both NHA (Fig. 3c–e) and U87 (Additional file 1: Figure S2C-E) models. Collectively, these results mechanistically linked 2-HG to the downregulation of PC and PE synthesis in IDHmut glioma cells.

HIF-1α downregulates CK and EK activity

Next, we looked for the molecular mechanism by which 2-HG downregulates PC and PE synthesis in IDHmut gliomas. HIF-1α has previously been reported to modulate CKα expression and PC levels in cancer [31, 32]. Furthermore, we and others previously demonstrated that HIF-1α levels are post-translationally stabilized in IDHmut gliomas as a result of 2-HG-mediated inhibition

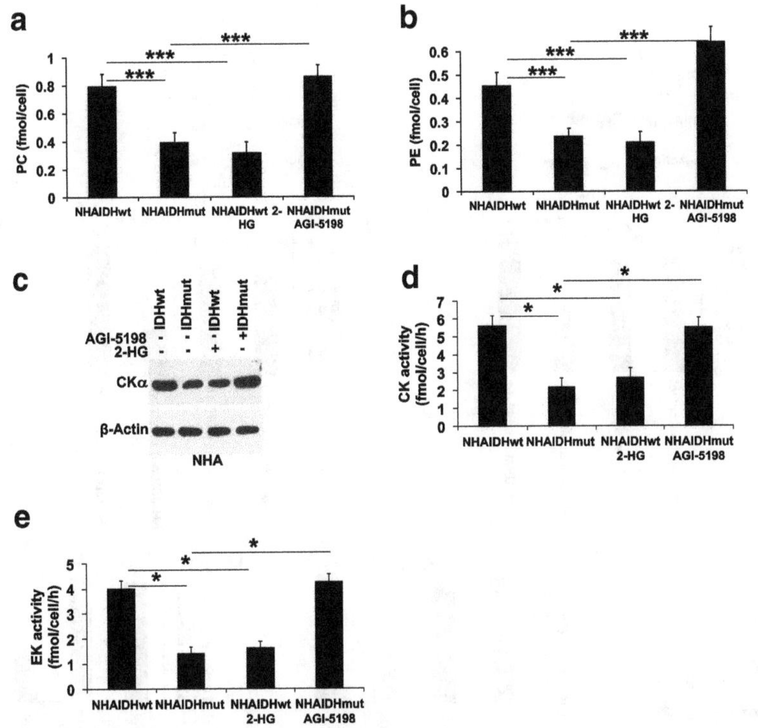

Fig. 3 2-HG is responsible for the downregulation of PC and PE synthesis in IDHmut glioma cells. PC (**a**), PE (**b**), CKα expression (**c**), CK activity (**d**), and EK activity (**e**) in NHAIDHwt cells, NHAIDHwt cells incubated with 2-HG, NHAIDHmut cells, and NHAIDHmut cells treated with AGI-5198

of the activity of the prolyl hydroxylases that target HIF-1α for degradation [30, 33–36]. Here, by examining HIF-1α levels in IDHwt cells treated with 2-HG and in IDHmut cells treated with AGI-5198, we confirmed that higher HIF-1α levels are linked to the presence of 2-HG in both NHA (Fig. 4a) and U87 (Additional file 1: Figure S3A) models. We then questioned whether HIF-1α was linked to PC and PE synthesis in our models. To this end, we silenced HIF-1α expression by RNA interference in both IDHwt and IDHmut cells (Fig. 4b and Additional file 1: Figure S3B). Silencing HIF-1α did not alter PC, PE, CKα expression, CK activity, or EK activity in IDHwt cells in both NHA (Fig. 4c–g) and U87 (Additional file 1: Figure S3C-G) models. In contrast, HIF-1α silencing restored PC, PE, CKα expression, CK activity, and EK activity to levels similar to those observed in IDHwt cells in both NHA (Fig. 4c–g) and U87 (Additional file 1: Figure S3C-G) models. We also established that treating IDHmut cells with 2-HG did not rescue the effects of HIF-1α silencing on PC (Additional file 1: Figure S4A-B), PE (Additional file 1: Figure S4C-D), CK activity (Additional file 1: Figure S4E-F), or EK activity (Additional file 1: Figure S4G-H). These results are in line with the observation that 2-HG stabilizes HIF-1α post-translationally [30, 33–36], while siRNA-mediated HIF-1α silencing occurs at the post-transcriptional level [37]. Taken together, these results suggest that 2-HG-mediated stabilization of HIF-1α downregulates CK activity and EK activity and thus leads to reduced PC and PE levels in IDHmut glioma cells.

Finally, 2-HG can alter gene expression in glioma cells via DNA hypermethylation [38, 39]. We, therefore, examined the methylome of IDHwt and IDHmut cells to determine whether the *CHKA*, *ETNK1*, or *ETNK2* genes were hypermethylated in our models. There was no significant difference in the $\Delta\beta$ value (difference in % methylation between IDHmut and IDHwt cells) of these genes in our NHA ($\Delta\beta = 0.02$, $p = 0.4$, probe cg27431247 for CHKA, $\Delta\beta = 0.01$, $p = 0.5$, probe cg25881344 for ETNK1, and $\Delta\beta = 0.03$, $p = 0.2$, probe cg08114257 for ETNK2) or U87 ($\Delta\beta = 0.04$, $p = 0.1$, probe cg27431247 for CHKA, $\Delta\beta = 0.03$, $p = 0.3$, probe cg25881344 for ETNK1, and $\Delta\beta = 0.01$, $p = 0.2$, probe cg08114257 for ETNK2) models. These results potentially rule out epigenetic effects of 2-HG on CK and EK expression in our models and suggest that the effect of 2-HG on PC and PE levels is primarily mediated by HIF-1α.

2-HG downregulates PC and PE synthesis in the BT54 patient-derived IDHmut glioma model

In order to confirm our findings in a clinically relevant IDHmut glioma model, we examined the BT54 patient-derived neurosphere model [19], which retains both IDHwt and IDHmut alleles and produces 2-HG [5, 19]. Consistent with our results in the genetically engineered

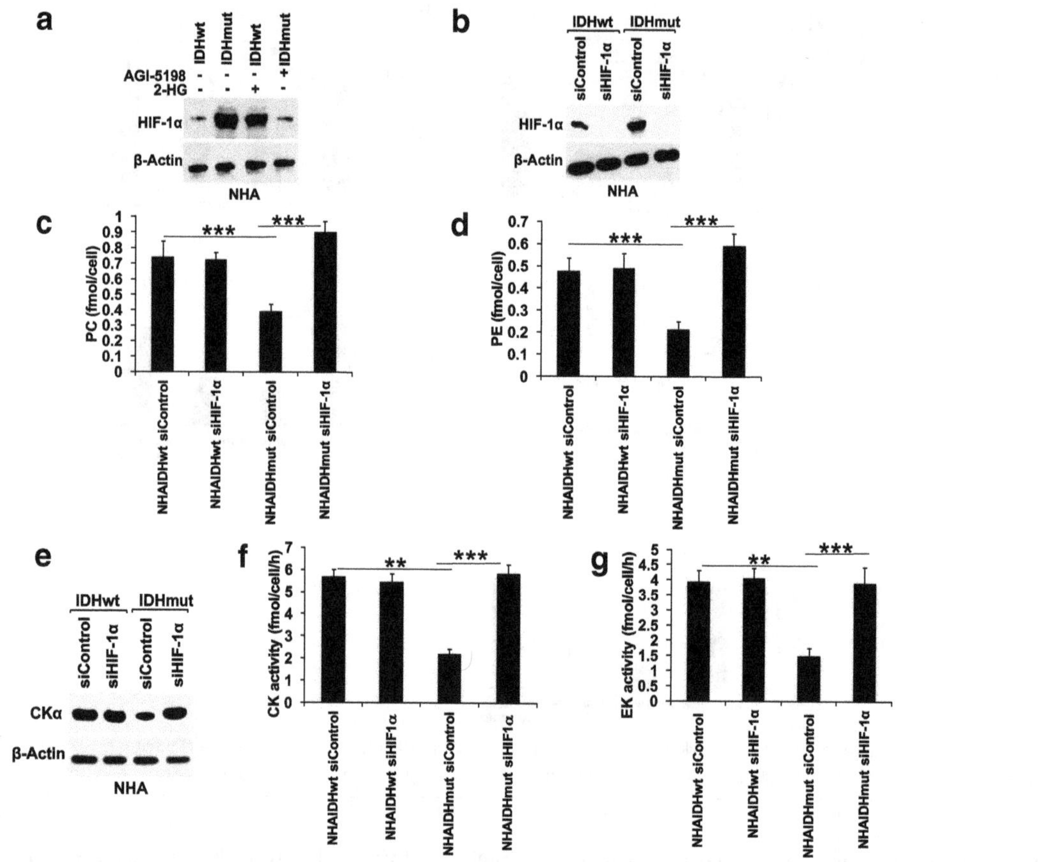

Fig. 4 HIF-1α downregulates PC and PE synthesis in IDHmut glioma cells. **a** Representative western blot showing the effect of 2-HG on HIF-1α in the NHA model. **b** Representative western blots showing silencing of HIF-1α in the NHA model. Effect of HIF-1α silencing on PC (**c**), PE (**d**), CKα expression (**e**), CK activity (**f**), and EK activity (**g**) in the NHA model

models, treating BT54 neurospheres with AGI-5198 increased PC, PE, CKα expression, CK activity, and EK activity (Fig. 5a–e), an effect that was associated with reduced HIF-1α levels (Fig. 5f). Importantly, silencing HIF-1α (Fig. 5g) increased PC, PE, CKα expression, CK activity, and EK activity (Fig. 5h–l), confirming the link between HIF-1α and downregulation of PC and PE synthesis in the clinically relevant BT54 model.

PC and PE levels are reduced in IDHmut gliomas in orthotopic tumor xenografts

Next, we examined PC and PE synthesis in U87IDHwt and U87IDHmut orthotopic tumor xenografts. We assessed extracts from tumors that had reached comparable sizes as determined by T2-weighted MR imaging (Fig. 6a). As shown in Fig. 6b, c, PC and PE levels were reduced in U87IDHmut tumors relative to U87IDHwt. Concomitantly, CKα expression (Fig. 6d and Additional file 1: Figure S5A), CK activity (Fig. 6e), and EK activity (Fig. 6f) were reduced in U87IDHmut tumors relative to U87IDHwt. As in the case of our cell models, these metabolic changes were accompanied by higher levels of HIF-1α in U87IDHmut tumors relative to U87IDHwt (Fig. 6g and Additional file 1: Figure S5B).

PC, PE, CKα expression, CK activity, and EK activity are reduced in IDHmut glioma patient biopsies

In order to determine whether our findings were relevant to human patients, we examined IDHwt and IDHmut glioma patient biopsies. Consistent with our results in cell and animal models, levels of PC and PE were reduced in IDHmut glioma patient biopsies relative to IDHwt (Fig. 7a, b). Concomitantly, CKα expression, CK activity, and EK activity were reduced in IDHmut patient biopsies relative to IDHwt (Fig. 7c–e) and this effect was accompanied by an increase in HIF-1α levels in IDHmut biopsies (Fig. 7f).

Finally, we also examined mRNA expression data for the CKα (*CHKA*) and EK genes (*ETNK1* and *ETNK2*) in low-grade (grade II and grade III) patient biopsy samples from The Cancer Genome Atlas (TCGA) database. As shown in Additional file 1: Figure S6A-B, the mean *z*-scores for *CHKA* and *ETNK2* mRNA expression showed a significant reduction in IDHmut glioma samples relative

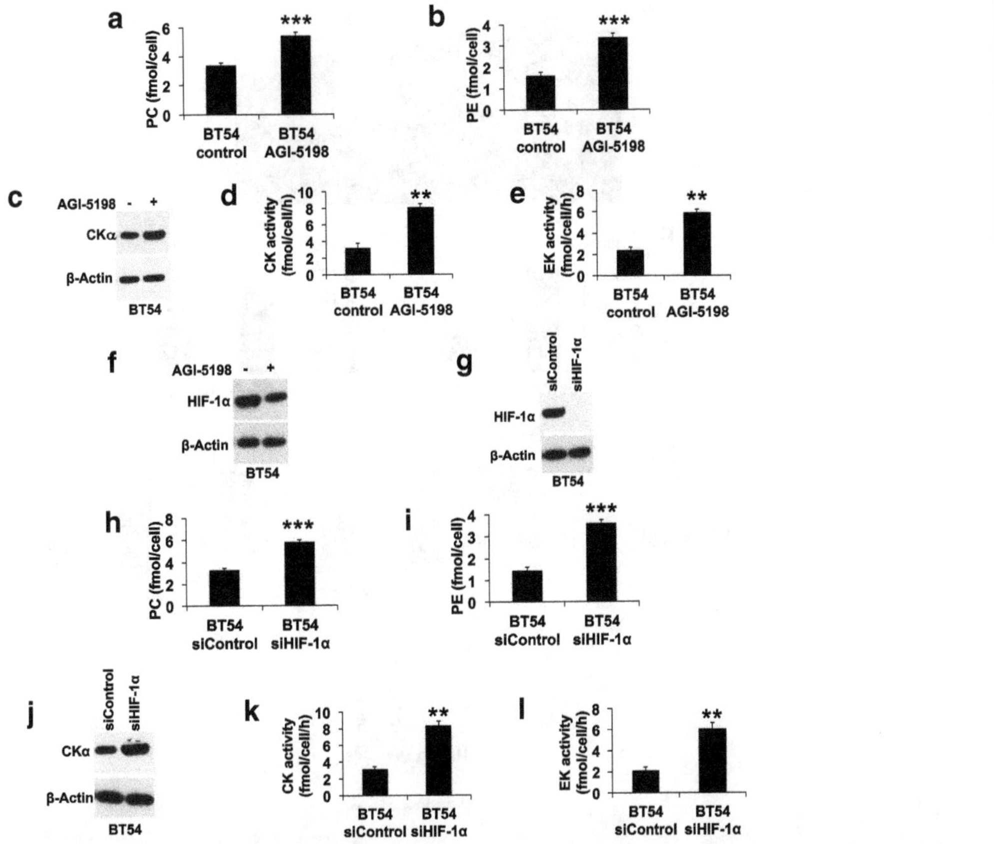

Fig. 5 2-HG, acting via HIF-1α, downregulates PC and PE synthesis in the BT54 patient-derived IDHmut glioma model. Effect of AGI-5198 on PC (**a**), PE (**b**), CKα expression (**c**), CK activity (**d**), EK activity (**e**), and HIF-1α (**f**) in the BT54 model. **g** Representative western blots showing silencing of HIF-1α in the BT54 model. Effect of HIF-1α silencing on PC (**h**), PE (**i**), CKα expression (**j**), CK activity (**k**), and EK activity (**l**) in the BT54 model

to IDHwt (0.21 in IDHwt to − 0.16 in IDHmut, $p < 0.0001$ for *CHKA* and 0.69 in IDHwt to − 0.12 in IDHmut, $p < 0.001$ for *ETNK2*). There was no significant difference in *ETNK1* mRNA expression (Additional file 1: Figure S6C, 0.11 in IDHwt vs. 0.29 in IDHmut, $p = 0.2$). We also examined DNA methylation for *CHKA, ETNK1*, and *ETNK2* genes within the IDHmut glioma population and, in line with the results in our cell models, found no correlation with mRNA *z*-scores (Pearson correlation coefficients of − 0.2 for *CHKA*, − 0.3 for *ETNK1*, and − 0.3 for *ETNK2*; Additional file 1: Figure S6d-f), suggesting that reduced *CHKA* and *ETNK2* mRNA expression in the IDHmut glioma patient samples was not the result of 2-HG-induced DNA hypermethylation at the promoters of these genes.

Discussion

In this study, we show that IDHmut gliomas downregulate PC and PE synthesis relative to IDHwt gliomas. This effect is mediated by 2-HG via HIF-1α stabilization and the subsequent downregulation of CK and EK or EK-like activity. Our finding that PC is reduced confirms our previous publication [11], and our results are also in line with the study by Reitman et al. who also showed reduced PC levels in IDHmut glioma cells relative to IDHwt [12]. Esmaeili et al. reported unchanged PC levels in IDHmut gliomas relative to IDHwt [13], but the same study showed a reduction in PE in IDHmut gliomas, consistent with our observations.

PC and PE are precursors in the synthesis of the phospholipids PtdCho and PtdE, which are structural components of cellular membranes [7]. Due to the higher demand for phospholipids associated with cell proliferation, tumor cells often upregulate phospholid biosynthesis [8, 28, 40]. In contrast, we recently demonstrated that 2-HG downregulates PtdCho and PtdE biosynthesis in IDHmut gliomas by inducing autophagic degradation of the endoplasmic reticulum (ER-phagy) [41]. Our observation that PC and PE levels are reduced in IDHmut gliomas is consistent with the reduction in PtdCho and PtdE levels. However, further studies are needed to assess whether the reduction in PC and PE levels induced by HIF-1α is mechanistically linked to the reduction in PtdCho and PtdE levels in IDHmut gliomas and, conversely, whether ER-phagy contributes to the reduction in PC and PE levels in IDHmut gliomas.

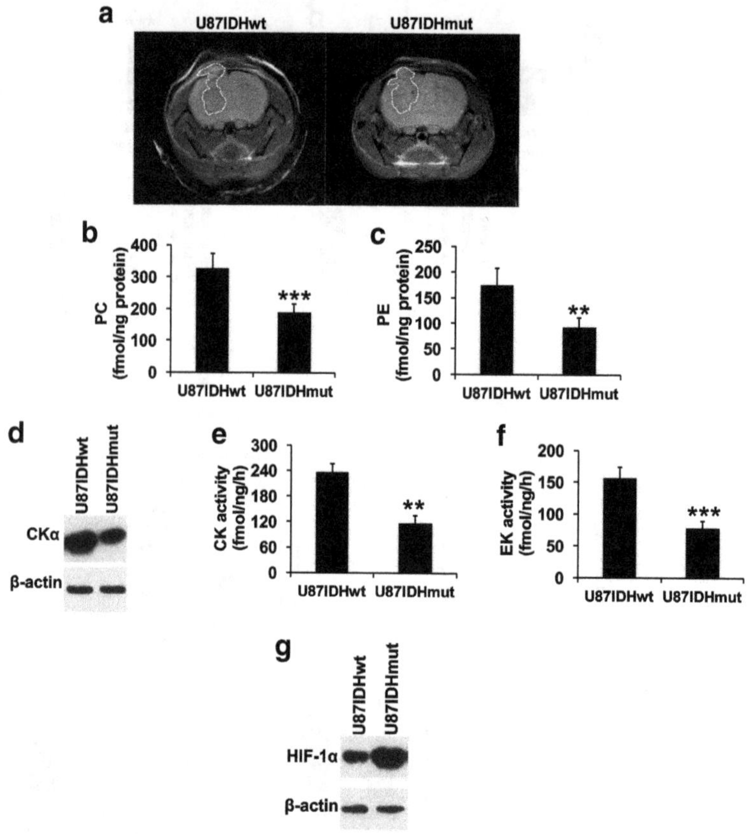

Fig. 6 PC and PE synthesis is downregulated in orthotopic IDHmut glioma xenografts. **a** Representative axial T2-weighted MR images of U87IDHwt and U87IDHmut orthotopic tumor-bearing mice. Tumor regions have been manually contoured in white. PC (**b**), PE (**c**), CKα expression (**d**), CK activity (**e**), EK activity (**f**), and HIF-1α (**g**) in U87IDHwt and U87IDHmut tumor xenografts

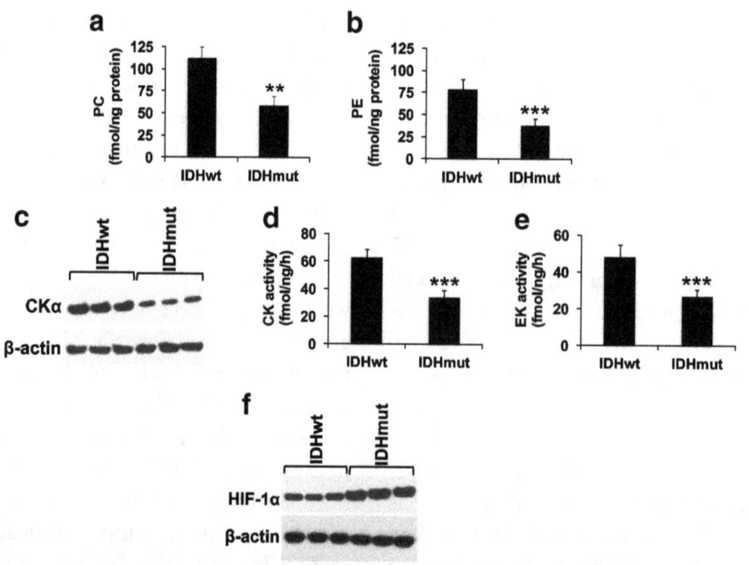

Fig. 7 PC and PE synthesis is downregulated in IDHmut glioma patient biopsies. PC (**a**), PE (**b**), CKα expression (**c**), CK activity (**d**), EK activity (**e**), and HIF-1α (**f**) in IDHwt and IDHmut glioma patient biopsies

We find that reduced CK activity is associated with reduced CKα expression in cell models, tumor xenografts, and patient biopsies. Importantly, CKα (*CHKA*) mRNA expression is reduced in IDHmut patient biopsies relative to IDHwt in the TCGA low-grade glioma dataset. These results are consistent with the central role of CKα in modulating PC levels in cancer [8–10]. CK catalyzes the first committed step in phosphatidylcholine biosynthesis which is the phosphorylation of free choline to PC [10, 42], and studies have shown that this reaction can be rate limiting in cancer cells [42, 43]. With regard to PE, the ethanolamine-specific EK enzymes encoded by the *ETNK1* and *ETNK2* genes mediate PE synthesis in mammalian cells [27, 28]. Although we were unable to detect expression of ETNK1 or ETNK2 in any of our samples using commercially available antibodies, it is important to note that ETNK2 mRNA levels are reduced in IDHmut patient biopsies relative to IDHwt in the TCGA dataset. Further studies are needed to confirm the molecular determinant of PE synthesis in IDHmut gliomas, but it is important to note that CK, which also possesses EK activity, could serve to phosphorylate ethanolamine to PE [9, 10, 44] in IDHmut gliomas.

Our study points to HIF-1α as the primary driver behind reduced CK and EK activity and thus PC and PE levels in IDHmut gliomas. Consistent with our observations, we found no evidence of methylation of the *CHKA*, *ETNK1*, and *ETNK2* genes in our models or in IDHmut glioma patient biopsies in the TCGA dataset, suggesting that 2-HG-induced DNA hypermethylation may not play a major role in downregulating CK and EK activity in IDHmut glioma cells. HIF-1α is a subunit of the HIF transcription factor that regulates expression of several genes involved in tumor proliferation, metabolism, and adaptation to hypoxic stress [45, 46]. In the context of phospholipid metabolism, HIF-1α has been linked to activation as well as repression of CK expression and activity [31, 32]. Furthermore, HIF-1α function can be regulated in a cell type- and context-dependent manner [47]. It is therefore possible that, in IDHmut gliomas, HIF-1α downregulates CK activity. With regard to EK, our study is the first to report downregulation of EK activity by HIF-1α. Further studies are needed to delineate the mechanism by which HIF-1α downregulates CK and EK activity in IDHmut gliomas.

Cellular HIF-1α levels are tightly regulated by post-translational degradation. Under normoxic conditions, HIF-1α is targeted for proteasomal degradation as a result of prolyl hydroxylation that is mediated by α-KG-dependent prolyl hydroxylases [45, 46]. Our finding that 2-HG stabilizes HIF-1α in IDHmut cells, even under normoxic conditions, is consistent with our previous publication [30] as well as previous reports by others indicating that 2-HG competitively inhibits prolyl hydroxylase activity, resulting in HIF-1α stabilization [33–36]. However, other studies have reported unchanged or lower HIF-1α levels in IDHmut gliomas relative to IDHwt [48, 49]. It should be noted that multiple α-KG-dependent prolyl hydroxylases are involved in HIF-1α hydroxylation [50] and the intracellular expression of these enzymes, as well as the efficacy with which 2-HG inhibits these enzymes, together with local levels of hypoxia, may vary, potentially accounting for the discrepancies in HIF-1α expression across different studies.

The complexity of factors affecting HIF-1α levels identifies a potential challenge in using PC and/or PE as imaging biomarkers of IDH status. Another potential confounder that could limit the utility of PC and PE is variability in 2-HG levels. Our results indicate that in IDHmut gliomas PC and PE are directly linked to the ongoing presence of 2-HG. However, a recent study has shown that a small proportion (~ 12%) of IDHmut gliomas spontaneously lose the IDHwt or IDHmut allele, thereby losing the ability to produce 2-HG, an effect that was also associated with progression to a higher grade tumor [51, 52]. Our results suggest that PC and PE synthesis would increase in these tumors. In addition, some ex vivo studies show a correlation between tumor cellularity and PC levels. Accordingly, and consistent with our findings, tissue samples from low-grade (WHO grades II and III) IDHmut gliomas that have undergone malignant progression to a higher cellularity, higher grade (grade IV), glioblastoma show an increase in PC levels and these levels are at least as high as those observed in primary IDHwt glioblastomas [53–55].

In the clinical setting, some in vivo ^{1}H-MRS studies suggest that tCho, normalized to creatine or to *N*-acetylaspartate, is higher in higher grade gliomas relative to low-grade [17, 56] and that these ratios could distinguish low-grade IDHmut gliomas from high-grade IDHwt glioblastomas [57, 58]. Most importantly, however, independent of IDH status, when compared to normal brain, normalized tCho is always elevated in the tumor region [59], and thus elevated tCho remains an important and useful indicator of tumor for patients with all brain tumor types [54, 59].

Conclusions

Our study establishes a role for 2-HG, acting via HIF-1α, in the downregulation of PC and PE synthesis in IDHmut gliomas. These results point to potential challenges in using PC and/or PE as indicators of tumoral IDH status. More importantly, our findings underscore the unusual metabolic reprogramming of IDHmut gliomas [3]. As mentioned, previous studies have identified other metabolic pathways that are reprogrammed differently in

IDHmut gliomas compared to IDHwt gliomas [3, 5, 6]. Here, we show, to our knowledge for the first time, oncometabolite-driven downregulation of choline and ethanolamine metabolism in cancer. Our findings thus expand our understanding of the unique metabolic reprogramming associated with the IDH1 mutation.

Abbreviations

2-HG: 2-Hydroxyglutarate; CK: Choline kinase; DMEM: Dulbecco's modified Eagle's medium; EK: Ethanolamine kinase; GPC: Glycerophosphocholine; GPE: Glycerophosphoethanolamine; HIF-1α: Hypoxia inducible factor-1α; IDH: Isocitrate dehydrogenase; IDHmut: Mutant isocitrate dehydrogenase 1; IDHwt: Wild-type isocitrate dehydrogenase 1; MRS: Magnetic resonance spectroscopy; NHA: Immortalized normal human astrocytes; PC: Phosphocholine; PE: Phosphoethanolamine; tCho: Total choline; WHO: World Health Organization; α-KG: α-Ketoglutarate

Acknowledgements

The authors thank Anne Marie Gillespie and Yunita Lim for the technical support.

Funding

This work was supported by the following grants: NIH R01CA172845 (SMR), NIH R01CA197254 (SMR), NIH R01CA154915 (SMR), FP7/2007-2013 REA600396 (JLI), SAF2014-59118-JIN (JLI), UCSF Brain Tumor Loglio Collective (SMR, ROP, JJP), NICO (SMR), UCSF Brain Tumor Research Center SPORE Tissue Core (P50CA97257) and UCSF Brain Tumor Research Center SPORE Career Development Grant (P50CA97257 to PV).

Authors' contributions

PV and SMR conceived the research and designed experiments. PV performed experiments and interpreted data. MR performed the in vivo experiments. JLI provided intellectual contributions to the design of experiments and interpretation of data. JJP conceived of patient biopsy studies and provided the patient samples. HAL, JGC, JJP, and ROP provided cell lines, reagents, and analytic tools. PV and SMR wrote the original manuscript. PV, MR, JLI, HAL, JGC, JJP, ROP, and SMR reviewed and commented on the manuscript. SMR, PV, and JLI secured funding for the manuscript. All authors read and approved the final manuscript.

Competing interests

The authors declare that they have no competing interests.

Author details

[1]Department of Radiology and Biomedical Imaging, University of California San Francisco, 1700 4th Street, Box 2532. Byers Hall 3rd Floor, Suite, San Francisco, CA 94143, USA. [2]Centro Nacional de Investigaciones Cardiovasculares (CNIC), Madrid, Spain. [3]CIBER de Enfermedades Respiratorias (CIBERES), Madrid, Spain. [4]Department of Cell Biology and Anatomy and Hotchkiss Brain Institute, University of Calgary, Calgary, Alberta, Canada. [5]Department of Clinical Neurosciences and Southern Alberta Cancer Research Institute, University of Calgary, Calgary, Alberta, Canada. [6]Department of Neurological Surgery, Helen Diller Research Center, University of California San Francisco, San Francisco, CA, USA.

References

1. Dang L, Su SM. Isocitrate dehydrogenase mutation and (R)-2-hydroxyglutarate: from basic discovery to therapeutics development. Annu Rev Biochem. 2017; https://doi.org/10.1146/annurev-biochem-061516-044732.
2. Wahl DR, Venneti S. 2-hydoxyglutarate: D/riving pathology in gLiomaS. Brain Pathol (Zurich, Switzerland). 2015;25:760–8. https://doi.org/10.1111/bpa.12309.
3. Viswanath P, Chaumeil MM, Ronen SM. Molecular imaging of metabolic reprograming in mutant IDH cells. Front Oncol. 2016;6:60. https://doi.org/10.3389/fonc.2016.00060.
4. Gatenby RA, Gillies RJ. Why do cancers have high aerobic glycolysis? Nat Rev Cancer. 2004;4:891–9. https://doi.org/10.1038/nrc1478.
5. Chesnelong C, Chaumeil MM, Blough MD, Al-Najjar M, Stechishin OD, Chan JA, et al. Lactate dehydrogenase A silencing in IDH mutant gliomas. Neuro-Oncology. 2014;16:686–95. https://doi.org/10.1093/neuonc/not243.
6. Viswanath P, Najac C, Izquierdo-Garcia JL, Pankov A, Hong C, Eriksson P, et al. Mutant IDH1 expression is associated with down-regulation of monocarboxylate transporters. Oncotarget. 2016;7:34942–55. https://doi.org/10.18632/oncotarget.9006.
7. Vance JE, Vance DE. Phospholipid biosynthesis in mammalian cells. Biochem Cell Biol. 2004;82:113–28. https://doi.org/10.1139/o03-073.
8. Cheng M, Bhujwalla ZM, Glunde K. Targeting phospholipid metabolism in cancer. Front Oncol. 2016;6:266. https://doi.org/10.3389/fonc.2016.00266.
9. Glunde K, Bhujwalla ZM, Ronen SM. Choline metabolism in malignant transformation. Nat Rev Cancer. 2011;11:835–48. https://doi.org/10.1038/nrc3162.
10. Arlauckas SP, Popov AV, Delikatny EJ. Choline kinase alpha—putting the ChoK-hold on tumor metabolism. Prog Lipid Res. 2016;63:28–40. https://doi.org/10.1016/j.plipres.2016.03.005.
11. Izquierdo-Garcia JL, Viswanath P, Eriksson P, Chaumeil MM, Pieper RO, Phillips JJ, et al. Metabolic reprogramming in mutant IDH1 glioma cells. PLoS One. 2015;10:e0118781. https://doi.org/10.1371/journal.pone.0118781.
12. Reitman ZJ, Jin G, Karoly ED, Spasojevic I, Yang J, Kinzler KW, et al. Profiling the effects of isocitrate dehydrogenase 1 and 2 mutations on the cellular metabolome. Proc Natl Acad Sci U S A. 2011;108:3270–5. https://doi.org/10.1073/pnas.1019393108.
13. Esmaeili M, Hamans BC, Navis AC, van Horssen R, Bathen TF, Gribbestad IS, et al. IDH1 R132H mutation generates a distinct phospholipid metabolite profile in glioma. Cancer Res. 2014;74:4898–907. https://doi.org/10.1158/0008-5472.can-14-0008.
14. Glunde K, Bhujwalla ZM. Metabolic tumor imaging using magnetic resonance spectroscopy. Semin Oncol. 2011;38:26–41. https://doi.org/10.1053/j.seminoncol.2010.11.001.
15. Gillies RJ, Morse DL. In vivo magnetic resonance spectroscopy in cancer. Annu Rev Biomed Eng. 2005;7:287–326. https://doi.org/10.1146/annurev.bioeng.7.060804.100411.
16. Glunde K, Penet MF, Jiang L, Jacobs MA, Bhujwalla ZM. Choline metabolism-based molecular diagnosis of cancer: an update. Expert Rev Mol Diagn. 2015;15:735–47. https://doi.org/10.1586/14737159.2015.1039515.
17. McKnight TR, Noworolski SM, Vigneron DB, Nelson SJ. An automated technique for the quantitative assessment of 3D-MRSI data from patients with glioma. J Magn Reson Imaging. 2001;13:167–77.
18. Daly PF, Lyon RC, Faustino PJ, Cohen JS. Phospholipid metabolism in cancer cells monitored by 31P NMR spectroscopy. J Biol Chem. 1987;262:14875–8.
19. Kelly JJ, Blough MD, Stechishin OD, Chan JA, Beauchamp D, Perizzolo M, et al. Oligodendroglioma cell lines containing t(1;19)(q10;p10). Neuro-Oncology. 2010;12:745–55. https://doi.org/10.1093/neuonc/noq031.
20. Ronen SM, Rushkin E, Degani H. Lipid metabolism in T47D human breast cancer cells: 31P and 13C-NMR studies of choline and ethanolamine uptake. Biochim Biophys Acta. 1991;1095:5–16.
21. Ward CS, Venkatesh HS, Chaumeil MM, Brandes AH, Vancriekinge M, Dafni H, et al. Noninvasive detection of target modulation following phosphatidylinositol 3-kinase inhibition using hyperpolarized 13C magnetic resonance spectroscopy. Cancer Res. 2010;70:1296–305. https://doi.org/10.1158/0008-5472.can-09-2251.
22. Gabellieri C, Beloueche-Babari M, Jamin Y, Payne GS, Leach MO, Eykyn TR. Modulation of choline kinase activity in human cancer cells observed by dynamic 31P NMR. NMR Biomed. 2009;22:456–61. https://doi.org/10.1002/nbm.1361.
23. Price ME, Cotton AM, Lam LL, Farre P, Emberly E, Brown CJ, et al. Additional annotation enhances potential for biologically-relevant analysis of the Illumina Infinium HumanMethylation450 BeadChip array. Epigenetics Chromatin. 2013;6:4. https://doi.org/10.1186/1756-8935-6-4.
24. Triche TJ Jr, Weisenberger DJ, Van Den Berg D, Laird PW, Siegmund KD. Low-level processing of Illumina Infinium DNA methylation beadarrays. Nucleic Acids Res. 2013;41:e90. https://doi.org/10.1093/nar/gkt090.
25. Gao J, Aksoy BA, Dogrusoz U, Dresdner G, Gross B, Sumer SO, et al. Integrative analysis of complex cancer genomics and clinical profiles using the cBioPortal. Sci Signal. 2013;6:pl1. https://doi.org/10.1126/scisignal.2004088.
26. Cerami E, Gao J, Dogrusoz U, Gross BE, Sumer SO, Aksoy BA, et al. The cBio cancer genomics portal: an open platform for exploring multidimensional cancer genomics data. Cancer Discov. 2012;2:401–4. https://doi.org/10.

1158%2F2159-8290.CD-12-0095 —The cBio Cancer Genomics Portal (http://cbioportal.org) is an open-access resource for interactive exploration of multidimensional cancer genomics data sets, currently providing access to data from more than 5,000 tumor samples from 20 cancer studies. The cBio Cancer Genomics Portal significantly lowers the barriers between complex genomic data and cancer researchers who want rapid, intuitive, and high-quality access to molecular profiles and clinical attributes from large-scale cancer genomics projects and empowers researchers to translate these rich data sets into biologic insights and clinical applications. Cancer Discov; 2(5); 401–4. ©2012 AACR.

27. Lykidis A, Wang J, Karim MA, Jackowski S. Overexpression of a mammalian ethanolamine-specific kinase accelerates the CDP-ethanolamine pathway. J Biol Chem. 2001;276:2174–9. https://doi.org/10.1074/jbc.M008794200.
28. Ridgway ND. Chapter 7—phospholipid synthesis in mammalian cells. Biochemistry of lipids, lipoproteins and membranes. 6th ed. Boston: Elsevier; 2016. p. 209–36.
29. Rohle D, Popovici-Muller J, Palaskas N, Turcan S, Grommes C, Campos C, et al. An inhibitor of mutant IDH1 delays growth and promotes differentiation of glioma cells. Science (New York, NY). 2013;340:626–30. https://doi.org/10.1126/science.1236062.
30. Izquierdo-Garcia JL, Viswanath P, Eriksson P, Cai L, Radoul M, Chaumeil MM, et al. IDH1 mutation induces reprogramming of pyruvate metabolism. Cancer Res. 2015;75:2999–3009. https://doi.org/10.1158/0008-5472.can-15-0840.
31. Glunde K, Shah T, Winnard PT Jr, Raman V, Takagi T, Vesuna F, et al. Hypoxia regulates choline kinase expression through hypoxia-inducible factor-1 alpha signaling in a human prostate cancer model. Cancer Res. 2008;68:172–80. https://doi.org/10.1158/0008-5472.can-07-2678.
32. Bansal A, Harris RA, DeGrado TR. Choline phosphorylation and regulation of transcription of choline kinase alpha in hypoxia. J Lipid Res. 2012;53:149–57. https://doi.org/10.1194/jlr.M021030.
33. Sasaki M, Knobbe CB, Itsumi M, Elia AJ, Harris IS, Chio II, et al. D-2-hydroxyglutarate produced by mutant IDH1 perturbs collagen maturation and basement membrane function. Genes Dev. 2012;26:2038–49. https://doi.org/10.1101/gad.198200.112.
34. Xu W, Yang H, Liu Y, Yang Y, Wang P, Kim SH, et al. Oncometabolite 2-hydroxyglutarate is a competitive inhibitor of alpha-ketoglutarate-dependent dioxygenases. Cancer Cell. 2011;19:17–30. https://doi.org/10.1016/j.ccr.2010.12.014.
35. Yalaza C, Ak H, Cagli MS, Ozgiray E, Atay S, Aydin HH. R132H mutation in IDH1 gene is associated with increased tumor HIF1-alpha and serum VEGF levels in primary glioblastoma multiforme. Ann Clin Lab Sci. 2017;47:362–4.
36. Zhao S, Lin Y, Xu W, Jiang W, Zha Z, Wang P, et al. Glioma-derived mutations in IDH1 dominantly inhibit IDH1 catalytic activity and induce HIF-1alpha. Science (New York, NY). 2009;324:261–5. https://doi.org/10.1126/science.1170944.
37. Wilson RC, Doudna JA. Molecular mechanisms of RNA interference. Annu Rev Biophys. 2013;42:217–39. https://doi.org/10.1146/annurev-biophys-083012-130404.
38. Lu C, Ward PS, Kapoor GS, Rohle D, Turcan S, Abdel-Wahab O, et al. IDH mutation impairs histone demethylation and results in a block to cell differentiation. Nature. 2012;483:474–8. https://doi.org/10.1038/nature10860.
39. Turcan S, Rohle D, Goenka A, Walsh LA, Fang F, Yilmaz E, et al. IDH1 mutation is sufficient to establish the glioma hypermethylator phenotype. Nature. 2012;483:479–83. https://doi.org/10.1038/nature10866.
40. Lykidis A, Jackowski S. Regulation of mammalian cell membrane biosynthesis. Prog Nucleic Acid Res Mol Biol. 2001;65:361–93.
41. Viswanath P, Radoul M, Izquierdo-Garcia JL, Ong WQ, Luchman HA, Cairncross JG, et al. 2-hydroxyglutarate-mediated autophagy of the endoplasmic reticulum leads to an unusual downregulation of phospholipid biosynthesis in mutant IDH1 gliomas. Cancer Res. 2018; https://doi.org/10.1158/0008-5472.can-17-2926.
42. Gibellini F, Smith TK. The Kennedy pathway—de novo synthesis of phosphatidylethanolamine and phosphatidylcholine. IUBMB Life. 2010;62:414–28. https://doi.org/10.1002/iub.337
43. Kent C. Regulation of phosphatidylcholine biosynthesis. Prog Lipid Res. 1990;29:87–105. https://doi.org/10.1016/0163-7827(90)90010-I.
44. Ishidate K. Choline/ethanolamine kinase from mammalian tissues. Biochim Biophys Acta. 1997;1348:70–8.
45. Semenza GL. HIF-1 mediates metabolic responses to intratumoral hypoxia and oncogenic mutations. J Clin Invest. 2013;123:3664–71. https://doi.org/10.1172/JCI67230.
46. Soni S, Padwad YS. HIF-1 in cancer therapy: two decade long story of a transcription factor. Acta Oncol. 2017;56:503–15. https://doi.org/10.1080/0284186X.2017.1301680
47. Dengler VL, Galbraith MD, Espinosa JM. Transcriptional regulation by hypoxia inducible factors. Crit Rev Biochem Mol Biol. 2014;49:1–15. https://doi.org/10.3109/10409238.2013.838205.
48. Williams SC, Karajannis MA, Chiriboga L, Golfinos JG, von Deimling A, Zagzag D. R132H-mutation of isocitrate dehydrogenase-1 is not sufficient for HIF-1alpha upregulation in adult glioma. Acta Neuropathol. 2011;121:279–81. https://doi.org/10.1007/s00401-010-0790-y.
49. Koivunen P, Lee S, Duncan CG, Lopez G, Lu G, Ramkissoon S, et al. Transformation by the (R)-enantiomer of 2-hydroxyglutarate linked to EGLN activation. Nature. 2012;483:484–8. https://doi.org/10.1038/nature10898.
50. Pappalardi MB, McNulty DE, Martin JD, Fisher KE, Jiang Y, Burns MC, et al. Biochemical characterization of human HIF hydroxylases using HIF protein substrates that contain all three hydroxylation sites. Biochem J. 2011;436:363–9. https://doi.org/10.1042/bj20101201.
51. Mazor T, Chesnelong C, Pankov A, Jalbert LE, Hong C, Hayes J, et al. Clonal expansion and epigenetic reprogramming following deletion or amplification of mutant IDH1. Proc Natl Acad Sci U S A. 2017;114:10743–8. https://doi.org/10.1073/pnas.1708914114.
52. Jin G, Reitman ZJ, Duncan CG, Spasojevic I, Gooden DM, Rasheed BA, et al. Disruption of wild-type IDH1 suppresses D-2-hydroxyglutarate production in IDH1-mutated gliomas. Cancer Res. 2013;73:496–501. https://doi.org/10.1158/0008-5472.can-12-2852.
53. Elkhaled A, Jalbert L, Constantin A, Yoshihara HA, Phillips JJ, Molinaro AM, et al. Characterization of metabolites in infiltrating gliomas using ex vivo (1)H high-resolution magic angle spinning spectroscopy. NMR Biomed. 2014;27:578–93. https://doi.org/10.1002/nbm.3097.
54. Jalbert LE, Elkhaled A, Phillips JJ, Neill E, Williams A, Crane JC, et al. Metabolic profiling of IDH mutation and malignant progression in infiltrating glioma. Sci Rep. 2017;7:44792. https://doi.org/10.1038/srep44792.
55. Miller BL, Chang L, Booth R, Ernst T, Cornford M, Nikas D, et al. In vivo 1H MRS choline: correlation with in vitro chemistry/histology. Life Sci. 1996;58:1929–35.
56. Yang D, Korogi Y, Sugahara T, Kitajima M, Shigematsu Y, Liang L, et al. Cerebral gliomas: prospective comparison of multivoxel 2D chemical-shift imaging proton MR spectroscopy, echoplanar perfusion and diffusion-weighted MRI. Neuroradiology. 2002;44:656–66. https://doi.org/10.1007/s00234-002-0816-9.
57. Zhang J, Zhuang DX, Yao CJ, Lin CP, Wang TL, Qin ZY, et al. Metabolic approach for tumor delineation in glioma surgery: 3D MR spectroscopy image-guided resection. J Neurosurg. 2016;124:1585–93. https://doi.org/10.3171/2015.6.jns142651.
58. Guo J, Yao C, Chen H, Zhuang D, Tang W, Ren G, et al. The relationship between Cho/NAA and glioma metabolism: implementation for margin delineation of cerebral gliomas. Acta Neurochir. 2012;154:1361–70; discussion 70. https://doi.org/10.1007/s00701-012-1418-x.
59. An Z, Tiwari V, Ganji SK, Baxter J, Levy M, Pinho MC, et al. Echo-planar spectroscopic imaging with dual-readout alternated gradients (DRAG-EPSI) at 7 T: application for 2-hydroxyglutarate imaging in glioma patients. Magn Reson Med. 2017; https://doi.org/10.1002/mrm.26884.

14

Cancer cell metabolic plasticity allows resistance to NAMPT inhibition but invariably induces dependence on LDHA

Natthakan Thongon[1], Chiara Zucal[1], Vito Giuseppe D'Agostino[1], Toma Tebaldi[1], Silvia Ravera[2], Federica Zamporlini[3], Francesco Piacente[4], Ruxanda Moschoi[5], Nadia Raffaelli[3], Alessandro Quattrone[1], Alessio Nencioni[4], Jean-Francois Peyron[5] and Alessandro Provenzani[1*]

Abstract

Background: Inhibitors of nicotinamide phosphoribosyltransferase (NAMPT), the rate-limiting enzyme in NAD^+ biosynthesis from nicotinamide, exhibit anticancer effects in preclinical models. However, continuous exposure to NAMPT inhibitors, such as FK866, can induce acquired resistance.

Methods: We developed FK866-resistant CCRF-CEM (T cell acute lymphoblastic leukemia) and MDA MB231 (breast cancer) models, and by exploiting an integrated approach based on genetic, biochemical, and genome wide analyses, we annotated the drug resistance mechanisms.

Results: Acquired resistance to FK866 was independent of NAMPT mutations but rather was based on a shift towards a glycolytic metabolism and on lactate dehydrogenase A (LDHA) activity. In addition, resistant CCRF-CEM cells, which exhibit high quinolinate phosphoribosyltransferase (QPRT) activity, also exploited amino acid catabolism as an alternative source for NAD^+ production, becoming addicted to tryptophan and glutamine and sensitive to treatment with the amino acid transport inhibitor JPH203 and with L-asparaginase, which affects glutamine exploitation. Vice versa, in line with their low QPRT expression, FK866-resistant MDA MB231 did not rely on amino acids for their resistance phenotype.

Conclusions: Our study identifies novel mechanisms of resistance to NAMPT inhibition, which may be useful to design more rational strategies for targeting cancer metabolism.

Keywords: NAMPT, Amino acid metabolism, Drug resistance, LDHA, QPRT

Background

The development of drug resistance during chemo- or targeted-therapies is a common event, which typically underlies disease relapse and is frequently associated with a poor prognosis. Drug resistance is usually classified as intrinsic (also known as primary) or acquired (also known as secondary), depending on whether it is already present in cancer cells at treatment onset or, rather, it eventually develops during treatment [1]. The molecular mechanisms responsible for drug resistance vary depending on the agent used, but some common mechanisms frequently do come into play [2]. These include activation of drug efflux pumps [3], mutations of the targeted protein [4, 5], activation of compensation/buffer mechanisms [6], and evasion of apoptosis [7, 8].

Nicotinamide phosphoribosyltransferase (NAMPT) is a key enzyme for NAD^+ production from nicotinamide, and NAMPT expression by a tumor predicts a poor prognosis [9] in colon cancer [10], gastric cancer [11], and lymphoma [12]. Therefore, NAMPT has been proposed as a viable cancer drug target, and many molecular agents have been developed that inhibit its enzymatic function, such as FK866, GNE618, and CHS-828 [13, 14]. Clinical trials showed a good tolerability for these drugs, with thrombocytopenia being the most common dose-limiting adverse event. Regrettably, no objective tumor remission in response to these NAMPT inhibitors was observed [15]. New NAMPT inhibitors are under development

* Correspondence: alessandro.provenzani@unitn.it
[1]Center For Integrative Biology (CIBIO), University of Trento, via Sommarive 9, Trento, Italy

which will hopefully overcome these limitations [16]. In addition, given the unique mode of action of NAMPT inhibitors, their association with other types of anticancer agents, such as chemotherapeutics, ibrutinib, bortezomib, tumor necrosis factor-related apoptosis-inducing ligand (TRAIL), and cyclosporine-A, has been proposed as a way to boost the efficacy of single treatments [17–22].

Yet, the key issue that limits the benefit of NAMPT inhibitors remains our limited understanding of the factors that determine cancer cell response to these agents vs. resistance across different cancer types [23]. Several NAD^+ biosynthetic pathways that are alternative to that controlled by NAMPT exist. The Preiss-Handler pathway for NAD^+ production utilizes nicotinic acid (NA) and requires the expression of nicotinic acid phosphoribosyltransferase (NAPRT) for the first enzymatic step to convert NA to nicotinic acid mononucleotide (NAMN) [19]. NAMPT inhibition is specifically effective in cancer cells in which NAPRT-mediated NAD^+ production is not functioning [24]. Treatment with NAMPT inhibitors combined with NA supplementation was proposed to allow the killing of NAPRT-deficient cancer cells while simultaneously protecting normal cells thanks to the ability of the latter, but not of the former, to exploit NA as NAD^+ precursor [25]. In addition, NAPRT silencing in a BRCA2-deficient cancer cell line exacerbated DNA damage in response to chemotherapeutics [26]. Acquired resistance to NAMPT inhibitors was also reported and was proposed to be mostly due to mutations in NAMPT itself, as in the case of HCT-116 colon cancer cells, which were induced to become resistant to CHS-828. A resistant clone exhibiting acquired resistance to CHS-828 was obtained by continuous cell exposure to increasing sub-lethal concentrations of the drug. Sequencing of the *NAMPT* gene in the CHS-828-resistant cell line revealed a single point mutation of amino acid 217 from glycine to arginine (G217R) [27]. Similarly, other mutations in the *NAMPT* gene (mapped to H191R, to D93del, and to Q388R) were also reported in resistant cell lines developed from HCT-116 and from NYH human small cell lung carcinoma cells and were found to confer drug resistance to other NAMPT inhibitors, such as FK866 and CHS-828. All of these mutations were found to structurally modify the inhibitor-binding pocket (G217R and H191R), preventing drug efficacy. The resistant cell lines showed tumorigenicity in mouse xenografts and in vivo resistance to NAMPT inhibitors [13]. Six mutations in the *NAMPT* gene were reported in GNE-618-resistant cells derived from rhabdosarcoma (RD), pancreatic cancer (MiaPaCa-2), and non-small cell lung cancer (NCI-H460) cells [28]. In addition to the previously identified G217R and D93del mutations, the new G217A, G217V, S165F, and S165Y mutations were reported as resistance-causing mutations in this study. Resistant cell lines were observed to be 10- to 1000-fold less sensitive to the NAMPT inhibitor GNE-618 as compared to the parental cells. Tumor xenografts established from NCI-H460 cells expressing the S165Y mutation were resistant to high doses of GNE-618 [28]. Notably, no cross-resistance to CHS-828 and FK866 was detected, suggesting that resistance to NAMPT inhibitors could be molecule-specific. Therefore, to date, tumor cell resistance to NAMPT inhibitors has been mostly ascribed to point mutations that are either proximal or distal to the enzyme substrate binding sites with the notable exception of one case of NAMPT inhibitor resistance, that was related to increased activity of the enzyme quinolinate phosphoribosyltransferase (QPRT), which mediates NAD^+ production from tryptophan [29].

One strategy to overcome drug resistance is to identify and target the specific vulnerabilities or addictions that arise in the cancer population. Here, we investigated the molecular mechanism leading to acquired FK866 resistance in two genetically different cancer cell lines, CCRF-CEM T-ALL cells, which are NAPRT-deficient, and MDA MB231 triple-negative breast cancer cells, which, vice versa, express an active NAPRT enzyme but lack QPRT (Table 1). Both cancer cell lines developed resistance to FK866, and interestingly, in both cases, acquired resistance was independent of mutations in *NAMPT* but rather relied on the activation of alternative metabolic pathways that compensated for low NAD(H) level (Fig. 1a). Interestingly, the compensatory mechanisms mediating resistance were found to be profoundly different in the two cell lines, inducing different types of vulnerabilities in the resistant cells and suggesting diversified pharmacological approaches to treat them. However, both types of resistant cells did exhibit a marked reliance on LDHA activity, thus pointing to this enzyme as a crucial crossroad for cancer cell survival and as a new anticancer target.

Table 1 Genetic differences between CCRF CEM and MDA MB231 cell lines

Gene expression	Peripheral blood (acute lymphoblastic) CCRF CEM	Breast (adenocarcinoma) MDA MB 231
NAMPT	Intermediate	High
NAPRT	–	High
QPRT	High	Very low
NRK	Low	Intermediate
LDH	Intermediate	Intermediate
*PTEN**	Mutation	–
*KRAS**	Mutation	Mutation
*TP53**	–	Mutation
*BRAF**	–	Mutation
CDKN2A*	–	Mutation

*Source: ATCC cell lines by gene mutation

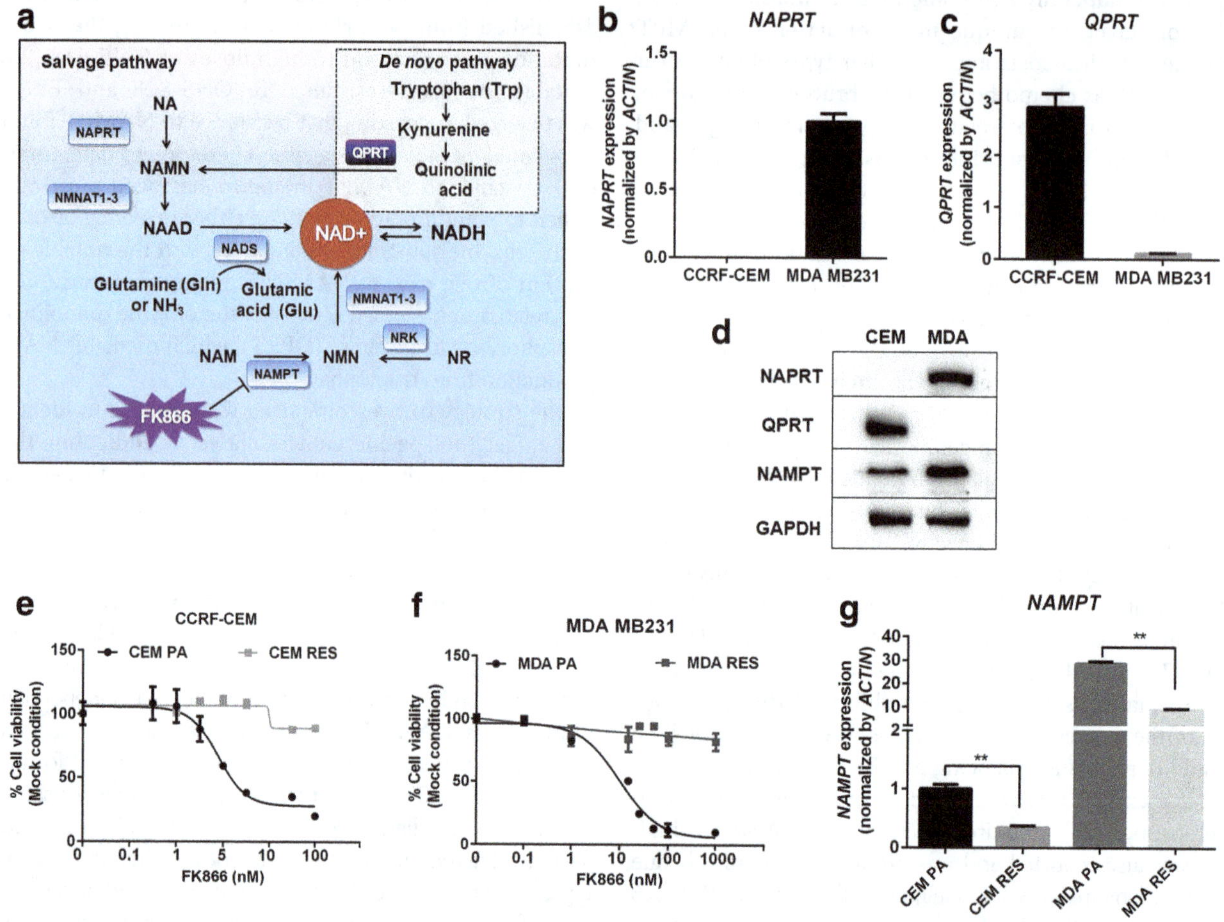

Fig. 1 Overview of NAD biosynthesis pathway and genetic differences in NAD(H) biosynthesis pathway between CCRF-CEM and MDA MB231 cell lines. **a** Schematic representation of salvage and de novo pathway of NAD biosynthesis. Pharmacological target of FK866 inhibiting NAMPT is displayed. Abbreviations: NAD, nicotinamide adenine dinucleotide; NA, nicotinic acid; NAMN, nicotinic acid mononucleotide; NAAD, nicotinic acid adenine dinucleotide; NAPRT, nicotinic acid phosphoribosyltransferase; NMNAT, nicotinamide mononucleotide adenylyltransferase; NADS, NAD synthase; NAM, nicotinamide; NMN, nicotinamide mononucleotide; NAMPT, nicotinamide phosphoribosyltransferase; NR, nicotinamide riboside; NRK, nicotinamide riboside kinase; QPRT, quinolinate phosphoribosyltransferase. **b**, **c** Expression of *NAPRT* and *QPRT* were determined in CCRF-CEM (CEM) and MDA MB231 (MDA) cell lines. **d** Western blot showing endogenous level of NAPRT, QPRT, and NAMPT in CEM and MDA cell lines. GAPDH was used as a loading control. **e**, **f** Sensitivity of CEM and MDA cells to FK866. CEM parental (CEM PA) and FK866-resistant CEM (CEM RES) cells (**e**) and MDA parental (MDA PA) and FK866-MDA resistant (MDA RES) cells (**f**) were exposed to various concentrations of FK866 (0.1–100 nM) for 48 h. Percentage of cell viability and EC50 were analyzed by MTT assay. **g** Downregulation of *NAMPT* in the resistant cells. Quantitative RT-PCR showing the expression of *NAMPT* in CEM PA, CEM RES, MDA PA, and MDA RES cells. *ACTIN* was used as a housekeeping gene

Methods

Cell culture and development of NAMPT-resistant cell models

Human acute lymphoblastic leukemia cells (CCRF-CEM) and human breast cancer cells (MDA MB231) were obtained from the Interlab Cell line Collection bank (ICLC HTL01002) and American Type Culture Collection (ATCC), respectively. CCRF-CEM (CEM) cells were maintained in RPMI 1640 (Invitrogen, Carlsbad, CA), and MDA MB231 (MDA) cells were maintained in DMEM supplemented with 10% fetal bovine serum (FBS, Lonza), 2 mM L-glutamine, and 100 U/ml penicillin-streptomycin (Lonza). They were cultured at 37 °C, 5% CO_2 incubator. NAMPT-resistant cell models were gradually developed by increasing the concentration of FK866 (sc-205325, Santa Cruz) up to 500 nM in both cell lines. Cell viability was determined by exclusion of 0.2% trypan blue. The FK866-resistant sublines, CEM RES and MDA RES, were maintained in the presence of 100 nM FK866 in the culture medium. A final 100-nM FK866-resistant subline (CEM RES) was used in all experiments.

In vitro cell viability and drug combination assays

CCRF-CEM and MDA MB231 cells were treated with FK866, CHS-828 (200484-11-3, Cayman Chemical), oligomycin A (75351, Sigma), 2-deoxyglucose (D8375, Sigma), GSK2837808A (GSK) (5189, Tocris), JPH203 (a selective L-type amino acid transporter), and L-asparaginase (11185, Sigma) for 48 h. JPH203 was kindly obtained from Dr.

Peyron [30]. In vitro drug sensitivity was assessed by the colorimetric methyl-thiazolyltetrazolium (MTT) assay (sigma), XTT proliferation kit (sigma), and OZBlue Cell Viability kit (OZbiosciences). Combination treatment of FK866 with JPH203 was performed and 48 h after combination treatment, Cell viability was determined using XTT assay (Invitrogen) and DAPI staining. Percentage of cell death was subjected for drug combination analysis as described by combination index (CI). CI was analyzed using CompuSyn software V1.0 by the method of Chou and Talalay [31]. CI < 1 indicates drug synergistic effect, CI > 1 indicates drug antagonistic effect, and CI = 1 indicates drug additive effect.

Determination of NAD(H), ATP levels, and rate of protein translation

Cells were treated with FK866 for 48 h. Intracellular NAD(H) and ATP content were assessed with a NAD/NADH-Glo (G9071, Promega) and CellTiter-Glo Luminescent Cell Viability Assay (G7571, Promega) according to the manufacturer's protocol. Fluorescence data were measured and normalized to protein concentration in the cell lysates (Bradford Reagent, Sigma). Rate of protein translation was analyzed by Click-iT AHA Alexa Fluor 488 Protein Synthesis Assay (Life Technologies) according to the manufacturer's protocol. Cells were treated with FK866 for 45 h and further incubated for 3H with 50 μM AHA in L-methionine-free medium (RPMI-1640 Medium, Sigma-Aldrich) containing the drug (or DMSO). After fixation and permeabilization, AHA incorporation was assessed by flow cytometry. 7-AAD Staining Solution (0.25 μg/sample) allowed the exclusion of non-viable cells. Flow cytometry experiments were carried out on two biological replicates, and statistics were based on acquisition of 50,000 events/sample.

For the HPLC analysis of NAD and NMN (nicotinamide mononucleotide), nucleotides were extracted by resuspending cell pellets in 0.4 M $HClO_4$. After 5 min on ice, samples were centrifuged at 16,000×g for 5 min. Pellets were resuspended in 100 μl formic acid, incubated 5 min at 37 °C, and used for the determination of the protein concentration (Bradford reagent). Supernatants were neutralized with 1 M K_2CO_3 and used for NAD and NMN determination. NAD was quantified by UV C18-HPLC under ion-pairing conditions [32]. NMN was first derivatized with acetophenone as described in [33] and then quantified by spectrofluorometric HPLC analysis as described in [32]. Values of NAD and NMN levels were referred to the protein concentration.

Western blot analysis

Amino acid depletion experiment was conducted in 20:80 mixture of normal RPMI-1640 (10% FBS + 2 mM L-glutamine) with Eagle's balanced salt solution (E3024; sigma) supplemented with 10% FBS. Cells were treated with FK866, JPH203, L-Asp, and indicated combinations for 24 h in the present or absent of amino acid supplementation including 2 mM L-glutamine (Sigma), 0.25 mM L-tryptophan (Sigma), 1× essential amino acid mixture (EAA) (Sigma), and 1× non-essential amino acid (NEAA) (Sigma). Samples were lysed in RIPA lysis buffer supplemented with Protease Inhibitor Cocktail (Thermo Scientific). Equal amounts of proteins were separated by SDS–PAGE. The antibodies used were the following: QPRT (TA501520) from OriGene; 4EBP1 (sc-6936), p-4EBP1(Ser 65/Thr 70; sc-12884), EIF4E (sc-9976), p-EIF4E (Ser209; sc-12885), MTOR (sc-8319), NAMPT(sc-130058), GAPDH (sc-32233), and LDHA (sc-137243) from Santa Cruz; NAPRT (ab-211529), EIF2A (ab26197), p-EIF2A (Ser 51; ab32157), and p-MTOR (Ser 2448; ab1093) from Abcam; and AMPKα (2603), p-AMPKα (Thr 172; 2531), ACTIN (3700), and CHOP (2895) from Cell Signaling. ACTIN and GAPDH were used as protein loading control. Densitometric analysis and normalization relative to control was conducted using ImageJ software. A representative western blot of three-independent biological experiments is shown.

shRNA and siRNA transfection

Lentiviral vector particles (LVPs) were generated in Lenti-HEK293 cells. Briefly, cells were co-transfected with a Δ891 and a VSV-G encoding vector along with a shRNA transfer lentiviral plasmid PLKO vector and a shNAPRT plasmid (a gift of Dr. Alessio Nencioni). Seventy-two hours post-transfection, viral supernatants were collected, filtrated, and performed quantification. MDA cells were stably transduced with shNAPRT, and selection of puromycin (2.5 μg/ml) was performed. Downregulation of LDHA in MDA cells was performed by transient transfection of siRNA of *LDHA* using INTERFERin in vitro siRNA/miRNA transfection reagent (Polyplus) for 48 h. Then, cells were treated with FK866 for 48 h.

RNA extraction and real-time PCR

Total RNA was extracted using RNA extraction kit (ZYMO research), and contaminant DNA was removed by RNase-Free DNase kit (ZYMO research). Synthesis of cDNA was carried out on RevertAid RT kit (K1691, Themoscientific). Real-time qPCR analyses were performed with triplicates using KAPA SYBR FAST Universal qPCR Kit on a CFX96 real-time PCR Detection system (Bio-Rad). Expression levels are always given relative to *ACTIN, 18S*, or *GAPDH.* Primer's sequences are provided in Additional file 1: Table S2.

Analysis of mitochondria functions and cellular compartment ATP production

Cells were costained with 100 nM MitoTracker™ CMTMRos Orange (Invitrogen) and DRAQ5 Fluorescent

Probe Solution (62251) (Thermo Scientific^{TM}) for 30 min. Mitochondria images, number, and intensity were acquired by PerkinElmer Operetta and analyzed by harmony analysis software. Loss functional mitochondria was monitored by the sensitivity to carbonilcyanide p-triflouromethoxyphenylhydrazone (FCCP).

Mitochondria and cytosolic ATP production

Cells were treated in triplicate with control (PBS), oligomycin A (10 μg/ml; Sigma), sodium iodoacetate (100 μM; Sigma), or both. Following a 1-h incubation at 37 °C, ATP levels were measured using the CellTiter-Glo Luminescent Cell Viability Assay (G7571, Promega) according to the manufacturer's protocol. Luminescence was then recorded on a Berthold Technologies Luminoscan. Oligomycin A is used to block ATP production by oxidative phosphorylation, and iodoacetate prevents the ATP production through glycolysis. The addition of both molecules is used to determine residual ATP levels which are subtracted for each condition.

Oxygen consumption measurements

Oxygen consumption was measured at 37 °C in a closed chamber, using an amperometric electrode (Unisense Microrespiration, Unisense A/S, Denmark). Two-hundred thousand cells were permeabilized with 0.03 mg/ml digitonin for 1 min, centrifuged for 9 min at 1000 rpm, and resuspended in a buffer containing 137 mM NaCl, 5 mM KCl, 0.7 mM KH2PO4, 25 mM Tris–HCl, pH 7.4, and 25 mg/ml ampicillin. The same solution was used in the oxymetric measurements; 10 mM pyruvate plus 5 mM malate were added to stimulate the pathway composed by complexes I, III, and IV. Then, 20 mM succinate was added to stimulate the pathway formed by complexes II, III, and IV. To observe the ADP-stimulated respiration rates, 0.08 mM ADP was added after pyruvate and malate or succinate addition. To verify whether oxygen consumption is really due to the electron transport chain 0.1 mM rotenone or 50 μM antimycin A, specific inhibitors of complex I or complex III were used (data not shown). The respiratory rates were expressed as nmol O/min/10^6 cells [34].

ATP synthase activity assay

To evaluate the ATP synthase activity, 100,000 cells were incubated for 10 min at 37 °C in a medium containing 10 mM Tris–HCl, pH 7.4, 100 mM KCl, 5 mM KH_2PO_4, 1 mM EGTA, 2.5 mM EDTA, 5 mM $MgCl_2$, 0.6 mM ouabain, and 25 mg/ml ampicillin. Afterward, ATP synthesis was induced by the addition of 10 mM pyruvate plus 5 mM malate or 20 mM succinate to stimulate the pathways composed by complexes I, III, and IV or complexes II, III, and IV, respectively. The reaction was monitored for 2 min, every 30 s, in a luminometer (GloMax® 20/20n Luminometer, Promega Italia, Milano, Italy), by the luciferin/luciferase chemiluminescent method, with ATP standard solutions between 10–8 and 10–5 M (luciferin/luciferase ATP bioluminescence assay kit CLSII, Roche, Basel, Switzerland). Data were expressed as nmol ATP produced/min/10^6 cells [35]. The oxidative phosphorylation efficiency (P/O ratio) was calculated as the ratio between the concentration of the produced ATP and the amount of consumed oxygen in the presence of respiring substrate and ADP. When the oxygen consumption is completed devoted to the energy production, the P/O ratio should be around 2.5 and 1.5 after pyruvate + malate or succinate addition, respectively [36].

Glucose consumption

Glucose consumption was evaluated by the hexokinase (HK) and glucose-6-phosphate dehydrogenase (G6PD) coupling system, following the reduction of NADP at 340 nm. The assay medium contained 100 mM Tris–HCl, pH 7.4, 2 mM ATP, 10 mM NADP, 2 mM MgCl2, 2 IU of hexokinase, and 2 IU of glucose-6-phosphate dehydrogenase. Data was normalized to the cell number and expressed as mM glucose consumed/10^6 cells [37].

Lactate release assay

Lactate concentration was assayed spectrophotometrically in the growth medium, following the reduction of NAD^+ at 340 nm. The assay medium contained 100 mM Tris–HCl (pH 8), 5 mM NAD^+, and 1 IU/ml of lactate dehydrogenase. Samples were analyzed before and after the addition of 4 μg of purified lactate dehydrogenase. Data was normalized to the cell number and expressed as mM lactate released/10^6 cells [37].

Glycolytic enzyme assays

All enzymatic assays were performed on 50 μg of total protein. The reaction mixtures used for the determination of each enzyme activity were prepared as follows [38]: hexokinase (HK, EC 2.7.1.1): 100 mM Tris–HCl, pH 7.4, 5 mM MgCl2, 200 mM glucose, 1 mM ATP, 0.91 mM NADP, and 0.55 IU/ml of glucose-6-phosphate dehydrogenase (G6PD); phosphofructokinase (PFK, EC 2.7.1.11): 100 mM Tris–HCl, pH 7.4, 2 mM MgCl2, 5 mM KCl, 2 mM fructose 6 phosphate, 1 mM ATP, 0.5 mM phosphoenolpyruvate (PEP), 40 μM rotenone, 0.2 mM NADH, and 2 IU/ml of pyruvate kinase plus lactate dehydrogenase; pyruvate kinase (PK, EC 2.7.1.40): 100 mM Tris–HCl, pH 7.6, 2.5 mM MgCl2, 10 mM KCl, 0.6 mM phosphoenolpyruvate, 40 μM rotenone, 0.2 mM NADH, 5 mM ADP, and 1 IU/ml of lactate dehydrogenase; and lactate dehydrogenase (LDH, EC 1.1.1.27): 100 mM Tris–HCl, pH 9, 5 mM pyruvate, 40 μM rotenone, and 0.2 mM NADH. Each enzymatic activity was expressed as mU/mg of total protein (micromoles/min/mg of protein).

Activity assay of NAD(H) biosynthetic enzymes

Pellets of about 20×10^6 cultured cells were homogenized with 0.25 ml buffer consisting of 50 mM Tris–HCl, pH 7.5, 0.15 M NaCl, 1 mM dithiothreitol (DTT), 1 mM phenylmethanesulfonyl fluoride, and 0.002 mg/ml each of leupeptin, antipain, chymostatin, and pepstatin. Homogenates were centrifuged at 20,000×*g* for 10 min at 4 °C, and the supernatants were used for the simultaneous assay of QAPRT, NAPRT, NAMPT, NRK, and NADS activities. NMNAT activity was assayed in the homogenates. The activities were measured by the coupled fluorometric assay [39]. Briefly, the products of the enzymes' catalyzed reactions, i.e., NMN, NAMN, and NAAD, were stoichiometrically converted to NAD^+ by using ancillary bacterial enzymes, and NAD^+ was quantified by a fluorometric cycling assay for QAPRT, NAPRT, NRK, and NAMPT activity determination [39]. NADS assay mixture contained 50 mM HEPES/KOH buffer, pH 7.5, 0.1 M KCl, 5 mM MgCl2, 10 mM KF, 4 mM ATP, 20 mM glutamine, 1 mM NAAD, and about 0.15 mg/ml cell lysate. A control mixture without NAAD was processed in parallel. NMNAT assay mixture consisted of 40 mM HEPES/KOH buffer, pH 7.5, 25 mM MgCl2, 10 mM KF, 0.06 mg/ml BSA, 1 mM DTT, 1 mM ATP, 1 mM NMN, and about 0.05 mg/ml cell homogenate. A control mixture without NMN was processed in parallel. Assay mixtures were incubated and processed for the quantitation of the formed NAD(H) as described in [39]. The enzymes' activity was referred to the protein concentration.

Flow cytometric cell cycle analysis

CCRF-CEM cells were treated with 10 and 20 μM GSK for 48 h, and they were incubated with the DNA-staining chemical propidium iodide (PI) (FITC/annexin V apoptosis detection kit; BD Pharmingen) for DNA content-based assessment of cell cycle distribution for 10 min. Cell cycle analysis was performed using flow cytometric. Twenty-four hours of cell starvation and 100 ng/ml Nocodazole were used as positive controls. Percentage of G1 phase, S phase, and G2 phase were analyzed using FACS.

Microarrays

Total RNA extracted from CEM RES cells was hybridized in quadruplicate on the Agilent Human GE 4x44K v2 Microarray (G2519F-026652) and compared with total RNA from parental cells. After quantile normalization and removal of low signals, differentially expressed genes were selected according to a double threshold on the log2 fold change (absolute value > 0.75) and moderated *t* test *p* value (< 0.05) calculated with the Limma package. Functional annotation enrichment analysis of the resulting lists of DEGs was performed with the clusterProfiler Bioconductor package. The significance of over-representation was determined using a *p* value threshold of 0.05. Gene ontology terms with less than 500 associated genes were used for the analysis. Microarray raw data are available on Gene Expression Omnibus under the following accession number: GSE96636.

Statistical analysis

Values are expressed as mean ± S.D. of three independent biological experiments conducted in technical triplicates. Student's *t* test or one-way ANOVA was employed to determined statistical significance between control and test groups. Values of $^*p < 0.05$, $^{**}p < 0.01$, and $^{***}p < 0.001$ were considered significant. Data were plotted by Graph prism 6 software.

Results

Generation of FK866-resistant cancer cell models

The absence of NAPRT in CCRF-CEM (CEM) cells and the low expression of QPRT in MDA MB231 (MDA) cells were found to be the main differences between the two cell lines with respect to their NAD^+ production apparatus (Fig. 1b–d). We developed FK866-resistant CEM and MDA cells by using a stepwise increase in FK866 concentration [8, 40] in both cases (Fig. 1e, f). FK866 concentration was increased over a 3-month period, and cells became increasingly resistant according to the dose used, suggesting the occurrence of a quick, clinically relevant, adaptation mechanism (Additional file 2: Figure S1A) [40]. The daughter resistant cells were then compared to the parental FK866-sensitive cells, assessing cell viability by MTT-based assays and by counting viable cells. FK866-resistant cells were kept under continuous exposure to FK866 during routine passages. The calculated EC_{50} after 48 h of treatment with FK866 was 9.8 μM for the resistant CCRF-CEM cells (CEM RES), whereas an EC_{50} of 4.4 nM could be estimated for the parental CEM (CEM PA) (about 2000-fold lower) (Fig. 1e, Additional file 2: Figure S1B). Moreover, CEM RES were still able to proliferate during a long-term (5-day) treatment with 500 nM FK866 (Additional file 2: Figure S1C). FK866-resistant MDA MB231 (MDA RES) cells were completely insensitive to FK866 (an EC_{50} could not be calculated), whereas parental cells showed an EC_{50} of 14.8 nM (Fig. 1f). *NAMPT* mRNA levels were higher in MDA cells as compared to CEM cells, and *NAMPT* expression significantly decreased in both resistant CEM and MDA (Fig. 1g). In the subsequent experiments, we aimed at identifying common mechanisms of resistance to NAMPT inhibition that could pinpoint novel therapeutic strategies.

Resistant CEM cells have lower NAD(H) levels than parental cells but do not show mutations in *NAMPT* coding sequence

Acquired resistance to FK866 was not specific for this compound. Instead, it was also observed in response to treatment with CHS-828, a second NAMPT inhibitor (Additional file 2: Figure S1D, E). In both FK866-resistant (CEM RES) and parental CEM (CEM PA), intracellular NAD(H) and ATP levels were measured after a 48-h treatment with FK866 to assess the effect of the drug. While in parental cells, FK866 strongly blunted intracellular ATP stores, in FK866-resistant CCRF-CEM, it had no effect on the nucleotide's levels (Fig. 2a and Additional file 2: Figure S1F). Interestingly, at baseline, NAD(H) levels in CEM RES were approximately 50% lower than those of untreated parental cells, likely due to the decreased expression of NAMPT. FK866 reduced intracellular NAD(H) amounts in both parental and CEM RES. However, the effect size was much bigger in CEM PA cells than in FK866-resistant cells (Fig. 2b, Additional file 2: Figure S1G). Similar to NAD(H), starting levels of NMN, the product of the NAMPT-catalyzed reaction from NAM, were also lower in CEM RES than in CEM PA cells. NMN decreased upon exposure to FK866 in both parental and resistant cells, even though the decrease was more pronounced in parental than in resistant cells (Additional file 2: Figure S1H). Incorporation of a modified alanine that can be fluorescently labeled (AHA) into nascent proteins after FK866 treatment revealed a decrease in protein synthesis in CEM PA, but not in resistant cells cultivated in the presence of 100 nM FK866 in the medium (Fig. 2c). Cell cycle analysis reported a small, but significant, increase in cycling cells in CEM RES (Additional file 2: Figure S1I).

To define the mechanism underlying acquired FK866 resistance in CEM cells, we first assessed a possible role of multi-drug resistance (MDR). However, treatment with inhibitors of drug efflux pumps, such as verapamil and cyclosporine A, failed to affect cell viability in FK866-resistant CEM exposed to FK866, thus excluding a role for MDR mechanisms in the acquired resistance to FK866 in these cells (Additional file 2: Figure S1J). We subsequently sequenced the *NAMPT* gene in both parental and resistant CEM cells. However, we did not observe any mutation in *NAMPT* coding region in both resistant and parental CEM [13]. By assaying the NAMPT enzymatic activity in the lysates from both cells, we found that it was downregulated by about 50% in the resistant model, in keeping with the lower expression of the protein (Figs. 1g and 2d).

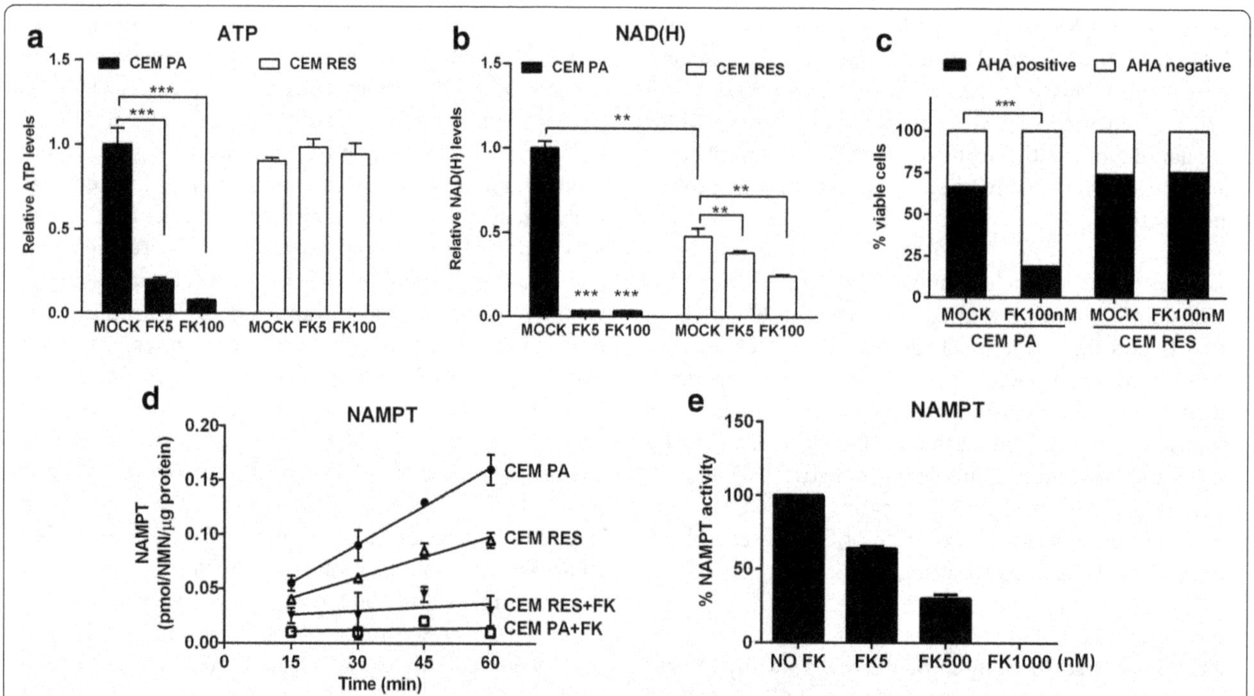

Fig. 2 Characterization of FK866-resistant cells. **a**, **b** Administration of FK866 decreases intracellular ATP and NAD(H) levels in CEM PA cells. CEM PA and CEM RES cells were treated with 5 and 100 nM FK866 for 48 h. Relative ATP and NAD(H) levels were normalized to number of viable cells. **c** FK866 inhibits global protein translation. CEM PA and CEM RES cells were treated with 100 nM FK866 for 48 h. Protein synthesis was monitored by Click-it chemistry based on the incorporation of an amino acid analog (AHA). The histogram quantifies FK866-induced protein synthesis arrest in the viable cell population. **d** Time course of the NAMPT enzymatic activity assayed in lysates from CEM PA and CEM RES cells. Assays were performed in the absence and in the presence of 1 μM FK866 in the reaction mixtures. **e** NAMPT enzymatic activity was analyzed in lysates from CEM RES cells in the absence and in the presence of the indicated FK866 concentrations. All data were conducted in three independent experiments with technical triplicates (*$p < 0.05$, **$p < 0.01$, ***$p < 0.001$ compared to Mock)

Notably, we did observe that NAMPT enzymatic activity was fully inhibited by 1 μM FK866 both in parental and resistant cells (Fig. 2d). Analysis of the dose-response sensitivity in the resistant model showed a 30 and 64% inhibition of the enzyme in the presence of 5 and 500 nM FK866, respectively (Fig. 2e). A 2-month FK866 washout of CEM RES only marginally affected their drug resistance (Additional file 2: Figure S2A, B), suggesting a stable genetic or epigenetic reprogramming as a mechanism underlying NAMPT inhibitor resistance.

CEM RES cells show constitutive alterations in metabolic pathways

To evaluate the effects of FK866 on gene expression, we profiled the transcriptome of parental vs. resistant CEM cells treated or not with the NAMPT inhibitor FK866 by microarrays. Using a double threshold on statistical significance (p value < 0.05) and log2 fold change (absolute value > 0.75), we identified 629 differentially expressed genes (DEGs, 285 upregulated and 344 downregulated) after FK866 treatment of parental cells (Fig. 3a, Additional file 3: Table S1). Functional annotation analyses of all DEGs highlighted the modulation of transcripts responsible for the epigenetic status of the cells. Specifically, we observed the enrichment of gene ontology (GO) categories associated with lysine acetylation; modulation of key epigenetic regulators, such as *ATF2*, *SIRT1*, and *SIRT3*; and transcription factors involved in energetic stress response and NAD(H) dependent enzymes. In addition, the enrichment of categories associated with cell response to DNA damage (*CHEK1*, *GADD45G*, *CHOP*) and modulation of apoptotic-converging signaling cascades suggested that FK866 caused toxic effects in parental cells (Fig. 3b, Additional file 3: Table S1). Exposure to FK866 of CEM RES did not induce significant changes in gene expression (about 150 DEGs, 66 upregulated and 96 downregulated), which is in line with the lack of effect of this agent on cell metabolism (Fig. 3c, Additional file 3: Table S1). Indeed, treatment of CEM RES did not activate the integrated stress response (ISR) as shown by the fact that 4EBP1 and EIF2A, two key proteins regulating translation initiation, did not change their phosphorylation status, suggesting that these pathways were not activated by FK866 treatment. Notably, AMPK, the AMP-regulated kinase sensing the cell energetic status and responding to stress, was constitutively phosphorylated in CEM RES, possibly suggesting that CEM RES rely on the activation of this kinase for overcoming the FK866 insult (Fig. 3d, e) [41]. *CHOP* expression also did not increase (Fig. 3f), thus showing that a key pro-apoptotic protein that became upregulated by FK866 in parental cells was not triggered in resistant cells by FK866 treatment. Direct comparison of untreated CEM RES vs. CEM PA highlighted major differences between the two samples. More than 5000 genes were differentially regulated (2354 upregulated, 2681 downregulated, Additional file 3: Table S1), a difference that clearly indicates a profound gene expression rewiring in resistant cells. According to a functional annotation of the transcripts undergoing major expression variations, strong differences were observed in metabolic pathways, such as glycolysis, oxidative phosphorylation (OXPHOS), NAD^+ biosynthesis, and amino acid transport (Fig. 3g, Additional file 3: Table S1). No indication of differential expression of drug efflux pumps was observed, confirming that a multi-drug resistance mechanism is unlikely to mediate FK866 resistance in CEM. Taken together, gene expression analysis of CEM RES suggested that cancer cells adapted to FK866-induced NAD(H) depletion by adopting profound changes in gene expression and by modulating their metabolic pathways. Therefore, we focused on these metabolic changes and assessed whether compensating metabolic mechanisms would be responsible for conferring resistance to FK866 and could possibly highlight vulnerabilities of the resistant cells.

CEM RES cells shift towards an aerobic glycolytic-based metabolism

We evaluated the degree of activation of glycolysis and of OXPHOS in CEM RES by measuring the level of ATP production in the mitochondria and in the cytoplasm, as well as the activity of key OXPHOS and glycolytic enzymes. Cytosolic ATP production increased by about 15% in resistant cells (Fig. 4a), although the energy production efficiency of both pathways of the mitochondrial respiratory chain, the one including complexes I, III, and IV and the one comprising complexes II, III, and IV, was reduced in CEM RES. In particular, the oxygen consumption rate (OCR) appeared significantly low only after succinate addition (Fig. 4b) that stimulates the pathway led by complex II, while ATP synthesis by Fo-F1 ATP synthase was impaired both in the presence of pyruvate + malate (which induces the complex I pathway) and with succinate (Fig. 4c). Parental and resistant cells showed a coupled OXPHOS as the P/O rate was within standard values [36]. The decrease in OXPHOS activity was paralleled by an increase in glucose consumption and in lactate production (Fig. 4d, e). The activities of the glycolytic enzymes, hexokinase (HK), phosphofructokinase (PFK), pyruvate kinase (PK), and lactate dehydrogenase (LDH), were all significantly increased in CEM RES as compared to the parental cells (Fig. 4f). Therefore, these data suggested that activation of aerobic glycolysis compensates for the decrease in OXPHOS observed in the resistant cells. We then evaluated whether FK866-resistant cells were addicted to glycolysis. We found that CEM RES were more sensitive to the glycolysis inhibitor 2-deoxyglucose, than parental cells, while no difference was observed when cells were treated with the OXPHOS inhibitor oligomycin A (Fig. 4g, h). Notably, consistent with the observed decrease

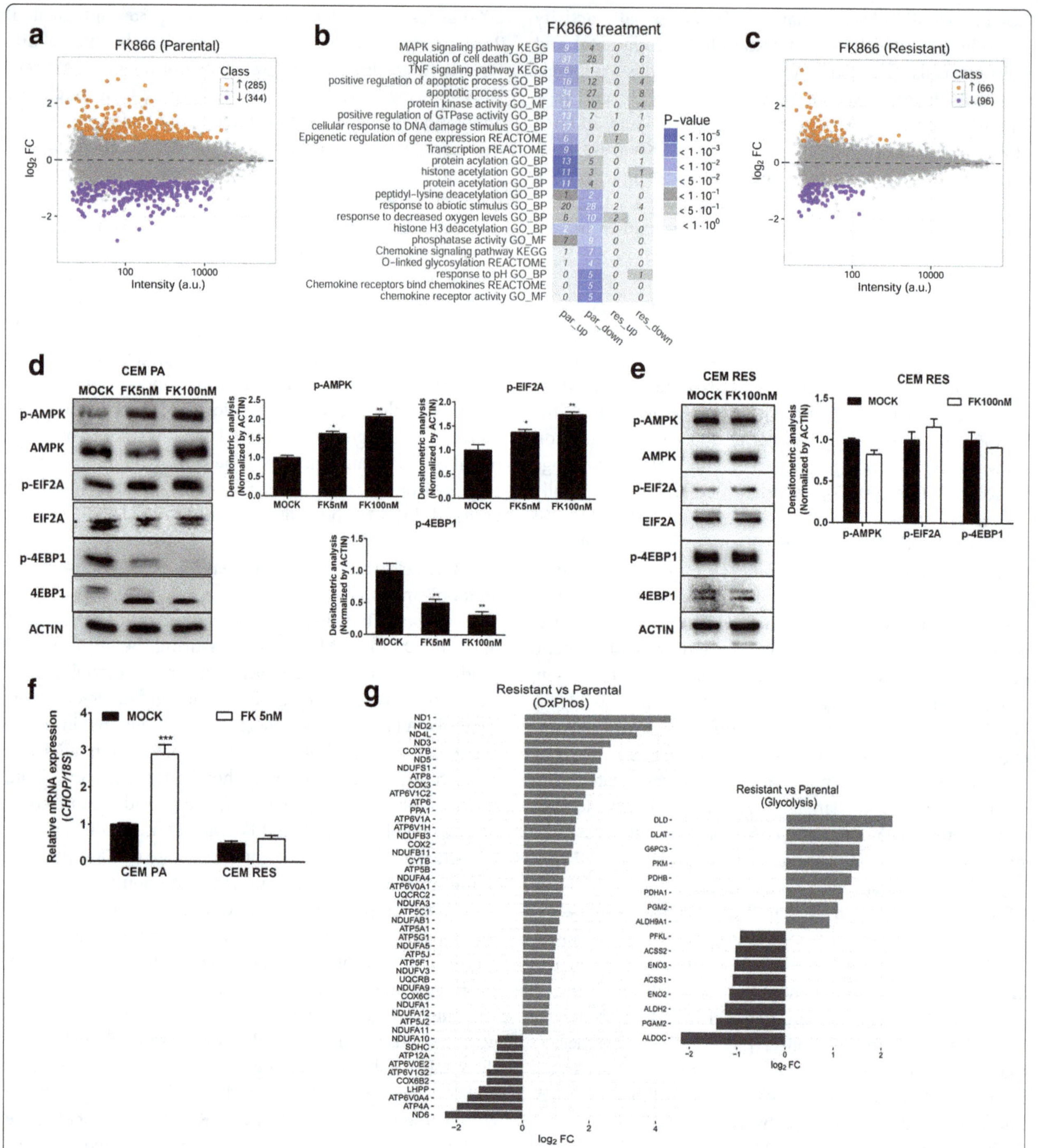

Fig. 3 (See legend on next page.)

(See figure on previous page.)
Fig. 3 Genome-wide analysis of gene expression in CCRF-CEM cells. **a** MA plot of transcriptome profiling in FK866-treated vs. untreated CEM PA cells. For each gene, the average $\log_{10}$ signal against the $\log_2$ fold change is plotted. Genes significantly up (orange)- or down (violet)-regulated upon FK866 treatment are highlighted. **b** Top enriched gene ontology (GO) terms and KEGG pathways among up- and downregulated genes upon FK866 treatment in CEM PA and CEM RES cells. The heatmap, colored according to enrichment *p* values, displays categories associated with lysine acetylation, modulation of key epigenetic regulators, and transcription factors involved in energetic stress response. The number of genes corresponding to each term is reported in each tile. **c** MA plot of transcriptome profiling in FK866-treated vs. untreated CEM RES cells. For each gene, the average $\log_{10}$ signal against the $\log_2$ fold change is plotted. **d** CEM PA cells were treated with 5 and 100 nM FK866 for 48 h. Western blot showing expression of AMPK, mTOR, 4EBP1, and EIF2A in CEM PA cells. **e** No translation inhibition and drug-induced energetic stress occurs upon FK866 treatment in the resistance. Western blot analysis of CEM RES cells treated 100 nM FK866 for 48 h. Quantitative data are expressed as relative expression to MOCK (normalized by ACTIN). **f** CEM RES cells treated with 5 nM FK866 for 48 h. Expression of *CHOP* was determined. Quantitative data were derived from three independent experiments and expressed as the mean ± S.D. (***$p < 0.001$). **g** Barplot displaying genes belonging to the enriched metabolic pathways OXPHOS and glycolysis (KEGG annotation) and with significantly altered expression between CEM PA and CEM RES cells

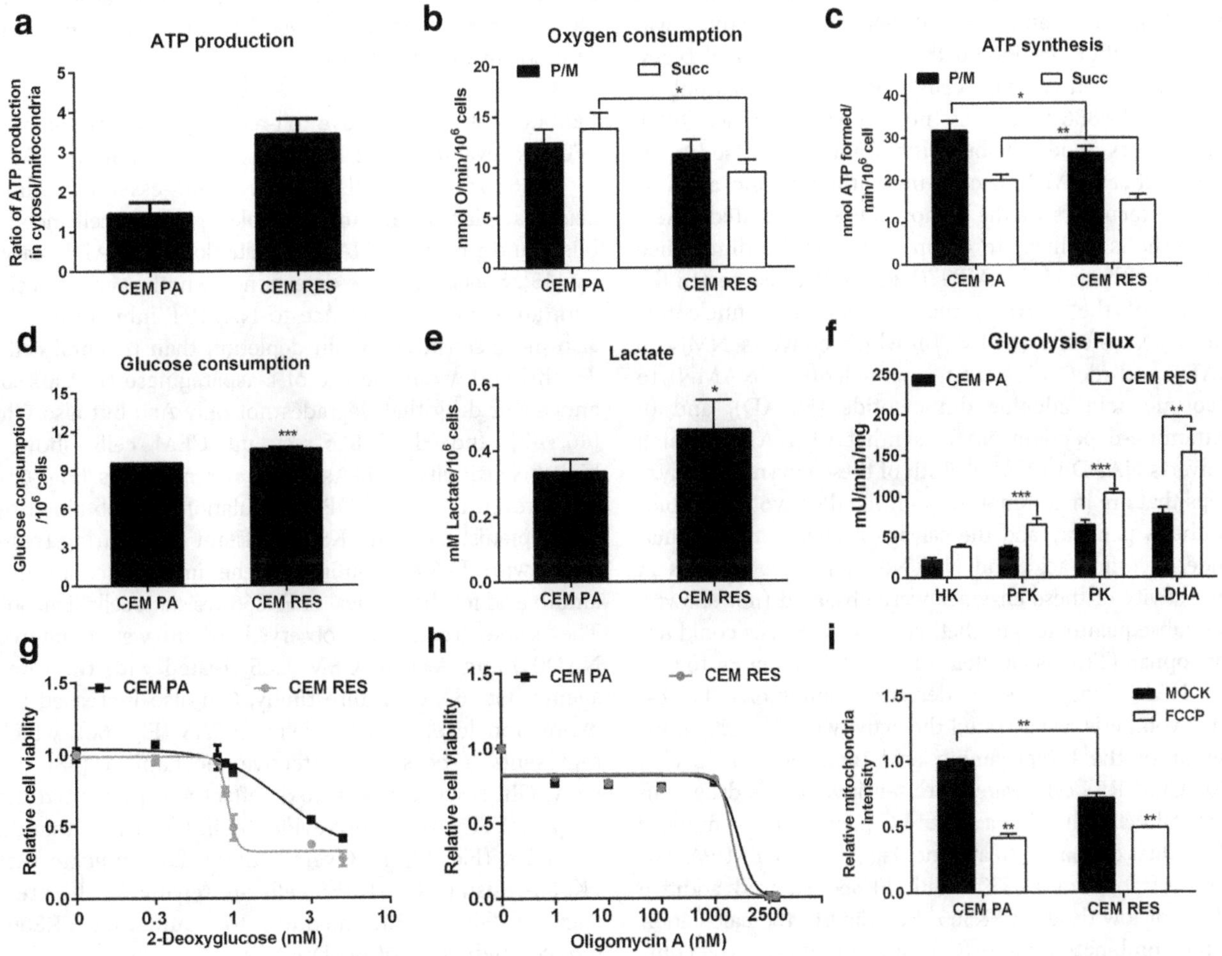

Fig. 4 Enhanced glycolysis dependency of CEM RES cells. **a** Production of ATP from mitochondria and glycolysis were measured in CEM PA and CEM RES cells. Ratio of ATP production in the cytosol/mitochondria is shown. **b–f** Metabolic enhanced towards glycolysis in CEM RES cells; CEM PA and CEM RES subclones at 10, 40, and 100 nM of FK866 were determined the aerobic metabolism, oxygen consumption (**b**), and ATP synthesis (**c**). Cells were analyzed in the presence of 5 mM pyruvate + 2.5 mM malate (P/M) or 20 mM succinate (Succ) to stimulate the pathways composed by complexes I, III, and IV or complexes II, III, and IV, respectively. To measure the glycolytic flux, glucose consumption (**d**), lactate production (**e**), and the activity of hexokinase (HK), 6-phospho-fructokinase (PFK), pyruvate kinase (PK), and lactate dehydrogenase (LDH) (**f**) were analyzed. **g–h** CEM PA and CEM RES cells were treated with 2-deoxyglucose (**g**) and oligomycin A (**h**) for 48 h. Relative cell viability is shown. **i** Analysis of mitochondria content was conducted in CEM PA and CEM RES cells. Cells were exposed to mitotracker staining. FCCB was used as a negative control. Data was shown as mean ± S.D. of three independent experiments with technical triplicates, *$p < 0.05$, **$p < 0.01$, and ***$p < 0.001$

in OXPHOS, the fluorescent signal produced by tetramethylrhodamine (TMRE), a dye whose incorporation into the mitochondria is driven by the strength of the mitochondrial transmembrane potential, was largely decreased in resistant cells (Fig. 4i). Therefore, CEM RES cells appear to compensate for the decrease in OXPHOS activity by increasing the activity of the glycolytic pathway and by shifting towards a Warburg-like metabolism.

CEM RES cells are sensitive to tryptophan deprivation

Thereafter, we measured the enzymatic activity of QPRT, NAPRT, and NRK (Fig. 1a), the enzyme converting nicotinamide riboside (NR) to NMN, in CEM cells to evaluate whether NAD^+ biosynthesis pathways alternative to the route controlled by NAMPT were exploited by CEM RES cells. As expected, no NAPRT activity was observed in both parental and resistant cells and no activity was measured after the FK866 treatment in both cell types. Interestingly, in resistant cells, NRK activity was not affected by FK866 treatment (not shown), whereas QPRT activity was modestly but significantly increased, suggesting that CEM RES cells may utilize amino acids as NAD^+ precursors via the de novo QPRT-mediated NAD^+ biosynthesis pathway to compensate for the diminished NAD^+ synthesis via NAMPT (Fig. 5a). We also tested the activity of the enzymes nicotinamide mononucleotide adenylyltransferase (NMNAT), which converts NMN to NAD^+ and nicotinic acid mononucleotide (NAMN) to nicotinic acid adenine dinucleotide (NAAD), and of glutamine-dependent NAD^+ synthetase (NADS), which converts NAAD to NAD+. Both of these enzymes catalyze steps that are in common to both the de novo NAD^+ biosynthesis pathway and the salvage routes from nicotinamide, nicotinic acid, and NR. No significant changes in the activity of these enzymes were observed (not shown). We subsequently tested whether CEM RES cells could use tryptophan (Trp) as an alternative NAD^+ precursor to sustain NAD^+ biosynthesis under stress conditions. To test this hypothesis, we assessed the activity of JPH203, an inhibitor of the L-type amino acid transporter 1 (LAT1) [30]. CEM RES cells were more sensitive to this drug than parental cells, showing a lower EC_{50} and a lower number of residual cells after treatment (Fig. 5b). In CEM PA, co-administration of JPH203 with FK866 showed additive effects at low doses of FK866 according to the calculation of the combination index (CI). In resistant cells, the combination of the two drugs had a synergistic effect in line with the higher efficacy of JPH203 in these cells than in parental cells (Fig. 5c). In amino acid deprivation experiments, CEM RES showed activation of the CHOP death pathway, indicating a fully active response of this stress-induced death pathway [41, 42]. Medium complementation with essential amino acids blocked CHOP activation while non-essential amino acids failed to do so (Fig. 5d). Therefore, CEM RES cells are sensitive to essential amino acid deprivation. Accordingly, co-treatment with JPH203 and FK866 activated the ATF4/CHOP death pathway, while this activation was prevented by tryptophan complementation, likely due to the competition of the amino acid with JPH203 for binding to LAT1 [43, 44] (Fig. 5e, f). Treatment with JPH203 and co-treatment with the two drugs caused a significant decrease in NAD(H) and ATP (Fig. 5g, h), showing the dependence of resistant cells on tryptophan metabolism for the production of these key metabolic molecules. Notably, the dependency on amino acid consumption appears to be caused by increased QPRT activity (Fig. 5a) and not by an increased expression of the LAT1 (Additional file 4: Figure S2C). Taken together, these data indicate that the development of FK866 resistance is associated with the addiction to at least one alternative mechanism of NAD^+ production, namely, via tryptophan/QPRT pathway.

CEM RES cells are sensitive to L-asparaginase treatment

We also evaluated the importance of L-glutamine (Gln) in FK866-resistant cells. Gln is a non-essential amino acid that plays a fundamental role in cancer cell metabolism and promotes NAD^+ production via NADS activity [45]. Specifically, we determined whether cancer cells with an acquired resistance to NAMPT inhibition were also more sensitive to Gln depletion than parental cells. To this end, we made use of L-asparaginase (L-Asp), an anticancer drug that degrades not only Asn but also Gln [46, 47]. Indeed, FK866-resistant CEM cells showed higher sensitivity to L-Asp than parental cells (Fig. 6a). The prevention of CHOP upregulation was obtained by Gln replenishment in FK866-resistant cells during treatment with L-Asp, confirming the importance of this amino acid for the survival of FK866-resistant cells (Fig. 6b). The same trend was observed when we monitored NAD(H) and ATP in CEM RES treated with the same agents (Fig. 6c, d). Interestingly, Gln also increased the expression level of the enzyme *ASNS* (Fig. 6e), which represents a possible protective mechanism [48]. Finally, Gln rescued L-Asp toxic effect and prevented the drop in ATP levels more evidently in CEM RES than in CEM PA (Fig. 6f, g). Overall, these data indicate that FK866-resistant CEM RES cells are relying on the presence of Gln in the medium to counteract FK866-induced reduction of NAD(H).

FK866-resistant MDA MB231 have lower endogenous NAD(H) levels than parental cells but do not shift towards aerobic glycolysis

Similar to CEM RES, FK866-resistant MDA MB231 (MDA RES) were completely insensitive to CHS-828, again showing the independence of their resistance mechanism from the type of NAMPT inhibitor (Additional file 2:

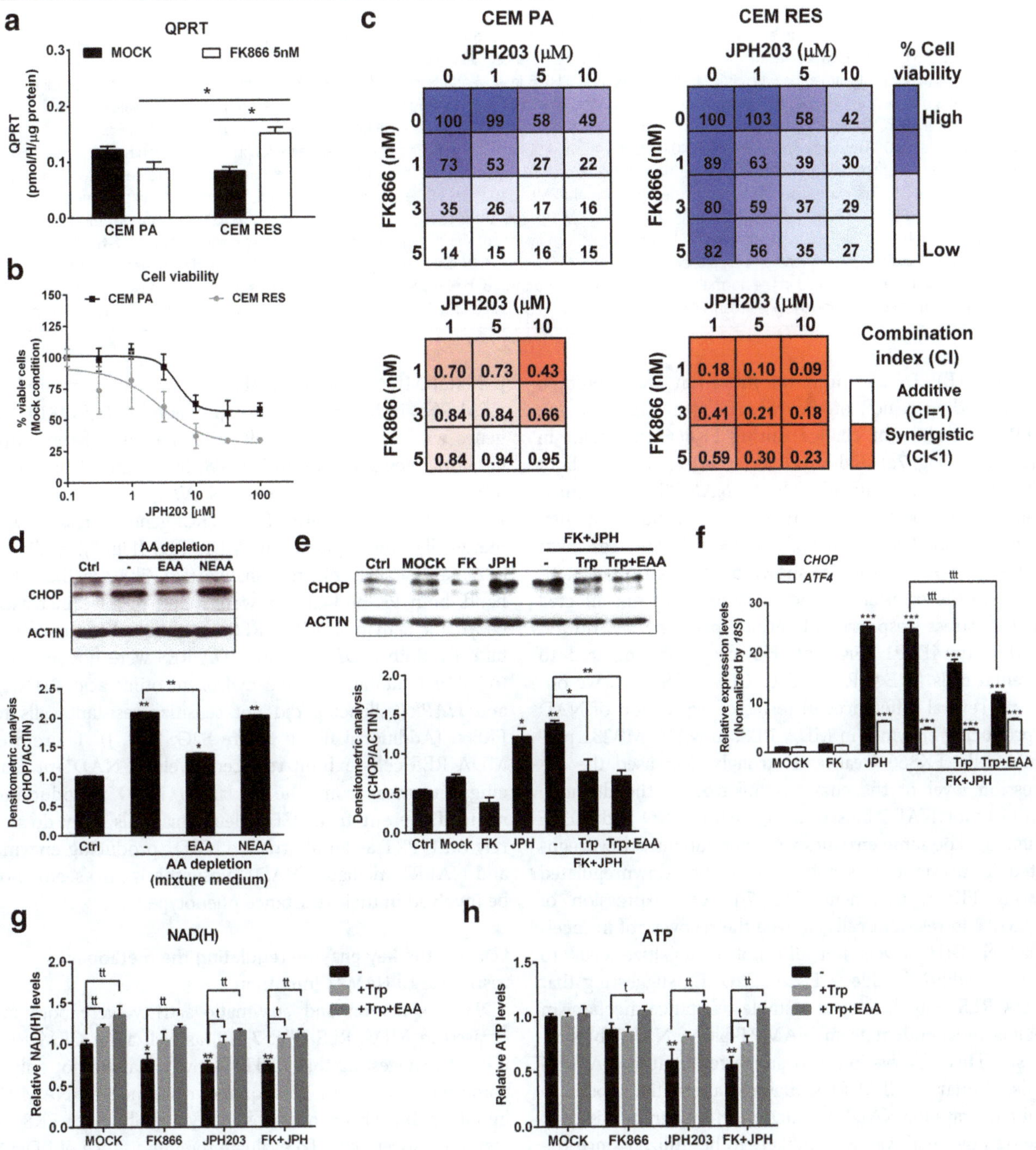

Fig. 5 (See legend on next page.)

(See figure on previous page.)
Fig. 5 Tryptophan was served as an alternative source for NAD production in the resistant cells. **a** CEM PA and CEM RES cells were treated with 5 nM FK866 for 48 h. QPRT enzymatic activity was determined. **b** Percentage of cell viability indicates the response of CEM PA and CEM RES cells to JPH203 (LAT1 inhibitor) at 48 h of treatment. **c** Synergistic effect of FK866 and JPH203 in CEM cells. Strong synergistic effect as detected by low value of combination index (CI < 1) is more evident in CEM RES compared to CEM PA. Percentage of cell viability and CI are shown in respect to DMSO. **d** Activation of CHOP by amino acid deprivation. Western blot depicts the level of CHOP in CEM RES cells. CEM RES cells were treated with normal RPMI-1640 (10% FBS + 2 mM L-glutamine) (lane1), 20:80 mixture of normal RPMI-1640 (10% FBS + 2 mM L-glutamine) with Eagle's balanced salt solution (10% FBS) (lanes 2–4) in the presence of essential amino acid (EAA) or non-essential amino acid (NEAA) for 24 h. **e** Tryptophan (Trp) rescues amino acid sensitized CEM RES cells to JPH203. This experiment was performed in normal RPMI-1640 (10% FBS + 2 mM L-glutamine) (lane 1) and mixture medium (lanes 2–6). CEM RES cells were treated with 5 nM FK866, 10 μM JPH203 (after O/N washout) or FK866 + JPH203. Supplementation of 0.25 mM tryptophan or 1× EAA was addressed to FK866 + JPH203 co-treatment. CHOP level was determined at 24 h after treatment. **f–h** CEM RES cells were treated with indicated conditions, and expression of *CHOP* and *ATF4* mRNA (**f**), NAD(H) level (**g**), and ATP level (**h**) were determined, respectively. Experiments in **a–c** were performed in the normal RPMI-1640 medium and in **d–h** were performed in the mixture medium. Data were plotted as mean ± S.D. from three independent experiments ($^{*}p < 0.05$, $^{***}p < 0.001$ compared to MOCK) and ($^{tt}p < 0.01$, $^{ttt}p < 0.001$ compared among treatments)

Figure S1E). In addition, no mutation was detected in the coding region of the *NAMPT* gene (not shown). ATP levels did not change during FK866 treatment in MDA RES (Fig. 7a), and NAD(H) level decreased to about 50% of the initial value likely due to NAMPT downregulation but did not drop as dramatically as it did in parental cells (Fig. 7b). The absence of toxicity of FK866 treatment in MDA RES cells was also shown by the continuous activation of the translation machinery that was not affected by the stress response inhibition mediated by EIF2A, AMPK, or 4EBP1 (Fig. 7c). However, as compared to parental cells (MDA PA) and to CEM RES cells, we observed several differences in terms of expression of NAD$^+$-producing enzymes in MDA RES. In MDA MB231 parental cells, FK866 treatment strongly decreased the expression level of the enzymes involved in the de novo pathway for NAD$^+$ biosynthesis, such as *IDO* and *KYNE* (Fig. 7d). The same enzymes were permanently downregulated in resistant cells and were further downregulated during FK866 treatment (Fig. 7d). Overexpression of NAMPT in resistant cells allowed the recovery of intracellular NAD(H) levels but did not re-sensitize cells to FK866 (Additional file 4: Figure S2D, E), suggesting that MDA RES cells developed a stable resistance mechanism that is independent from NAMPT-based NAD$^+$ biosynthesis. This observation also suggested that MDA RES cells, similar to CEM RES, may use alternative biochemical pathways for NAD$^+$ production. However, in this case, the de novo pathway was unlikely to be utilized since the enzymes involved in this metabolic route were found to be downregulated compared to the parental cells. In line with these findings, MDA RES cells did not show an increased sensitivity to amino acid deprivation, including tryptophan, as shown by their response to JPH203 (Fig. 7e). In addition, MDA RES also failed to show an increased sensitivity to 2-deoxyglucose, to L-Asp, and to oligomycin A (Fig. 7f–h), indicating the absence of a shift towards a Warburg-like metabolism or dependencies on specific amino acids. No difference in mitochondrial transmembrane potential (TMRE signal) was detected between parental MDA and MDA RES (Fig. 7i). As compared to CEM RES, in MDA RES, the expression level of OXPHOS genes was either unchanged, as in the case of the mitochondrial genes *COX3* and *ATP8*, or affected to a much lesser extent, as in the case of *ND1* (Fig. 7j, Fig. 3g, Additional file 4: Figure S2F). *HK2* gene expression was marginally downregulated in MDA RES (Fig. 7j), while its enzymatic activity did not change (Fig. 7k). On the other hand, both PK and LDHA were found to have increased enzymatic activity in MDA RES as compared to the parental cells. Both MDA PA and MDA RES were not sensitive to NAPRT inhibition with 2-hydroxynicotinic acid (2HNA), and *NAPRT* silencing did not sensitize resistant cells to FK866 (Additional file 4: Figure S2G, H, I, J). Therefore, MDA RES cells exhibit reduced levels of NAD$^+$-producing enzymes from the de novo NAD$^+$ production route. Different from CEM leukemia cells, they do not rely on QPRT as an alternative NAD$^+$-producing enzyme and NAPRT-mediated NAD$^+$ biosynthesis also seems not be involved in their resistance phenotype.

LDHA is the key enzyme regulating the metabolic resistance to NAMPT inhibition

LDHA expression and enzymatic activity were both increased in MDA RES (Fig. 7j, k), as well as in CEM RES (Fig. 4f), suggesting that LDHA activity may be not only a common mechanism of acquired resistance to NAMPT inhibition but also a new possible vulnerability of FK866-resistant cancer cells. To evaluate the importance of LDHA in the resistance of both cell models, we treated our cell lines with the LDH inhibitor GSK2837808A (GSK). When using GSK as a single agent, we observed a marginal increase in sensitivity in CEM RES compared to parental cells (Fig. 8a) and a decrease in ATP and NAD(H) levels (Fig. 8b, c). In cell cycle experiments, we found that GSK induced a strong accumulation in the S and in the G2/M phases of the cell cycle in CEM RES cells (Fig. 8d, e) [49]. At the molecular level, GSK activated the ATF4/CHOP-dependent pro-apoptotic pathway and decreased lactate production (Fig. 8f and Additional file 5: Figure S3A). GSK

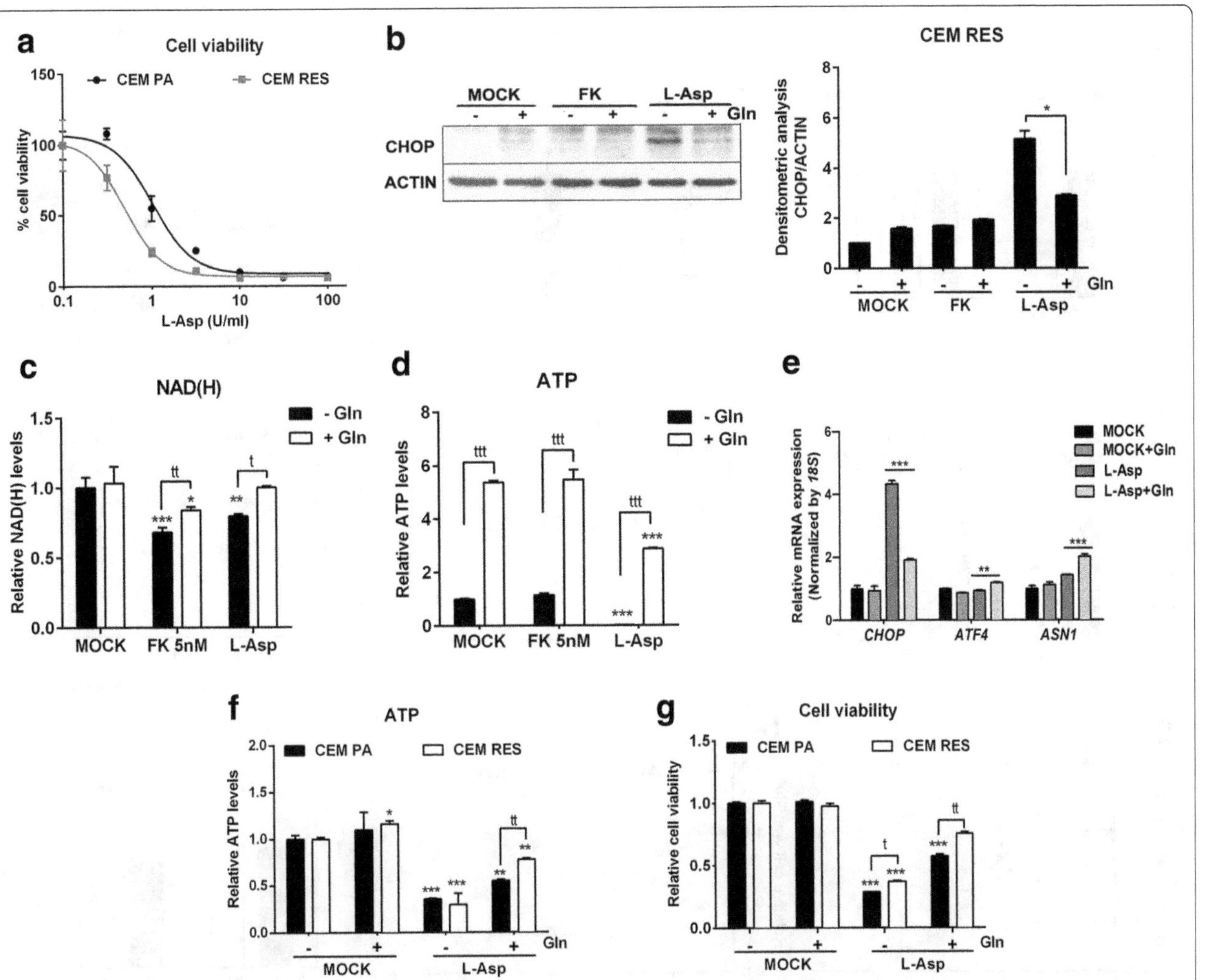

Fig. 6 The resistant cells are sensitive to L-asparaginase. **a** CEM PA and CEM RES cells were treated with L-asparaginase (L-Asp) for 48 h. This experiment was performed in normal RPMI-1640 (10% FBS + 2 mM L-glutamine). Percentage of cell viability was determined. **b** CEM RES cells were treated with 5 nM FK866 and 3 U/ml L-Asp in the presence or absence of Gln supplementation. Twenty-four hours post-treatment, western blot analysis of CHOP expression was conducted. **c, d** CEM RES cells were treated with 5 nM FK866 and 3 U/ml L-Asp in the presence or absence of Gln supplementation. Twenty-four hours post-treatment, NAD(H) (**c**) and ATP level (**d**) were measured. **e** CEM RES cells were treated with 3 U/ml L-Asp in the presence and absence of Gln supplementation for 24 h. Expression of *CHOP*, *ATF4*, and *ASNS* were determined. Expression of *18S* was served as a housekeeping gene. **f, g** CEM PA and CEM RES cells were treated with 3 U/ml L-Asp in the presence and absence of Gln exposure for 24 h. ATP level (**f**) and cell viability (**g**) were measured. Experiments in **b–g** were performed in 20:80 mixture of normal RPMI-1640 (10% FBS + 2 mM L-glutamine) with Eagle's balanced salt solution (10% FBS). Data were plotted as mean ± S.D. from three independent experiments with technical triplicates ($^{*}p < 0.05$, $^{**}p < 0.01$, $^{***}p < 0.001$ compared to MOCK) and ($^{tt}p < 0.01$, $^{ttt}p < 0.001$ compared among treatments)

also decreased *LDHA* expression (Fig. 8g), in addition to blunting its enzymatic activity, and effectively re-sensitized CEM RES cells to FK866 in co-treatment experiments as shown by an additive ATP decrease (Fig. 8h). MDA RES cells showed a similar but not identical response to GSK treatment. Specifically, MDA RES were more sensitive than the parental population to GSK treatment at high doses (Fig. 9a, b). GSK effectively reduced the acidity of the medium both in MDA PA and in MDA RES (Additional file 5: Figure S3B). By itself, GSK did not decrease NAD(H) levels and it did not activate the ATF4/CHOP apoptotic pathway in MDA RES (Fig. 9c, Additional file 5: Figure S3C, D). However, it effectively re-sensitized MDA RES cells to FK866 in co-treatment experiments (Fig. 9d). To prove the relevance of LDHA in determining resistance to FK866, we silenced it by RNA interference with siRNAs (Additional file 5: Figure S3E, F) and exposed the cells to FK866 treatment. Indeed, LDHA silencing phenocopied the effect of GSK treatment by reducing ATP but not NAD(H) levels, decreasing lactate production and medium acidity (Additional file 5: Figure S3G, H, I). In response to *LDHA* silencing, FK866 also activated the pro-apoptotic ATF/CHOP pathway (Fig. 9e, f), which is in line with the synergistic effect observed during

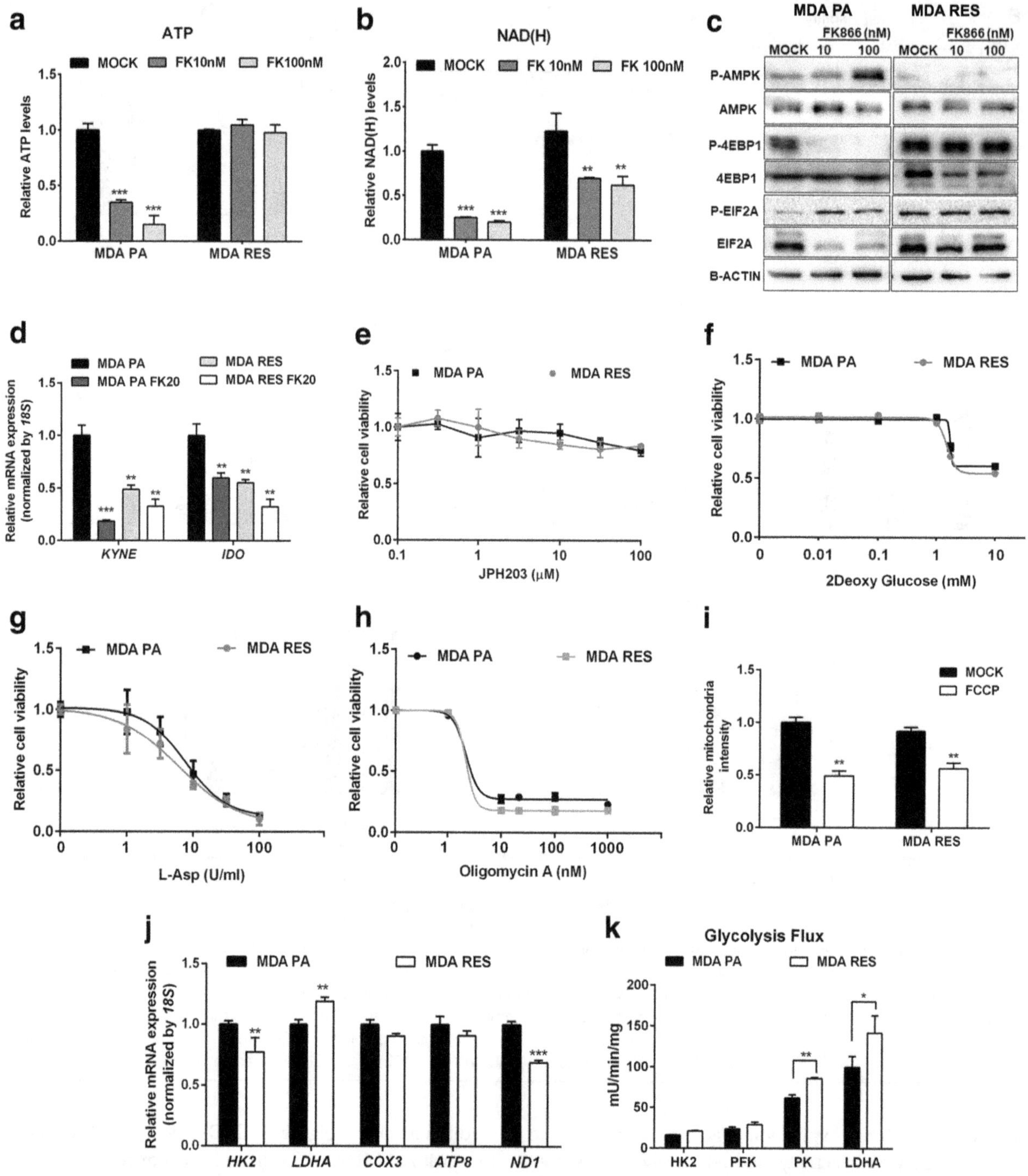

Fig. 7 Characterization of MDA MB231 and FK866-resistant MDA MB231 cells. **a**, **b** MDA MB231 parental (MDA PA) and resistant cells (MDA RES) cells were treated with 10 and 100 nM FK866 for 48 h. ATP (**a**) and NAD(H) (**b**) levels were measured. **c** Western blot showing no alter in translation inhibition in MDA RES along with FK866 treatment in respect to MDA PA. Protein expression from total lysates were determined by detecting with indicated antibodies. B-ACTIN was used as a loading control. **d** MDA PA and MDA RES cells were treated with 20 nM FK866 for 48 h. Expression of *KYNE* and *IDO*, genes involved in the de novo pathway for NAD^+ synthesis, were evaluated. **e**–**h** Relative cell viability of CEM PA and CEM RES cells treated with JPH203 (**e**), 2-deoxyglucose (**f**), L-Asp (**g**), and oligomycin A (**h**) for 48 h was displayed. **i** Analysis of mitochondria content. MDA PA and MDA RES cells were exposed to mitotracker staining. FCCB was used as a negative control. **j** Expression of genes involved in glycolysis and OXPHOS pathway were determined in MDA PA and MDA RES cells. Expression of *18S* was served as a housekeeping gene. **k** Enhanced LDHA activity in the resistance. Enzymatic activity of glycolysis pathway was measured in MDA PA and MDA RES cells. Data were plotted as mean ± S.D. from three biological experiments with technical triplicates (*$p < 0.05$, **$p < 0.01$, ***$p < 0.001$)

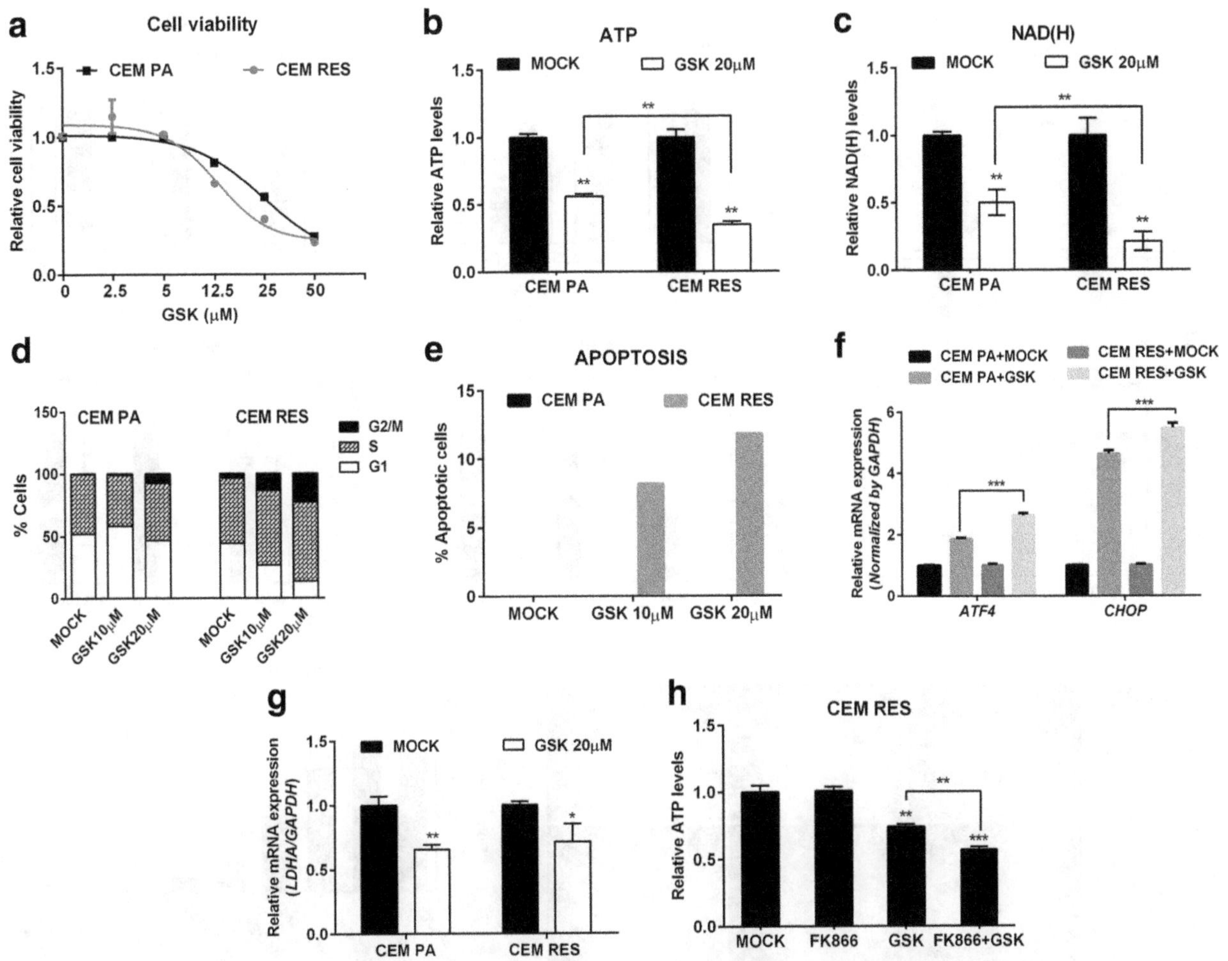

Fig. 8 LDHA regulates metabolic resistance in CEM cells. **a** CEM PA and CEM RES cells were treated with LDH inhibitor (GSK) for 48 h. Relative cell viability was analyzed using MTT assay in respect to Mock. **b**, **c** CEM PA and CEM RES cells were treated with 20 μM GSK for 48 h; ATP (**b**) and NAD(H) (**c**) levels were determined. **d**, **e** CEM PA and CEM RES cells were treated with 10 and 20 μM GSK for 48 h. Cell cycle analysis and percentage of apoptotic cell were determined, respectively. **f**, **g** CEM PA and CEM RES cells were treated with 20 μM GSK for 48 h; quantitative RT-PCR of *ATF4/CHOP* (**f**) and *LDHA* (**g**) was determined, respectively. Expression of *GAPDH* was used as a housekeeping gene. **h** Synergistic effect of FK866 and GSK was detected by a strong reduction of ATP level in CEM RES cells. ATP level was measured in CEM RES cells treated with 5 nM FK866, 20 μM GSK, and co-treatment between FK866 and GSK for 48 h. All data were represent as mean ± S.D. from three independent experiments (*$p < 0.05$, **$p < 0.01$, ***$p < 0.001$)

co-treatment with GSK. In MDA PA, GSK potentiated FK866's ability to reduce the clonogenic capacity of these cells. MDA RES cells were sensitive only to the co-treatment with GSK and FK866 but were fully resistant to the single treatments (Fig. 9g). Therefore, overall, these data indicate that LDHA plays a pivotal role in the metabolic rewiring that underlies cancer cells' acquired resistance to NAMPT inhibition in our models.

Discussion

In this study, we applied a selection strategy to obtain T-ALL and triple-negative breast cancer cells that are resistant to the NAMPT inhibitor FK866 and essentially observed that the metabolic plasticity of cancer cells allows them to escape the toxic insult of this drug after protracted exposure. According to their different initial genetic background, the two cell lines that we utilized for our study, CCRF-CEM and MDA-MB231, exploit different mechanisms to synthesize NAD^+: the T-ALL cell line, CCRF-CEM, was found not to express NAPRT but expressed QPRT, and their resistance phenotype reflected the ability to exploit amino acid catabolism, on the one hand, and an increase in their glycolytic flow and LDHA activity, on the other. The triple-negative breast cancer cell line, MDA MB231, was found to express NAPRT, to have low levels of QPRT, and to primarily rely on LDHA activity for its resistance to FK866. Importantly, in both cell models, cancer cell death appeared to occur via reactivation of the EIF2A/ATF4/CHOP pathway (Fig. 10).

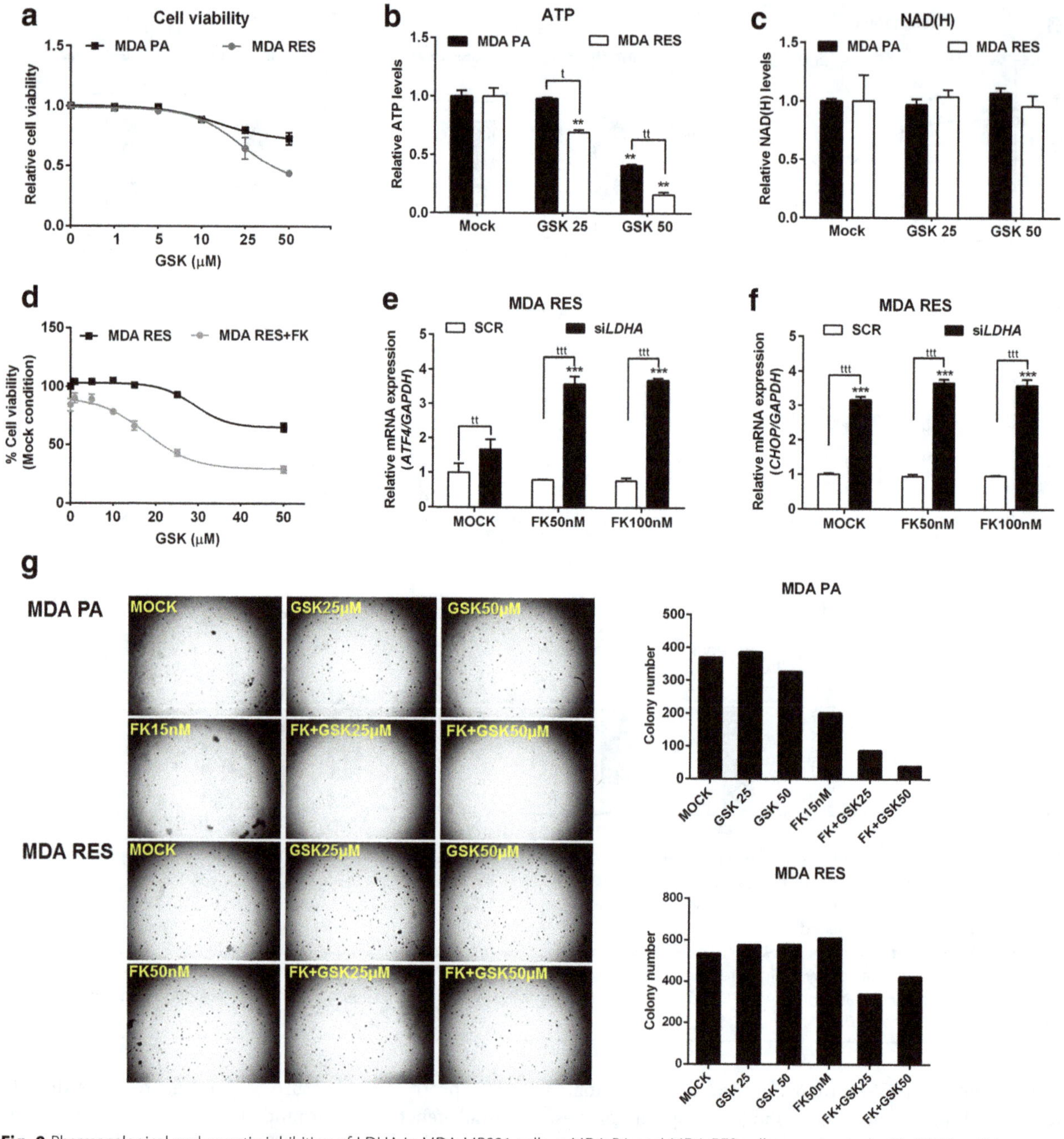

Fig. 9 Pharmacological and genetic inhibition of LDHA in MDA MB231 cells. **a** MDA PA and MDA RES cells were treated with GSK for 48 h. Relative cell viability was analyzed. **b**, **c** MDA PA and MDA RES cells were treated with 25 and 50 μM GSK for 48 h; ATP (**b**) and NAD(H) (**c**) levels were determined, respectively. **d** Synergistic effect of FK866 and GSK inhibits cell growth in MDA RES cells. MDA RES cells were treated with various concentrations of GSK and co-treatment with 20 nM FK866 for 48 h. Percentage of cell viability was determined. **e, f** Downregulation of *LDHA* by siRNA was performed in MDA RES cells. Twenty-four hours after silencing, MDA RES cells were treated with GSK for 48 h. Expression levels of *ATF4* (**e**) and *CHOP* (**f**) were evaluated. Expression of *GAPDH* was used as a housekeeping gene. All data were represent as mean ± S.D. from three independent experiments (*$p < 0.05$, **$p < 0.01$, ***$p < 0.001$). **g** MDA PA and MDA RES cells were performed anchorage-independent growth (colony formation assay) in soft agar along with indicated concentrations of FK866 and GSK treatment for 21 days. A representative colony formation experiment was illustrated and colony number was counted by operetta

Chronic exposure to an anticancer agent frequently leads to the development of resistance [1, 2], and this notion also applies to metabolic drugs [50]. In the case of NAMPT inhibitors, most of the mechanisms of resistance described so far consist in mutations in the enzyme itself with consequent loss of protein/drug interaction [28]. In our models, we found that the acquisition of resistance to the NAMPT inhibitor FK866 was not caused by mutations in *NAMPT*

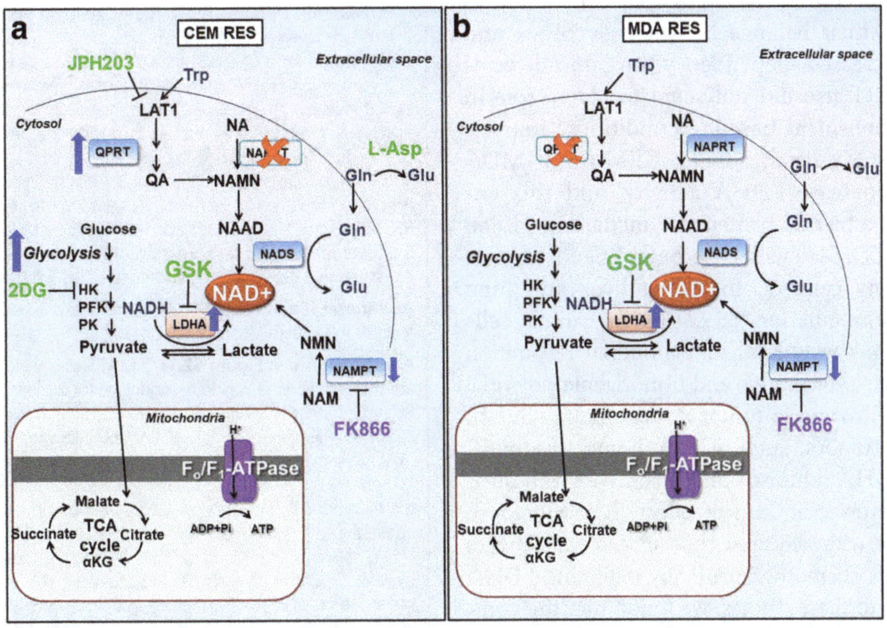

Fig. 10 Schematic representation of different metabolic responses in acquiring FK866 resistance in CEM RES (**a**) and MDA RES (**b**) cells. CEM RES cells are NAPRT-negative and QPRT-positive cells and appear to increase the de novo pathway for NAD production. The metabolic resistance of CEM is more dependent on glycolysis and LDHA activity whereas MDA RES shows very low level of QPRT and primarily rely on LDHA activity for its resistance to FK866. The small molecules having a pro-death pharmacological effect are indicated in green. Abbreviations: NAD, nicotinamide adenine dinucleotide; NA, nicotic acid; NAMN, nicotinic acid mononucleotide; NAAD, nicotinic acid adenine dinucleotide, NAPRT, nicotinic acid phosphoribosyltransferase; NMNAT, nicotinamide mononucleotide adenylyltransferase; NADS, NAD synthase; NAM, nicotinamide; NMN, nicotinamide mononucleotide; NAMPT, nicotinamide phosphoribosyltransferase; NR, nicotinamide riboside; NRK, nicotinamide riboside kinase; QPRT, quinolinate phosphoribosyltransferase; HK, hexokinase; PFK, phosphofructokinase; PK, pyruvate kinase; LDH, lactate dehydrogenase; Gln, glutamine; Glu, glutamic acid; GSK, LDHA inhibitor; 2DG, 2-deoxyglucose; JPH, JPH203; L-Asp, L-asparaginase; GSK, GSK2837808A; LAT1, L-type amino acid transporter 1

but rather reflected by a metabolic rewiring. Our selection protocol was based on the quick adaptation of resistant cells to small drug increases [40], reducing at minimum the possibility to introduce gross genetic rearrangements and thus favoring the escape of pre-existing resistant cells [8]. Notably, we found that the acquisition of resistance to FK866 exposed new, specific cell vulnerabilities. At the molecular level, FK866-resistant cancer cells were found to effectively prevent the activation of the EIF2A/ATF4/CHOP pathway that promotes cell death [41, 51, 18]. Microarray gene expression analyses supported by biochemical evaluations of metabolites (Fig. 4f) suggested that FK866-resistant T-ALL cells pushed glycolysis at the expenses of OXPHOS (Fig. 3g), rendering resistant cells more susceptible to anti-glycolytic drugs (Fig. 4g). In addition, the need to produce NAD^+ via an alternative biochemical path (in a context in which NAPRT is not expressed) (Fig. 1a, c) translated into a dependency on amino acids such as tryptophan and glutamine. Notably, a dependency on QPRT activity was recently observed in human fibrosarcoma cells with acquired resistant to NAMPT inhibition that still presented a point mutation in the NAMPT enzyme [29]. We specifically investigated tryptophan and glutamine for their role in acquired resistance to NAMPT inhibitors. Tryptophan is the NAD^+ precursor utilized in the "de novo" NAD^+ biosynthesis pathway. We observed that T-ALL cells that are resistant to FK866 rely on tryptophan for NAD^+ production, which indicated a possible metabolic vulnerability of these cells. JPH203, an inhibitor of amino acid transport, was shown to possess anticancer activity both in vitro and in vivo against HT-29 tumors transplanted in nude mice [44, 52] and to cause apoptosis in YD-38 human oral cancer cells [53]. In our hands, this compound induced CHOP activation in FK866-resistant CCRF-CEM cells. Interestingly, the same was found to hold true for Gln [54], another amino acid involved in the production of NAD^+, not as an NAD^+ precursor but rather as a nitrogen donor in the reaction catalyzed by the enzyme NAD synthetase (*NADS*). Gln degradation by L-Asp also activated CHOP and potentiated FK866 activity in FK866-resistant CCRF-CEM. Thus, essential amino acid utilization emerges as an alternative source for NAMPT-independent NAD^+ production in FK866-resistant T-ALL cells. The triple-negative breast cancer model represented by MDA MB231 cells expresses NAPRT, an enzyme that was previously associated to resistance to FK866 [55]. In this model, we observed different mechanisms of acquired resistance to FK866. Specifically, as compared to parental cells, MDA RES cells failed to show changes in their balance between glycolysis and OXPHOS or increased dependency on amino acids (Fig. 7e–h). NAPRT also did not seem to play a role in MDA RES metabolism in baseline conditions. Importantly, both FK866-resistant CCRF-CEM and MDA MB231 showed increase LDHA activity, and this enzyme emerged as a pivotal protein for mediating FK866 resistance. High *LDHA* levels have been linked to poor prognosis in many cancers, including liver and lung cancer [56]. Downregulation of *LDHA* in cancer cells by siRNA or shRNA stimulates mitochondrial respiration and reduces cellular proliferative and tumorigenic potential in cancer cells in vitro and in tumor xenografts [57–59]. In highly glycolytic tumors, such as lymphoma, the combination of an LDHA inhibitor and a NAMPT inhibitor resulted in a synergistic anticancer effect [60]. Moreover, breast cancer cells with acquired resistance to taxol were re-sensitized to this chemotherapeutic by inhibiting LDHA [61]. Consistent with these studies, we found that the combination of FK866 with GSK was highly effective against FK866-resistant CCRF-CEM. LDHA silencing in MDA RES cells increased their sensitivity to FK866 as shown by CHOP/ATF4 activation. Thus, targeting LDHA together with NAMPT may offer novel opportunities for selective killing of cancer cells, particularly in cancer types that are addicted to aerobic glycolysis for survival.

Conclusions

In conclusion, our data show that FK866 treatment can lead to the development of different mechanisms of acquired resistance. Such mechanisms depend on the original metabolic profile of the tumor, including the pattern of expression of NAD^+-producing enzymes, such as NAPRT or QPRT, since the latter can come into play for compensating for chronic NAMPT inhibition, ensuring that sufficient NAD^+ is produced for a cancer cell to survive. Closely monitoring the metabolic adaptations of a tumor to NAMPT inhibition could be useful to inform therapeutic decisions. In this context, LDHA inhibitors should be considered for further evaluation in clinical trials as drugs capable of reverting resistance to NAMPT inhibitors.

Additional files

Additional file 1: Table S2. List of RT-PCR primer sequences. (XLS 34 kb)

Additional file 2: Figure S1. A Dose-dependent resistant to FK866; CEM PA and CEM RES cells at 100 nM of FK866 were treated with various concentrations of FK866 for 48 h. Percentage of cell viability was conducted by MTT assay and analyzed in respect to DMSO treatment. B CEM PA and CEM RES 100 nM cells were treated with 5 or 100 nM of FK866 for 72 h. Percentage of viable and dead cells was evaluated by DAPI staining and analyzed in respect to DMSO. C CEM RES cells were insensitive to long-term treatment of FK866; cells were grown in the present of 500 nM FK866 for 5 days. Percentage of cell viability was measured by 0.2% trypan blue staining. D, E Resistant cells were insensitive to another NAMPT inhibitor (CHS-828). CEM and MDA cells were treated with CHS-828 for 48 h. Percentage of cell viability was analyzed. F-H CEM PA and CEM RES cells were treated with 5 nM FK866 for 48 h. Amount of ATP (represent as energy charge), NAD+, and NMN levels were evaluated through HPLC analysis and referred to the protein content. I Cell cycle analysis was conducted in CEM PA and CEM RES cells by FACS analysis. J No involvement of multi-drug resistance mechanism in the resistant CEM model; CEM PA and CEM RES cells were treated with 2.5 nM FK866, 5 μM cyclosporin A (CsA), 5 μM verapamil, and combination of FK866 with CsA or verapamil for 48 h. Relative cell viability was accessed by MTT assay. (PDF 1757 kb)

Additional file 3: Table S1. List of gene expression from genome wide analysis in CCRF-CEM cells. (XLSX 44303 kb)

Additional file 4: Figure S2. A CEM RES cells were maintained in the absence of FK866 (a washout condition) for 2 months as referred to CEM RES WO; then, they were re-exposed to 100 nM FK866 for 96 h. Relative ATP level was measured. B CEM PA, CEM RES with FK866 (CEM RES), and CEM RES-washed out FK866 (CEM WO FK) cells were re-exposed to 100 nM FK866 for 48 h. Relative ATP levels were measured at 48 h after the treatment. C Expression of L-type amino acid transporter 1 (LAT1) in parental and resistant cells. Expression of LAT1 in CCRF-CEM and MDA MB231 cells was determined by CD98 staining and the analysis was performed by FACS. D–E MDA PA and MDA RES cells were transiently transfected with two different NAMPT overexpressed plasmids (NAMPT1 and NAMPT2) or empty vector (PBP). Twenty-four hours after transfection, cells were treated with 20 and 40 nM FK866 for 48 h. NAD(H) levels (D) and cell viability (E) were determined. F Expression of gene involved glycolysis and OXPHOS pathways in CEM PA and CEM RES cells. G MDA PA and MDA RES cells were treated with a NAPRT inhibitor (2-HNA) for 48 h. Relative cell viability compared to untreated control was evaluated by OZBlue Cell Viability kit. H Stable downregulation of *NAPRT* cell lines were obtained from transduction of lentiviral vector contained sh*NAPRT*. Western blot depicts decrease in NAPRT levels of sh*NAPRT* MDA cells. GAPDH was used as a loading control. I–J Stable sh*NAPRT* MDA PA and MDA RES cell lines were treated with 20 nM FK866 in MDA PA and 100 nM FK866 in MDA RES for 48 h. Relative ATP (I) and NAD(H) levels (J) compared to MOCK were determined (*$p < 0.05$, **$p < 0.01$ compared to MOCK). (PDF 2199 kb)

Additional file 5: Figure S3. A MDA PA and MDA RES cells were treated with 25 and 50 μM GSK for 48 h. Lactate production was determined. B Reduction of acidity was observed in GSK treatments. MDA PA and MDA RES cells were treated with various concentrations of GSK (0.1–50 μM) for 48 h. A decrease of acidity was visualized by changing of medium colors from red to yellow (basic to acidic). C, D Expression of *ATF* and *CHOP* mRNA along with 25 μM GSK treatment for 48 h in MDA. E Western blot showing downregulation of LDHA level in LDHA silencing MDA cells conducted by siRNA. ACTIN was used as a loading control. F FK866 decreased *LDHA* mRNA levels. MDA RES cells were transiently transfected with siLDHA. Twenty-four hours after silencing, cells were treated with 50 and 100 nM FK866 for 48 h. Expression of *LDHA* was detected. G–I MDA PA and MDA RES cells were transiently transfected with siLDHA. Forty-eight hours post transfection, ATP (G), NAD(H) (H), and lactate production (I) were measured (*$p < 0.05$, **$p < 0.01$, ***$p < 0.001$). (PDF 2727 kb)

Abbreviations

2HNA: 2-Hydroxynicotinic acid; CEM PA: Parental CCRF-CEM cells; CEM RES: FK866-resistant CCRF-CEM cells; CEM: CCRF-CEM cells; DEGs: Differentially expressed genes; GSK: LDH inhibitor GSK2837808A; HK: Hexokinase; L-Asp: L-Asparaginase; LAT1: L-type amino acid transporter 1; LDHA: Lactate dehydrogenase A; LVP: Lentiviral vector particle; MDA RES: FK866-resistant MDA MB231 cells; MDA PA: Parental MDA MB231 cells; MDR: Multi-drug resistance; NA: Nicotinic acid; NAMN: Nicotinic acid mononucleotide; NAMPT: Nicotinamide phosphoribosyltransferase; NAPRT: Nicotinic acid phosphoribosyltransferase; OCR: Oxygen consumption rate; OXPHOS: Oxidative phosphorylation; PFK: Phosphofructokinase; PK: Pyruvate kinase; QPRT: Quinolinate phosphoribosyltransferase; TMRE: Tetramethylrhodamine; TRAIL: Tumor necrosis factor-related apoptosis-inducing ligand; Trp: Tryptophan

Acknowledgements
We thank Johanna Chiche (C3M-U1065, Nice, France) for setting up the OXPhos/glycolysis ATP production assay, Mickaël Ohana for the helpful discussion about the NAD^+ metabolism, and Hitoshi Endou (JPharma, Yokohama, Japan) and Michael F Wempe (University of Colorado, Aurora, CO, USA) for providing the JPH203.

Funding
The following support was received: CIBIO intramural start-up to AP, MFAG AIRC #17153 to AP, IG AIRC #17736 to AN, US Dept. of Defense BCRP BC161452P1 to AN, and IBSA Foundation to FP.

Authors' contributions
NT, AN, NR, AQ, JFP, and AP conceived and supervised the study. NT, CZ, VDA, FP, and RM performed the cell-based studies. TT performed the bioinformatics analyses. SR and FZ performed the biochemical experiments. NT, CZ, AN, and AP wrote the manuscript. All authors read and approved the final manuscript.

Competing interests
The authors declare that they have no competing interests.

Author details
[1]Center For Integrative Biology (CIBIO), University of Trento, via Sommarive 9, Trento, Italy. [2]Department of Pharmacy, Biochemistry Laboratory, University of Genova, Genova, Italy. [3]Department of Agricultural, Food and Environmental Sciences, Polytechnic University of Marche, Ancona, Italy. [4]Department of Internal Medicine, University of Genoa, Genoa, Italy. [5]Université Côte d'Azur, Centre Méditerranéen de Médecine Moléculaire (C3M), INSERM U1065, Nice, France.

References

1. Holohan C, Van Schaeybroeck S, Longley DB, Johnston PG. Cancer drug resistance: an evolving paradigm. Nat. Rev. Cancer. 2013;13:714–26.
2. Housman G, Byler S, Heerboth S, Lapinska K, Longacre M, Snyder N, et al. Drug resistance in cancer: an overview. Cancers (Basel). 2014;6:1769–92.
3. Szakács G, Paterson JK, Ludwig JA, Booth-Genthe C, Gottesman MM. Targeting multidrug resistance in cancer. Nat Rev Drug Discov. 2006;5:219–34.
4. Sharma SV, Bell DW, Settleman J, Haber DA. Epidermal growth factor receptor mutations in lung cancer. Nat Rev Cancer. 2007;7:169–81.
5. Watson PA, Arora VK, Sawyers CL. Emerging mechanisms of resistance to androgen receptor inhibitors in prostate cancer. Nat Rev Cancer. 2015;15:701–11.
6. Vouri M, Hafizi STAM. Receptor tyrosine kinases in cancer drug resistance. Cancer Res. 2017;77:2775–8.
7. Micheau O, Shirley S, Dufour F. Death receptors as targets in cancer. Br J Pharmacol. 2013;169:1723–44.
8. Latorre E, Tebaldi T, Viero G, Spartà AM, Quattrone A, Provenzani A. Downregulation of HuR as a new mechanism of doxorubicin resistance in breast cancer cells. Mol Cancer. 2012;11:13.
9. Hufton SE, Moerkerk PT, Brandwijk R, de Bruïne AP, Arends JW, Hoogenboom HRA. Profile of differentially expressed genes in primary colorectal cancer using suppression subtractive hybridization. FEBS Lett. 1999;463:77–82.
10. Van Beijnum JR, Moerkerk PTM, Gerbers AJ, De Bruïne AP, Arends J-W, Hoogenboom HR, et al. Target validation for genomics using peptide-specific phage antibodies: a study of five gene products overexpressed in colorectal cancer. Int J Cancer. 2002;101:118–27.
11. Bi T-Q, Che X-M, Liao X-H, Zhang D-J, Long H-L, Li H-J, et al. Overexpression of Nampt in gastric cancer and chemopotentiating effects of the Nampt inhibitor FK866 in combination with fluorouracil. Oncol Rep. 2011;26:1251–7.
12. Olesen UH, Hastrup N, Sehested M. Expression patterns of nicotinamide phosphoribosyltransferase and nicotinic acid phosphoribosyltransferase in human malignant lymphomas. APMIS. 2011;119:296–303.
13. Olesen UH, Petersen JG, Garten A, Kiess W, Yoshino J, Imai S-I, et al. Target enzyme mutations are the molecular basis for resistance towards pharmacological inhibition of nicotinamide phosphoribosyltransferase. BMC Cancer. 2010;10:677.
14. Kim M-K, Lee JH, Kim H, Park SJ, Kim SH, Kang GB, et al. Crystal structure of visfatin/pre-B cell colony-enhancing factor 1/nicotinamide phosphoribosyltransferase, free and in complex with the anti-cancer agent FK-866. J Mol Biol. 2006;362:66–77.
15. Holen K, Saltz LB, Hollywood E, Burk K, Hanauske A-R. The pharmacokinetics, toxicities, and biologic effects of FK866, a nicotinamide adenine dinucleotide biosynthesis inhibitor. Investig New Drugs. 2008;26:45–51.
16. Xu T-Y, Zhang S-L, Dong G-Q, Liu X-Z, Wang X, Lv X-Q, et al. Discovery and characterization of novel small-molecule inhibitors targeting nicotinamide phosphoribosyltransferase. Sci Rep. 2015;5:10043.
17. Cea M, Cagnetta A, Acharya C, Acharya P, Tai Y-T, Yang C, et al. Dual NAMPT and BTK targeting leads to synergistic killing of Waldenström Macroglobulinemia cells regardless of MYD88 and CXCR4 somatic mutation status. Clin Cancer Res. 2016;22:6099–109.
18. Cagnetta A, Caffa I, Acharya C, Soncini D, Acharya P, Adamia S, et al. APO866 increases antitumor activity of cyclosporin-A by inducing mitochondrial and endoplasmic reticulum stress in leukemia cells. Clin Cancer Res. 2015;21:3934–45.
19. Roulston A, Shore GC. New strategies to maximize therapeutic opportunities for NAMPT inhibitors in oncology. Mol Cell Oncol. 2016;3:e1052180.
20. Pogrebniak A, Schemainda I, Azzam K, Pelka-Fleischer R, Nüssler V, Hasmann M. Chemopotentiating effects of a novel NAD biosynthesis inhibitor, FK866, in combination with antineoplastic agents. Eur J Med Res. 2006;11:313–21.
21. Cagnetta A, Cea M, Calimeri T, Acharya C, Fulciniti M, Tai Y-T, et al. Intracellular NAD^+ depletion enhances bortezomib-induced anti-myeloma activity. Blood. 2013;122:1243–55.
22. Zoppoli G, Cea M, Soncini D, Fruscione F, Rudner J, Moran E, et al. Potent synergistic interaction between the Nampt inhibitor APO866 and the apoptosis activator TRAIL in human leukemia cells. Exp Hematol. 2010;38:979–88.
23. Xiao Y, Kwong M, Daemen A, Belvin M, Liang X, Hatzivassiliou G, et al. Metabolic response to NAD depletion across cell lines is highly variable. Tan M, editor. PLoS One 2016;11:e0164166.
24. Duarte-Pereira S, Pereira-Castro I, Silva SS, Correia MG, Neto C, da Costa LT, et al. Extensive regulation of nicotinate phosphoribosyltransferase (NAPRT) expression in human tissues and tumors. Oncotarget. 2015;7:1973–83.
25. Cerna D, Li H, Flaherty S, Takebe N, Coleman CN, Yoo SS. Inhibition of nicotinamide phosphoribosyltransferase (NAMPT) activity by small molecule GMX1778 regulates reactive oxygen species (ROS)-mediated cytotoxicity in a p53- and nicotinic acid phosphoribosyltransferase1 (NAPRT1)-dependent manner. J Biol Chem. 2012;287:22408–17.
26. Piacente F, Caffa I, Ravera S, Sociali G, Passalacqua M, Vellone VG, et al. Nicotinic acid phosphoribosyltransferase regulates cancer cell metabolism, susceptibility to NAMPT inhibitors and DNA repair. Cancer Res. 2017;canres.3079.2016.
27. Watson M, Roulston A, Bélec L, Billot X, Marcellus R, Bédard D, et al. The small molecule GMX1778 is a potent inhibitor of NAD+ biosynthesis: strategy for enhanced therapy in nicotinic acid phosphoribosyltransferase 1-deficient tumors. Mol Cell Biol. 2009;29:5872–88.
28. Wang W, Elkins K, Oh A, Ho Y-C, Wu J, Li H, et al. Structural basis for resistance to diverse classes of NAMPT inhibitors. Xu W, editor. PLoS One 2014;9:e109366.
29. Guo J, Lam LT, Longenecker KL, Bui MH, Idler KB, Glaser KB, et al. Identification of novel resistance mechanisms to NAMPT inhibition via the de novo NAD(+) biosynthesis pathway and NAMPT mutation. Biochem Biophys Res Commun. 2017;491:681–6.
30. Rosilio C, Nebout M, Imbert V, Griessinger E, Neffati Z, Benadiba J, et al. L-type amino-acid transporter 1 (LAT1): a therapeutic target supporting growth and survival of T-cell lymphoblastic lymphoma/T-cell acute lymphoblastic leukemia. Leukemia. 2015;29:1253–66.
31. Chou T-C. Drug combination studies and their synergy quantification using the Chou-Talalay method. Cancer Res. 2010;70:440–6.
32. Mori V, Amici A, Mazzola F, Di Stefano M, Conforti L, Magni G, et al. Metabolic profiling of alternative NAD biosynthetic routes in mouse tissues. de Crécy-Lagard V, editor. PLoS One 2014;9:e113939.
33. Sociali G, Raffaghello L, Magnone M, Zamporlini F, Emionite L, Sturla L, et al. Antitumor effect of combined NAMPT and CD73 inhibition in an ovarian cancer model. Oncotarget. 2016;7:2968–84.
34. Ravera S, Vaccaro D, Cuccarolo P, Columbaro M, Capanni C, Bartolucci M, et al. Mitochondrial respiratory chain complex I defects in Fanconi anemia complementation group A. Biochimie. 2013;95:1828–37.

36. Hinkle PC. P/O ratios of mitochondrial oxidative phosphorylation. Biochim Biophys Acta. 2005;1706:1–11.
37. Colla R, Izzotti A, De Ciucis C, Fenoglio D, Ravera S, Speciale A, et al. Glutathione-mediated antioxidant response and aerobic metabolism: two crucial factors involved in determining the multi-drug resistance of high-risk neuroblastoma. Oncotarget. 2016;7:70715–37.
38. Ravera S, Dufour C, Cesaro S, Bottega R, Faleschini M, Cuccarolo P, et al. Evaluation of energy metabolism and calcium homeostasis in cells affected by Shwachman-Diamond syndrome. Sci Rep. 2016;6:25441.
39. Zamporlini F, Ruggieri S, Mazzola F, Amici A, Orsomando G, Raffaelli N. Novel assay for simultaneous measurement of pyridine mononucleotides synthesizing activities allows dissection of the NAD(+) biosynthetic machinery in mammalian cells. FEBS J. 2014;281:5104–19.
40. McDermott M, Eustace AJ, Busschots S, Breen L, Crown J, Clynes M, et al. In vitro development of chemotherapy and targeted therapy drug-resistant cancer cell lines: a practical guide with case studies. Front Oncol. 2014;4:40.
41. Zucal C, D'Agostino VG, Casini A, Mantelli B, Thongon N, Soncini D, et al. EIF2A-dependent translational arrest protects leukemia cells from the energetic stress induced by NAMPT inhibition. BMC Cancer. 2015;15:855.
42. Averous J, Bruhat A, Jousse C, Carraro V, Thiel G, Fafournoux P. Induction of CHOP expression by amino acid limitation requires both ATF4 expression and ATF2 phosphorylation. J Biol Chem. 2004;279:5288–97.
43. Cormerais Y, Giuliano S, LeFloch R, Front B, Durivault J, Tambutté E, et al. Genetic disruption of the multifunctional CD98/LAT1 complex demonstrates the key role of essential amino acid transport in the control of mTORC1 and tumor growth. Cancer Res. 2016;76:4481–92.
44. Oda K, Hosoda N, Endo H, Saito K, Tsujihara K, Yamamura M, et al. L-type amino acid transporter 1 inhibitors inhibit tumor cell growth. Cancer Sci. 2010;101:173–9.
45. Altman BJ, Stine ZE, Dang CV. From Krebs to clinic: glutamine metabolism to cancer therapy. Nat Rev Cancer. 2016;16:619–34.
46. Samudio I, Konopleva M. Asparaginase unveils glutamine-addicted AML. Blood. 2013;122:3398–400.
47. Willems L, Jacque N, Jacquel A, Neveux N, Maciel TT, Lambert M, et al. Inhibiting glutamine uptake represents an attractive new strategy for treating acute myeloid leukemia. Blood. 2013;122:3521–32.
48. Balasubramanian MN, Butterworth EA, Kilberg MS. Asparagine synthetase: regulation by cell stress and involvement in tumor biology. Am J Physiol Endocrinol Metab. 2013;304:E789–99.
49. Zhai X, Yang Y, Wan J, Zhu R, Wu Y. Inhibition of LDH-A by oxamate induces G2/M arrest, apoptosis and increases radiosensitivity in nasopharyngeal carcinoma cells. Oncol Rep. 2013;30:2983–91.
50. Zhao Y, Butler EB, Tan M. Targeting cellular metabolism to improve cancer therapeutics. Cell Death Dis. 2013;4:e532.
51. Rozpedek W, Pytel D, Mucha B, Leszczynska H, Diehl JA, Majsterek I. The role of the PERK/eIF2α/ATF4/CHOP signaling pathway in tumor progression during endoplasmic reticulum stress. Curr Mol Med. 2016;16:533–44.
52. Wempe MF, Rice PJ, Lightner JW, Jutabha P, Hayashi M, Anzai N, et al. Metabolism and pharmacokinetic studies of JPH203, an L-amino acid transporter 1 (LAT1) selective compound. Drug Metab Pharmacokinet Elsevier. 2012;27:155–61.
53. Yun D-W, Lee SA, Park M-G, Kim J-S, Yu S-K, Park M-R, et al. JPH203, an L-type amino acid transporter 1-selective compound, induces apoptosis of YD-38 human oral cancer cells. J Pharmacol Sci. 2014;124:208–17.
54. Zhang J, Pavlova NN, Thompson CB. Cancer cell metabolism: the essential role of the nonessential amino acid, glutamine. EMBO J. 2017;36:1302–15.
55. Hara N, Yamada K, Shibata T, Osago H, Hashimoto T, Tsuchiya M. Elevation of cellular NAD levels by nicotinic acid and involvement of nicotinic acid phosphoribosyltransferase in human cells. J Biol Chem. 2007;282:24574–82.
56. Hermes A, Gatzemeier U, Waschki B, Reck M. Lactate dehydrogenase as prognostic factor in limited and extensive disease stage small cell lung cancer—a retrospective single institution analysis. Respir Med. 2010;104:1937–42.
57. Xie H, Hanai J-I, Ren J-G, Kats L, Burgess K, Bhargava P, et al. Targeting lactate dehydrogenase—a inhibits tumorigenesis and tumor progression in mouse models of lung cancer and impacts tumor-initiating cells. Cell Metab. 2014;19:795–809.
58. Billiard J, Dennison JB, Briand J, Annan RS, Chai D, Colón M, et al. Quinoline 3-sulfonamides inhibit lactate dehydrogenase A and reverse aerobic glycolysis in cancer cells. Cancer Metab. 2013;1:19.
59. Wang ZY, Loo TY, Shen JG, Wang N, Wang DM, Yang DP, et al. LDH-A silencing suppresses breast cancer tumorigenicity through induction of oxidative stress mediated mitochondrial pathway apoptosis. Breast Cancer Res Treat. 2012;131:791–800.
60. Le A, Cooper CR, Gouw AM, Dinavahi R, Maitra A, Deck LM, et al. Inhibition of lactate dehydrogenase A induces oxidative stress and inhibits tumor progression. Proc Natl Acad Sci U S A. 2010;107:2037–42.
61. Zhou M, Zhao Y, Ding Y, Liu H, Liu Z, Fodstad O, et al. Warburg effect in chemosensitivity: targeting lactate dehydrogenase-A re-sensitizes taxol-resistant cancer cells to taxol. Mol Cancer. 2010;9:33.

Permissions

All chapters in this book were first published in C&M, by BioMed Central; hereby published with permission under the Creative Commons Attribution License or equivalent. Every chapter published in this book has been scrutinized by our experts. Their significance has been extensively debated. The topics covered herein carry significant findings which will fuel the growth of the discipline. They may even be implemented as practical applications or may be referred to as a beginning point for another development.

The contributors of this book come from diverse backgrounds, making this book a truly international effort. This book will bring forth new frontiers with its revolutionizing research information and detailed analysis of the nascent developments around the world.

We would like to thank all the contributing authors for lending their expertise to make the book truly unique. They have played a crucial role in the development of this book. Without their invaluable contributions this book wouldn't have been possible. They have made vital efforts to compile up to date information on the varied aspects of this subject to make this book a valuable addition to the collection of many professionals and students.

This book was conceptualized with the vision of imparting up-to-date information and advanced data in this field. To ensure the same, a matchless editorial board was set up. Every individual on the board went through rigorous rounds of assessment to prove their worth. After which they invested a large part of their time researching and compiling the most relevant data for our readers.

The editorial board has been involved in producing this book since its inception. They have spent rigorous hours researching and exploring the diverse topics which have resulted in the successful publishing of this book. They have passed on their knowledge of decades through this book. To expedite this challenging task, the publisher supported the team at every step. A small team of assistant editors was also appointed to further simplify the editing procedure and attain best results for the readers.

Apart from the editorial board, the designing team has also invested a significant amount of their time in understanding the subject and creating the most relevant covers. They scrutinized every image to scout for the most suitable representation of the subject and create an appropriate cover for the book.

The publishing team has been an ardent support to the editorial, designing and production team. Their endless efforts to recruit the best for this project, has resulted in the accomplishment of this book. They are a veteran in the field of academics and their pool of knowledge is as vast as their experience in printing. Their expertise and guidance has proved useful at every step. Their uncompromising quality standards have made this book an exceptional effort. Their encouragement from time to time has been an inspiration for everyone.

The publisher and the editorial board hope that this book will prove to be a valuable piece of knowledge for researchers, students, practitioners and scholars across the globe.

List of Contributors

Nathan J. Lanning and Andre N. Leon
California State University, Los Angeles, 5151 State University Drive, Los Angeles, CA 90032, USA

Joshua P. Castle, Elizabeth A. Tovar and Carrie R. Graveel
Van Andel Research Institute, 333 Bostwick Ave, NE, Grand Rapids, MI 49503, USA

Jeffrey P. MacKeigan
Van Andel Research Institute, 333 Bostwick Ave, NE, Grand Rapids, MI 49503, USA
College of Human Medicine, Michigan State University, 15 Michigan St. NE, Grand Rapids, MI 49503, USA

Simar J. Singh, Amandeep Sanghera and Fabian V. Filipp
Systems Biology and Cancer Metabolism, Program for Quantitative Systems Biology, University of California Merced, 2500 North Lake Road, Merced, CA 95343, USA

Manan M. Mehta, Samuel E. Weinberg, Elizabeth M.Steinert, Krishan Chhiba, Harris R. Perlman, Paul Bryce and Navdeep S. Chandel
Department of Medicine, Northwestern University Feinberg School of Medicine, McGaw Pavilion, Rm. M-334, 240 East Huron Street, Chicago, IL 60611, USA

Carlos Alberto Martinez
Department of Biochemistry and Molecular Genetics, Northwestern University Feinberg School of Medicine, Chicago, IL 60611, USA

Peng Gao
Metabolomics Core Facility, Northwestern University Robert H. Lurie Comprehensive Cancer Center, Chicago, IL 60611, USA

Nissim Hay
Department of Biochemistry and Molecular Genetics, University of Illinois at Chicago, Chicago, IL 60607, USA

Parmanand Malvi, Balkrishna Chaube, Shivendra Vikram Singh, Naoshad Mohammad, Maleppillil Vavachan Vijayakumar, Snahlata Singh, Surbhi Chouhan and Manoj Kumar Bhat
National Centre for Cell Science, Savitribai Phule Pune University Campus, Ganeshkhind, Pune 411 007, India

Catharina Bartmann, Katrin Bahlke, Jana Willingstorfer, Maria Strunz, Achim Wöckel, Michaela Kapp and Ulrike Kämmerer
Department of Obstetrics and Gynaecology, University Hospital of Würzburg, Josef-Schneider-Str. 4, 97080 Würzburg, Germany

Sudha R. Janaki Raman, Jessica Flöter and Almut Schulze
Department of Biochemistry and Molecular Biology, Theodor-Boveri-Institute, Biocenter, University of Würzburg, 97070 Würzburg, Germany

Rainer J. Klement
Department of Radiotherapy and Radiation Oncology, Leopoldina Hospital, 97422 Schweinfurt, Germany

Cholpon S. Djuzenova
Department of Radiotherapy, University Hospital of Würzburg, 97080 Würzburg, Germany

Christoph Otto
Experimental Surgery, Department of General, Visceral, Vascular, and Pediatric Surgery, University Hospital of Würzburg, 97080 Würzburg, Germany

Ashley R. Maiuri
Medical Sciences, Indiana University School of Medicine, Bloomington,Indiana, USA

Heather M. O'Hagan
Medical Sciences, Indiana University School of Medicine, Bloomington,Indiana, USA
Indiana University Melvin and Bren Simon Cancer Center, Indianapolis, Indiana, USA

Hongde Li, Barry D. Stein and Jason M. Tennessen
Department of Biology, Indiana University, Bloomington, Indiana, USA

Jason W. Locasale
Duke Cancer Institute, Duke University School of Medicine, Durham, NC 27710, USA
Duke Molecular Physiology Institute, Duke University School of Medicine, Durham, NC 27710, USA
Department of Pharmacology and Mehrmohamadi et al. Cancer & Metabolism (2017) 5:8 Page 12 of 13 Cancer Biology, Duke University School of Medicine, Durham, NC 27710, USA

Mahya Mehrmohamadi
Duke Cancer Institute, Duke University School of Medicine, Durham, NC 27710, USA
Duke Molecular Physiology Institute, Duke University School of Medicine, Durham, NC 27710, USA
Department of Pharmacology and Mehrmohamadi et al. Cancer & Metabolism (2017) 5:8 Page 12 of 13 Cancer Biology, Duke University School of Medicine, Durham, NC 27710, USA
Department of Molecular Biology and Genetics, Field of Genetics, Genomics and Development, Cornell University, Ithaca, NY 14853, USA

Seong Ho Jeong
Department of Molecular Biology and Genetics, Field of Genetics, Genomics and Development, Cornell University, Ithaca, NY 14853, USA

Costas Koufaris and Roland Nilsson
Cardiovascular Medicine Unit, Department of Medicine, Karolinska Institutet, SE-171 76 Stockholm, Sweden
Division of Cardiovascular Medicine, Karolinska University Hospital, SE-171 76 Stockholm, Sweden
Center for Molecular Medicine, Karolinska Institutet, SE-171 76 Stockholm, Sweden

Shili Xu, Arthur Catapang and Hanna M. Doh
Department of Molecular and Medical Pharmacology, David Geffen School of Medicine, University of California, Los Angeles, Los Angeles, CA 90095, USA

Harvey R. Herschman
Department of Molecular and Medical Pharmacology, David Geffen School of Medicine, University of California, Los Angeles, Los Angeles, CA 90095, USA
Department of Biological Chemistry, David Geffen School of Medicine, University of California, Los Angeles, Los Angeles, CA 90095, USA
Crump Institute for Molecular Imaging, David Geffen School of Medicine, University of California, Los Angeles, Los Angeles, CA 90095, USA
Jonsson Comprehensive Cancer Center, David Geffen School of Medicine, University of California, Los Angeles, Los Angeles, CA 90095, USA
Molecular Biology Institute, David Geffen School of Medicine, University of California, Los Angeles, Los Angeles, CA 90095, USA

Daniel Braas
Department of Molecular and Medical Pharmacology, David Geffen School of Medicine, University of California, Los Angeles, Los Angeles, CA 90095, USA
UCLA Metabolomics Center, David Geffen School of Medicine, University of California, Los Angeles, Los Angeles, CA 90095, USA

Thomas G. Graeber
Department of Molecular and Medical Pharmacology, David Geffen School of Medicine, University of California, Los Angeles, Los Angeles, CA 90095, USA
UCLA Metabolomics Center, David Geffen School of Medicine, University of California, Los Angeles, Los Angeles, CA 90095, USA
Crump Institute for Molecular Imaging, David Geffen School of Medicine, University of California, Los Angeles, Los Angeles, CA 90095, USA
Jonsson Comprehensive Cancer Center, David Geffen School of Medicine, University of California, Los Angeles, Los Angeles, CA 90095, USA

Jason T. Lee
Department of Molecular and Medical Pharmacology, David Geffen School of Medicine, University of California, Los Angeles, Los Angeles, CA 90095, USA

Crump Institute for Molecular Imaging, David Geffen School of Medicine, University of California, Los Angeles, Los Angeles, CA 90095, USA
Jonsson Comprehensive Cancer Center, David Geffen School of Medicine, University of California, Los Angeles, Los Angeles, CA 90095, USA

Robert Damoiseaux
Department of Molecular and Medical Pharmacology, David Geffen School of Medicine, University of California, Los Angeles, Los Angeles, CA 90095, USA
California NanoSystems Institute, David Geffen School of Medicine, University of California, Los Angeles, Los Angeles, CA 90095, USA

Linsey Stiles and Orian Shirihai
Division of Endocrinology, Department of Medicine, David Geffen School of Medicine, University of California, Los Angeles, Los Angeles, CA 90095, USA

Jack Mottahedeh
Department of Molecular, Cell & Developmental Biology, University of California Los Angeles, Los Angeles, CA, USA

Michael C. Haffner
Sidney Kimmel Comprehensive Cancer Center at Johns Hopkins, Baltimore, MD, USA
Department of Pathology, Johns Hopkins University School of Medicine, Baltimore, MD, USA

David A. Elashoff
Department of Medicine Statistics Core, University of California Los Angeles, Los Angeles, CA, USA
Jonsson Comprehensive Cancer Center, University of California Los Angeles, Los Angeles, CA, USA

Himisha Beltran
Department of Medicine, Division of Medical Oncology, Weill Cornell Medicine, New York, NY, USA
Englander Institute for Precision Medicine, Weill Cornell Medicine, New York, NY, USA

Matthew Garrett
Department of Neurosurgery, and the Interdepartmental Program in the Neurosciences, University of California, Los Angeles, CA 90095, USA

Linda M. Liau
Department of Neurosurgery, and the Interdepartmental Program in the Neurosciences, University of California, Los Angeles, CA 90095, USA
Jonsson Comprehensive Cancer Center, UCLA, Room 379 Neuroscience Research Building, 635 Charles E. Young Dr. South, Los Angeles, CA 90095, USA

Jantzen Sperry
Department of Molecular and Medical Pharmacology, David Geffen School of Medicine, UCLA, Room 379 Neuroscience Research Building, 635 Charles E. Young Dr. South, Los Angeles, CA 90095, USA

Weihong Yan
Department of Chemistry and Biochemistry, UCLA, Los Angeles, USA

Jack Mottahedeh
Department of Psychiatry and Biobehavioral Sciences and Semel Institute for Neuroscience & Human Behavior, UCLA, Room 379 Neuroscience Research Building, 635 Charles E. Young Dr. South, Los Angeles, CA 90095, USA

Giovanni Coppola
Department of Psychiatry and Biobehavioral Sciences and Semel Institute for Neuroscience & Human Behavior, UCLA, Room 379 Neuroscience Research Building, 635 Charles E. Young Dr. South, Los Angeles, CA 90095, USA
Department of Neurology, UCLA, Los Angeles, USA

Esther A. Zaal, Wei Wu and Celia R. Berkers
Biomolecular Mass Spectrometry and Proteomics, Bijvoet Center for Biomolecular Research and Utrecht Institute of Pharmaceutical Sciences, Utrecht University, Padualaan 8, 3584 CH Utrecht, The Netherlands

Gerrit Jansen
Amsterdam Rheumatology and Immunology Center—Location VUMC, VU University Medical Center, Amsterdam, The Netherlands

Sonja Zweegman
Department of Hematology, VU University Medical Center, Amsterdam, The Netherlands

Jacqueline Cloos
Department of Hematology, VU University Medical Center, Amsterdam, The Netherlands
Pediatric Oncology/Hematology, VU University Medical Center, Amsterdam, The Netherlands

Dipti Athavale, Surbhi Chouhan, Shyamananda Singh Mayengbam, Snahlata Singh and Manoj Kumar Bhat
Laboratory No.6, National Centre for Cell Science, Savitribai Phule Pune University Campus, Ganeshkhind, Pune 411 007, India

Vimal Pandey
Laboratory No. 6, National Centre for Cell Science, Savitribai Phule Pune University Campus, Ganeshkhind, Pune 411 007, India
Present address: Laboratory of Neuroscience, Department of Biotechnology & Bioinformatics, School of Life Sciences, University of Hyderabad, Hyderabad, Telangana 500046, India

Pavithra Viswanath, Marina Radoul and Sabrina M. Ronen
Department of Radiology and Biomedical Imaging, University of California San Francisco, 1700 4th Street, Byers Hall 3rd Floor, Suite, San Francisco, CA 94143, USA

Jose Luis Izquierdo-Garcia
Centro Nacional de Investigaciones Cardiovasculares (CNIC), Madrid, Spain
CIBER de Enfermedades Respiratorias (CIBERES), Madrid, Spain

Hema Artee Luchman
Department of Cell Biology and Anatomy and Hotchkiss Brain Institute, University of Calgary, Calgary, Alberta, Canada

J. Gregory Cairncross
Department of Clinical Neurosciences and Southern Alberta Cancer Research Institute, University of Calgary, Calgary, Alberta, Canada

Russell O. Pieper and Joanna J. Phillips
Department of Neurological Surgery, Helen Diller Research Center, University of California San Francisco, San Francisco, CA, USA

Natthakan Thongon, Chiara Zucal, Vito Giuseppe D'Agostino, Toma Tebaldi, Alessandro Quattrone and Alessandro Provenzani
Center For Integrative Biology (CIBIO), University of Trento, via Sommarive 9, Trento, Italy

Silvia Ravera
Department of Pharmacy, Biochemistry Laboratory, University of Genova, Genova, Italy

Federica Zamporlini and Nadia Raffaelli
Department of Agricultural, Food and Environmental Sciences, Polytechnic University of Marche, Ancona, Italy

Alessio Nencioni and Francesco Piacente
Department of Internal Medicine, University of Genoa, Genoa, Italy

Jean-Francois Peyron and Ruxanda Moschoi
Université Côte d'Azur, Centre Méditerranéen de Médecine Moléculaire (C3M), INSERM U1065, Nice, France

Index

www.ingramcontent.com/pod-product-compliance
Lightning Source LLC
LaVergne TN
LVHW080655210926
848485LV00003B/379